T0259569

Lipid Disorders: A Multidisciplinary Approach

Editorial Advisor

JOEL J. HEIDELBAUGH

ELSEVIER

1600 John F. Kennedy Boulevard ● Suite 1800 ● Philadelphia, Pennsylvania, 19103-2899

http://www.theclinics.com

CLINICS COLLECTIONS
ISSN 2352-7986, ISBN-13: 978-0-323-42820-0

Editor: John Vassallo (j.vassallo@elsevier.com)
Developmental Editor: Patrick Manley (p.manley@elsevier.com)

Clinics Collections (ISSN 2352-7986) is published by Elsevier Inc., 360 Park Avenue South, New York, NY 10010-1710. Business and editorial offices: 1600 John F. Kennedy Boulevard, Suite 1800, Philadelphia, PA 19103-2899. **POSTMASTER:** Send address changes to *Clinics Collections*, Elsevier Health Sciences Division, Subscription Customer Service, 3251 Riverport Lane, Maryland Heights, MO 63043. **Customer Service: Telephone: 1-800-654-2452** (U.S. and Canada); **1-314-447-8871** (outside U.S. and Canada). **Fax: 314-447-8029. E-mail: journalscustomerserviceusa@elsevier.com** (for print support); **journalsonlinesupport-usa@ elsevier.com** (for online support).

Reprints. For copies of 100 or more of articles in this publication, please contact the Commercial Reprints Department, Elsevier Inc., 360 Park Avenue South, New York, NY 10010-1710. Tel.: 212-633-3874; Fax: 212-633-3820; E-mail: reprints@elsevier.com.

Contributors

EDITORIAL ADVISOR

JOEL J. HEIDELBAUGH, MD, FAAFP, FACG
Clinical Associate Professor, Departments of Family Medicine and Urology; Clerkship Director, University of Michigan Medical School, Ann Arbor; Ypsilanti Health Center, Ypsilanti, Michigan

AUTHORS

BHAVIN B. ADHYARU, MS, MD
Assistant Professor, Division of General Internal Medicine and Geriatrics, Department of Medicine, Emory University School of Medicine, Atlanta, Georgia

KAWTAR ALKHALLOUFI, MD
Howard University College of Medicine, Washington, DC

KRISTEN M.J. AZAR, RN, MSN, MPH
Palo Alto Medical Foundation Research Institute, Palo Alto, California

JUAN J. BADIMON, PhD
Cardiovascular Institute, Icahn School of Medicine at Mount Sinai, New York, New York

CHRISTIE M. BALLANTYNE, MD, FACC, FACP, FAHA, FNLA
Chief, Sections of Cardiovascular Research and Cardiology; Professor of Medicine, Department of Medicine; Professor of Genetics, Baylor College of Medicine; Director of the Center for Cardiovascular Disease Prevention, Houston Methodist DeBakey Heart and Vascular Center, Houston, Texas

BRUCE BARRETT, MD, PhD
Professor, Department of Family Medicine, University of Wisconsin, Madison, Wisconsin

SETH J. BAUM, MD
Division of Medicine, Charles E. Schmidt College of Biomedical Science, Florida Atlantic University, Boca Raton, Florida

OZLEM BILEN, MD
Medical Resident, Department of Medicine, Baylor College of Medicine, Houston, Texas

VERA BITTNER, MD, MSPH, FNLA
Division of Cardiovascular Disease, Department of Medicine, University of Alabama at Birmingham, Birmingham, Alabama

MICHAEL B. BOFFA, PhD
Associate Professor, Department of Chemistry and Biochemistry, University of Windsor, Windsor, Ontario, Canada

VICTORIA ENCHIA BOUHAIRIE, MD
Clinical Fellow in Endocrinology, Division of Endocrinology, Metabolism, and Lipid Research, Department of Medicine, Washington University School of Medicine, St Louis, Missouri

ELIOT A. BRINTON, MD, FAHA, FNLA
Director, Atherometabolic Research, Utah Foundation for Biomedical Research; President, Utah Lipid Center, Salt Lake City, Utah

ANDREW CLARK, MD, MA, FRCP
Department of Cardiology, Hull York Medical School, Castle Hill Hospital, Kingston-upon-Hull, United Kingdom

JOHN G.F. CLELAND, MD, PhD, FRCP, FESC, FACC
National Heart and Lung Institute, Royal Brompton and Harefield Hospitals, Imperial College, London, United Kingdom

LISANDRO D. COLANTONIO, MD, MSc
Department of Epidemiology, University of Alabama at Birmingham, Birmingham, Alabama

JUDITH S. CURRIER, MD, MSc
Division of Infectious Diseases, Department of Medicine, David Geffen School of Medicine, University of California, Los Angeles, Los Angeles, California

MICHAEL DAVIDSON, MD
Section of Cardiology, University of Chicago, Chicago, Illinois

MICHAEL DEMYEN, MD
Assistant Professor, Department of Medicine, Rutgers New Jersey Medical School, Newark, New Jersey

MARY R. DICKLIN, PhD
Metabolic Sciences, Midwest Center for Metabolic & Cardiovascular Research, Glen Ellyn, Illinois

ALISON B. EVERT, MS, RD, CDE
Coordinator, Diabetes Education Programs, Diabetes Care Center, University of Washington Medical Center, Seattle, Washington

STEPHEN P. FORTMANN, MD
Kaiser Permanente Center for Health Research, Portland, Oregon

GREGORY C. GARDNER, MD, FACP
Gilliland-Henderson Professor of Medicine, Division of Rheumatology, University of Washington, Seattle, Washington

EDWARD A. GILL, MD, FASE, FAHA, FACC, FACP, FNLA
Professor of Medicine, Division of Cardiology; Adjunct Professor of Radiology, UW Department of Medicine; Director of Harborview Medical Center Echocardiography, University of Washington School of Medicine; Clinical Professor of Diagnostic Ultrasound, Seattle University, Seattle, Washington

ANNE CAROL GOLDBERG, MD
Associate Professor of Medicine, Division of Endocrinology, Metabolism, and Lipid Research, Department of Medicine, Washington University School of Medicine, St Louis, Missouri

ARPETA GUPTA, MD
Fellow, Division of Endocrinology, Diabetes, and Bone Diseases, Icahn School of Medicine at Mount Sinai, New York, New York

KATHERINE G. HASTINGS, BA
Stanford University School of Medicine, Stanford, California

HARVEY S. HECHT, MD, FACC, FSCCT
Associate Director of Cardiovascular Imaging, Department of Cardiology, Mount Sinai Medical Center; Professor of Medicine, Icahn School of Medicine at Mount Sinai, New York, New York

KATE HUTCHINSON, MBChB
Department of Cardiology, Hull York Medical School, Castle Hill Hospital, Kingston-upon-Hull, United Kingdom

TERRY A. JACOBSON, MD
Director, Lipid Clinic and Cardiovascular Risk Reduction Program; Professor, Department of Medicine, Emory University School of Medicine, Atlanta, Georgia

PHILIP K. JOHNSON, BS
Department of Cardiology, Boston Children's Hospital; Department of Pediatrics, Harvard Medical School, Boston, Massachusetts

EYAL KEDAR, MD
Senior Fellow in Rheumatology, Division of Rheumatology, University of Washington, Seattle, Washington

THEODOROS KELESIDIS, MD, PhD
Division of Infectious Diseases, Department of Medicine, David Geffen School of Medicine, University of California, Los Angeles, Los Angeles, California

MARLYS L. KOSCHINSKY, PhD
Dean, Faculty of Science; and Professor, Department of Chemistry and Biochemistry, University of Windsor, Windsor, Ontario, Canada

KENT B. LEWANDROWSKI, MD
Associate Chief of Pathology; Director of Pathology, Laboratories and Molecular Medicine, Division of Laboratory Medicine, Massachusetts General Hospital; Professor of Pathology, Department of Pathology, Harvard Medical School, Boston, Massachusetts

KEVIN C. MAKI, PhD
Metabolic Sciences, Midwest Center for Metabolic & Cardiovascular Research, Glen Ellyn, Illinois

CAMILIA R. MARTIN, MD, MS
Associate Director, NICU, Department of Neonatology; Director for Cross-Disciplinary Research Partnerships; Assistant Professor of Pediatrics; Division of Translational Research, Beth Israel Deaconess Medical Center, Harvard Medical School, Boston, Massachusetts

VANI NIMBAL, MPH
Palo Alto Medical Foundation Research Institute, Palo Alto, California

LATHA P. PALANIAPPAN, MD, MS
Stanford University School of Medicine, Stanford, California

PIERPAOLO PELLICORI, MD
Department of Cardiology, Hull York Medical School, Castle Hill Hospital, Kingston-upon-Hull, United Kingdom

YASHASHWI POKHAREL, MD, MSCR
Clinical Postdoctoral Fellow, Section of Cardiovascular Research, Department of Medicine, Baylor College of Medicine; Center for Cardiovascular Disease Prevention, Methodist DeBakey Heart and Vascular Center, Houston, Texas

NIKOLAOS T. PYRSOPOULOS, MD, PhD, MBA, FACP, AGAF
Associate Professor of Medicine; Director of Gastroenterology and Hepatology; Medical Director Liver Transplantation, Rutgers New Jersey Medical School, University Hospital, Newark, New Jersey

JIA PU, PhD
Palo Alto Medical Foundation Research Institute, Palo Alto, California

FREDERICK J. RAAL, MBBCh, MMED, PhD
Department of Medicine, Faculty of Health Sciences, University of the Witwatersrand, Johannesburg, South Africa

JASON A. RICCO, MD, MPH
Research Fellow, Department of Family Medicine, University of Wisconsin, Madison, Wisconsin

MICHAEL C. RIDDELL, PhD
Professor and Graduate Program Director, Muscle Health Research Center, School of Kinesiology and Health Science, Bethune College, York University, Toronto, Ontario, Canada

ROBERT ROMANELLI, PhD
Palo Alto Medical Foundation Research Institute, Palo Alto, California

ROBERT S. ROSENSON, MD
Cardiovascular Institute, Icahn School of Medicine at Mount Sinai, New York, New York

JOSEPH RUDOLF, MD
Division of Laboratory Medicine, Department of Pathology, Resident Pathologist, Massachusetts General Hospital, Harvard Medical School, Boston, Massachusetts

CARLOS G. SANTOS-GALLEGO, MD
Cardiovascular Institute, Icahn School of Medicine at Mount Sinai, New York, New York

AMITA SINGH, MD
Section of Cardiology, University of Chicago, Chicago, Illinois

DONALD A. SMITH, MD, MPH, FACP, FNLA, FACE
Associate Professor of Medicine and Preventive Medicine, Icahn School of Medicine at Mount Sinai, New York, New York

EVAN A. STEIN, MD, PhD
Metabolic and Atherosclerosis Research Center, Cincinnati, Ohio

MARGARET L. WALLACE, PharmD, BCACP
Research Fellow, Department of Family Medicine, University of Wisconsin, Madison, Wisconsin

ELIZABETH A. WEEDIN, DO
Section of General Obstetrics and Gynecology, Department of Obstetrics and Gynecology, University of Oklahoma Health Sciences Center, Oklahoma City, Oklahoma

ROBERT WILD, MD, MPH, PhD
Section of Reproductive Endocrinology and Infertility, Department of Obstetrics and Gynecology, University of Oklahoma Health Sciences Center, Oklahoma City, Oklahoma

DON WILSON, MD, FNLA
Department of Pediatric Endocrinology, Cook Children's Medical Center, Fort Worth, Texas

ALAN H.B. WU, PhD
Clinical Chemistry Laboratory, Department of Laboratory Medicine, San Francisco General Hospital, University of California, San Francisco, California

JUSTIN P. ZACHARIAH, MD, MPH
Department of Cardiology, Boston Children's Hospital; Department of Pediatrics, Harvard Medical School, Boston, Massachusetts

BEINAN ZHAO, MS
Palo Alto Medical Foundation Research Institute, Palo Alto, California

Contents

> Increased total serum cholesterol and low-density lipoprotein cholesterol
> concentrations are associated with atherosclerosis and risk for myocardial
> infarction and stroke. Those who have high cholesterol with other factors
> that predispose them to cardiovascular disease should be treated with
> cholesterol-lowering medications. The pathophysiology of hyperlipidemia
> is important in the proper selection of drug therapy. Patients who have
> increased cholesterol synthesis should be medicated with drugs that
> reduce in vivo cholesterol production, whereas those who have increased
> dietary absorption of cholesterol should be treated with drugs that inhibit
> dietary absorption. Sterol-based biomarkers are available to assess the
> cause of hypercholesterolemia and may have an impact on therapeutic
> selection.

> This article reconciles the classic view of high-density lipoproteins (HDL)
> associated with low risk for cardiovascular disease (CVD) with recent
> data (genetics studies and randomized clinical trials) casting doubt over
> the widely accepted beneficial role of HDL regarding CVD risk. Although
> HDL cholesterol has been used as a surrogate measure to investigate
> HDL function, the cholesterol content in HDL particles is not an indicator
> of the atheroprotective properties of HDL. Thus, more precise measures
> of HDL metabolism are needed to reflect and account for the beneficial
> effects of HDL particles. Current and emerging therapies targeting HDL
> are discussed.

> Coronary heart disease is a common and costly epidemic in the Western
> world. Intensive study has led to a deeper understanding of the pathogen-
> esis of coronary disease and risk stratification. Traditional risk factor
> assessment has focused on parameters derived from the Framingham
> Heart Study (age, hypertension, cholesterol, family history, and cigarette
> smoking). New emerging risk factors, both biological and genetic, are
> reshaping the understanding of heart disease and the approach to risk
> stratification. As these emerging assays become more standardized,

automated, and inexpensive to perform, they are becoming increasingly important tools in the assessment and treatment of coronary heart disease.

Elevated plasma concentrations of lipoprotein(a) (Lp[a]) are an emerging risk factor for the development of coronary heart disease (CHD). Recent genetic and epidemiologic data have provided strong evidence for a causal role of Lp(a) in CHD. Despite these developments, which have attracted increasing interest from clinicians and basic scientists, many unanswered questions persist. The true pathogenic mechanism of Lp(a) remains a mystery. Significant uncertainty exists concerning the appropriate use of Lp(a) in the clinical setting. No therapeutic intervention remains that can specifically lower plasma Lp(a) concentrations, although the list of compounds that lower Lp(a) and LDL continues to expand.

Hereditary dyslipidemias are often underdiagnosed and undertreated, yet with significant health implications, most importantly causing preventable premature cardiovascular diseases. The commonly used clinical criteria to diagnose hereditary lipid disorders are specific but are not very sensitive. Genetic testing may be of value in making accurate diagnosis and improving cascade screening of family members, and potentially, in risk assessment and choice of therapy. This review focuses on using genetic testing in the clinical setting for lipid disorders, particularly familial hypercholesterolemia.

Familial hypercholesterolemia is a common, inherited disorder of cholesterol metabolism that leads to early cardiovascular morbidity and mortality. It is underdiagnosed and undertreated. Statins, ezetimibe, bile acid sequestrants, niacin, lomitapide, mipomersen, and low-density lipoprotein (LDL) apheresis are treatments that can lower LDL cholesterol levels. Early treatment can lead to substantial reduction of cardiovascular events and death in patients with familial hypercholesterolemia. It is important to increase awareness of this disorder in physicians and patients to reduce the burden of this disorder.

Lipids and Pharmacotherapy

Although the past 4 decades have been the most productive in transitioning from an low-density lipoprotein cholesterol (LDL-C) hypothesis to demonstration of clinical benefit, cardiovascular disease remains a major cause of mortality and morbidity. It is fortunate that most of the effective lipid-lowering drugs, the statins, have become generic and inexpensive. However, there remains a large unmet medical need for new and effective agents that are also well tolerated and safe, especially for patients unable to either tolerate statins or achieve optimal LDL-C on current therapies. It is likely that the agents discussed in this review will fill that need.

Amita Singh and Michael Davidson

Many lipid-lowering drugs improve cardiovascular (CV) outcomes. However, when therapies have been studied in addition to statins, it has been challenging to show an additional clinical benefit in terms of CV event reduction, although overall safety seems acceptable. This debate has been complicated by recent guidelines that emphasize treatment with high-potency statin monotherapy. Combination therapy allows more patients to successfully reach their ideal lipid targets. Further testing of novel therapies may introduce an era of potent low-density lipoprotein decrease without dependence on statins, but until then, they remain the mainstay of therapy.

Michael Demyen, Kawtar Alkhalloufi, and Nikolaos T. Pyrsopoulos

Lipid-lowering therapy is increasingly being used in patients for a variety of diseases, the most important being secondary prevention of cardiovascular disease. Many lipid-lowering drugs carry side effects that include elevations in hepatic function tests and liver toxicity. In many cases, these drugs are not prescribed or they are underprescribed because of fears of injury to the liver. This article attempts to review key trials with respect to the hepatotoxicity of these drugs. Recommendations are also provided with respect to the selection of low-risk patients and strategies to lower the risk of hepatotoxicity when prescribing these medications.

Lipids and Heart Disease

Margaret L. Wallace, Jason A. Ricco, and Bruce Barrett

The purpose of this article is to update the primary care community on the evidence and guidelines for cardiovascular disease screening in a general-risk adult population, with the goal of assisting clinicians in developing an evidence-based approach toward screening. This article discusses global risk assessment and screening strategies, including blood pressure, lipids, C-reactive protein, homocysteine, coronary artery calcium score, carotid intima-media thickness, ultrasound of the abdominal aorta, and electrocardiography.

Arpeta Gupta and Donald A. Smith

The 2013 American College of Cardiology/American Heart Association Guideline on the Treatment of Blood Cholesterol to Reduce Atherosclerotic Cardiovascular Risk in Adults and Guideline on the Assessment of

Cardiovascular Risk were released in mid-November 2013. This article explains the guidelines, the risk equations, and their derivations, and addresses criticisms so that practicing physicians may be more comfortable in using the guidelines and the risk equations to inform patients of their atherosclerotic cardiovascular risk and choices to reduce that risk. The article also addresses patient concerns about statin safety if lifestyle changes have been insufficient to reduce their risk.

This review discusses the 2013 American College of Cardiology (ACC)/American Heart Association (AHA) Guideline on the Treatment of Blood Cholesterol to Reduce Atherosclerotic Cardiovascular Risk in Adults and compares it with the 2014 National Lipid Association (NLA) Recommendations for Patient-Centered Management of Dyslipidemia. The review discusses some of the distinctions between the guidelines, including how to determine a patient's atherosclerotic cardiovascular disease risk, the role of lipoprotein treatment targets, the importance of moderate- and high-intensity statin therapy, and the use of nonstatin therapy in light of the IMProved Reduction of Outcomes: Vytorin Efficacy International Trial (IMPROVE-IT) trial.

Mendelian randomization data strongly suggest that hypertriglyceridemia (HTG) causes atherosclerotic cardiovascular disease (ASCVD), and so triglyceride (TG) level–lowering treatment in HTG is now more strongly recommended to address the residual ASCVD risk than has been the case in (generally earlier) published guidelines. Fibrates are the best-established agents for TG level lowering and are generally used as first-line treatment of TG levels greater than 500 mg/dL. Statins are the best-established agents for ASCVD prevention, and so are usually used as first-line treatment of TG levels less than 500 mg/dL.

Interventions for coronary artery disease in heart failure have not been successful. It seems unlikely that coronary events play no role in the progression of heart failure and the ultimate demise of the patient. Meta-analysis suggests no benefit of fibrates in cardiovascular disease or heart failure. Polyunsaturated fats have equal benefit in cardiovascular disease. Two large trials of statins found no effect on mortality, but one trial found a reduction in morbidity. Retrospective analyses suggest that patients with milder disease might retain the benefit observed with statins in patients with coronary disease who do not have heart failure. Differences among statins may exist.

Lisandro D. Colantonio and Vera Bittner

About one-half of individuals with an acute myocardial infarction have a low-density lipoprotein cholesterol level of less than 100 mg/dL at the time of occurrence, but remain at risk for recurrent events. This residual risk is likely mediated by multiple factors, including burden of atherosclerosis, residual dyslipidemia, nonlipid risk factors, and suboptimal implementation of lifestyle therapy and evidence-based pharmacologic therapy. This article reviews management options for this high-risk population.

Alison B. Evert and Michael C. Riddell

Diabetes now affects more than 29 million Americans, and more than 9 million of these people do not know they have diabetes. In adults, type 2 diabetes accounts for about 90% to 95% of all diagnosed cases of diabetes and is the focus of this article. Lifestyle intervention is part of the initial treatment as well as the ongoing management of type 2 diabetes. Lifestyle intervention encompasses a healthful eating plan, physical activity, and often medication to assist in achievement of glucose, lipid, and blood pressure goals. Patient education and self-care practices are also important aspects of disease management.

Lipids and Chronic Disease

Kevin C. Maki, Mary R. Dicklin, and Seth J. Baum

A statin is first-line drug therapy for dyslipidemia. Clinical trial data suggest there is an increase in the incidence of new-onset type 2 diabetes mellitus with statin use. The National Lipid Association (NLA) Statin Diabetes Safety Task Force concluded that the cardiovascular benefit of statin therapy outweighs the risk for developing diabetes. The NLA panel advocated following the standards of care from the American Diabetes Association for screening and diagnosis of diabetes, and emphasized the importance of lifestyle modification. This article summarizes NLA's review of the evidence, expanding it to include recent results, and outlines the clinical recommendations.

Eyal Kedar and Gregory C. Gardner

Rheumatologic manifestations of hyperlipidemia and lipid-associated arthritis are rarely seen in the rheumatologist's office. On the other hand, a rheumatologist may be the clinician who identifies and initiates proper therapy for disorders related to hyperlipidemia when the musculoskeletal manifestations of these syndromes are recognized. In this article both the joint and tendon manifestations are reviewed, including the lesser known lipid liquid crystal form of arthritis. The relationship between gout and hyperuricemia is briefly discussed, as are the autoimmune manifestations of lipid-lowering therapy.

Lipids and Pediatrics

Challenges remain in optimizing the delivery of fatty acids to attain their nutritional and therapeutic benefits in neonatal health. In this review, knowledge about placental transfer of fatty acids to the developing fetus is summarized, the potential role and mechanisms of fatty acids in enhancing neonatal health and minimizing morbidities is outlined, the unique considerations for fatty acid delivery in the preterm population are defined, and the research questions are proposed that need to be addressed before new standards of care are adopted at the bedside for the provision of critical fatty acids to preterm infants.

The National Heart, Lung and Blood Institute Expert Panel Integrated Guidelines promote the prevention of cardiovascular disease (CVD) events by encouraging healthy behaviors in all children, screening and treatment of children with genetic dyslipidemias, usage of specific lifestyle modifications, and limited administration of lipid pharmacotherapy in children with the highest CVD risk. These recommendations place children in the center of the fight against future CVD. Pediatric providers may be in a position to shift the focus of CVD prevention from trimming multiple risk factors to cutting out the causes CVD.

Lipids and Women's Health

Recent studies have revealed evidence that poorly controlled cholesterol, triglycerides, and their metabolites during pregnancy may be associated with cardiometabolic dysfunction and have significant detrimental fetal and maternal vascular consequences. Cardiometabolic dysfunction during pregnancy may not only contribute to long-term effects of the mother and child's vascular health but also potentially create cardiovascular risk for generational offspring. This article provides updates on this rapidly expanding and multifaceted topic and reviews new insight regarding why recognition of this disordered maternal cholesterol and triglyceride metabolism is likely to have long-term effect on the increasing atherosclerotic burden of the burgeoning population.

Understanding opportunities to reduce dyslipidemia before, during, and after pregnancy has major implications for cardiovascular disease risk prevention for the entire population. The best time to screen for dyslipidemia is before pregnancy or in the early antenatal period. The differential diagnosis of hypertriglyceridemia in pregnancy is the same as in nonpregnant women except that clinical lipidologists need to be aware of the potential obstetric complications associated with hypertriglyceridemia. Dyslipidemia discovered during pregnancy should be treated with diet and exercise intervention, as well as glycemic control if indicated. A complete lipid profile assessment during each trimester of pregnancy is recommended.

Special Considerations

The pathogenesis of atherosclerosis in human immunodeficiency virus (HIV)-infected individuals is incompletely understood and appears to be multifactorial. Proatherogenic changes in blood and tissue lipids are associated with an increased risk of cardiovascular disease among HIV-infected subjects, and these changes may be both quantitative (dyslipidemia) and qualitative. In view of the pivotal role of dyslipidemia in the process of atherosclerosis, the increased incidence of dyslipidemia in HIV-infected individuals, and the emerging role of lipid abnormalities in systemic pathophysiologic processes such as immune activation, we review the contributions of dyslipidemia to cardiovascular risk in HIV infection.

Coronary artery calcium scanning (CAC) is the most powerful prognosticator of cardiac risk in the asymptomatic primary prevention population, far exceeding the role of risk factor–based paradigms. The primary utility of risk factors is to identify treatable targets for risk reduction after risk has been determined by CAC. Serial calcium scanning to evaluate progression of calcified plaque is useful for determining the response to treatment. The 2013 cholesterol treatment guidelines understate the value of CAC scanning for atherosclerotic disease risk assessment.

This article reviews racial/ethnic differences in dyslipidemia—prevalence of dyslipidemia, its relation to coronary heart disease (CHD) and stroke mortality rates, response to lipid-lowering agents, and lifestyle modification. Asian Indians, Filipinos, and Hispanics are at higher risk for dyslipidemia, which is consistent with the higher CHD mortality rates in these groups. Statins may have greater efficacy for Asians, but the data are mixed. Lifestyle modifications are recommended. Culturally-tailored prevention and intervention should be provided to the minority populations with elevated risk for dyslipidemia and considerably more research is needed to determine the best approaches to helping specific subgroups.

Preface

Clinics Review Articles have been a part of the physicians', nurses', and residents' library for nearly 100 years. This trusted resource covers more than 50 medical disciplines each year, producing thousands of articles focused on the most current concepts and techniques in medicine. This collection of articles, devoted to lipid disorders, draws from this *Clinics* database to provide multidisciplinary teams with practical clinical advice on the therapies and comorbidities of these highly prevalent conditions.

A multidisciplinary perspective is key to effective team-based management. Featured articles from the *Cardiology Clinics, Heart Failure Clinics, Endocrinology and Metabolism Clinics of North America, Medical Clinics of North America, Clinics in Laboratory Medicine, Clinics in Liver Disease,* and *Primary Care: Clinics in Office Practice* reflect the wide range of clinicians who manage patients with lipid disorders.

I encourage you to share this volume with your colleagues in hopes that it may promote more collaboration, new perspectives, and informed, effective care for your patients.

Joel J. Heidelbaugh, MD, FAAFP, FACG
Ypsilanti, MI, USA
June 2015

http://dx.doi.org/10.1016/j.ccol.2015.05.001
2352-7986/15/$ – see front matter © 2015 Published by Elsevier Inc.

Biomarkers for Cholesterol Absorption and Synthesis in Hyperlipidemic Patients
Role for Therapeutic Selection

Alan H.B. Wu, PhD

KEYWORDS

- Statins • Ezetimibe • Campesterol • Lathosterol • β-Sitosterol • Squalene
- Desmosterol • Cholestanol

KEY POINTS

- Hypercholesterolemia is caused by increased rate of synthesis or absorption from the diet.
- Biomarkers of increased synthesis include squalene, desmosterol, and lathosterol.
- Biomarkers of increased absorption include campesterol, β-sitosterol, and cholestanol.
- Statins are most effective when used in patients with increased synthesis.
- Cholesterol absorption drugs, such as ezetimibe, are most effective in patients with increased absorption.

INTRODUCTION

Increased total serum cholesterol and low-density lipoprotein (LDL) cholesterol concentrations are associated with atherosclerosis and risk for myocardial infarction and stroke. International guidelines, such as from the National Cholesterol Education Program, have established cutoff concentrations for total and LDL cholesterol that identify individuals at moderate and high risk for future adverse cardiac events.[1] Individuals with a borderline cholesterol concentration with few or no other risk factors are at moderate risk and should undergo modifications in their diet, exercise, and smoking habits. Those who have high cholesterol with other factors that predisposes them to cardiovascular disease are at the highest risk should be treated with cholesterol-lowering medications. The pathophysiology of hyperlipidemia is important in the proper selection of drug therapy. Patients who have increased cholesterol synthesis should be medicated with drugs that reduce *in vivo* cholesterol production, whereas

This article originally appeared in Clinics in Laboratory Medicine, Volume 34, Issue 1, March 2014.

Clinical Chemistry Laboratory, Department of Laboratory Medicine, San Francisco General Hospital, University of California, San Francisco, 1001 Potrero Avenue, San Francisco, CA 94110, USA

E-mail address: wualan@labmed2.ucsf.edu

those who have increased dietary absorption of cholesterol should be treated with drugs that inhibit dietary absorption. Sterol-based biomarkers are available to assess the cause of hypercholesterolemia and may have an impact on therapeutic selection.

BIOMARKERS OF CHOLESTEROL SYNTHESIS AND ABSORPTION
Cholesterol Synthesis Pathway

Cholesterol produced in mammalian cells originates from acetate. The important steps are shown in **Fig. 1**.[2] Acetate is converted to 3-hydroxy-3-methyl-glutaryl-CoA (HMG) by HMG-CoA synthase and then to mevalonate by HMG-CoA reductase. The class of statin drugs reduces cholesterol synthesis by inhibiting this important rate-limiting step. In the absence of statins, mevalonate is converted to squalene and then to lanosterol. Subsequently, there are two different pathways that convert lanosterol to cholesterol. In the Bloch pathway, lanosterol is converted to desmosterol. In the Kandutsch-Russell pathway, lanosterol is first converted to lathosterol, then 7-dehydrocholesterol, and finally cholesterol. The intermediate metabolites squalene, lathosterol, and desmosterol are used as biomarkers to evaluate cholesterol synthesis. High concentrations of these markers indicate increased in vivo production. The value of measuring cholesterol precursors depends on the presumption that the serum or plasma concentrations of these biomarkers are proportional to their formation in the synthetic pathway. Bjorkhem and colleagues[3] showed that there was a linear relationship between absolute total serum lathosterol concentration and hepatic HMG-CoA reductase activity ($r = 0.82$). In this study, the correlation of enzyme activity to desmosterol and squalene was weaker ($r = 0.50$ and 0.20, respectively).

Mechanism of Cholesterol Absorption

The manner by which cholesterol is absorbed from lumen has been studied extensively. According to Wang,[4] intestinal cholesterol originates from dietary absorption, the bile, and intestinal epithelial slothing. Collectively, these sources contribute roughly 2000 mg/day. A western diet contributes about 300 to 500 mg of this total by absorption through the duodenum and proximal jejunum. The cholesterol forms micelles in conjunction with bile salts, phospholipids, and monoglycerides. Micelles formation facilitates transport of cholesterol to the brush border of the small intestines. There, cholesterol is removed from the micelles and monomeric unesterified cholesterol is passed through to enterocytes through the Niemann-Pick C1-like (NPC1) transporter. Once absorbed, cholesterol is esterified by CoA:cholesterol acyltransferase. Efflux from the enterocyte seems to be mediated by intestinal ATP-binding cassette transporters (ABC) G5 and G8 proteins. There are genetic variances of this protein that results in the hyperabsorption of cholesterol.[5]

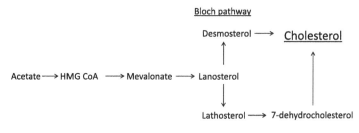

Fig. 1. Cholesterol synthesis pathways.

Hypercholesterolemia caused by increased dietary absorption can be assessed by the measurement of plant sterols, such as β-sitosterol and campesterol. These phytosterols have a role in supporting membrane structure for plants in a similar way to the role of cholesterol in animals. When present in the diet, these endogenous compounds inhibit cholesterol absorption, because they both compete for incorporation into micelles.[6] Plant steroids are more hydrophobic resulting in a higher affinity to these structures. Measurement of serum β-sitosterol and campesterol concentrations, when normalized to total cholesterol, is a surrogate for assessing cholesterol absorption.

Ezetimibe is a cholesterol absorption inhibitor approved by the Food and Drug Administration for treating patients with hypercholesterolemia.[7] Ezetimibe is metabolized to ezetimibe glucuronide, which is more active than the parent drug. Both the parent and metabolite are located within the brush border of the intestinal villi, where they block the entry of cholesterol into the enterocytes. The mode of action for ezetimide and the glucuronide is the inhibition of the NPC1-like transporter.[8] In a pig model, the administration of ezetimibe resulted in upregulation of the NPC1 transporter in the jejunum in a compensatory response to the depletion of cholesterol in the intestines.[9] Nevertheless, the ezetimibe present is able to inhibit the extra NPC1 transporter expression. There is no effect of ezetimide on the ABC G5 or G8 enterocyte efflux transport.

Analytical Analysis of Cholesterol Synthesis and Absorption Biomarkers

The analysis of endogenous cholesterol precursor molecules and phytosteroids can be performed by gas-chromatography/mass spectrometry.[10] Samples require hydrolysis of endogenous triglycerides to glycerol and free fatty acids by saponification with hydroxides. Sterol results are expressed in absolute terms in micromoles per liter or normalized to 100 mmol of sterol per mole of total cholesterol. The overall precision ranges from 8% to 10%. Recently, liquid chromatography tandem mass spectrometry (LC-MS/MS) has been developed.[11] LC-MS/MS assays have higher analytical sensitivity and precision than gas-chromatography/mass spectrometry and are more amendable to on-line extractions. There are currently no assays cleared by the US Food and Drug Administration. Therefore, all testing is conducted under the Clinical Laboratory Improvement Amendment under the auspice of a "Laboratory Developed Test." A Food and Drug Administration cleared test might be possible if an immunoassay can be constructed, but raising specific antibodies to these sterols is highly unlikely given that they exist in all mammalian species and their chemical structure is conserved. Cholesterol absorption and synthesis biomarkers are available through commercial Clinical Laboratory Improvement Amendment-certified reference laboratories.

The biologic variation for hypercholesterol biomarkers has recently been measured. The intraindividual variation for β-sitosterol, campesterol, and lathosterol was slightly higher than for traditional cholesterol biomarkers including total, high-density lipoprotein, and LDL cholesterol.[11] The index of individuality for novel sterol biomarkers was low (<0.6), indicating that reference intervals based on a population are of little value. Accordingly, these markers are best used to establish the cause of hypercholesterolemia, selecting the most appropriate therapy, and monitoring the success of lipid-lowering drugs. Serial testing is needed to establish an individual's homeostatic set point and to evaluate the success of lipid-lowering medications.

Table 1 shows the mean concentration of cholesterol synthesis and absorption markers studied from different therapeutic trials.[12–15] Although these results are not "reference limits," these mean values are within the decision limits listed by reference

Table 1
Mean values for cholesterol synthesis and absorption markers

Squalene		Desmosterol		Lathosterol		Campesterol		β-Sitosterol		Cholestanol		Ref
M	W	M	W	M	W	M	W	M	W	M	W	
38	40	59	54	114	110	225	215	168	160	126	122	12
ND	ND	37	31	123	111	143	157	89	99	ND	ND	13
ND	ND	37	33	117	110	150	144	91	90	ND	ND	13
35	35	74	77	132	140	201	184	158	132	135	134	14
34	36	72	75	110	129	232	221	169	168	144	143	14
ND	ND	ND	ND	ND	ND	200	207	121	135	162	158	15
Mean												
36	37	56	54	119	120	192	188	133	131	142	139	

Mean results are shown. Results are expressed as 10^2 mmol/mol of cholesterol.
Abbreviation: ND, no data.
Data from Expert Panel on Detection, Evaluation, and Treatment of High Blood Cholesterol in Adults (Adult Treatment Panel III). Third Report of the National Cholesterol Education Program (NCEP) Expert Panel on Detection, Evaluation, and Treatment of High Blood Cholesterol in Adults. Final Report. Circulation 2002;106:3143–421.

laboratories offering these tests. Individuals with hypercholesterolemia who have values exceeding the means for cholesterol synthesis markers (squalene, desmosterol, and lathosterol) and/or absorption markers (campesterol, β-sitosterol, and cholethanol) are candidates for lipid-lowering medications, such as the statins and ezetimibe, respectively.

CHOLESTEROL ABSORPTION AND SYNTHESIS MARKERS AS RISK FACTORS FOR CORONARY HEART DISEASE

The suggestion that cholesterol absorption markers might have value as a cardiovascular risk assessment marker was based on the observation in patients with a complete mutation in either the ABC G5 or G6 gene.[16] These individuals developed a profound increase in sitosterol and total cholesterol caused by increased absorption and decreased biliary excretion. "Sitosterolemia" is an autosomal-recessive trait where sitosterol concentrations are increased by 10- to 20-fold. Individuals with sitosterolemia have advance and premature atherosclerosis with a high incidence of cardiovascular disease caused by deposition of cholesterol into the coronary arteries. Xanthomas are also evident in these patients.

Clinical trials involving cholesterol synthesis markers and the incidence of heart disease have produced mixed results. In two preliminary early studies involving small numbers of subjects, Rajaratnam and colleagues[17] and Sudhop and colleagues[18] showed that campesterol and β-sitosterol were higher in cases of these trials (N = 48 and 27, respectively) than matched control subjects (N = 61 and 28, respectively). In the Framingham Offspring Study of participants with coronary heart disease, Matthan and coworkers[13] showed that subjects who had a greater than or equal to 50% carotid stenosis (N = 155) had higher ratios of campesterol, β-sitosterol, and cholestanol to cholesterol than control subjects (N = 414). These findings were not confirmed by later and larger studies. No difference in the ratio of campesterol and β-sitosterol was seen in the EPIC-Norfolk study of 373 cases with coronary artery disease against 758 control subjects,[19] the Dallas Heart study of 1032 subjects with atherosclerosis as determined by electron-beam tomography against 1792 control subjects,[20] or the PROSPER of 223 cases with a coronary heart disease event and 257 control subjects.[14]

There is little disagreement in the literature regarding the concentration of cholesterol synthesis markers in heart disease versus control subjects. There was no difference in lathosterol levels versus control subjects in the PROSPER, EPIC-Norfolk, and Dallas Heart trials.[14,19,20] In the Framingham Offspring Trial, desmosterol and lathosterol values were actually higher in control subjects than in the cases. It can be concluded from these studies that cholesterol absorption and synthesis markers are not independent risk biomarkers beyond the traditional lipid tests of cholesterol and LDL cholesterol.

In most of these trials, the total, LDL, and high-density lipoprotein cholesterol concentration were matched between the study and control groups. Individuals who had hypercholesterolemia were at high risk independent to the mechanism for the high lipid levels. That there was no difference in cholesterol absorption and synthesis tests between groups may indicate that control subjects are also at risk and will likely benefit from lipid-lowering medications. There is no debate regarding the benefits of lipid-lowering therapy among patients with hypercholesterolemia. If National Cholesterol Education Program recommendations suggest the at-risk individual should be treated with drugs, the critical important question is determining the type of medication or combination that is most likely to be effective.

The value of measurement of cholesterol absorption and synthesis markers may be in the identification of individuals who are refractory to either statins or cholesterol absorption inhibitors. In a meta-analysis of nearly 30,000 patients, Josan and colleagues[21] showed that roughly 50% of individuals on intense statin monotherapy did not achieve an LDL-cholesterol that reached a target goal of 77 mg/dL. Although these data suggested use of combination therapy to treat these patients, these authors were unable to address the efficacy of this approach. Currently, there have been no studies to compare clinical success of using cholesterol absorption and synthesis markers in therapeutic selection when triaged according to these novel biomarkers. However, there are data demonstrating the effect of statins and cholesterol absorption drugs on lowering the concentrations of these biomarkers in addition to total and LDL cholesterol. If biomarkers that indicate the mechanism of hypercholesterolemia are reduced after treatment, clinical outcomes might also be expected to improve.

Ezetimibe and other cholesterol-lowering drugs were approved years after statins were put into clinical practice. They are marketed to be used in conjunction with statins to improve statin efficacy in lowering LDL cholesterol, and as an alternative for individuals who are statin intolerant because of the presence of liver dysfunction and myalgia. Although all medications have some side effects and potential for drug-drug interactions, ezetimibe intolerance or resistance has not been described. However, if overproduction is the cause for hypercholesterolemia and not hyperabsorption, ezetimibe treatment alone will likely be ineffective, and other types of lipid-lowering medications would be indicated. To date, there are no clinical trials where therapeutic selection is based on results of cholesterol synthesis and plant steroids biomarkers. It is unlikely that these studies will be conducted because all of these drugs are in the postmarket phase and there is insufficient economic incentive to cost justify such trials by the pharmaceutical industry.

EFFECT OF LIPID-LOWERING DRUGS ON CHOLESTEROL SYNTHESIS AND ABSORPTION

There is a considerable amount of data demonstrating that the concentrations of β-sitosterol, campesterol, and lathosterol are altered with administration of statins and ezetimide alone and in combination. **Table 2** summarizes the changes in cholesterol synthesis markers caused by statin use. **Table 3** summaries the changes in cholesterol absorption markers caused by ezetimide. In both tables the effect of statins on absorption biomarkers and the effect of ezetimide on synthesis biomarkers are also given where such data are available.

In one of the earlier studies, Reihner and colleagues[22] showed that 20 mg twice a day of pravastatin reduced the concentration of lathosterol by 63%. Subsequent studies have confirmed that the magnitude of decline ranges from 5% to 76% (**Table 2**).[14,22–25] This is despite the use of different types of statins and inhibitors and varying dosing. One of these studies showed that the decrease in desmosterol was considerably less at 11% to 12% than lathosterol at 50% to 56%.[14] There is disagreement as to the effect statins have on cholesterol absorption biomarkers. Although no studies have shown a significant decrease in campesterol and β-sitosterol, one study showed no change.[23] In this study, polygenic and familial combined hyperlipidemia were studied. There was no change in absorption markers in the polygenic, and a modest increase seen in familial patients but not to the extent that other investigators had seen and the delta change did not exceed the biologic variation of these markers.[11] This is in contrast to all of the other studies cited in this work that showed an increase.[14,24,25] The existing statin regimen may be appropriate for those

Table 2
Change in cholesterol balance tests caused by statin use[a]

Study Condition	ΔDesmosterol	ΔLathosterol	ΔAbsorption Markers	Ref
Pravastatin, 20 mg	—	−63%	NA	22
Pravastatin, 20 mg w/CAD	−12%	−50%	+48% campesterol, +25% β-sitosterol	14
Pravastatin, 20 mg w/o CAD	−11%	−56%	+51% campesterol, +26% β-sitosterol	
20 mg sim or 10 atorvast PHC	—	−45%	−6% campesterol, −2% β-sitosterol	23
20 mg sim or 10 atorvast FHC	—	−63%	+26% campesterol, +14% β-sitosterol	
Rouvastatin, 40 mg	—	−64%	+52% campesterol, +57% β-sitosterol	24
Atorvastatin, 80 mg	—	−68%	+72% campesterol, +96% β-sitosterol	
Atorvastatin, 40 mg[b]	—	−76%	+65% campesterol, +70% β-sitosterol	25

Abbreviations: CAD, coronary artery disease; FHC, familial hypercholesterolemia; PHC, polygenic cholesterolemia.
[a] Expressed as 10^2 mmol/mol cholesterol except where indicated.
[b] Expressed in μmol/L.

individuals in whom there was no subsequent change in absorption biomarkers. In contrast, investigators who have demonstrated that campesterol and β-sitosterol concentrations have increased after statin treatment suggest that this is a compensatory mechanism toward cholesterol concentration within the enterocyte of the brush border. Tremblay and coworkers[25] showed that cholesterol depletion stimulates the transcription of the NPC1-like transporter. Perhaps individuals exhibiting this phenotype would benefit from the addition of ezetimide to their statin regimen.

A similar but inverse situation is observed for patients treated with ezetimide alone. Results are summarized in **Table 3**.[18,26–29] There is a consistent 20% to 50% decline in campesterol and β-sitosterol, with no increase in lathosterol in one study[26] and a significant 50% increase in other studies.[18,27–29] As with statins, use of ezetimibe may cause some compensatory upregulation in the cholesterol synthesis pathway.

Table 3
Change in cholesterol absorption tests caused by ezetimibe use[a]

Study Condition	ΔCampesterol	ΔSitosterol	ΔCholestanol	ΔSynthesis	Ref
Ezetimibe, 10 mg[b]	−48%	−41%	—	+53% lathosterol	18
Ezetimibe, 10 mg[b]	−51%	−44%	—	0% lathosterol	26
Ezetimibe, 10 mg	−24%	−21%	—	+37% lathosterol	27
Ezetimibe, 10 mg + statins	—	−52%	—	+83% lathosterol	28
Ezetimibe, 10 mg ± statins[b]	−46%	−39%	−7%	+51% lathosterol	29

[a] Expressed as 10^2 mmol/mol cholesterol except where indicated.
[b] Expressed in μmol/L.

In a pig model, Telford and colleagues[9] duplicated this phenotype by showing that an ezetimibe dose in pigs equivalent to 10 mg in humans resulted in a 91% decrease in campesterol, 90% decrease in β-sitosterol, and 65% increase in lathosterol. Importantly, the addition of simvastatin to ezetimibe resulted in a return of lathosterol concentrations back to the baseline. These data may provide some scientific basis for using both drugs to treat patients who behave in this manner.

PROPOSED CLINICAL USE OF CHOLESTEROL ABSORPTION AND SYNTHESIS TESTS

Routine measurements of biomarkers of cholesterol absorption and synthesis have not yet been endorsed by international guidelines. Although the pathophysiology seems sound, the benefits of therapeutic selection based on these markers remains to be determined. There is ample documentation that lipid lowering does improve clinical outcomes. If a patient on statins does not exhibit a reduction in total and LDL cholesterol, it is possible that the mechanism for the hypercholesterolemia is caused by increased absorption, which could have been predicted by measurement of lathosterol before drug treatment, and verified as the mechanism after failure. Although the mechanism can be inferred post hoc (ie, unaltered postadministration lipid analysis), a priori assessment of cholesterol synthesis status could avoid the time, effort, and expense necessary to initiate an ineffective drug. A proposed algorithm for the use of these tests is shown in **Fig. 2**. Testing for increased cholesterol absorption or synthesis is conducted for individuals with hypercholesterolemia (eg, >200 mg/dL). Ezetemibe is recommended for those who have an increase in β-sitosterol and campesterol alone, whereas a statin is recommended for those who have an isolated increase in lathosterol. Combination therapy is reserved for patients with initial increases in both types of biomarkers. Those who have mildly high cholesterol with

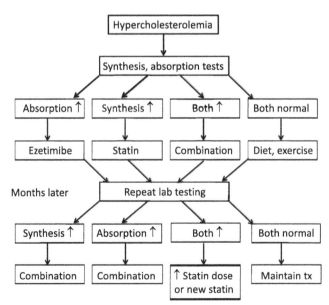

Fig. 2. Proposed therapy based on results of cholesterol synthesis and absorption biomarkers. See text for discussion. Note that this algorithm has not been validated by any clinical trial nor is it endorsed by any clinical practice guidelines. It is presented for discussion purposes only. tx, treatment.

no other risk factors and no increase in β-sitosterol, campesterol, or lathosterol can be treated with modifications of diet and exercise. After a few months of therapy, the cholesterol absorption and synthesis tests are repeated. Patients on ezetimibe who have normal β-sitosterol and campesterol but now have high lathosterol as a consequence should be treated with the addition of a statin (combination therapy). There are medications available that have combined these classes of drugs into a single pill. Patients on statins who have normal lathosterol but now have high β-sitosterol and campesterol as a consequence should be treated with the addition of ezetimibe. If combination therapy was originally used because both synthesis and absorption markers were increased, the alternative is to increase the dose of statins or choose an alternate statin. There are no data regarding the use of increased ezetimide dosing to lower cholesterol. The existing therapy should be maintained in individuals who have normal levels of synthesis and absorption markers (see **Fig. 2**).

REFERENCES

1. Expert Panel on Detection, Evaluation, and Treatment of High Blood Cholesterol in Adults (Adult Treatment Panel III). Third Report of the National Cholesterol Education Program (NCEP) Expert Panel on Detection, Evaluation, and Treatment of High Blood Cholesterol in Adults. Final Report. Circulation 2002;106:3143–421.
2. Liscum L. Cholesterol biosynthesis. In: Vance DE, Vance JE, editors. Biochemistry of lipids, lipoproteins and membranes. 4th edition. Amsterdam: Elsevier; 2002. p. 409–31.
3. Bjorkhem I, Miettinen T, Reihner E, et al. Correlation between serum levels of some cholesterol precursors and activity of HMG-CoA reducatase in human liver. J Lipid Res 1987;27:1137–43.
4. Wang DQ. New concepts of mechanisms of intestinal cholesterol absorption. Ann Hepatol 2003;2(3):113–21.
5. Hubacek JA, Berge KE, Cohen JC, et al. Mutations in ATP-cassette binding protein G5 (ABCG5) and G8 (ABCG8) causing sitosterolemia. Hum Mutat 2001;18: 359–60.
6. Baumgartner S, Mensink RP, Plat J. Plant sterols and stanols in the treatment of dysplipidemia: new insights into targets and mechanisms related to cardiovascular risk. Curr Pharm Des 2011;17:922–32.
7. Catapano AL. Ezetimibe: a selective inhibitor of cholesterol absorption. Eur Heart J 2001;3(Suppl):E6–10.
8. Singh P, Saxena R, Srinivas G, et al. Cholesterol biosynthesis and homeostatsis in regulation of the cell cycle. PLoS One 2013;8:e58833. http://dx.doi.org/10.1371/journal.pone.0059933.
9. Telford DE, Sutherland BG, Edwards JY, et al. The molecular mechanisms underlying the reduction of LDL apoB-100 by ezetimibe plus simvastatin. J Lipid Res 2007;48:699–708.
10. Matthan NR, Raeini-Sarjaz M, Lichtenstein HA, et al. Deuterium uptake and plasma cholesterol precursor levels correspond as methods for measurement of endogenous cholesterol synthesis in hypercholesterolemic women. Lipids 2000;35:1037–44.
11. Wu AH, Ruan W, Todd J, et al. Biological variation of β-sitosterol, campesterol, and lathosterol as cholesterol absorption and synthesis biomarkers. Clin Chim Acta, in press.
12. Matthan NR, Lei Z, Pencina M, et al. Sex-specific differences in the predictive value of cholesterol homeostatic markers and 10-year cardiovascular disease

event rate in Framingham Offspring Study participants. J Am Heart Assoc 2013; 2:e005066. http://dx.doi.org/10.1161/JAHA. 112.005066.

13. Matthan NR, Pencina M, laRocque JM, et al. Alterations in cholesterol absorption/synthesis markers characterize Framingham Offspring Study participants with CHD. J Lipid Res 2009;50:1927–35.

14. Matthan NR, Resteghinini N, Robertson M, et al. Cholesterol absorption and synthesis markers in individuals with and without a CHD event during pravastatin therapy: insights from the PROSPER Trial. J Lipid Res 2010;51:202–9.

15. Van Himbergen TM, Otokozawa S, Matthan NR, et al. Familial combined hyperlipidemia is associated with alterations in the cholesterol synthesis pathway. Arterioscler Thromb Vasc Biol 2010;30:113–20.

16. Salen G, Shefer S, Nguyen L, et al. Sitosterolemia. J Lipid Res 1992;33:945–55.

17. Rajaratnam RA, Gylling H, Miettinen TA. Independent association of serum squalene and noncholesterol sterols with coronary artery disease in postmenopausal women. J Am Coll Cardiol 2000;35:1185–91.

18. Sudhop T, Lutjohann D, Kodal A, et al. Inhibition of intestinal cholesterol absorption by ezetimibe humans. Circulation 2002;106:1943–8.

19. Pinedo S, Vissers MN, von Bergmann K, et al. Plasma levels of plant steros and the risk of coronary artery disease: the prospective EPIC-Norfolk Population Study. J Lipid Res 2007;48:139–44.

20. Wilund KR, Yu L, Xu F, et al. Plant sterol levels are not associated with atherosclerosis in mice and men. Arterioscler Thromb Vasc Biol 2004;24:1–7.

21. Josan K, Majumdar SR, McAlister FA. The efficacy and safety of intensive statin therapy: a meta-analysis of randomized trials. CMAJ 2008;178:576–84.

22. Reihner E, Rudling M, Stahlberg D, et al. Influence of pravastatin, a specific inhibitor of HMG-CoA reductase, on hepatic metabolism of cholesterol. N Engl J Med 1990;323:224–8.

23. Lupattelli G, Siepi D, De Vuono S, et al. Cholesterol metabolism differs after statin therapy according to the type of hyperlipidemia. Life Sci 2012;90:846–50.

24. van Himbergen TM, Matthan NR, Resteghini NA, et al. Comparison of the effects of maximal dose atorvastatin and rosuvastatin therapy on cholesterol synthesis and absorption markers. J Lipid Res 2009;50:730–9.

25. Tremblay AJ, Lamarche B, Lemelin V, et al. Atorvastatin increases intestinal expression of NPC1L1 in hyperlipidemic men. J Lipid Res 2011;52:558–65.

26. Lutjohann D, von Bergmann K, Sirah W, et al. Long-term efficacy and safety of ezetimibe 10 mg in patients with homozygous sitosterolemia: a 2-year, open lapel extension study. Int J Clin Pract 2008;62:1499–510.

27. Salen G, von Bergmann K, Lutjohann D, et al. Ezetimibe effectively reduces plasma plant sterols in patients with sitosterolemia. Circulation 2004;108:966–71.

28. Thongtang N, Lin J, Schaefer EJ, et al. Effects of ezetimibe added to statin therapy on markers of cholesterol absorption and synthesis and LDL-C lowering in hyperlipidemic patients. Atherosclerosis 2012;225:388–96.

29. Kishimoto M, Sugiyama T, Osame K, et al. Efficacy of ezetimibe as monotherapy or combination therapy in hyperchoelsterolemic patients with and without diabetes. J Med Invest 2011;58:86–94.

Beginning to Understand High-Density Lipoproteins

Carlos G. Santos-Gallego, MD, Juan J. Badimon, PhD, Robert S. Rosenson, MD*

KEYWORDS

- High-density lipoprotein • Apolipoprotein A-I • High-density lipoprotein particles
- Reverse cholesterol transport • Atherosclerosis • Niacin • Fibrates
- Cholesteryl ester transfer protein inhibitor

KEY POINTS

- High-density lipoprotein (HDL) cholesterol (HDL-C) has been considered to reduce the risk for atherosclerotic cardiovascular disease (CVD).
- Contradictory evidence has appeared in the last years, including the lack of inverse association between HDL-C and CVD risk in the presence of very low levels of low-density lipoprotein cholesterol (LDL-C), and the failure of novel pharmacologic strategies targeting increases in HDL-C.
- Cholesterol implicated in the reverse cholesterol transport contributes only 5% of all the clinically measured HDL-C; therefore, HDL-C levels (or the change in them) are not a precise parameter for adequately assessment of the contribution of HDL to CVD risk.
- The cholesterol content of HDL does not represent many important HDL functions that are related to CVD risk, such as antioxidant, anti-inflammatory, antiapoptotic, and vasorelaxant properties. Therefore, a need exists to move beyond HDL-C as a surrogate for the beneficial actions of HDL.
- HDL particle concentration is a better biomarker than HDL-C, because it predicts CVD risk even after adjusting for HDL-C and also in the presence of very low levels of LDL-C.

INTRODUCTION

For the last 60 years, high-density lipoproteins (HDL) have been widely considered to reduce the risk for cardiovascular disease (CVD); in fact, the cholesterol carried by HDL (HDL-C) has earned the moniker of "good cholesterol". This concept has led to the development of several pharmacologic strategies aiming to raise HDL-C to reduce

This article originally appeared in Endocrinology and Metabolism Clinics, Volume 43, Issue 4, December 2014.

Disclosures: None (C.G. Santos-Gallego, J.J. Badimon); Grant/Research Support: AstraZeneca, Amgen, Hoffman-LaRoche, Sanofi; Consultant/Advisor: Aegerion, Amgen, Astra Zeneca, Eli Lilly, Janssen, LipoScience, Novartis, Regeneron, Sanofi; Equity Interests/Stock Options: LipoScience, (R.S. Rosenson).

Cardiovascular Institute, Icahn School of Medicine at Mount Sinai, One Gustave Levy Place, Box 1030, New York, NY 10029, USA
* Corresponding author.
E-mail address: robert.rosenson@mssm.edu

CVD risk. The proposition that HDL protects against the development of cardiovascular diseases is based on several robust and consistent observations: (1) numerous human population studies have shown that the plasma concentrations of both HDL-C and the major HDL apolipoprotein (apo), apoA-I, are independent, inverse predictors of the risk of having a CVD event (**Table 1**). Moreover, low HDL-C remains predictive of increased CVD, even when low-density lipoprotein (LDL) cholesterol (LDL-C) has been reduced to low levels by treatment with statins[1]; (2) HDL have several well-documented functions with the potential to protect against cardiovascular disease (see later discussion); (3) interventions that increase the concentration of HDL inhibit the development and progression of atherosclerosis in several animal models[2–4]; and (4) in proof-of-concept studies in humans, intravenous infusions of reconstituted HDL (rHDL) consisting of apoA-I complexed with phospholipids promote regression of coronary atheroma as assessed by intravascular ultrasonography.[5,6]

However, the hypothesis that HDL-C and apoA-I directly confer biological protection against atherosclerosis has never been proved. The same is true for the hypothesis that raising HDL-C or apoA-I levels will result in reduced CVD risk. In fact, several recent lines of evidence have questioned HDL-C and apoA-I as relevant therapeutic targets. First, a recent study showed that some genetic variants that raise HDL-C levels are not associated with a proportionally lower risk of myocardial infarction.[7] Second, a subanalysis of the JUPITER trial has shown that HDL-C and apoA-I were associated with reduced CVD risk among patients in the placebo arm, but that this association was lost among people on rosuvastatin 20 mg achieving very low levels of LDL-C.[8] Third, data from population studies and from a meta-analysis have suggested that changes in HDL-C levels after initiation of lipid-modifying therapy are not independently associated with CVD risk.[9,10] Finally, recent clinical trials have shown that HDL-C–raising pharmacologic therapy increases HDL-C levels but does not reduce CVD events (eg, AIM-HIGH[11] and HPS-THRIVE[12] for niacin, dal-OUTCOMES[13] for dalcetrapib, ACCORD[14] for fenofibrate).

This review attempts to reconcile the beneficial effects of HDL metabolism on CVD risk with the more recent studies, which seem to cast a shadow on the future of HDL by formulating a comprehensive hypothesis that includes both facts. Finally, current and future pharmacologic strategies targeting HDL are discussed.

COMPOSITION OF THE HIGH-DENSITY LIPOPROTEIN PARTICLES

A crucial distinction must be made between HDL-C (ie, the amount of cholesterol carried by the HDL) and the HDL particle (HDL-P, the individual molecule containing proteins and lipids—specifically cholesterol but also other types of lipids). The levels of HDL-C do not necessarily reflect the concentration of HDL-P because HDL-P can be fully or only partially loaded with cholesterol. This distinction is key to shedding light on the recent seeming "failings" of the protective role of HDL-C in CVD.

HDL-P is a complex and heterogeneous assembly of proteins, lipids, and micro-RNAs (miRNA).

- *Proteome composition of HDL-P.* Approximately 75% of the protein content of HDL is apoA-I, which serves as the primary protein scaffolding on which the lipid cargo-carrying particle is built. Each HDL particle contains 2 to 5 molecules of apoA-I,[15,16] so apoA-I levels provide no indication of the HDL-P concentration. Other protein components of HDL are apoA-II, apoA-IV, apoA-V, apoE, apoJ, apoM, lecithin-cholesterol acyl transferase (LCAT), cholesteryl ester transfer protein (CETP), and the antioxidant enzymes paroxonase 1 (PON-1) and glutathione selenoperoxidase.

Table 1
Epidemiologic studies suggesting an inverse relationship between HDL-C concentrations and CVD risk

Study	Population	Methods	Results
Tromsø Heart Study[179]	6595 males, age 20–49 y	Population screening, followed for 2 y	HDL-C level was inversely correlated with CV risk. HDL-C was 3 times better than non–HDL-C for CVD risk prediction
Framingham Heart Study[180]	1605 patients, age 49–82 y	16 groups stratified by HDL and TC levels, followed for 12 y	High levels of HDL-C were shown to correlate with lower incidences of CHD for all levels of TC (1 mg/dL increase in HDL correlated with 2%–3% decrease in CHD risk)
MRFIT (Multiple Risk Factor – Intervention Trial)[181]	5792 males with elevated CHD risk factors, age 35–57 y	Risk factor modification vs no intervention, followed for 7 y	No change in HDL levels; no significant difference in CHD mortality
Lipid Research Clinics Coronary Primary Prevention Trial[182]	1808 males with hyperlipidemia, age 30–69 y	Lipid-lowering diet + placebo vs cholestyramine, followed for 7 y	In both the drug and placebo groups, a 1 mg/dL increase in HDL was associated with a 3.4%–5.5% reduction in primary CHD events
Prospective Cardiovascular Munster (PROCAM)[183]	19,698 volunteers (4559 males between 40 and 64 y were analyzed)	Followed for 6 y	Subjects with HDL <35 mg/dL showed a 4 times greater CV risk
Israeli Ischemic Heart Disease Study (Gouldbort)[184]	8565 males, age >42 y	4 groups stratified by HDL and TC levels, followed for 21 y	Subgroups with low HDL-C had a 35% higher CV mortality rate than those groups with high HDL-C (even after adjusting by age and other CV risk factors)
Atherosclerosis Risk in Communities (ARIC) Study[185]	12,339 participants, age 45–64 y	Followed for 10 y	Inverse relation between HDL-C and CV risk. Risk prediction by HDL-C seems to be greater in females than in males
Prospective Epidemiological Study of Myocardial Infarction (PRIME)[186]	10,592 volunteers, age 50–59 y	Prospective cohort study, followed for 5 y	A significant (P<.0001) linear increase in relative CVD risk was observed for HDL-C decrease. The levels of apoA-I were also predictive.

Abbreviations: ApoA-I, apolipoprotein A-I; CHD, coronary heart disease; CV, cardiovascular; CVD, cardiovascular disease; TC, total cholesterol.
Data from Refs.[179–186]

- *Lipidome composition of the HDL-P.* The lipid composition of HDL-P is also rich, because it mainly contains cholesteryl esters (CE) but also other lipids such as free cholesterol (FC), triglycerides (TG), and phospholipids (PL). PL and FC form the surface lipid monolayer of HDL-P, while CE and TG build the hydrophobic lipid core. Of interesting, PL quantitatively predominate in the HDL lipidome (accounting for 20%–30% of total HDL mass), followed by CE (14%–18%), TG (3%–6%), and FC (3%–5%).[17] The lysophospholipid sphingosine-1-phosphate (S1P) is also predominantly carried by the HDL-P, and has recently been demonstrated to specifically possess antiatherosclerotic effects.[18–20]
- *micro RNA (miRNA)* are small ($\sim$22 nucleotides), noncoding RNA, which bind to partially complementary sites primarily found in the 3'-untranslated region of target mRNAs and which inhibit gene expression via induction of mRNA degradation. Although miRNAs act intracellularly, they can be exported in exosomes and microparticles. Recently, HDL-P have been discovered to transport miRNA,[21] and HDL-P are much more enriched in miRNA than LDL particles (LDL-P). Furthermore, HDL-mediated delivery of miRNAs to recipient cells was demonstrated to be dependent on scavenger receptor class B type I (SR-BI).[21] Moreover, HDL-P are much more enriched than LDL-P in miRNA,[22] and miR-223, miR-126, and miR-92 are detected with the higher number of copies.[22] Preliminary reports suggested that the human HDL-miRNA profile of normal subjects is significantly different from that of CVD patients,[21] but data seem contradictory.[22]

Molar differences in the content of major proteins and lipid constituents of HDL cause considerable heterogeneity of HDL as delineated by electron microscopy (shape), ultracentrifugation (density), gel filtration, polyacrylamide gel electrophoresis, nuclear magnetic resonance spectroscopy (size), charge (agarose gel electrophoresis), or affinity (apolipoprotein composition); unfortunately, there is overlap between the proposed HDL subclasses defined by the various isolation methods. To homogenize the concepts and facilitate communication, the authors have previously proposed a uniform standardized nomenclature[23] of 5 HDL subclasses according to size that allows clinicians and scientists to be consistent in their definitions.

OVERVIEW OF HIGH-DENSITY LIPOPROTEIN METABOLIC PATHWAYS: REVERSE CHOLESTEROL TRANSPORT

The purpose of this review is to propose an explanation about the discordant later results with HDL as a therapeutic target. Therefore, the metabolism of HDL is only succinctly summarized (**Fig. 1**; for a more detailed explanation, see Refs.[24–26]).

In contrast to LDL, HDL requires a maturation process. ApoA-I is expressed and secreted predominantly by the liver (70%) and also by the small intestine (30%). Lipid-free apoA-I rapidly obtains small amounts of PL[25] (very small HDL [HDL-VS] in the standardized nomenclature, also called pre-β migrating HDL). These HDL-VS bind to adenosine triphosphate (ATP)-binding cassette transporter A1 (ABCA1) on liver, intestine, or macrophages, thus acquiring FC, increasing its lipid content and becoming discoid-shaped larger HDL particles (small HDL [HDL-S]).

LCAT catalyzes the transfer of an acyl group from lecithin to FC and generates hydrophobic CE, which migrate to the core of HDL-P thus leading to the formation of spherical mature particles (medium HDL [HDL-M] in the standardized nomenclature). Mature HDL-M bind with receptors ATP-binding cassette transporter G1 (ABCG1) and SR-BI, which are responsible for additional cholesterol efflux to mature HDL particles, further increasing the size and CE content of the now buoyant and

Increase Preβ-HDL and ApoA-I

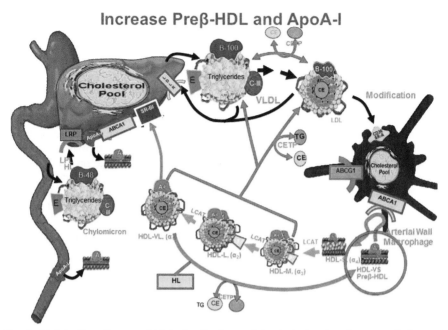

Fig. 1. Metabolic pathways of high-density lipoprotein cholesterol and reverse cholesterol transport in humans. ABCA1, adenosine triphosphate (ATP)-binding cassette transporter A1; ABCG1, ATP-binding cassette transporter G1; Apo, apolipoprotein; CE, cholesteryl ester; CETP, cholesteryl ester transfer protein; HDL, high-density lipoprotein (-VS, very small; -S, small; -M, medium; -L, large; -VL, very large); HL, hepatic lipase; LCAT, lecithin-cholesterol acyl transferase; LDLR, low-density lipoprotein receptor; LPL, lipoprotein lipase; LRP, lipoprotein receptor–related protein; TG, triglycerides; VLDL, very low-density lipoprotein. (*Courtesy of* H. Bryan Brewer Jr, MD, Washington, DC, and Robert S. Rosenson, MD, New York, NY.)

spherical HDL particle (large HDL [HDL-L] and very large HDL [HDL-VL] in the standardized nomenclature).

The reverse cholesterol transport (RCT) loop is closed with CE delivery to the liver by 2 different mechanisms. First, HDL-L and HDL-VL are selectively taken up in the liver by means of hepatic SR-BI receptors, thus completing cholesterol return to the liver. In addition, CETP transfers CE from HDL particles to TG-rich lipoproteins (very low-density lipoprotein [VLDL] and LDL); cholesterol finally reaches the liver when LDL-P are taken up by the liver via the LDL receptor.

There is functional heterogeneity among the different HDL particles. HDL-S and HDL-VS particles are most efficient in interacting with the ABCA1 to promote cholesterol efflux from cells, whereas HDL-L and HDL-VL are the most efficient in interacting with liver SR-BI for delivery of cholesterol to the liver.[23] HDL-M particles are the ones most interactive with ABCG1 to promote cellular cholesterol efflux.[23] Specifically, HDL-VS seem to be very active; in fact, delipidated HDL or apoA-I Milano complexed with phospholipids (which can be assimilated to HDL-VS) have been shown to promote regression of coronary atherosclerosis.[5,6] Therefore, because some HDL-P are more effective than others at cholesterol efflux, the number and size of the HDL-P (ie, the capacity to accept more cholesterol) seems to be much more relevant for HDL antiatherosclerotic effects than the absolute concentration of HDL-C.

Only 3% to 5% of the mass of HDL-P, however, is derived from macrophage cholesterol efflux.[25] Thus, the fraction of cholesterol in HDL-P specifically corresponding to macrophage cholesterol efflux (ie, responsible for the antiatherosclerotic effect of HDL) is very small and most likely does not change HDL-C levels.[25] Therefore, HDL-C concentrations may be either an insensitive or ineffective method to quantify cholesterol changes in the vascular macrophages that have been proposed to reduce CVD events.

However, the use of multiple static measures of the pool size of HDL-C is likely an inadequate approach for the characterization of a dynamic process such as the aforementioned RCT and HDL metabolism. For these reasons, different experimental models for assessing the dynamic macrophage RCT have been developed.[25,27] At present, in vivo quantification of macrophage RCT can only be determined in animal models (murine model of intraperitoneal injection of macrophages loaded with tritium-labeled cholesterol) or through kinetic modeling of isotope dilution.[25,27] Clinically, ex vivo assays have been used to assess the capacity of individual patient serum and HDL specimens to remove cholesterol from cultured cholesterol-loaded macrophages (either J774 mouse macrophages or THP-1 human macrophages). Relative contributions of the efflux pathways in murine macrophages are as follows: ABCA1, 35%; aqueous diffusion, 35%; ABCG1, 21%; and SR-BI, 9%. In cholesterol-loaded human macrophages, the relative contributions of these pathways to cholesterol efflux are different; the ABCA1 pathway remains predominant, but ABCG1 does not contribute to efflux, and the SR-BI pathway is relatively more important.[25] A recent study reported that the capacity of individual patient serum to stimulate cholesterol efflux from J774 macrophages has a strong inverse association with angiographically quantified coronary artery disease (CAD) that was statistically independent of HDL-C or apoA-I levels.[28,29] Regarding carotid territories, cholesterol efflux capacity is also inversely associated with carotid intima-media thickness (cIMT),[28] with increasing carotid stenosis[30] and with more advanced carotid plaque morphology.[30] This result confirms that the functionality of HDL-P (determined by the size and concentration of HDL-P), but not the levels of HDL-C, is the main determinant of the beneficial effect of HDL. Surprisingly, some investigators have reported that an increased cholesterol efflux was paradoxically associated with a higher rate of CVD events[29]; however, one should consider that the overall number of events was low, and the definitive answer to the relationship of cholesterol efflux capacity to CVD events awaits much larger prospective cohort analyses.

ATHEROPROTECTIVE EFFECTS OF HIGH-DENSITY LIPOPROTEIN CHOLESTEROL INDEPENDENT OF REVERSE CHOLESTEROL TRANSPORT

Besides its cholesterol efflux capacity, HDL is well known to possess additional salutary effects including anti-inflammatory, antioxidant, antiapoptotic, and antithrombotic actions, and vasorelaxant, antidiabetic, and infarct-size–reducing properties. These pleiotropic actions may potentially contribute to the benefits conveyed by HDL. These mechanisms that involve the HDL proteome and lipidome have been extensively reviewed elsewhere.[15,31]

Anti-inflammatory Properties

Aside from RCT, the next best recognized HDL function is anti-inflammatory regulation. In contrast to its important positive effect on RCT, lipid-poor apoA-I does not possess several of the endothelial cell–protective and anti-inflammatory activities of HDL-C that are mediated by binding to SR-BI.[32] HDL reduces the expression of adhesion molecules and inflammatory markers in macrophages and endothelial cells.[33] HDL reduces tumor necrosis factor (TNF)-mediated induction of cell adhesion molecules (vascular [VCAM-1] and intercellular [ICAM-1]) both in cell culture[34] and in vivo models of atherosclerosis. HDL also inhibits the synthesis of monocyte chemo-attractant protein 1, responsible for recruitment of monocytes, dendritic cells, and T lymphocytes to sites of inflammation. Moreover, apoA-I treatment modulates macro-phage polarization from an M1 (proinflammatory) to an M2 (anti-inflammatory) pheno-type.[35] HDL also interacts with circulating leukocytes to limit inflammation through an ABCA1-dependent mechanism (for instance, apoA-I can inhibit adhesion through CD11b).[36]

HDL and the ATP-binding cassette transporters act at the level of hematopoietic stem cells (HSCs) to suppress HSC proliferation and the production of monocytes and neutrophils. HDL interacts with ABCA1/ABCG1 to promote cholesterol efflux in the bone marrow and to control levels and signaling of interleukin (IL)-3/granulocyte macrophage colony–stimulating factor. If HDL is lowered or ABCA1/ABCG1 is absent, there is excessive proliferation of HSC in hypercholesterolemia, resulting in monocy-tosis.[37] However, this HSC proliferation can be suppressed with liver X-receptor ago-nists. IL-23–mediated HSC mobilization from the bone marrow and extramedullary hematopoiesis in the spleen also result in monocytosis, but can also be prevented by increased HDL.[38]

Endothelial-Protective and Vasodilating Effects

HDL-C enhances production of nitric oxide (NO) from endothelial NO synthase (eNOS) through SR-BI activation[39] and can reverse the oxidized LDL-mediated decrease in NO production. SR-BI colocalizes with eNOS in the caveolae of endothelial cells, and interaction with HDL-C directly activates eNOS. ABCG1 is also needed in this pro-cess.[40] HDL-C is also capable of inducing eNOS synthesis, thus favoring vasorelaxa-tion.[19] Although apoA-I plays the major role, HDL-associated S1P may stimulate eNOS through activation of the lysophospholipid receptor S1P-I in endothelial cells.[19]

Ex vivo, HDL increases NO-mediated vasorelaxation in aortic ring preparations.[40] Moreover, HDL favors endothelial cell proliferation and migration by means of SR-BI,[41] which results in normalization of the dysfunctional atherosclerotic endothelium. Recombinant HDL (rHDL) enhances endothelial function in vivo in humans with normal cholesterol levels[42] and in individuals with low HDL-C levels.[43] Injection of HDL from healthy subjects into diabetic patients increased endothelial NO production, dimin-ished endothelial oxidant stress, enhanced endothelium-dependent vasodilation, and promoted endothelial progenitor cell–mediated repair.[44]

Antiapoptotic Actions

HDL attenuates TNF-α–induced[45] and oxidized LDL-induced[46] apoptosis of endothe-lial cells and macrophages by activating the Akt pathway and inhibiting proapoptotic Bax. HDL has been demonstrated to also inhibit apoptosis in macrophages through a pathway involving ABCA1 and ABCG1[47]; this action is crucial because apoptotic macrophages release metalloproteinases and cytokines, which cause plaque desta-bilization. S1P, which is mainly carried in the plasma by HDL, also possesses antia-poptotic properties.[48]

Antithrombotic Effects

Low levels of HDL-C have been associated with increased arterial and venous[49] thrombotic events. Intravenous infusion of apoA-I decreases acute thrombus forma-tion in an in vivo rat model of thrombogenesis.[50] The antithrombotic properties of HDL have been attributed to (1) increased NO production[39]; (2) enhanced prostacyclin synthesis (both apoA-I and lipids in HDL stimulate cyclooxygenase-2, the key enzyme in prostacyclin pathway) and simultaneous decrease in thromboxane A_2 synthesis; (3) moreover, large HDL particles can act as a surface on which the ability of activated protein C or S to cleave active factor V is enhanced[51] (thus inhibiting thrombin generation); (4) HDL has direct antiplatelet effects—in humans, infusion of reconstituted HDL decreases collagen-, adenosine diphosphate-, or thrombin-induced platelet aggregation[52]; (5) HDL shows some fibrinolytic properties because it upregulates tissue plasminogen activator.[53]

Antidiabetic Effects

HDL also potentially exerts antidiabetic effects. First, HDL directly improves β-cell insulin secretion through ABCA1 and ABCG1; in fact, deletion of ABCA1 in both mice[54] and humans (Tangier disease[55]) results in glucose intolerance. Moreover, cholesterol accumulation in β cells reduces insulin secretion, a phenomenon that can be rescued by β-cell cholesterol unloading, either by HDL-related RCT or the cholesterol-depleting agent methyl-β-cyclodextrin.[56] An acute infusion of reconstituted HDL increased plasma insulin levels and reduced plasma glucose levels in patients with type 2 diabetes (T2DM).[57] HDL also improves insulin sensitivity; interestingly, HDL activates adenosine monophosphate kinase via ABCA1 in endothelial cells, adipose tissue, and skeletal muscle,[56] and also increases glucose uptake in primary cultured myocytes from diabetic patients.[57] In fact, depletion of apoA-I in mice resulted in impaired glucose tolerance, whereas apoA-I overexpression increased insulin sensitivity.[58] Finally, reconstituted HDL infusion inhibited fasting-induced lipolysis and fatty acid oxidation both in vitro and in vivo in T2DM patients.[59]

Myocardial Ischemia-Reperfusion Injury

Another beneficial effect (although not directly related to atherosclerosis) is that HDL reduces myocardial ischemia-reperfusion (I/R) injury. HDL reduces the size of infarction in an I/R model; this effect is related to the presence of S1P.[60] Plasma HDL and reconstituted HDL have been shown to directly reduce infarct size ex vivo in isolated rat hearts[61,62] or in vivo in rabbit models.[63] In fact, elevated HDL-C reduces the risk and extent of PCI-related myocardial infarction and improves the long-term prognosis in patients.[64]

HIGH-DENSITY LIPOPROTEIN DYSFUNCTION

HDL loses its beneficial properties in certain pathologic situations (eg, acute situations such as acute-phase response[65] or influenza A infection,[66] or chronic conditions such as CVD[15] or diabetes[67]), which has been termed dysfunctional HDL.

In CVD, leukocyte myeloperoxidase (MPO) has also been associated with the generation of dysfunctional HDL, with proinflammatory properties.[68] Circulating HDL (with at least 2 apoA-I molecules in each particle) readily diffuses into the artery wall, specifically within MPO-enriched atherosclerotic lesions. MPO binds to one apoA-I α helix in that HDL particle, and promotes site-specific oxidative modification at residue Trp72 of the contralateral apoA-I helix.[69] In contrast to circulating HDL, most apoA-I in atheroma is not associated with the HDL particle; lipid-poor apoA-I in atheroma is cross-linked and oxidized at Trp72, thus resulting in a dysfunctional HDL particle, which is both proinflammatory and shows reduced ability to promote cholesterol efflux via ABCA1.[69] This oxTrp72–apoA-I can diffuse back to the plasma; in fact, the concentration of plasma oxTrp72–apoA-I is directly correlated with CVD, even after adjusting for HDL-C and conventional risk factors.[69] Furthermore, MPO-mediated oxidation fails to polarize macrophages from M1 into M2 phenotype[35] and also renders apoA-I unable to mediate beneficial changes in the composition of atherosclerotic plaques[35] (ie, MPO-oxidized apoA-I does not shift plaques into a less vulnerable and more stable phenotype).

Diabetes also causes HDL dysfunction, especially through nonenzymatic glycation of HDL-P. (1) Nonenzymatic glycation of apoA-I reduces ABCA1-dependent cholesterol efflux[70] and the HDL-mediated activation of LCAT.[70] (2) The usual HDL-induced inhibition of endothelial VCAM-1 expression is lost in HDL from diabetic patients, thus favoring the adhesion of macrophages to activated endothelial cells[44,71,72] and reducing the anti-inflammatory activity of HDL. (3) HDL from diabetic patients loses its vasorelaxant effects, owing to a reduced ability to stimulate endothelial NO production (thus decreasing endothelial-dependent vasodilation), and also mitigates endothelial progenitor cell–mediated endothelial repair.[73] (4) HDL from diabetic patients activates proapoptotic pathways while failing to activate antiapoptotic proteins in endothelial cells.[72]

There are other mechanisms explaining dysfunctional HDL in CVD. Chronic inflammation (atherosclerosis is also considered a chronic inflammatory status) elevates serum amyloid A (SAA) protein,[74] and SAA displaces apoA-I from the surface of HDL, thus generating free apoA-I, which is cleared faster by the kidney. Furthermore, oxidative stress is enhanced in CVD, which both reduces the levels of PON-1[75] and selectively oxidizes amino acid residues in apoA-I (such as Met, Cys, Tyr, and Lys), with the final result being a decrease in the antioxidant capacity of HDL particles.

Chronic kidney disease (CKD) is associated with low HDL-C and increased CVD. Two different studies have focused on the HDL proteome in renal disease. CKD patients undergoing dialysis have increased levels of the acute-phase inflammatory proteins SAA, lipoprotein-associated phospholipase A_2, apoC-III, antitrypsin, retinol-binding protein 4, and transthyretin in HDL, along with decreases in phospholipid and increases in TG content.[76,77] These changes correspond with impaired cholesterol efflux function[76] and impaired anti-inflammatory properties.[77] The decrease in PON-1 and glutathione peroxidase explains the lower antioxidant function; interestingly, the reduction in antioxidant activity of HDL is a predictor of CVD and overall mortality in CKD patients on dialysis.[78] These studies are suggestive of a link between HDL dysfunction and increased CVD risk in CKD.

The changes in lipid content also contribute to HDL dysfunction. The altered phospholipid composition of HDL results in an elevated sphingomyelin to phosphatidylcholine ratio, which increases HDL-P surface rigidity[79] (a key determinant of antioxidant activity of HDL)[80] and impairs HDL-P functionality. Moreover, diabetic dyslipoproteinemia is characterized by hypertriglyceridemia and low levels of HDL-C, with TG-enriched HDL resulting from a CETP-mediated interchange of TG from TG-rich lipoproteins to HDL-L/HDL-VL. A low CE/TG ratio indicates unstable HDL particles, which are rapidly cleared from the circulation, further decreasing HDL-P.

BEGINNING TO UNDERSTAND HIGH-DENSITY LIPOPROTEINS: WHY IS THE HIGH-DENSITY LIPOPROTEIN HYPOTHESIS SEEMINGLY FAILING?

As explained earlier, several modern studies have cast a shadow on the beneficial effect of HDL on CVD risk. Here a comprehensive hypothesis is formulated that may explain the atheroprotective effects of HDL assessed in both the "classical" and "modern" studies, which slightly curb enthusiasm for HDL. The authors propose that the focus on a surrogate measurement of HDL functionality, such as HDL-C, or the cholesterol content of HDL-P is not an accurate indicator of the beneficial properties of HDL. Thus, the focus should be more on quantitative measurement of

HDL (eg, HDL-P) and certain validated HDL functions (macrophage cholesterol efflux, antioxidant and anti-inflammatory properties), which truly reflect and are responsible for the actual beneficial effects of HDL. For instance, the relationship between HDL-C and CVD risk is partially confounded by the association between low HDL-C and high levels of LDL-P. In fact, data from the Framingham Offspring Study[81] demonstrate a significant disconnect between LDL-C and LDL-P in patients with low HDL-C levels; thus implying that a substantial portion of the excess CVD risk of patients with low HDL-C stems from an unrecognized excess of small, dense LDL-P containing less cholesterol than normal, which raises the issue of low HDL-C as a marker of atherogenic lipoproteins. It is recognized that HDL-C, apoA-I, and HDL-P are static mass-based measurements, and thus cannot represent a dynamic functional process such as RCT (or the anti-inflammatory, antiapoptotic, and antioxidant effects of HDL).

As previously stated, 4 recent lines of evidence have questioned HDL-C and apoA-I as relevant therapeutic targets. All of these drawbacks of the HDL hypothesis can be explained with the newly formulated hypothesis.

1. *Problem:* A recent study showed that some genetic variants in the endothelial lipase (EL) gene that raise HDL-C levels are not associated with a proportionally lower risk of myocardial infarction.[7]

   Possible explanation: The clinical relevance of HDL-P explains the results of this genetic analysis. Mutations resulting in reduced EL activity only increase HDL-C without actually increasing HDL-P; thus, patients with low EL activity may have higher levels of HDL-C but lower levels of HDL-P, which does not translate into reduced CVD risk.[7] On the contrary, the mutations resulting in reduced phospholipid transfer protein activity translate into reduced CVD risk because they result in an increased number of HDL-P.[82]

2. *Problem:* A subanalysis of the JUPITER trial has shown that HDL-C and apoA-I were associated with reduced CVD risk only among patients in the placebo arm. This beneficial association was lost among people on rosuvastatin 20 mg achieving very low levels of LDL-C.[8]

   Possible explanation: First of all, the JUPITER results are not supported by the Clinical Outcomes Utilizing Revascularization and Aggressive Drug Evaluation (COURAGE) trial; in fact, on-trial HDL-C levels in COURAGE at 6 months were associated with increased CVD risk after 4 years in the subgroup of 2193 patients who achieved LDL-C levels of 70 mg/dL or less[83] (although one must take into account that this analysis did not adjust for LDL-P or apoB). However, even only considering the JUPITER results one must take into account the clinical relevance of HDL-C versus HDL-P. Most importantly, as previously explained, HDL-P concentration has emerged as a predictor of CVD risk that may be superior to that of HDL-C in both population studies[84–86] and randomized clinical trials of lipid-modifying therapies.[87,88] In the Multi-Ethnic Study of Atherosclerosis (MESA), HDL-C was not associated with cIMT after adjusting for HDL-P and LDL-P; however, low HDL-P predicted higher risk of elevated cIMT regardless of HDL-C level,[85] even after adjusting for LDL-P. This finding is supported by a subanalysis of the Veterans Affair High-Density Lipoprotein Intervention Trial (VA-HIT)[87]; HDL-VS particles (with high capacity to accept cholesterol) were predictors of lower CVD risk (odds ratio [OR] 0.71, 95% confidence interval [CI] 0.60–0.84, $P<.01$), whereas the lower risk associated with HDL-M concentration was weaker (OR 0.82, 95% CI 0.70–0.96, $P<.02$), and for HDL-L/HDL-VL particles (with low capacity to regain cholesterol) it was nonsignificant. In fact, a recent analysis of the

JUPITER trial has shown that, even though HDL-C did not predict CVD risk in statin-treated patients, HDL-P did predict CVD risk in all patients (placebo and statin), even after adjusting for HDL-C levels.[88]

3. *Problem:* A recent meta-analysis and some population studies suggest that changes in HDL-C levels after initiation of lipid-modifying therapy are not independently associated with CVD risk.[9,10]

    Possible explanation: Only 5% of the total cholesterol carried by HDL-P is derived from macrophage cholesterol efflux,[25] so HDL-C may be an insensitive method for quantification of the antiatherosclerotic properties of HDL. Moreover, HDL-C does not represent many important HDL functions that are related to CVD risk, such as antioxidant, anti-inflammatory, antiapoptotic, and vasorelaxant properties. Therefore, HDL-C levels (or the change in them) may not be the proper parameter to assess adequately the contribution of HDL to CVD risk.

4. *Problem:* Recent clinical trials have shown that HDL-C–raising pharmacologic therapy increases HDL-C levels but does not reduce CVD events (eg, AIM-HIGH[11] and HPS2-THRIVE for niacin,[12] dal-OUTCOMES[13] for dalcetrapib, ACCORD[14] for fenofibrate).

    Possible explanation: Strategies that increase HDL-C without expanding the pool of HDL-P with its rich proteome/lipidome do not seem to be effective. First of all, the combination of statin and niacin does not increase the number of HDL-P[89,90] (niacin treatment in AIM-HIGH raised HDL-C by 29% but did not improve cholesterol efflux or the HDL anti-inflammatory properties[91]). Furthermore, dalcetrapib increases the CE cargo of each HDL-P but without effectively increasing the level of HDL-P. Fenofibrate (as used in the Action to Control Cardiovascular Risk in Diabetes [ACCORD] trial) has not been shown to increase the concentration of HDL-P; conversely, gemfibrozil (which reduced CVD risk in the VA-HIT trial[92]) is the rare example of a therapy raising the concentration of HDL-P (10%) and HDL-VS/HDL-S particles (21%). In addition, the methodological concerns about AIM-HIGH, HPS2-THRIVE, and ACCORD may have also played a role (see later discussion).

NONPHARMACOLOGIC STRATEGIES THAT POSITIVELY BENEFIT HIGH-DENSITY LIPOPROTEINS
Aerobic Exercise

Regular aerobic exercise moderately increases HDL-C by about 5%[93,94] (with increases in HDL-VL or HDL-L by 11%[95]). A minimum energy expenditure of 900 kcal per week (or 120 min/wk) from physical activity was required to elicit changes in HDL-C.[94] Exercise duration per session was the most important element of an exercise prescription, more so than exercise intensity or duration. A meta-analysis of 25 studies estimated that for energy expended above this threshold, there existed a dose-response relationship; every 10-minute prolongation of exercise per session (ie, above 120 min/wk) was associated with a 1.4-mg/dL increase in HDL-C.[94] Exercise was more effective in raising HDL-C in subjects with initially total cholesterol levels greater than 220 mg/dL or if the body mass index was less than 28 kg/m[2].[94] In the first month of exercising the anti-inflammatory effects of HDL-C predominated; in fact after only 3 weeks of exercise, although HDL-C levels did not change, HDL-C preferentially converted to an anti-inflammatory state.[96] The exercise-induced improvements in HDL-C are mediated by exercise-induced increases in lipoprotein lipase (LPL) activity; interestingly, inactivity per se reduces LPL activity and, even just by reducing time spent in sedentary activities, the LPL activity is increased and HDL-C levels elevated.[97] Moreover, overweight patients who exercise and diet experience more HDL-C elevation than patients only on diet.[98]

Weight Loss

Weight loss has favorable effects on the lipoprotein profile. In obese patients, the loss of only 1 kg is associated with a 0.35 mg/dL increase in HDL-C concentration.[99] Weight loss of 5% to 10% of body weight results in approximately a 15% reduction in LDL-C, a 20% decrease in triglycerides, and an 8% to 10% increase in HDL-C.[100] Because LPL levels are reduced in acute caloric restriction but are greatly increased with established weight loss,[101] subjects actively losing weight experience an early and transient phase of HDL-C reduction and then HDL-C levels increase proportionally to weight loss when the weight is stabilized.[99,102] In 34 morbid obese patients, bariatric surgery was accompanied by a 20% decrease in weight, a 14% increase in HDL-C levels, a 42% raise in HDL-L particles, and an improvement in cholesterol efflux through ABCG1 and SR-BI.[103]

Alcohol Intake

Moderate alcohol intake (30–40 g daily, roughly 2 drinks in males and 1 in females) increases HDL-C levels by 5% to 15% and decreases CVD risk.[104–106] It seems to be ethanol per se that causes this modification in lipid profile, thus all alcoholic drinks can increase HDL-C.[106] In a recent meta-analysis of more than 16,000 patients, there was a J-shaped curve of alcohol consumption versus all-cause and CVD mortality[107] (maximal protection 18% and 22%, respectively); in another meta-analysis there was reduced CVD mortality in light (32% reduction) and moderate (38% reduction) drinking.[108] Notwithstanding, the benefits of alcohol consumption must be balanced against the risks (potential abuse, dependence, caloric intake, and heavy alcohol intake being associated with increased all-cause and CVD mortality[109]).

Tobacco Cessation

Among nonsmokers and light, moderate, and heavy smokers, a significant dose-response effect was present for HDL-C (reduction of 4.6%, 6.3%, and 8.9% for light, moderate, and heavy smokers compared with nonsmokers) and apoA-I (reduction of 0%, 3.7%, and 5.7% for light, moderate, and heavy smokers compared with non-smokers).[110] Tobacco cessation increases HDL-C concentrations (by 4 mg/dL in men and 6 mg/dL in women), apoA-I levels,[111] and HDL-P (especially HDL-L),[111] as early as 2 weeks after cessation.[112]

Diets

Mediterranean diet and diets rich in polyunsaturated free fatty acids (nuts, olive oil, and fatty fish such as salmon, trout, or sardines) increase HDL-C levels by approximately 3 mg/dL.[113] The PREDIMED study demonstrated that Mediterranean diet supplemented with olive oil or nuts increased HDL-C by 2.5 mg/dL in comparison with a traditional low-fat diet,[114] while also reducing LDL-C by 4 to 6 mg/dL and TG (only in the nut-supplemented arm) by 7 mg/dL. Furthermore, a Mediterranean diet caused a switch of the lipid profile to a less atherogenic pattern, with an increase in the number of HDL-P, especially of HDL-L,[115] and a decrease in LDL-P, specifically of the small, oxidized LDL-P in the nut-supplemented arm.[115] Most importantly, a Mediterranean diet reduced carotid atheroma burden[116] and CVD mortality.[117] Consumption of saturated fat reduces the anti-inflammatory potential of HDL and impairs arterial endothelial function. By contrast, the anti-inflammatory activity of HDL improves after consumption of polyunsaturated fat.[118] Even the specific consumption of fatty fish (fish containing high quantities of omega-3 polyunsaturated fatty acids, such as trout, salmon, tuna, or sardines) did not affect HDL-C, but increased HDL-P and shifted the distribution of HDL-P to a less atherogenic profile.[119]

Diets with low glycemic index both increase HDL-C levels[120,121] and improve HDL anti-inflammatory properties[96] while also reducing TG. In fact, considering glycemic index as a continuous variable, a reduction in HDL-C concentration of -0.06 mmol/L per 15-unit increase in glycemic index in the diet was reported.[121] However, achieving nutrient adequacy via food-based dietary recommendations is difficult for an absolutely strict low–glycemic index diet because of limitations in foods allowed (eg, milk, fruits, and whole grains). Thus, long-term safety studies of this dietary pattern are needed before recommendations can be made.

PHARMACOLOGIC THERAPY TO RAISE HIGH-DENSITY LIPOPROTEIN CHOLESTEROL CONCENTRATIONS
Statins

In addition to LDL-C lowering, statins also do have a small effect on HDL-C levels. In a meta-analysis of 32,258 patients, it was shown that this increase was dose and statin dependent, with HDL-C increases ranging from 2.3% to 7.9%.[122] This effect did not correlate with the effect size of the LDL-C reduction. In fact, baseline HDL-C and TG levels were the best independent predictors of statin-induced HDL-C elevations.[122] Rosuvastatin exerts the most potent effect in increasing both HDL-C and HDL-P, an essential parameter regarding HDL functionality, as discussed earlier. In a double-blind study of 318 patients with metabolic syndrome, rosuvastatin increased HDL-P by 15% and HDL-C by 10% compared with placebo, and was more effective than atorvastatin in increasing both HDL-C and HDL-P.[123] Moreover, rosuvastatin increased both HDL-C and HDL-P in all patients, while atorvastatin was predominantly effective in patients with high baseline TG levels.[123]

This effect is partly due to a mild increase in apoA-I synthesis[124] and a reduction in CETP activity.[125] In addition, statin therapy seems to improve the effects of HDL on cholesterol efflux through SR-BI but not through ABCA1. Specifically, treatment with atorvastatin was accompanied by a dose-dependent increase in cholesterol efflux from hepatoma cells, an experimental model already validated for the SR-BI receptor.[126] Conversely, in J774 cells (an experimental model validated for ABCA1 receptor), incubation with statins reduced ABCA1-mediated cholesterol efflux to HDL,[127] which may be mediated by a statin-induced increase in miR-33 expression, thus reducing ABCA1 expression. However, whether such statin effects demonstrated under cell culture conditions are relevant in vivo remains unknown.

Fibrates

Fibrates, the agonists of the peroxisome proliferator–activated receptor α (PPAR-α), raise HDL-C levels by 10% to 20% while they reduce TG by 20% to 50% and LDL-C by 10% to 20%. It must be reiterated that gemfibrozil is the rare example of a drug that increases the level of HDL-C (by 7%) and, even more importantly, the concentration of HDL-P (by 21%).[87] Their mechanism of action is multiple.[128] Fibrates slightly increase the expression of apoA-I, ABCA1, and SR-BI, which directly causes an increase in HDL-C. Fibrates also decrease TG (by reducing VLDL synthesis and by activating LPL), leading to decreased CETP activity and thereby indirectly raising HDL-C. Therefore, TG reduction is an indirect way of increasing HDL-C, and the higher the baseline levels of TG, the more marked is the increase in HDL-C levels.

Several studies have been performed to assess the efficacy of fibrates on CVD end points, but the exact significance remains elusive. Positive results for gemfibrozil were reported from trials of participants with low HDL-C and high cholesterol and elevated TG levels. The primary-prevention Helsinki Heart Study showed a 34% reduction in CVD events with an 11% increase in HDL-C[129]; the benefits were more pronounced in the subgroup with TG greater than 200 mg/dL and HDL-C less than 42 mg/dL, in which there was a 72% reduction in CVD events.[130] However, as LDL-C was also decreased by 11%, these results could be attributed to LDL-C reduction. The secondary-prevention VA-HIT[92] clinical trial was the first trial to demonstrate that an increase in HDL-C concentrations reduced CVD events in patients. As LDL-C levels were identical in both study groups, the 22% reduction in CVD events could only be attributed to the gemfibrozil-mediated 7% increase in HDL-C levels. Of note, gemfibrozil treatment raised the concentration of total HDL-P (10%) and HDL-VS/HDL-S particles (21%); in fact the concentrations of these HDL-P achieved with gemfibrozil were significant, independent, inversely related predictors of new CVD events (OR 0.71, 95% CI 0.61–0.81, $P = .03$).

By contrast, the Bezafibrate Infarction Prevention (BIP)[131] and Fenofibrate Intervention and Event Lowering in Diabetes (FIELD)[132] clinical trials did not show a reduction in CVD events in the overall study population, but did reduce the primary composite end point in the prespecified subgroup with TG greater than 200 mg/dL and HDL-C less than 35 mg/dL.

Previously mentioned studies compared the effect of fibrate monotherapy with that of placebo. Only 2 studies (ACCORD and FIRST) investigated the effect of statin/fibrate therapy versus statin/placebo. For ethical reasons, all future novel lipid-lowering therapies for CVD event reduction will be started in conjunction with statins. The ACCORD lipid trial[14] studied in 5518 T2DM patients the combination of statin and fibrate versus statin/placebo; there were no significant differences in CVD events in the overall population but fibrates again decreased CVD events in the prespecified subgroup with TG greater than 204 mg/dL and HDL-C less than 40 mg/dL. The FIRST study[133] investigated fenofibrate/atorvastatin versus atorvastatin/placebo in patients with type IIb dyslipidemia and with controlled LDL-C. There was no difference in progression of cIMT between both groups; in post hoc analysis, the fenofibrate arm was favored in patients older than 60 years, with previous CVD, severe CVD (higher cIMT), and high TG. It must be emphasized that not all fibrates are created equal; unlike gemfibrozil,[87] fenofibrate has not been shown to increase the concentration of HDL-P, thereby not improving HDL metabolism. For a review of all the trials, see **Table 2** and other publications.[26] There is, therefore, solid evidence that fibrates significantly reduced CVD events when compared with placebo in subgroups of patients with reduced HDL-C and elevated TG, whereas there was no benefit observed in the subgroups without these characteristics or when combined with statin therapy.

Niacin

Niacin (vitamin B_3, at doses of 1–1.5 g) is the most effective therapy thus far for raising HDL-C. It increases HDL-C by 20% to 35%, reduces LDL-C by 15% to 20%, and reduces TG by 30% to 50%, while also decreasing lipoprotein(a). Of interest, niacin treatment does not increase the number of HDL-P but increases HDL-C exclusively, owing to an increase in the size of the HDL-P.[90] Niacin treatment also seemed to improve the cholesterol efflux and anti-inflammatory, antioxidant, vasorelaxant, and endothelial-protective effects of HDL-C in diabetic patients.[73,89]

Niacin initially showed consistent benefits in several small-scale clinical trials with and without statins using as outcome both clinical and imaging end points (atherosclerosis burden). For a review of all the trials, see **Table 2** and other publications.[26] However, great controversy has arisen over the last 2 years with the premature end of seemingly definitive trials combining statin and niacin therapy, namely the Atherothrombosis Intervention in Metabolic Syndrome with Low HDL/High Triglycerides: Impact on Global Health Outcomes[11] (AIM-HIGH) and the Heart Protection Study–2-Treatment of HDL to Reduce the Incidence of Vascular Events (HPS-2 THRIVE), both showing lack of effect of niacin treatment added to statins using CVD outcomes as primary end points. The AIM-HIGH study randomized 3300 statin-naïve patients who achieved LDL-C of less than 80 mg/dL on simvastatin + ezetimibe to a 3-year follow-up under additional 2 g of niacin or placebo, but failed to demonstrate a difference in CVD events between both arms. HPS-2 THRIVE enrolled 25,673 patients (32% with diabetes) with a follow-up of 4 years randomized to simvastatin + placebo or simvastatin/niacin/laropiprant (niacin causes flushing by binding to the PGD2 receptor and laropiprant inhibits this receptor, thus mitigating flushing), but also failed to demonstrate a difference in CVD events. Moreover, the niacin arm was associated with a 3.7% absolute increase in diabetes complications and a 1.8% absolute increase in new diagnoses of diabetes (25% increased risk of new-onset diabetes).

The design of both clinical trials may offer an initial possible explanation about the lack of effect of niacin. Several peculiarities of the AIM-HIGH study design limit its interpretation: (1) patients in the placebo arm received much higher doses of statins and ezetimibe (in a vain attempt to match the LDL-C levels between both arms); (2) small quantities of niacin (200 mg daily) were given to the placebo arm to maintain the double-blind status (regarding flushing), which explains why HDL-C increased 5 mg/dL in the placebo arm—thus, at the end of the study HDL-C levels were very similar (44 mg/dL in statin/niacin arm, 40 mg/dL in the statin/placebo arm); (3) the early termination of AIM-HIGH may have obscured a potential late benefit (eg, in VA-HIT the difference appeared after 3 years of follow-up); (4) it enrolled a very low-risk population (baseline LDL-C 71 mg/dL, TG 161 mg/dL, before randomization); (5) it is an underpowered trial (the REVEAL trial enrolled 30,000 patients and HPS-THRIVE enrolled 25,000, whereas AIM-HIGH enrolled only 3300 patients). Some additional comments should also be noted regarding HPS2-THRIVE. (1) The study only compared statin/placebo with statin/niacin/laropiprant, so it is certainly plausible that laropiprant is not really biologically inert, and plausible that some (or most) of the off-target effects observed in this trial may be related to laropiprant as opposed to niacin. In fact, mice knocked-out for PGD2 receptor exhibit accelerated atherosclerosis and thrombogenesis.[134] This issue could only have been addressed with a 2 × 2 factorial design. (2) The studied sample does not represent the actual population most susceptible to benefit from niacin treatment because it was at a very low risk (baseline LDL-C 62 mg/dL, HDL-C almost normal 44 mg/dL, TG 125 mg/dL, total cholesterol 128 mg/dL); it is highly unlikely that in real life clinicians would consider prescribing 2 g of niacin + laropiprant to patients with similar lipid profiles. (3) There was a large population heterogeneity because greater than 10,000 patients were recruited in China, and Asians are known both not to raise HDL-C by much in response to niacin and not to tolerate niacin or high-dose statins. Nevertheless, with 2 large outcome clinical trials being prematurely terminated for futility, niacin is unlikely to become a significant player in CVD risk-reduction strategies.

Additional hypotheses may explain the failure of niacin in this context. First and foremost, the combination of statin and niacin does not increase the number of HDL-P.[89,90] Therefore, strategies that increase HDL-C without expanding the pool

Table 2
Main randomized clinical trials involving HDL-C-raising drugs with their clinical and imaging end points

Study	Drugs	Patients Receiving Treatment, No./Total (%)	Elevation in HDL-C Levels (%)	Follow-up (y)	Outcomes
Nicotinic Acid					
Clinical outcomes studies					
CDP, 1975	Niacin	1119/8341 (13.4)	NR	6	Decreased (15%) nonfatal MI
CDP Follow-up, 1986	Niacin	1119/8341 (13.4)	NR	15	Decreased (11%) death
Stockholm, 1988	Niacin + clofibrate	279/555 (50.3)	NR	5	Decreased (26%) death; decreased (36%) CAD death
HATS, 2001	Niacin + simvastatin	38/160 (23.8)	26	3	Decreased (90%) first death, MI, stroke, or revascularization
AFREGS, 2005	Niacin + gemfibrozil + cholestyramine	71/143 (49.7)	36	2.5	Decreased (13%) composite clinical outcome of angina, MI, TIA, stroke, death, and CV procedures; decreased focal coronary stenosis (secondary outcome)
AIM-HIGH, 2011[11]	Niacin + simvastatin	1718/3414 (50.3)	25 (12)	3	No difference in primary end point (MI, coronary death, hospitalized, revascularization)
HPS2-THRIVE, 2013	Niacin + laropiprant	12,838/25,673 (50)	13	3.9	No difference in primary end point (coronary event, stroke, revascularization)
Imaging studies					
CLAS I, 1987	Niacin + colestipol	94/188 (50.0)	37	2	Decreased coronary atherosclerosis
CLAS II, 1990	Niacin + colestipol	75/138 (54.3)	37	4	Decreased coronary atherosclerosis
FATS, 1990	Niacin + colestipol	48/146 (32.9)	43	2.5	Decreased coronary atherosclerosis; decreased death, MI, or revascularization (secondary outcome)
CLAS Fem, 1991	Niacin + colestipol	80/162 (49.4)	38	2	Decreased femoral atherosclerosis

CLAS IMT; 1993	Niacin + colestipol	39/78 (50.0)	38	4	Decreased carotid IMT (regression also observed at years 1 and 2)
SCRIP, 1994	Niacin + colestipol + gemfibrozil + lovastatin + aggressive lifestyle modification	145/300 (48.3)	12	4	Decreased coronary atherosclerosis; decreased frequency of new coronary lesion formation
ARBITER 2, 1994	Niacin + statin	87/167 (52.1)	21	1	No progression in atherosclerosis (carotid IMT)
ARBITER 3, 1996	Niacin + statin	87/167 (52.1)	23	2	Decreased carotid IMT
ARBITER 6, 2009	Niacin + statin vs ezetimibe + statin	187/336 (55.6), only 208 had follow-up study at 14 mo	18.4	14 mo	Decreased carotid IMT
Oxford Niacin Study, 2009	Niacin + statin	71	23	1	Decreased carotid wall area, as per MRI
NIA plaque, 2013[190]	Niacin + statin	145	6	1.5	No change on carotid wall volume, as per MRI
Fibrates					
Clinical outcomes studies					
Newcastle, 1971	Clofibrate	244/497 (49.1)	NR	5	Decreased (33%) MI
Edinburgh, 1971	Clofibrate	350/717 (48.8)	NR	6	Decreased (62%) death; decreased (53%) MI
CDP, 1975	Clofibrate: 1.6 g	1103/8341 (13.2)	NR	6	Nonsignificant decrease (9%) in nonfatal MI or CAD death ($P>.05$)
WHO Cooperative Trial, 1978	Clofibrate: 1.6 g	5331/15,745 (33.9)	NR	5.3	Increased (47%) death; Decreased (20%) incidence of CAD (mainly due to decreased [25%] nonfatal MI)
WHO Follow-up, 1984	Clofibrate: 1.6 g	5331/15,745 (33.9)	NR	13	Nonsignificant increase (11%) in death ($P>.05$)
HHS, 1987[129]	Gemfibrozil: 1200 mg	2051/4081 (50.3)	11	5	Decreased nonfatal MI or CAD death (34%, $P<.02$)

(continued on next page)

Table 2
(continued)

Study	Drugs	Patients Receiving Treatment, No./Total (%)	Elevation in HDL-C Levels (%)	Follow-up (y)	Outcomes
VA-HIT, 1999[92]	Gemfibrozil: 1200 mg	1264/2531 (49.9)	6	5.1	Decreased nonfatal MI or CAD death (22%, $P = .006$)
BIP, 2000[131]	Bezafibrate: 400 mg	1548/3090 (50.1)	18	6.2	Nonsignificant decrease in nonfatal MI or CAD death (9%, $P>.24$) Significant decrease if baseline TG >200 and HDL <35 (42%, $P = .02$)
LEADER; 2002	Bezafibrate: 400 mg	783/1568 (46.9)	11	5	Nonsignificant decrease (4%) in CAD and stroke ($P>.05$) Decreased (40%) nonfatal MI (secondary outcome)
FIELD, 2005[132]	Fenofibrate: 200 mg	4895/9795 (50.0)	1.2	5	Nonsignificant decrease (11%) in CAD death or nonfatal MI ($P = .16$) 24% decrease in nonfatal MI ($P = .01$) Nonsignificant increase in total mortality (19%, $P = .22$)
ACCORD[14]	Fenofibrate	2765/5518 (50.0)	1.8	4.7	No decrease in primary end point (major CV events) and secondary end points (major coronary events, stroke, CV mortality)
Imaging studies					
BECAIT, 1996[187]	Bezafibrate	42/92 (45.7)	9	5	Decreased progression of CAD
LOCAT, 1997[188]	Gemfibrozil	197/395 (49.9)	21	2.7	Decreased progression of CAD
DAIS, 2001[189]	Fenofibrate	207/418 (49.5)	8	3	Decreased progression of CAD in patients with DM

CETP Inhibitors

Clinical outcomes studies

Study	Agent	N (%)			Findings
ILLUMINATE, 2007[141]	Torcetrapib + atorvastatin	7533/15,067 (50)	72	1	25% increase in CV events (P = .001); increased death (58%).
Dalcetrapib, DAL-Outcome[13]	Dalcetrapib + statin	7938/15,871 (50)	40	1	No difference in coronary event + coronary death + stroke

Imaging studies

Study	Agent	N (%)			Findings
ILLUSTRATE, 2007[142]	Torcetrapib + atorvastatin	591/1188 (49.7)	61	2	No decrease in coronary atherosclerosis progression, as per IVUS
RADIANCE 1, 2007[97]	Torcetrapib + atorvastatin	450/904 (49.8)	54	2	No decrease in carotid atherosclerosis progression by IMT
RADIANCE 2, 2007[98]	Torcetrapib + atorvastatin	377/752 (50)	63	1.8	No change in maximum intima-media thickness
dal-PLAQUE[151]	Dalcetrapib + statin	64/130 (49.8)	31	2	No decrease in carotid wall (MRI) or macrophage infiltration (PET)

Therapies Specifically Increasing HDL-P

Study	Agent	N (%)			Findings
ApoA-I Milano, 2003[5]	ETC-216 (Apo A-I Milano + PL)	45/57 (78.9)	NR	5 wk	Decreased coronary atheroma volume on IVUS
ERASE, 2007[6]	Reconstituted HDL (CSL-111)	111/183 (60.7)	NR	6 wk	No decrease in coronary atheroma volume on IVUS
Waksmann et al,[171] 2010	Autologous delipidated HDL	14/28 (50)	NR	2 wk	HDL-VS increased from 5% to 80% Atheroma volume was reduced by 12% (P = .2)
ASSURE, 2014[157]	Resverlogix	240/323 (75)	NR	26 wk	Reduction of 0.6% in atheroma volume as per IVUS (P = .08), which was significant if high CRP. Less vulnerability as per VH

Abbreviations: AHA, American Heart Association; CAD, coronary artery disease; CETP, cholesteryl ester transfer protein; CHD, coronary heart disease; CRP, C-reactive protein; CV, cardiovascular; DM, diabetes mellitus; HDL-P, high-density lipoprotein particles; HDL-VS, very small high-density lipoprotein; IMT, intima-media thickness; IVUS, intravascular ultrasonography; MI, myocardial infarction; MRI, magnetic resonance imaging; NR, not reported; PET, positron emission tomography; PL, phospholipids; TG, triglycerides; TIA, transient ischemic attack; VH, virtual histology; WHO, World Health Organization.

Adapted from Santos-Gallego CG, Rosenson RS. Role of HDL in those with diabetes. Curr Cardiol Rep 2014;16(8):512; with permission.

of HDL with its rich proteome/lipidome may not be an effective strategy. It is possible that shedding of atheroprotective proteins with niacin may result in a less functional HDL-P that does not improve cholesterol efflux or HDL anti-inflammatory properties,[91] thus providing a mechanistic hypothesis for these disappointing results. In addition, niacin treatment (without concomitant statin treatment) moderately enhances the capacity of serum HDL to promote cholesterol efflux from cholesterol-loaded THP-1 macrophages,[89] but statin therapy reduces cholesterol efflux through an miR-33–mediated decrease in ABCA1 expression.[127] Because all patients in both trials were actually treated with niacin on the background of statin therapy, the atheroprotective properties attributed to niacin may not be the same in statin-treated patients as those reported for niacin monotherapy.

Cholesteryl Ester Transfer Protein Inhibitors

Certain Japanese subjects with very high HDL-C levels attributable to low CETP activity were reported in 1989.[135] This discovery was the rationale for the development of several CETP inhibitors, including torcetrapib, dalcetrapib, anacetrapib, and evacetrapib. The first epidemiologic studies suggested that polymorphisms resulting in low CETP activity were associated with reduced progression of atherosclerosis,[136] but a longer follow-up of the same population contradicted this initial finding, showing more CVD events in those individuals[137]; since then, the evidence about the role of CETP is at best contradictory.[138,139] Torcetrapib was a promising agent because it increased HDL-C by 60%.[140] Unexpectedly, torcetrapib exhibited deleterious effects in humans. The Investigation of Lipid Level Management to Understand its Impact in Atherosclerotic Events (ILLUMINATE) clinical trial was a clinical outcomes trial studying the effect of torcetrapib on clinical events in 15,067 patients (45% with diabetes)[141]; it showed a significant increase in both CVD mortality and all-cause mortality despite an HDL-C increase of 72% and LDL-C decreases of 25%, while the 3 imaging studies confirmed atherosclerosis progression (using both intravascular ultrasonography [IVUS][142] and cIMT[143,144]).

The cause of this excess in mortality has been the subject of much debate, with 2 different hypotheses aiming to explain this unexpected finding. The first theory relies on the CETP inhibition strategy per se being deleterious because it increases HDL-C levels by increasing the cholesterol content within the HDL-P, not by increasing the concentration of HDL-P (thus not expanding HDL lipidome/proteome and not augmenting the HDL-VS, the main acceptors for macrophage cholesterol efflux). The second hypothesis is that CETP inhibition strategy is safe and useful (even some preliminary reports suggest that torcetrapib modestly improves the cholesterol efflux to HDL-L/HDL-VL[145,146]), but there was unexpected off-target toxicity of the specific molecule torcetrapib. In fact, torcetrapib resulted in activation of the renin-angiotensin-aldosterone system, increases in natremia, reductions in kalemia, and increases in blood pressure (in some patients up to 15 mm Hg)[141]; this vasopressor effect is driven by adrenal aldosterone and cortisol release in addition to endothelin-1 upregulation,[147] and in vitro studies showed that torcetrapib induced aldosterone and cortisol release from adrenocortical cells.[148] In support of this hypothesis, it is noteworthy that no effect on blood pressure or aldosterone levels was observed for dalcetrapib, anacetrapib, or evacetrapib, and that there is no association between CETP gene polymorphisms and blood pressure in 67,687 individuals.[149]

Dalcetrapib is the second CETP inhibitor tested in clinical trials. It increases HDL-C by 34%[150] but has demonstrated no improvement in CVD outcomes (although it was not harmful) in dal-OUTCOMES[13] in 15,781 patients, no reduction of atherosclerosis burden as evaluated by magnetic resonance imaging (MRI) or in plaque macrophage content as assessed by positron emission tomography in dal-PLAQUE,[151] and no improvement in endothelial function as per flow-mediated dilation in dal-VESSEL.[152] In the dal-ACUTE study, whereas HDL-C was increased by one-third, apoA-I and cholesterol efflux were increased by less than one-tenth,[153] further supporting the concept of dissociation between improvements in HDL function and HDL-C levels. This fact reinforces the previously explained notion that therapies that increase HDL-C without expanding the pool of HDL with its rich proteome/lipidome do not seem to be an effective strategy.

The Determining the Efficacy and Tolerability of CETP Inhibition with Anacetrapib (DEFINE) clinical trial[154] was performed to investigate the safety and efficacy of anacetrapib in 1623 patients with high CVD risk. After 76 weeks, anacetrapib increased HDL-C by 138% and reduced LDL-C by 40%, without any increase in CVD events or any sign of toxicity[154]; interestingly, anacetrapib treatment enhanced cholesterol efflux to HDL and the anti-inflammatory properties of HDL.[89] The Randomized EValuation of the Effects of Anacetrapib Through Lipid-modification (REVEAL HPS-3 TIMI 55) trial will be the outcomes clinical trial assessing the effectiveness of anacetrapib 100 mg in clinical practice in CVD patients in combination with statins; more than 30,000 patients have been enrolled, the follow-up is 4 years, and completion is expected by 2017. An interesting aspect of anacetrapib is the 40% reduction in LDL-C, so it is possible that anacetrapib improves CVD outcomes, but it will be difficult to demonstrate if this beneficial effect is due to the effect on HDL metabolism or to the additional lowering of LDL-C.

Evacetrapib is the most recent CETP inhibitor to be developed. Evacetrapib increased HDL-C by 129% (in monotherapy) or 88% (in combination with statins) and reduced LDL-C by 36% and 14%, respectively. The Assessment of Clinical Effects of Cholesteryl Ester Transfer Protein Inhibition With Evacetrapib in Patients at a High-Risk for Vascular Outcomes (ACCELERATE) phase III outcome trial is currently recruiting an estimated 11,000 patients at high CVD risk to be randomized to either evacetrapib 130 mg or placebo in addition to optimal lipid-lowering treatment.

Emerging Therapies Specifically Targeting the Concentration of High-Density Lipoprotein Particles

There is solid evidence that therapeutic strategies that increase HDL-C without expanding the pool of HDL-P are not effective in reducing CVD events. Therefore, there is an urgent need to develop new treatments that increase the concentration of HDL-P.

Resverlogix

Resverlogix (RVX-208) is a small molecule that acts as an apoA-I upregulator. The bromodomain and extra terminal (BET) protein inhibits apoA-I transcription; resverlogix inhibits BET, leading to enhanced apoA-I gene transcription and thus increased apoA-I synthesis. Resverloglix increased apoA-I mRNA expression, de novo apoA-I synthesis, and nascent HDL in vitro in hepatic cell culture; resverlogix also increased serum apoA-I by 60% and HDL-C levels by 97% in vivo in adult green monkeys, while simultaneously increasing cholesterol efflux via ABCA1, ABCG1, and SR-BI.[155] In an initial human study with 18 healthy volunteers, RVX-208 treatment increased apoA-I by 10%, HDL-C by 10%, cholesterol efflux by 11%, and HDL-VS by 42%.[155] However, these promising results were only moderately confirmed in the subsequent ASSERT study involving 299 statin-treated patients; RVX-208 showed a dose-dependent increase on apoA-I levels and HDL-C, with maximum increases of 5.6% and 8.3%, respectively.[156] HDL-P only increased by 5% (HDL-VS by 4%), which may not be enough to translate into improvements in CVD outcomes. In fact, the very recent ASSURE clinical trial did not show clear benefits. A total of 324 patients with CVD and HDL-C less than 39 mg/dL were randomized to RVX-208 for 26 weeks or placebo. There was no statistically significant difference in the primary end point (−0.6% change in percent atheroma volume as determined by IVUS, $P = .08$), but there was nonetheless significant reduction of atheroma in patients with high levels of C-reactive protein and also less vulnerability of the atheroma plaque as assessed by virtual histology.[157]

Apolipoprotein A-I Milano

ApoA-I Milano is a molecular variant of apoA-I characterized by the Arg(173)→Cys substitution caused by a rare point mutation (R173C), which allows for disulfide dimer formation and subsequent increase in the antioxidant properties of the thiol groups. The discovery that subjects from the Italian village of Limone sul Garda with very low plasma HDL-C levels (10–15 mg/dL) exhibited paradoxically low CVD risk led to the hypothesis that apoA-I Milano could be a more functional and beneficial variant of apoA-I.[158,159] In experimental animal models, apoA-I Milano has been shown to regress atherosclerosis in mice[160] and rabbits,[161] to change the atheroma plaque into a less vulnerable phenotype,[161] to reduce in-stent restenosis,[162] and to exhibit antithrombotic[50] and vasoprotective[163] properties. These beneficial effects have been initially confirmed in human patients. First, 47 patients immediately after acute coronary syndrome (ACS) received 5 weekly injections of apoA-I Milano, and IVUS revealed plaque regression of 4.5%.[5] Another study with injection of reconstituted HDL-C with apoA- I Milano was associated with reverse coronary remodeling and reduced atheroma burden.[164]

Direct infusion of recombinant high-density lipoprotein

Direct infusion of rHDL (a combination of apoA-I and phospholipids) has been shown to improve RCT[165] and to be endothelially protective.

1. In a human trial, Effect of rHDL on Atherosclerosis – Safety and Efficacy (ERASE),[6] 183 ACS patients received 4 once-weekly intravenous infusions of rHDL (CSL-111) containing apoA-I isolated from healthy humans combined with soybean phosphatidylcholine; atheroma burden by IVUS was the primary end point. There was an improvement in atheroma burden after rHDL compared with baseline; however, the treatment did not result in a significant change in atheroma volume compared with placebo, and there was a high percentage of liver abnormalities. Based on the results of CSL-111, a second-generation compound (CSL-112) is in development. In 44 patients with established CVD, CSL-112 increased the concentrations of HDL-P (especially HDL-VS), apoA-I, and HDL-C, while also elevating the cholesterol efflux capacity from macrophages.[166]

2. CER-001 is an engineered lipoprotein particle mimicking pre-β HDL (HDL-VS) and consisting of a combination of recombinant human apoA-I and 2 phospholipids. The CHI-SQUARE study failed to show a difference between placebo and CER-001 in the end point of nominal change in atheroma volume assessed with IVUS.[167] Two very recent proof-of-concept studies show that CER-001 had a statistically significant reduction in the carotid atheroma burden assessed by MRI in patients with homozygous familial hypercholesterolemia (MODE,[168] 23 patients) and hypoalphalipoproteinemia (SAMBA,[169] 7 patients).

Infusions of autologous delipidated high-density lipoproteins

Infusion of autologous delipidated HDL is another novel and promising strategy to positively affect HDL-P. Plasma from patients is collected and extracorporeally subjected to a process that selectively removes lipid from HDL; the resulting lipid-poor HDL, which resemble the apoA-I/phospholipid rHDL described in the previous section, are subsequently reinfused back into the patient. This strategy decreased diet-induced atherosclerosis in cynomolgus monkeys.[170] In an initial clinical trial with ACS patients, 7 once-weekly injections of autologous delipidated HDL reduced plaque volume by 12%, whereas placebo increased plaque volume by 3%. This difference was not statistically significant ($P = .2$) owing to the small sample size (only 28 patients). The concentration of HDL-VS increased in the delipidated arm by 28-fold (from an initial 5.6% to an impressive 79.8%), and this increase in the pool of HDL-P likely explains the impressive reduction in IVUS-determined atheroma burden.[171] Further larger studies that use this approach are currently being planned.

Apolipoprotein A-I mimetic peptides

ApoA-I mimetic peptides are 18-amino-acid peptides, which do not have sequence homology with apoA-I (containing 243 amino acids) but mimic the secondary helix-like structure of apoA-I without sharing primary amino acid homology. ApoA-I mimetic peptides are smaller than native recombinant apoA-I and are therefore easier to produce, a characteristic that is of particular interest for drug development. Several compounds have been developed by replacing a variable number of nonpolar amino acids with phenylalanine (F) or alanine (A) residues.

1. Intravenous L-4F inhibited lesion formation in diet-induced atherosclerosis in mice,[172] but did not increase HDL-C or change the anti-inflammatory properties of HDL in human patients.[173]
2. D-4F is the same peptide as L-4F, but is synthesized from all D-amino acids instead of L-amino acids, which confers resistance to intestinal peptidases, thereby allowing oral administration; in fact, oral D-4F protected mice from diet-induced atherosclerosis.[174] In humans, the administration of a single dose of D-4F to CVD patients did not elevate HDL-C but did improve the anti-inflammatory properties of HDL.[175]
3. To overcome the barrier of the cost of chemically synthesizing these peptides, a new variety of tomato genetically overexpressing the apoA-I mimetic 6F has been developed,[176] which also decreases atherosclerosis in a murine model.[176]
4. FX-5A is based on the initial compound 5A; intravenous administration of 5A complexed with phospholipids increased HDL-C, improved both cholesterol efflux and HDL anti-inflammatory capacity, and reduced atherosclerosis in an animal model.[177]
5. ETC-642 is an apoA-I mimetic peptide that has demonstrated reduced atherosclerosis in animal models, and has been shown to be comparable with human apoA-I with regard to cholesterol efflux and anti-inflammatory effects.[178]

SUMMARY

HDL were widely considered to be beneficial regarding CVD because there is an inverse correlation between HDL-C levels and CVD risk, because HDL exert atheroprotective effects in vitro and in animal models, and because initial proof-of-concept studies in humans show that infusion of HDL reduces atherosclerosis. However, recent data question HDL-C as a relevant therapeutic target because genetic and population studies have not universally shown the usual inverse correlation between HDL-C and CVD risk, and because clinical trials have not demonstrated a reduction in CVD risk with certain HDL-related pharmacologic therapies.

The main problem is that sensitive in vivo markers of HDL function are lacking. Given that the amount of cholesterol carried by an HDL particle is not likely to confer atheroprotection, serum HDL-C levels (or the change in them) may not be the proper parameter for assessment of the contribution of HDL to CVD risk. Besides, static measurements, such as HDL-C or apoA-I, do not accurately reflect a dynamic process such as RCT. Therefore, too much emphasis has been placed on HDL-C as a surrogate marker of HDL metabolism/action, when in fact HDL-C is a poor marker of HDL function. Thus, research should focus on more sensitive markers of HDL metabolism that truly reflect and are responsible for the actual beneficial effects of HDL, such as the concentration of HDL-P.

Finally, therapeutic strategies that increase HDL-C without expanding the pool of HDL-P, with its rich proteome/lipidome, do not seem to be an effective strategy to reduce CVD risk. Ongoing discussion of this topic should have some impact on the basic research about HDL metabolism and on the current and emerging therapies targeting HDL.

REFERENCES

1. Barter P, Gotto AM, LaRosa JC, et al. HDL cholesterol, very low levels of LDL cholesterol, and cardiovascular events. N Engl J Med 2007;357(13):1301–10.
2. Badimon JJ, Badimon L, Fuster V. Regression of atherosclerotic lesions by high density lipoprotein plasma fraction in the cholesterol-fed rabbit. J Clin Invest 1990;85(4):1234–41.
3. Badimon JJ, Badimon L, Galvez A, et al. High density lipoprotein plasma fractions inhibit aortic fatty streaks in cholesterol-fed rabbits. Lab Invest 1989;60(3):455–61.
4. Rubin EM, Krauss RM, Spangler EA, et al. Inhibition of early atherogenesis in transgenic mice by human apolipoprotein AI. Nature 1991;353(6341):265–7.
5. Nissen SE, Tsunoda T, Tuzcu EM, et al. Effect of recombinant ApoA-I Milano on coronary atherosclerosis in patients with acute coronary syndromes: a randomized controlled trial. JAMA 2003;290(17):2292–300.
6. Tardif JC, Gregoire J, L'Allier PL, et al. Effects of reconstituted high-density lipoprotein infusions on coronary atherosclerosis: a randomized controlled trial. JAMA 2007;297(15):1675–82.
7. Voight BF, Peloso GM, Orho-Melander M, et al. Plasma HDL cholesterol and risk of myocardial infarction: a mendelian randomisation study. Lancet 2012; 380(9841):572–80.
8. Ridker PM, Genest J, Boekholdt SM, et al. HDL cholesterol and residual risk of first cardiovascular events after treatment with potent statin therapy: an analysis from the JUPITER trial. Lancet 2010;376(9738):333–9.
9. Ray K, Wainwright NW, Visser L, et al. Changes in HDL cholesterol and cardiovascular outcomes after lipid modification therapy. Heart 2012;98(10):780–5.
10. Briel M, Ferreira-Gonzalez I, You JJ, et al. Association between change in high density lipoprotein cholesterol and cardiovascular disease morbidity and mortality: systematic review and meta-regression analysis. BMJ 2009;338:b92.
11. Boden WE, Probstfield JL, Anderson T, et al. Niacin in patients with low HDL cholesterol levels receiving intensive statin therapy. N Engl J Med 2011; 365(24):2255–67.
12. Landray MJ, Haynes R, Hopewell JC, et al. Effects of extended-release niacin with laropiprant in high-risk patients. N Engl J Med 2014;371(3):203–12.
13. Schwartz GG, Olsson AG, Abt M, et al. Effects of dalcetrapib in patients with a recent acute coronary syndrome. N Engl J Med 2012;367(22):2089–99.

14. Ginsberg HN, Elam MB, Lovato LC, et al. Effects of combination lipid therapy in type 2 diabetes mellitus. N Engl J Med 2010;362(17):1563–74.
15. Rosenson RS, Brewer HB Jr, Ansell B, et al. Translation of high-density lipoprotein function into clinical practice: current prospects and future challenges. Circulation 2013;128(11):1256–67.
16. Davidson WS, Silva RA, Chantepie S, et al. Proteomic analysis of defined HDL subpopulations reveals particle-specific protein clusters: relevance to antioxidative function. Arterioscler Thromb Vasc Biol 2009;29(6):870–6.
17. Toth PP, Barter PJ, Rosenson RS, et al. High-density lipoproteins: a consensus statement from the National Lipid Association. J Clin Lipidol 2013;7(5):484–525.
18. Nofer JR, Bot M, Brodde M, et al. FTY720, a synthetic sphingosine 1 phosphate analogue, inhibits development of atherosclerosis in low-density lipoprotein receptor-deficient mice. Circulation 2007;115(4):501–8.
19. Nofer JR, van der Giet M, Tolle M, et al. HDL induces NO-dependent vasorelaxation via the lysophospholipid receptor S1P3. J Clin Invest 2004;113(4): 569–81.
20. Poti F, Simoni M, Nofer JR. Atheroprotective role of high-density lipoprotein (HDL)-associated sphingosine-1-phosphate (S1P). Cardiovasc Res 2014;103: 395–404.
21. Vickers KC, Palmisano BT, Shoucri BM, et al. MicroRNAs are transported in plasma and delivered to recipient cells by high-density lipoproteins. Nat Cell Biol 2011;13(4):423–33.
22. Wagner J, Riwanto M, Besler C, et al. Characterization of levels and cellular transfer of circulating lipoprotein-bound microRNAs. Arterioscler Thromb Vasc Biol 2013;33(6):1392–400.
23. Rosenson RS, Brewer HB Jr, Chapman MJ, et al. HDL measures, particle heterogeneity, proposed nomenclature, and relation to atherosclerotic cardiovascular events. Clin Chem 2011;57(3):392–410.
24. Santos-Gallego CG, Ibanez B, Badimon JJ. HDL-cholesterol: is it really good? Differences between apoA-I and HDL. Biochem Pharmacol 2008;76(4):443–52.
25. Rosenson RS, Brewer HB Jr, Davidson WS, et al. Cholesterol efflux and atheroprotection: advancing the concept of reverse cholesterol transport. Circulation 2012;125(15):1905–19.
26. Santos-Gallego CG, Torres F, Badimon JJ. The beneficial effects of HDL-C on atherosclerosis: rationale and clinical results. Clinical Lipidol 2011;6(2):181–208.
27. Santos-Gallego CG, Giannarelli C, Badimon JJ. Experimental models for the investigation of high-density lipoprotein-mediated cholesterol efflux. Curr Atheroscler Rep 2011;13(3):266–76.
28. Khera AV, Cuchel M, de la Llera-Moya M, et al. Cholesterol efflux capacity, high-density lipoprotein function, and atherosclerosis. N Engl J Med 2011;364(2): 127–35.
29. Li XM, Tang WH, Mosior MK, et al. Paradoxical association of enhanced cholesterol efflux with increased incident cardiovascular risks. Arterioscler Thromb Vasc Biol 2013;33(7):1696–705.
30. Doonan RJ, Hafiane A, Lai C, et al. Cholesterol efflux capacity, carotid atherosclerosis, and cerebrovascular symptomatology. Arterioscler Thromb Vasc Biol 2014; 34(4):921–6.
31. Camont L, Lhomme M, Rached F, et al. Small, dense high-density lipoprotein-3 particles are enriched in negatively charged phospholipids: relevance to cellular cholesterol efflux, antioxidative, antithrombotic, anti-inflammatory, and antiapoptotic functionalities. Arterioscler Thromb Vasc Biol 2013;33(12):2715–23.

32. Feig JE, Hewing B, Smith JD, et al. High-density lipoprotein and atherosclerosis regression: evidence from preclinical and clinical studies. Circ Res 2014;114(1): 205–13.

33. Nicholls SJ, Dusting GJ, Cutri B, et al. Reconstituted high-density lipoproteins inhibit the acute pro-oxidant and proinflammatory vascular changes induced by a periarterial collar in normocholesterolemic rabbits. Circulation 2005;111(12): 1543–50.

34. Cockerill GW, Rye KA, Gamble JR, et al. High-density lipoproteins inhibit cytokine-induced expression of endothelial cell adhesion molecules. Arterioscler Thromb Vasc Biol 1995;15(11):1987–94.

35. Hewing B, Parathath S, Barrett T, et al. Effects of native and myeloperoxidase-modified apolipoprotein a-I on reverse cholesterol transport and atherosclerosis in mice. Arterioscler Thromb Vasc Biol 2014;34(4):779–89.

36. Murphy AJ, Woollard KJ, Hoang A, et al. High-density lipoprotein reduces the human monocyte inflammatory response. Arterioscler Thromb Vasc Biol 2008; 28(11):2071–7.

37. Murphy AJ, Akhtari M, Tolani S, et al. ApoE regulates hematopoietic stem cell proliferation, monocytosis, and monocyte accumulation in atherosclerotic lesions in mice. J Clin Invest 2011;121(10):4138–49.

38. Westerterp M, Gourion-Arsiquaud S, Murphy AJ, et al. Regulation of hematopoietic stem and progenitor cell mobilization by cholesterol efflux pathways. Cell Stem Cell 2012;11(2):195–206.

39. Yuhanna IS, Zhu Y, Cox BE, et al. High-density lipoprotein binding to scavenger receptor-BI activates endothelial nitric oxide synthase. Nat Med 2001;7(7): 853–7.

40. Tall AR. Cholesterol efflux pathways and other potential mechanisms involved in the athero-protective effect of high density lipoproteins. J Intern Med 2008; 263(3):256–73.

41. Seetharam D, Mineo C, Gormley AK, et al. High-density lipoprotein promotes endothelial cell migration and reendothelialization via scavenger receptor-B type I. Circ Res 2006;98(1):63–72.

42. Spieker LE, Sudano I, Hurlimann D, et al. High-density lipoprotein restores endothelial function in hypercholesterolemic men. Circulation 2002;105(12): 1399–402.

43. Bisoendial RJ, Hovingh GK, Levels JH, et al. Restoration of endothelial function by increasing high-density lipoprotein in subjects with isolated low high-density lipoprotein. Circulation 2003;107(23):2944–8.

44. Besler C, Heinrich K, Rohrer L, et al. Mechanisms underlying adverse effects of HDL on eNOS-activating pathways in patients with coronary artery disease. J Clin Invest 2011;121(7):2693–708.

45. Sugano M, Tsuchida K, Makino N. High-density lipoproteins protect endothelial cells from tumor necrosis factor-alpha-induced apoptosis. Biochem Biophys Res Commun 2000;272(3):872–6.

46. Suc I, Escargueil-Blanc I, Troly M, et al. HDL and ApoA prevent cell death of endothelial cells induced by oxidized LDL. Arterioscler Thromb Vasc Biol 1997;17(10): 2158–66.

47. Yvan-Charvet L, Pagler TA, Seimon TA, et al. ABCA1 and ABCG1 protect against oxidative stress-induced macrophage apoptosis during efferocytosis. Circ Res 2010;106(12):1861–9.

48. Kontush A, Therond P, Zerrad A, et al. Preferential sphingosine-1-phosphate enrichment and sphingomyelin depletion are key features of small dense HDL3

particles: relevance to antiapoptotic and antioxidative activities. Arterioscler Thromb Vasc Biol 2007;27(8):1843–9.

49. Deguchi H, Pecheniuk NM, Elias DJ, et al. High-density lipoprotein deficiency and dyslipoproteinemia associated with venous thrombosis in men. Circulation 2005;112(6):893–9.

50. Li D, Weng S, Yang B, et al. Inhibition of arterial thrombus formation by ApoA1 Milano. Arterioscler Thromb Vasc Biol 1999;19(2):378–83.

51. Griffin JH, Kojima K, Banka CL, et al. High-density lipoprotein enhancement of anticoagulant activities of plasma protein S and activated protein C. J Clin Invest 1999;103(2):219–27.

52. Calkin AC, Drew BG, Ono A, et al. Reconstituted high-density lipoprotein attenuates platelet function in individuals with type 2 diabetes mellitus by promoting cholesterol efflux. Circulation 2009;120(21):2095–104.

53. Mineo C, Deguchi H, Griffin JH, et al. Endothelial and antithrombotic actions of HDL. Circ Res 2006;98(11):1352–64.

54. Brunham LR, Kruit JK, Pape TD, et al. Beta-cell ABCA1 influences insulin secretion, glucose homeostasis and response to thiazolidinedione treatment. Nat Med 2007;13(3):340–7.

55. Vergeer M, Brunham LR, Koetsveld J, et al. Carriers of loss-of-function mutations in ABCA1 display pancreatic beta-cell dysfunction. Diabetes Care 2010;33(4):869–74.

56. Drew BG, Rye KA, Duffy SJ, et al. The emerging role of HDL in glucose metabolism. Nat Rev Endocrinol 2012;8(4):237–45.

57. Drew BG, Duffy SJ, Formosa MF, et al. High-density lipoprotein modulates glucose metabolism in patients with type 2 diabetes mellitus. Circulation 2009;119(15):2103–11.

58. Han R, Lai R, Ding Q, et al. Apolipoprotein A-I stimulates AMP-activated protein kinase and improves glucose metabolism. Diabetologia 2007;50(9):1960–8.

59. Drew BG, Carey AL, Natoli AK, et al. Reconstituted high-density lipoprotein infusion modulates fatty acid metabolism in patients with type 2 diabetes mellitus. J Lipid Res 2011;52(3):572–81.

60. Theilmeier G, Schmidt C, Herrmann J, et al. High-density lipoproteins and their constituent, sphingosine-1-phosphate, directly protect the heart against ischemia/reperfusion injury in vivo via the S1P3 lysophospholipid receptor. Circulation 2006;114(13):1403–9.

61. Calabresi L, Rossoni G, Gomaraschi M, et al. High-density lipoproteins protect isolated rat hearts from ischemia-reperfusion injury by reducing cardiac tumor necrosis factor-alpha content and enhancing prostaglandin release. Circ Res 2003;92(3):330–7.

62. Rossoni G, Gomaraschi M, Berti F, et al. Synthetic high-density lipoproteins exert cardioprotective effects in myocardial ischemia/reperfusion injury. J Pharmacol Exp Ther 2004;308(1):79–84.

63. Marchesi M, Booth EA, Rossoni G, et al. Apolipoprotein A-IMilano/POPC complex attenuates post-ischemic ventricular dysfunction in the isolated rabbit heart. Atherosclerosis 2008;197(2):572–8.

64. Sattler KJ, Herrmann J, Yun S, et al. High high-density lipoprotein-cholesterol reduces risk and extent of percutaneous coronary intervention-related myocardial infarction and improves long-term outcome in patients undergoing elective percutaneous coronary intervention. Eur Heart J 2009;30(15):1894–902.

65. Van Lenten BJ, Hama SY, de Beer FC, et al. Anti-inflammatory HDL becomes pro-inflammatory during the acute phase response. Loss of protective effect

of HDL against LDL oxidation in aortic wall cell cocultures. J Clin Invest 1995; 96(6):2758–67.

66. Van Lenten BJ, Wagner AC, Nayak DP, et al. High-density lipoprotein loses its anti-inflammatory properties during acute influenza A infection. Circulation 2001;103(18):2283–8.

67. Morgantini C, Natali A, Boldrini B, et al. Anti-inflammatory and antioxidant properties of HDLs are impaired in type 2 diabetes. Diabetes 2011;60(10):2617–23.

68. Zheng L, Nukuna B, Brennan ML, et al. Apolipoprotein A-I is a selective target for myeloperoxidase-catalyzed oxidation and functional impairment in subjects with cardiovascular disease. J Clin Invest 2004;114(4):529–41.

69. Huang Y, Didonato JA, Levison BS, et al. An abundant dysfunctional apolipoprotein A1 in human atheroma. Nat Med 2014;20:193–203.

70. Hoang A, Murphy AJ, Coughlan MT, et al. Advanced glycation of apolipoprotein A-I impairs its anti-atherogenic properties. Diabetologia 2007;50(8):1770–9.

71. Ansell BJ, Navab M, Hama S, et al. Inflammatory/antiinflammatory properties of high-density lipoprotein distinguish patients from control subjects better than high-density lipoprotein cholesterol levels and are favorably affected by simvastatin treatment. Circulation 2003;108(22):2751–6.

72. Riwanto M, Rohrer L, Roschitzki B, et al. Altered activation of endothelial anti- and proapoptotic pathways by high-density lipoprotein from patients with coronary artery disease: role of high-density lipoprotein-proteome remodeling. Circulation 2013;127(8):891–904.

73. Sorrentino SA, Besler C, Rohrer L, et al. Endothelial-vasoprotective effects of high-density lipoprotein are impaired in patients with type 2 diabetes mellitus but are improved after extended-release niacin therapy. Circulation 2010; 121(1):110–22.

74. Choudhury RP, Leyva F. C-Reactive protein, serum amyloid A protein, and coronary events. Circulation 1999;100(15):e65–6.

75. Nobecourt E, Jacqueminet S, Hansel B, et al. Defective antioxidative activity of small dense HDL3 particles in type 2 diabetes: relationship to elevated oxidative stress and hyperglycaemia. Diabetologia 2005;48(3):529–38.

76. Holzer M, Birner-Gruenberger R, Stojakovic T, et al. Uremia alters HDL composition and function. J Am Soc Nephrol 2011;22(9):1631–41.

77. Weichhart T, Kopecky C, Kubicek M, et al. Serum amyloid A in uremic HDL promotes inflammation. J Am Soc Nephrol 2012;23(5):934–47.

78. Kalantar-Zadeh K, Kopple JD, Kamranpour N, et al. HDL-inflammatory index correlates with poor outcome in hemodialysis patients. Kidney Int 2007;72(9): 1149–56.

79. de Souza JA, Vindis C, Hansel B, et al. Metabolic syndrome features small, apolipoprotein A-I-poor, triglyceride-rich HDL3 particles with defective anti-apoptotic activity. Atherosclerosis 2008;197(1):84–94.

80. Zerrad-Saadi A, Therond P, Chantepie S, et al. HDL3-mediated inactivation of LDL-associated phospholipid hydroperoxides is determined by the redox status of apolipoprotein A-I and HDL particle surface lipid rigidity: relevance to inflammation and atherogenesis. Arterioscler Thromb Vasc Biol 2009;29(12):2169–75.

81. Otvos JD, Jeyarajah EJ, Cromwell WC. Measurement issues related to lipoprotein heterogeneity. Am J Cardiol 2002;90(8A):22i–9i.

82. Vergeer M, Boekholdt SM, Sandhu MS, et al. Genetic variation at the phospholipid transfer protein locus affects its activity and high-density lipoprotein size and is a novel marker of cardiovascular disease susceptibility. Circulation 2010;122(5):470–7.

83. Acharjee S, Boden WE, Hartigan PM, et al. Low levels of high-density lipoprotein cholesterol and increased risk of cardiovascular events in stable ischemic heart disease patients: a post-hoc analysis from the COURAGE Trial (Clinical Outcomes Utilizing Revascularization and Aggressive Drug Evaluation). J Am Coll Cardiol 2013;62(20):1826–33.
84. Kuller LH, Grandits G, Cohen JD, et al. Lipoprotein particles, insulin, adiponectin, C-reactive protein and risk of coronary heart disease among men with metabolic syndrome. Atherosclerosis 2007;195(1):122–8.
85. Mackey RH, Greenland P, Goff DC Jr, et al. High-density lipoprotein cholesterol and particle concentrations, carotid atherosclerosis, and coronary events: MESA (multi-ethnic study of atherosclerosis). J Am Coll Cardiol 2012;60(6): 508–16.
86. Akinkuolie AO, Paynter NP, Padmanabhan L, et al. High-density lipoprotein particle subclass heterogeneity and incident coronary heart disease. Circ Cardiovasc Qual Outcomes 2014;7(1):55–63.
87. Otvos JD, Collins D, Freedman DS, et al. Low-density lipoprotein and high-density lipoprotein particle subclasses predict coronary events and are favorably changed by gemfibrozil therapy in the Veterans Affairs High-Density Lipoprotein Intervention Trial. Circulation 2006;113(12):1556–63.
88. Mora S, Glynn RJ, Ridker PM. High-density lipoprotein cholesterol, size, particle number, and residual vascular risk after potent statin therapy. Circulation 2013; 128(11):1189–97.
89. Yvan-Charvet L, Kling J, Pagler T, et al. Cholesterol efflux potential and antiinflammatory properties of high-density lipoprotein after treatment with niacin or anacetrapib. Arterioscler Thromb Vasc Biol 2010;30(7):1430–8.
90. Airan-Javia SL, Wolf RL, Wolfe ML, et al. Atheroprotective lipoprotein effects of a niacin-simvastatin combination compared to low- and high-dose simvastatin monotherapy. Am Heart J 2009;157(4):687.e1–8.
91. Khera AV, Patel PJ, Reilly MP, et al. The addition of niacin to statin therapy improves high-density lipoprotein cholesterol levels but not metrics of functionality. J Am Coll Cardiol 2013;62(20):1909–10.
92. Rubins HB, Robins SJ, Collins D, et al. Gemfibrozil for the secondary prevention of coronary heart disease in men with low levels of high-density lipoprotein cholesterol. Veterans Affairs High-Density Lipoprotein Cholesterol Intervention Trial Study Group. N Engl J Med 1999;341(6):410–8.
93. Kraus WE, Houmard JA, Duscha BD, et al. Effects of the amount and intensity of exercise on plasma lipoproteins. N Engl J Med 2002;347(19):1483–92.
94. Kodama S, Tanaka S, Saito K, et al. Effect of aerobic exercise training on serum levels of high-density lipoprotein cholesterol: a meta-analysis. Arch Intern Med 2007;167(10):999–1008.
95. Kelley GA, Kelley KS. Aerobic exercise and HDL2-C: a meta-analysis of randomized controlled trials. Atherosclerosis 2006;184(1):207–15.
96. Roberts CK, Ng C, Hama S, et al. Effect of a short-term diet and exercise intervention on inflammatory/anti-inflammatory properties of HDL in overweight/obese men with cardiovascular risk factors. J Appl Physiol (1985) 2006;101(6):1727–32.
97. Hamilton MT, Hamilton DG, Zderic TW. Role of low energy expenditure and sitting in obesity, metabolic syndrome, type 2 diabetes, and cardiovascular disease. Diabetes 2007;56(11):2655–67.
98. Wood PD, Stefanick ML, Williams PT, et al. The effects on plasma lipoproteins of a prudent weight-reducing diet, with or without exercise, in overweight men and women. N Engl J Med 1991;325(7):461–6.

99. Dattilo AM, Kris-Etherton PM. Effects of weight reduction on blood lipids and lipoproteins: a meta-analysis. Am J Clin Nutr 1992;56(2):320–8.

100. Van Gaal LF, Mertens IL, Ballaux D. What is the relationship between risk factor reduction and degree of weight loss. Eur Heart J Suppl 2005;7(Suppl L):L21–6.

101. Schwartz RS, Brunzell JD. Increase of adipose tissue lipoprotein lipase activity with weight loss. J Clin Invest 1981;67(5):1425–30.

102. Weisweiler P. Plasma lipoproteins and lipase and lecithin:cholesterol acyltransferase activities in obese subjects before and after weight reduction. J Clin Endocrinol Metab 1987;65(5):969–73.

103. Aron-Wisnewsky J, Julia Z, Poitou C, et al. Effect of bariatric surgery-induced weight loss on SR-BI-, ABCG1-, and ABCA1-mediated cellular cholesterol efflux in obese women. J Clin Endocrinol Metab 2011;96(4):1151–9.

104. Gaziano JM, Buring JE, Breslow JL, et al. Moderate alcohol intake, increased levels of high-density lipoprotein and its subfractions, and decreased risk of myocardial infarction. N Engl J Med 1993;329(25):1829–34.

105. Valmadrid CT, Klein R, Moss SE, et al. Alcohol intake and the risk of coronary heart disease mortality in persons with older-onset diabetes mellitus. JAMA 1999;282(3):239–46.

106. Mukamal KJ, Conigrave KM, Mittleman MA, et al. Roles of drinking pattern and type of alcohol consumed in coronary heart disease in men. N Engl J Med 2003; 348(2):109–18.

107. Costanzo S, Di Castelnuovo A, Donati MB, et al. Alcohol consumption and mortality in patients with cardiovascular disease: a meta-analysis. J Am Coll Cardiol 2010;55(13):1339–47.

108. Mukamal KJ, Chen CM, Rao SR, et al. Alcohol consumption and cardiovascular mortality among U.S. adults, 1987 to 2002. J Am Coll Cardiol 2010;55(13): 1328–35.

109. Klatsky AL, Friedman GD, Siegelaub AB. Alcohol and mortality. A ten-year Kaiser-Permanente experience. Ann Intern Med 1981;95(2):139–45.

110. Craig WY, Palomaki GE, Haddow JE. Cigarette smoking and serum lipid and lipoprotein concentrations: an analysis of published data. BMJ 1989;298(6676): 784–8.

111. Richard F, Marecaux N, Dallongeville J, et al. Effect of smoking cessation on lipoprotein A-I and lipoprotein A-I: A-II levels. Metabolism 1997;46(6):711–5.

112. Maeda K, Noguchi Y, Fukui T. The effects of cessation from cigarette smoking on the lipid and lipoprotein profiles: a meta-analysis. Prev Med 2003;37(4): 283–90.

113. Esposito K, Marfella R, Ciotola M, et al. Effect of a Mediterranean-style diet on endothelial dysfunction and markers of vascular inflammation in the metabolic syndrome: a randomized trial. JAMA 2004;292(12):1440–6.

114. Estruch R, Martinez-Gonzalez MA, Corella D, et al. Effects of a Mediterranean-style diet on cardiovascular risk factors: a randomized trial. Ann Intern Med 2006;145(1):1–11.

115. Damasceno NR, Sala-Vila A, Cofan M, et al. Mediterranean diet supplemented with nuts reduces waist circumference and shifts lipoprotein subfractions to a less atherogenic pattern in subjects at high cardiovascular risk. Atherosclerosis 2013;230(2):347–53.

116. Sala-Vila A, Romero-Mamani ES, Gilabert R, et al. Changes in ultrasound-assessed carotid intima-media thickness and plaque with a Mediterranean diet: a substudy of the PREDIMED trial. Arterioscler Thromb Vasc Biol 2014; 34(2):439–45.

117. Estruch R, Ros E, Salas-Salvado J, et al. Primary prevention of cardiovascular disease with a Mediterranean diet. N Engl J Med 2013;368(14):1279–90.
118. Nicholls SJ, Lundman P, Harmer JA, et al. Consumption of saturated fat impairs the anti-inflammatory properties of high-density lipoproteins and endothelial function. J Am Coll Cardiol 2006;48(4):715–20.
119. Lankinen M, Kolehmainen M, Jaaskelainen T, et al. Effects of whole grain, fish and bilberries on serum metabolic profile and lipid transfer protein activities: a randomized trial (Sysdimet). PLoS One 2014;9(2):e90352.
120. Frost G, Leeds AA, Dore CJ, et al. Glycaemic index as a determinant of serum HDL-cholesterol concentration. Lancet 1999;353(9158):1045–8.
121. Ford ES, Liu S. Glycemic index and serum high-density lipoprotein cholesterol concentration among us adults. Arch Intern Med 2001;161(4):572–6.
122. Barter PJ, Brandrup-Wognsen G, Palmer MK, et al. Effect of statins on HDL-C: a complex process unrelated to changes in LDL-C: analysis of the VOYAGER Database. J Lipid Res 2010;51(6):1546–53.
123. Rosenson RS, Otvos JD, Hsia J. Effects of rosuvastatin and atorvastatin on LDL and HDL particle concentrations in patients with metabolic syndrome: a randomized, double-blind, controlled study. Diabetes Care 2009;32(6):1087–91.
124. Schaefer JR, Schweer H, Ikewaki K, et al. Metabolic basis of high density lipoproteins and apolipoprotein A-I increase by HMG-CoA reductase inhibition in healthy subjects and a patient with coronary artery disease. Atherosclerosis 1999;144(1):177–84.
125. Chapman MJ, Le Goff W, Guerin M, et al. Cholesteryl ester transfer protein: at the heart of the action of lipid-modulating therapy with statins, fibrates, niacin, and cholesteryl ester transfer protein inhibitors. Eur Heart J 2010;31(2):149–64.
126. Guerin M, Egger P, Soudant C, et al. Dose-dependent action of atorvastatin in type IIB hyperlipidemia: preferential and progressive reduction of atherogenic apoB-containing lipoprotein subclasses (VLDL-2, IDL, small dense LDL) and stimulation of cellular cholesterol efflux. Atherosclerosis 2002;163(2):287–96.
127. Niesor EJ, Schwartz GG, Suchankova G, et al. Statin decrease in transporter ABC A1 expression via miR33 induction may counteract cholesterol efflux by high-density lipoproteins raised with the cholesteryl ester transfer protein modulator dalcetrapib. American College of Cardiology 2013 Scientific Sessions. San Francisco, California. March 9-11, 2013.
128. Staels B, Dallongeville J, Auwerx J, et al. Mechanism of action of fibrates on lipid and lipoprotein metabolism. Circulation 1998;98(19):2088–93.
129. Frick MH, Elo O, Haapa K, et al. Helsinki Heart Study: primary-prevention trial with gemfibrozil in middle-aged men with dyslipidemia. Safety of treatment, changes in risk factors, and incidence of coronary heart disease. N Engl J Med 1987;317(20):1237–45.
130. Manninen V, Tenkanen L, Koskinen P, et al. Joint effects of serum triglyceride and LDL cholesterol and HDL cholesterol concentrations on coronary heart disease risk in the Helsinki Heart Study. Implications for treatment. Circulation 1992;85(1):37–45.
131. Bezafibrate Infarction Prevention (BIP) Study. Secondary prevention by raising HDL cholesterol and reducing triglycerides in patients with coronary artery disease. Circulation 2000;102(1):21–7.
132. Scott R, O'Brien R, Fulcher G, et al. Effects of fenofibrate treatment on cardiovascular disease risk in 9,795 individuals with type 2 diabetes and various components of the metabolic syndrome: the Fenofibrate Intervention and Event Lowering in Diabetes (FIELD) study. Diabetes Care 2009;32(3):493–8.

133. Davidson MH, Rosenson RS, Maki KC, et al. Effects of fenofibric acid on carotid intima-media thickness in patients with mixed dyslipidemia on atorvastatin therapy: randomized, placebo-controlled study (FIRST). Arterioscler Thromb Vasc Biol 2014;34(6):1298–306.

134. Song WL, Stubbe J, Ricciotti E, et al. Niacin and biosynthesis of PGD(2)by platelet COX-1 in mice and humans. J Clin Invest 2012;122(4):1459–68.

135. Inazu A, Brown ML, Hesler CB, et al. Increased high-density lipoprotein levels caused by a common cholesteryl-ester transfer protein gene mutation. N Engl J Med 1990;323(18):1234–8.

136. Kuivenhoven JA, Jukema JW, Zwinderman AH, et al. The role of a common variant of the cholesteryl ester transfer protein gene in the progression of coronary atherosclerosis. The Regression Growth Evaluation Statin Study Group. N Engl J Med 1998;338(2):86–93.

137. Regieli JJ, Jukema JW, Grobbee DE, et al. CETP genotype predicts increased mortality in statin-treated men with proven cardiovascular disease: an adverse pharmacogenetic interaction. Eur Heart J 2008;29(22):2792–9.

138. Vasan RS, Pencina MJ, Robins SJ, et al. Association of circulating cholesteryl ester transfer protein activity with incidence of cardiovascular disease in the community. Circulation 2009;120(24):2414–20.

139. Ritsch A, Scharnagl H, Eller P, et al. Cholesteryl ester transfer protein and mortality in patients undergoing coronary angiography: the Ludwigshafen Risk and Cardiovascular Health study. Circulation 2010;121(3):366–74.

140. Brousseau ME, Schaefer EJ, Wolfe ML, et al. Effects of an inhibitor of cholesteryl ester transfer protein on HDL cholesterol. N Engl J Med 2004;350(15):1505–15.

141. Barter PJ, Caulfield M, Eriksson M, et al. Effects of torcetrapib in patients at high risk for coronary events. N Engl J Med 2007;357(21):2109–22.

142. Nissen SE, Tardif JC, Nicholls SJ, et al. Effect of torcetrapib on the progression of coronary atherosclerosis. N Engl J Med 2007;356(13):1304–16.

143. Bots ML, Visseren FL, Evans GW, et al. Torcetrapib and carotid intima-media thickness in mixed dyslipidaemia (RADIANCE 2 study): a randomised, double-blind trial. Lancet 2007;370(9582):153–60.

144. Kastelein JJ, van Leuven SI, Burgess L, et al. Effect of torcetrapib on carotid atherosclerosis in familial hypercholesterolemia. N Engl J Med 2007;356(16):1620–30.

145. Yvan-Charvet L, Matsuura F, Wang N, et al. Inhibition of cholesteryl ester transfer protein by torcetrapib modestly increases macrophage cholesterol efflux to HDL. Arterioscler Thromb Vasc Biol 2007;27(5):1132–8.

146. Bellanger N, Julia Z, Villard EF, et al. Functionality of postprandial larger HDL2 particles is enhanced following CETP inhibition therapy. Atherosclerosis 2012; 221(1):160–8.

147. Simic B, Hermann M, Shaw SG, et al. Torcetrapib impairs endothelial function in hypertension. Eur Heart J 2012;33(13):1615–24.

148. Hu X, Dietz JD, Xia C, et al. Torcetrapib induces aldosterone and cortisol production by an intracellular calcium-mediated mechanism independently of cholesteryl ester transfer protein inhibition. Endocrinology 2009;150(5):2211–9.

149. Sofat R, Hingorani AD, Smeeth L, et al. Separating the mechanism-based and off-target actions of cholesteryl ester transfer protein inhibitors with CETP gene polymorphisms. Circulation 2010;121(1):52–62.

150. de Grooth GJ, Kuivenhoven JA, Stalenhoef AF, et al. Efficacy and safety of a novel cholesteryl ester transfer protein inhibitor, JTT-705, in humans: a randomized phase II dose-response study. Circulation 2002;105(18):2159–65.

151. Fayad ZA, Mani V, Woodward M, et al. Safety and efficacy of dalcetrapib on atherosclerotic disease using novel non-invasive multimodality imaging (dal-PLAQUE): a randomised clinical trial. Lancet 2011;378(9802):1547–59.
152. Luscher TF, Taddei S, Kaski JC, et al. Vascular effects and safety of dalcetrapib in patients with or at risk of coronary heart disease: the dal-VESSEL randomized clinical trial. Eur Heart J 2012;33(7):857–65.
153. Ray KK, Ditmarsch M, Kallend D, et al. The effect of cholesteryl ester transfer protein inhibition on lipids, lipoproteins, and markers of HDL function after an acute coronary syndrome: the dal-ACUTE randomized trial. Eur Heart J 2014; 35(27):1792–800.
154. Cannon CP, Shah S, Dansky HM, et al. Safety of anacetrapib in patients with or at high risk for coronary heart disease. N Engl J Med 2010;363(25):2406–15.
155. Bailey D, Jahagirdar R, Gordon A, et al. RVX-208: a small molecule that increases apolipoprotein A-I and high-density lipoprotein cholesterol in vitro and in vivo. J Am Coll Cardiol 2010;55(23):2580–9.
156. Nicholls SJ, Gordon A, Johansson J, et al. Efficacy and safety of a novel oral inducer of apolipoprotein a-I synthesis in statin-treated patients with stable coronary artery disease a randomized controlled trial. J Am Coll Cardiol 2011; 57(9):1111–9.
157. Puri R, Kataoka Y, Wolski K, et al. Effects of an apolipoprotein A-1 inducer on progression of coronary atherosclerosis and cardiovascular events in patients with elevated inflammatory markers. American College of Cardiology 2014 Scientific Sessions. Washington, DC. March 29-31, 2014.
158. Franceschini G, Sirtori CR, Capurso A 2nd, et al. A-IMilano apoprotein. Decreased high density lipoprotein cholesterol levels with significant lipoprotein modifications and without clinical atherosclerosis in an Italian family. J Clin Invest 1980;66(5):892–900.
159. Sirtori CR, Calabresi L, Franceschini G, et al. Cardiovascular status of carriers of the apolipoprotein A-I(Milano) mutant: the Limone sul Garda study. Circulation 2001;103(15):1949–54.
160. Shah PK, Nilsson J, Kaul S, et al. Effects of recombinant apolipoprotein A-I(Milano) on aortic atherosclerosis in apolipoprotein E-deficient mice. Circulation 1998;97(8):780–5.
161. Ibanez B, Vilahur G, Cimmino G, et al. Rapid change in plaque size, composition, and molecular footprint after recombinant apolipoprotein A-I Milano (ETC-216) administration: magnetic resonance imaging study in an experimental model of atherosclerosis. J Am Coll Cardiol 2008;51(11):1104–9.
162. Kaul S, Rukshin V, Santos R, et al. Intramural delivery of recombinant apolipoprotein A-IMilano/phospholipid complex (ETC-216) inhibits in-stent stenosis in porcine coronary arteries. Circulation 2003;107(20):2551–4.
163. Kaul S, Coin B, Hedayiti A, et al. Rapid reversal of endothelial dysfunction in hypercholesterolemic apolipoprotein E-null mice by recombinant apolipoprotein A-I(Milano)-phospholipid complex. J Am Coll Cardiol 2004;44(6):1311–9.
164. Nicholls SJ, Tuzcu EM, Sipahi I, et al. Relationship between atheroma regression and change in lumen size after infusion of apolipoprotein A-I Milano. J Am Coll Cardiol 2006;47(5):992–7.
165. Eriksson M, Carlson LA, Miettinen TA, et al. Stimulation of fecal steroid excretion after infusion of recombinant proapolipoprotein A-I. Potential reverse cholesterol transport in humans. Circulation 1999;100(6):594–8.
166. Gille A, D'Andrea D, Easton R, et al. CSL112, a novel formulation of human apolipoprotein A-I, dramatically increases cholesterol efflux capacity in patients

with stable atherothrombotic disease: a multicenter, randomized, double-blind, placebo-controlled, ascending-dose study. Circulation 2013;128:A15780.

167. Tardif JC, Ballantyne CM, Barter P, et al. Effects of the high-density lipoprotein mimetic agent CER-001 on coronary atherosclerosis in patients with acute coronary syndromes: a randomized trial. Eur Heart J 2014. [Epub ahead of print].

168. Hovingh GK, Stroes ES, Gaudet D. Effects of CER-001 on carotid atherosclerosis by 3TMRI in homozygous familial hypercholesterolaemia (HOFH): the modifying orphan disease evaluation (MODE) study. European Atherosclerosis Society Scientific Meeting 2014. Madrid, Spain, June 2, 2014.

169. Kootte RS, Smits LP, van der Valk FM. Recombinant human apolipoprotein-A-I prebeta-HDL (CER-001) promotes reverse cholesterol transport and reduces carotid wall thickness in patients with genetically determined low HDL. European Atherosclerosis Society Scientific Meeting 2014. Madrid, Spain, June 2, 2014.

170. Sacks FM, Rudel LL, Conner A, et al. Selective delipidation of plasma HDL enhances reverse cholesterol transport in vivo. J Lipid Res 2009;50(5):894–907.

171. Waksman R, Torguson R, Kent KM, et al. A first-in-man, randomized, placebo-controlled study to evaluate the safety and feasibility of autologous delipidated high-density lipoprotein plasma infusions in patients with acute coronary syndrome. J Am Coll Cardiol 2010;55(24):2727–35.

172. Garber DW, Datta G, Chaddha M, et al. A new synthetic class A amphipathic peptide analogue protects mice from diet-induced atherosclerosis. J Lipid Res 2001;42(4):545–52.

173. Watson CE, Weissbach N, Kjems L, et al. Treatment of patients with cardiovascular disease with L-4F, an apo-A1 mimetic, did not improve select biomarkers of HDL function. J Lipid Res 2011;52(2):361–73.

174. Navab M, Anantharamaiah GM, Hama S, et al. Oral administration of an Apo A-I mimetic Peptide synthesized from D-amino acids dramatically reduces atherosclerosis in mice independent of plasma cholesterol. Circulation 2002;105(3):290–2.

175. Bloedon LT, Dunbar R, Duffy D, et al. Safety, pharmacokinetics, and pharmacodynamics of oral apoA-I mimetic peptide D-4F in high-risk cardiovascular patients. J Lipid Res 2008;49(6):1344–52.

176. Chattopadhyay A, Navab M, Hough G, et al. A novel approach to oral apoA-I mimetic therapy. J Lipid Res 2013;54(4):995–1010.

177. Tabet F, Remaley AT, Segaliny AI, et al. The 5A apolipoprotein A-I mimetic peptide displays antiinflammatory and antioxidant properties in vivo and in vitro. Arterioscler Thromb Vasc Biol 2010;30(2):246–52.

178. Iwata A, Miura S, Zhang B, et al. Antiatherogenic effects of newly developed apolipoprotein A-I mimetic peptide/phospholipid complexes against aortic plaque burden in Watanabe-heritable hyperlipidemic rabbits. Atherosclerosis 2011;218(2):300–7.

179. Miller NE, Thelle DS, Forde OH, et al. The Tromso Heart Study. High-density lipoprotein and coronary heart-disease: a prospective case-control study. Lancet 1977;1(8019):965–8.

180. Castelli WP, Garrison RJ, Wilson PW, et al. Incidence of coronary heart disease and lipoprotein cholesterol levels. The Framingham Study. JAMA 1986;256(20):2835–8.

181. Multiple risk factor intervention trial. Risk factor changes and mortality results. Multiple Risk Factor Intervention Trial Research Group. JAMA 1982;248(12):1465–77.

182. Lipid Research Clinics Program. JAMA 1984;252(18):2545–8.
183. Assmann G, Schulte H, von Eckardstein A, et al. High-density lipoprotein cholesterol as a predictor of coronary heart disease risk. The PROCAM experience and pathophysiological implications for reverse cholesterol transport. Atherosclerosis 1996;124(Suppl):S11–20.
184. Goldbourt U, Yaari S, Medalie JH. Isolated low HDL cholesterol as a risk factor for coronary heart disease mortality. A 21-year follow-up of 8000 men. Arterioscler Thromb Vasc Biol 1997;17(1):107–13.
185. Sharrett AR, Ballantyne CM, Coady SA, et al. Coronary heart disease prediction from lipoprotein cholesterol levels, triglycerides, lipoprotein(a), apolipoproteins A-I and B, and HDL density subfractions: The Atherosclerosis Risk in Communities (ARIC) Study. Circulation 2001;104(10):1108–13.
186. Luc G, Bard JM, Ferrieres J, et al. Value of HDL cholesterol, apolipoprotein A-I, lipoprotein A-I, and lipoprotein A-I/A-II in prediction of coronary heart disease: the PRIME Study. Prospective Epidemiological Study of Myocardial Infarction. Arterioscler Thromb Vasc Biol 2002;22(7):1155–61.
187. Ericsson CG, Hamsten A, Nilsson J, et al. Angiographic assessment of effects of bezafibrate on progression of coronary artery disease in young male postinfarction patients. Lancet 1996;347(9005):849–53.
188. Frick MH, Syvanne M, Nieminen MS, et al. Prevention of the angiographic progression of coronary and vein-graft atherosclerosis by gemfibrozil after coronary bypass surgery in men with low levels of HDL cholesterol. Lopid Coronary Angiography Trial (LOCAT) Study Group. Circulation 1997;96(7):2137–43.
189. Effect of fenofibrate on progression of coronary-artery disease in type 2 diabetes: the Diabetes Atherosclerosis Intervention Study, a randomised study. Lancet 2001;357(9260):905–10.
190. Sibley CT, Vavere AL, Gottlieb I. MRI-measured regression of carotid atherosclerosis induced by statins with and without niacin in a randomised controlled trial: the NIA plaque study. Heart 2013;99(22):1675–80.

Cholesterol, Lipoproteins, High-sensitivity C-reactive Protein, and Other Risk Factors for Atherosclerosis

Joseph Rudolf, MD, Kent B. Lewandrowski, MD*

KEYWORDS

- Laboratory medicine • Cardiac markers • Biomarkers • Atherosclerosis
- Lipoprotein • Cholesterol biomarker • High-sensitivity CRP • Apolipoprotein E

KEY POINTS

- Intensive study has led to a deeper understanding of the pathogenesis of coronary disease and risk stratification in recent decades.
- Traditional risk factor assessment has focused on parameters derived from the Framingham Heart Study (age, hypertension, cholesterol, family history, and cigarette smoking).
- New emerging risk factors, both biological and genetic, are reshaping the understanding of heart disease and the approach to risk stratification.

INTRODUCTION

Coronary heart disease (CHD) is a common and costly epidemic in the Western world. According to statistics compiled by the American Heart Association there is a 7% prevalence of coronary artery disease (CAD) in adults 20 years of age and older.[1] In 2008, 1 in every 6 deaths in the United States was attributable to CHD, resulting in approximately 400,000 deaths nationwide.[1] The direct cost of care for patients with cardiovascular disease and stroke is estimated to exceed US$170 billion per year.[1]

Significant progress has been made in the understanding of the pathogenesis of CHD and its treatment since the identification of the first cardiovascular risk factors in the Framingham Heart Study. Although there are proven laboratory tests for the assessment of cardiovascular risk and effective means of modifying cardiovascular risk factors, understanding of the pathophysiology of CHD is still incomplete. The American Heart Association laid out ambitious goals for the year 2020, "to improve

This article originally appeared in Clinics in Laboratory Medicine, Volume 34, Issue 1, March 2014.
The authors have no conflicts of interest.
Division of Laboratory Medicine, Department of Pathology, Massachusetts General Hospital, Harvard Medical School, 55 Fruit Street, Boston, MA 02114-2696, USA
* Corresponding author.
E-mail address: klewandrowski@partners.org

the cardiovascular health of all Americans by 20%, while reducing deaths from cardiovascular diseases and stroke by 20%."[2] Reaching this goal will require more aggressive efforts to expand conventional risk assessment and treatment to the general population, along with the implementation of a new generation of laboratory tests focusing on novel biomarkers of cardiovascular risk and genetic screening.

PATHOGENESIS OF ATHEROSCLEROSIS

The pathogenic manifestation of atherosclerotic disease involves the development of raised intimal lesions in affected arteries filled with a lipid core, known as atheromas. Atheromas cause morbidity and mortality via multiple mechanisms, including obstruction of luminal blood flow, rupture of atheromatous plaques leading to thrombosis, and the facilitation of aneurysmal formation predisposing patients to vessel rupture.[3]

To date, many risk factors for cardiovascular disease have been identified, including both constitutional and modifiable risk factors (**Box 1**). Of the constitutional risk factors, family history is the single most important risk factor, implicating a strong role for a genetic contribution to cardiovascular risk. Other important nonmodifiable risk factors have been implicated in the form of both age and gender, whereby cardiovascular risk increases with age and premenopausal women have a markedly decreased risk compared with men. Modifiable risk factors include serum lipid levels, hypertension, cigarette smoking, and diabetes mellitus.[3]

At the cellular level, the development of atherosclerosis is described by the response to injury hypothesis. This hypothesis states that atherosclerosis results from the "chronic inflammatory and healing response of the arterial wall to endothelial damage and lesion progression occurs through the interaction of modified lipoproteins, monocyte-derived macrophages, and T lymphocytes with normal cellular constituents of the arterial wall."[4] Inflammation plays a role at all stages of atherosclerosis. Endothelial damage resulting from the deposition of lipoproteins in vessel walls triggers the release of inflammatory mediators. These inflammatory mediators attract monocytes, which engulf deposited lipoproteins leading to the transformation of

---

Box 1
CHD risk factors

CHD risk factors

    Age

    Men greater than or equal to 45 years of age or women greater than or equal to 55 years of age

    Family history of premature CHD

    Current cigarette smoking

    Hypertension

    Low high-density lipoprotein

    High low-density lipoprotein

CHD risk equivalents

    Other atherosclerotic disease (peripheral arterial disease, abdominal aortic aneurysm, carotid artery disease)

    Diabetes

    Multiple CHD risk factors and 10-year Framingham Risk Score greater than 20%

macrophages into foam cells. Foam cells secrete C-reactive protein, activating local endothelial cells to attract leukocytes. Leukocytes then promote the proliferation of smooth muscle cells and the production of extracellular matrix. The net result is increased intimal thickness, which, under continued inflammation-mediated endothelial injury, promotes additional lipid accumulation and further expansion of the atheroma.[3]

THE ROLE OF LIPOPROTEINS

Lipoprotein particles are the biological mediators of cholesterol and triglyceride transport. Although lipoproteins exist in a spectrum of sizes and vary in their specific surface protein compositions, they share a common structure consisting of a hydrophobic core of triglycerides and cholesterol esters surrounded by a hydrophilic phospholipid shell.[5]

Subclasses of lipoproteins are defined by the size and density of the lipoprotein's core lipids. The subclasses are broadly divided into high-density lipoprotein (HDL), intermediate-density lipoprotein (IDL), low-density lipoprotein (LDL), and very-low-density lipoprotein (VLDL) (**Table 1**). LDL is responsible for the transport of cholesterol to tissues and has long been considered to be the most significant atherogenic lipoprotein.[5] Among the LDL particles, the smallest and densest particles are the most atherogenic because of their ability to easily penetrate the subendothelial space.[6] Working in opposition to LDL, HDL is responsible for the process of reverse cholesterol transport, whereby cholesterol is mobilized from peripheral tissues and returned to the liver for excretion.[7] HDL has thus been termed good cholesterol.

TREATMENT GOALS

The dominant consensus document for the treatment of hypercholesterolemia for the modification of atherosclerotic risk is published by an expert panel from the National Institutes of Health's National Cholesterol Education Program (NCEP).[8] The third in the series of NCEP guidelines, the NCEP's Adult Treatment Panel III (ATP-III) establishes formulas for CHD risk assessment based on modifiable and nonmodifiable risk factors and evidence-based guidelines for lifestyle and pharmacologic intervention. The ATP-III presents goals for traditional serum biomarkers and establishes LDL as the major therapeutic target for reducing cardiovascular risk (**Table 2**).[8]

The ATP-III's approach to pharmacologic intervention in heart disease is based on the 10-year Framingham Risk Score (FRS). The FRS is calculated from a patient's age, gender, total cholesterol, HDL cholesterol, smoking status, and blood pressure. The 10-year FRS is then converted to one of 3 ATP-III categories: greater than 20% (including known CHD and risk equivalents including diabetes mellitus), 10% to 20%, and less than 10%. Patients are then treated based on their FRS risk score,

Table 1
Lipoprotein structure and content (in order of decreasing size)

	Content	Apolipoproteins
Chylomicron	Triglyceride > cholesterol ester	Apo B
VLDL	Triglyceride > cholesterol ester	Apo B, Apo C, Apo E
IDL	Cholesterol ester > triglyceride	Apo B, Apo E
LDL	Cholesterol ester > triglyceride	Apo B
HDL	Cholesterol ester > triglyceride	Apo AI, Apo AII

Table 2
Serum biomarker ranges and classification per the ATP-III

Total cholesterol (mg/dL)	Desirable <200		Borderline 200–239	High ≥240	
LDL (mg/dL)	Optimal <100	Near Optimal 100–129	Borderline 130–159	High 160–189	Very High ≥190
HDL (mg/dL)	Low <40			High ≥60	
Triglycerides (mg/dL)	Normal <150		Borderline High 150–199	High	Very High ≥500

with LDL being the primary treatment target (**Table 3**). Interventions include attempts to affect modifiable risk factors including hypertension, cigarette use, obesity, and diet, as well as pharmacologic interventions, most notably with statins. The algorithm for calculating FRS acknowledges the observation that cardiovascular disease event risk increases with age. If all other variables are constant, treating a total cholesterol of 240 mg/dL in a 60-year-old patient seems to yield a more substantial risk reduction than treating a 30-year-old patient with the same profile. However, this assumes that the patient has a 10-year life expectancy (**Table 4**). A patient more than 80 years of age may not live long enough to achieve the benefits of risk reduction when weighed against the cost and side effects of therapy, whereas the life expectancy of a 30-year-old is many decades, which shows the importance of early intervention.

Although the FRS depends in part on HDL for its calculation, the ATP-III does not define secondary guidelines for treatment of HDL once LDL goals have been met. In particular, the document does not address goals for HDL, even though each increase of 1 mg/dL HDL corresponds with a decreased risk of cardiovascular disease of 2% to 3%.[9] In comparison, a 40-mg/dL decrease in LDL is associated with 24% decrease in cardiovascular disease risk.[10] Even in patients with an LDL less than 70 mg/dL, the therapeutic target for patients with established CHD, HDL remains an independent predictor of cardiovascular death.[10] This observation, along with the discovery of a series of novel markers of cardiovascular risk in the 10 years since the ATP-III's publication, argues for a reassessment of the guidelines for calculating and treating cardiovascular disease.

LIPOPROTEIN ANALYSIS

Standard automated methods for the measurement of lipoprotein fractions couple enzymatic methods with spectrophotometric measurement to produce values for 3 primary analytes: total cholesterol, HDL, and triglycerides. LDL is then calculated from these primary analytes by the Friedewald equation ([LDL cholesterol] = [total cholesterol] − [HDL cholesterol] − [triglyceride]/5).[5] Although these assays are

Table 3
LDL treatment targets according to risk

10 y Risk (%)	LDL Goal (mg/Dl)
>20	<100
10–20	<130
<10 (≥2 risk factors)	<130
<10 (0–1 risk factors)	<160

Table 4
Ten-year risk calculations based on age

Age (y)	Total Cholesterol (mg/dL)	Smoking	HDL (mg/dL)	HTN	10-y Risk (%)	10-y Risk After Cholesterol Intervention (%)
30	240	No	50	No	<1	<1
40	240	No	50	No	2	1
50	240	No	50	No	6	2
60	240	No	50	No	10	6
70	240	No	50	No	14	11
80	240	No	50	No	16	17

standardized, calculated LDL (LDL-c) by the Friedewald equation is inaccurate at high triglyceride levels. There are also concerns about the linearity of the Friedewald calculation at the low range of LDL.[11] Methods for direct LDL measurement are now available. These methods perform better at high triglyceride levels (>400 mg/dL). However, it has yet to be established whether directly measured LDL values compare equivalently with established, and prospectively validated, calculated values.[7] Older traditional methods for the direct evaluation of lipoprotein subfractions are cumbersome, involving ultracentrifugation followed by optical or enzymatic methods for quantification.[12] Newer, more automated assays for the direct measurement of LDL have become available for routine use. Nonetheless, most clinical laboratories still perform calculated LDL values on most patients.[11]

In recent years, new approaches for quantifying serum lipoprotein content have been proposed and validated. The most promising of these quantification methods has been the apolipoprotein B (ApoB)/apolipoprotein AI (ApoAI) ratio.[13] ApoB100 is the signature capsular protein of LDL, whereas ApoAI is the signature capsular protein of HDL. Each lipoprotein carries only a single apolipoprotein type. Thus, a measurement of the number of ApoAI molecules is a direct proxy for the number of HDL molecules, whereas the measurement of ApoB is a direct proxy of LDL levels. With the realization that atherogenesis is a function of the number of lipoprotein molecules in circulation, with smaller molecules being more atherogenic than larger molecules, it is clear that the ApoB/ApoAI ratio adds prognostic information beyond traditional assays that measure the concentration of lipoproteins only.[6] The ApoB/ApoAI ratio is superior to traditional methods in patients with a normal calculated LDL.[13] Although the adoption of apolipoprotein measurement in clinical practice has been slow in the United States, Canadian guidelines have recommended its use as far back as 2003.[14] In their 2012 update, the Canadian guidelines recommend ApoB measurement as a valid alternative for cardiovascular risk assessment and treatment.[15] According to the guidelines, intermediate-risk patients (10-year FRS of 10%–19%) with ApoB levels of greater than or equal to 1.2 g/L and all high-risk patients (10-year FRS ≥20%) should be treated to a therapeutic target of less than or equal to 0.80 g/L.[15] In addition to its prognostic value, the ApoB and ApoAI assays are precise and internationally standardized, making them an attractive approach for risk assessment.[13] Most clinical laboratories already have the technical capability and equipment to perform the immunonephelometric or immunoturbidimetric assays necessary to implement ApoB/ApoAI screening.[16] However, these assays are more expensive than conventional cholesterol screening and are not as automated.

Methods for the determination of LDL particle number by nuclear magnetic resonance (NMR) spectroscopy have also been developed. NMR yields more precision than ApoB measurements and provides additional information in the form of quantified lipoprotein subclasses, some of which may assist in cardiovascular risk assessment.[17] NMR facilitates excellent discrimination by interrogating and quantifying the terminal methyl groups on individual lipoprotein subclasses, each of which emits a characteristic NMR spectrum.[17] Despite the additional subclass information provided by lipoprotein NMR, the technique is considered to be less attractive than ApoB/ApoAI measurement in the current environment because it is more expensive, difficult to automate, and difficult to scale up for high-volume automated testing.[16,17] Although the cost will likely decrease in the future, it is unclear whether NMR will be able accommodate the capacity necessary for routine lipid screening, which is performed an estimated 216,000,000 times a year in the United States alone.[17]

NOVEL BIOMARKERS

Because of its long latency and robust strategies for primary prevention, cardiovascular disease is a promising area for the development of novel soluble biomarkers for risk assessment and to guide treatment.[18] Current risk factor prediction and approaches for intervention have led to reduced morbidity and mortality of CHD. However, the success of preventive measures depends on the ability to accurately assess an individual patient's risk.[6] In patients with known cardiovascular disease, diabetes, or kidney disease, atherosclerotic risk based on calculated LDL provides adequate insight.[6] However, it is known that patients with the same calculated LDL concentration can have different risks for cardiovascular disease, suggesting that LDL is a necessary but not sufficient means of calculating cardiovascular risk.[6,19]

In 2007, investigators Morrow and de Lemos[20] proposed criteria for evaluating new cardiovascular biomarkers. They suggested that the benchmarks for biomarkers include that they be easily measured, add prognostic information not available by other current markers, and have implications for patient management.[20] An important addition to these criteria is that a biomarker must be able to distinguish disease states from nondisease states with great resolution to be helpful in risk stratification.[18]

Many potential biomarkers have been proposed in the decade since the most recent ATP-III guidelines were released. Although many association studies have been undertaken to evaluate proposed biomarkers, few have been tested in randomized controlled trials to investigate their use in primary prevention.[18] Cardiovascular disease is a complex biological phenomenon and it is likely that cardiovascular risk modeling will require an equally complex approach. Individual biomarkers vary in the type of cardiovascular event that they help to predict, and it is increasingly clear that no single marker is sensitive or specific enough to predict the sum total risk of cardiovascular disease in isolation.[18] However, even small incremental improvements in the prediction of cardiovascular risk will translate into significant health gains given the high prevalence of cardiovascular disease.[6] Biomarkers for cardiovascular risk are emerging at a steady rate and there is hope that the summation of multiple factors will help to better quantify cardiovascular risk.

HIGH-SENSITIVITY C-REACTIVE PROTEIN

One of the most promising and well-studied emerging biomarkers is high-sensitivity C-reactive protein (hs-CRP). Keen interest in CRP as a cardiovascular risk marker emerged through the increasing understanding of the role of inflammation in the pathogenesis of cardiovascular disease. CRP is an acute phase reactant and member of the pentraxin family.[21] Secreted in response to interleukin-6, CRP plays a role in the innate immune system response through the opsonization of bacteria and the activation of complement.[3] CRP is secreted by foam cells sequestered in the intima of atherosclerotic lesions and activates local endothelial cells to induce a prothrombotic state, markedly increasing the adhesiveness of leukocytes to damaged endothelium.[3]

More than 20 studies to date have shown the value of hs-CRP in the prediction of cardiovascular disease in a variety of populations.[22] Most studies have reported that the increased risk associated with high hs-CRP levels (generally those more than 2 mg/L) are independent of known classic cardiovascular risk factors, are relevant in a magnitude similar to other established risk factors such as hypertension, and increase in a graded manner.[23] Increased hs-CRP levels have also been shown to be strong predictors of incident cardiovascular events including myocardial infarction, stroke, sudden cardiac death, and peripheral vascular disease in seemingly healthy adults.[24]

Initial studies showed that patients treated with statins and who had low LDL and low hs-CRP had better outcomes than treated patients with low LDL and high hs-CRP levels.[25] The landmark hs-CRP trial was the Justification of the Use of Statins in Primary Prevention (JUPITER) trial.[26,27] The JUPITER trial was the first prospective study to show the benefit of hs-CRP screening.[27] Patients with LDL values less than 130 mg/dL but hs-CRP levels greater than or equal to 2 mg/L were treated with resuvastatin or placebo and followed for primary cardiovascular events. Incident cardiovascular events were reduced by 44% and all-cause mortality was decreased by 20%.[22] The trial was stopped early at 1.9 years because of the magnitude of these findings.[28] These reductions were all seen in patients who would have been predicted as low or intermediate risk when scored by the ATP-III. The 5-year number needed to treat (NNT) associated with the JUPITER trial was calculated to be 25, which compares favorably with the NNT for many other interventions.[22]

CRP has long been used as a laboratory assay for quantitating inflammation, but only recently became a realistic marker of cardiovascular disease risk assessment with the advent of high-sensitivity assays. Traditional assays for CRP had a lower linear range of approximately 5 mg/L; this is insufficient for measuring cardiac risk, which necessitates accurate measurement in the 1 mg/L range.[24] At 5 mg/L CRP lacked the sensitivity to be used in the stratification of cardiovascular risk.[24] The development of high-sensitivity screening assays has allowed accurate CRP measurement at less than 1 mg/L, enabling its use in cardiovascular disease screening (**Fig. 1**).

In many ways CRP is an ideal analyte. It is stable over long periods of time, shows little diurnal variation, and can be inexpensively measured with high-sensitivity assays.[29] CRP has a constant half-life such that the degree of increase in CRP levels

Test name	Result	Ref Range	Units	Completed
ⓔ CRP, High Sensitivity	0.2	N/A	mg/L	07/12/2013 14:51
	Reference Range: Quintile 1 Lowest Risk <0.7 mg/L Quintile 2 Low Risk 0.7-1.1 mg/L Quintile 3 Moderate Risk 1.2-1.9 mg/L Quintile 4 High Risk 2.0-3.8 mg/L Quintile 5 Highest Risk >3.8 mg/L When the result is >15.0 mg/L, risk analysis may be confounded by recent or acute inflammatory disease. In these cases, the risk for coronary heart disease can not be provided. A repeat specimen, taken two weeks after resolution of any acute inflammatory condition may allow provision of coronary risk information.			

Fig. 1. Sample hs-CRP report with reference quintiles.

is directly proportional to the degree of inflammation.[18] There also seems to be no significant variations in CRP by race or gender, so gender-specific or ethnic-specific cutoffs are not necessary.[24] In addition, although CRP tends to increase with age, there seems to be no significant variation between the ages of 20 and 70 years, which is an important range for risk stratification.[24]

CRP has high intraindividual variation and varies markedly in the setting of asymptomatic inflammation or subclinical infection.[24] Given this high variability, the use of a single CRP measurement for the purpose of risk stratification is likely to result in the misclassification of many individuals.[30] Therefore it is necessary to get at least 2 CRP measurements to establish an accurate baseline for a patient to prevent risk misclassification.[31]

Based on the compelling evidence, tentative recommendations have been issued by various sources for the use of hs-CRP in screening. The JUPITER group suggested that hs-CRP measurement may be useful for stratification in of men greater than or equal to 50 years of age and women greater than or equal to 60 years of age with normal LDL in whom statin therapy is not clearly indicated (for example, those patients with an intermediate risk score by ATP-III guidelines).[22] In addition, they recommend screening at an earlier age in patients with a family history of cardiovascular disease.[22] Most trials have recommended using 2 mg/L as an hs-CRP cutoff for intervention, but critics of the JUPITER trial and hs-CRP have recommended that better stratification is achieved with cutoffs of less than 1 mg/L and greater than 3 mg/L because of the intraindividual variation in measurement.[30] Although a lack of consensus regarding the use of hs-CRP exists and hs-CRP will almost certainly not be used as a sole marker of cardiovascular risk assessment, it is a clear independent prognosticator of cardiovascular disease and has management implications for low-risk to intermediate-risk patients who may benefit from statin therapy. As such, it is likely to become a standard component of cardiovascular screening in selected patient populations.

APOLIPOPROTEIN-ASSOCIATED PHOSPHOLIPASE A2

Another novel biomarker that has received substantial attention in recent years is apolipoprotein-associated phospholipase A2 (Lp-PLA2). The enzyme Lp-PLA2 is a member of the phospholipase A family.[32] Produced by monocytes, lymphocytes, and mast cells, Lp-PLA2 participates in the hydrolysis of oxidized LDLs mediating proatherogenic and inflammatory processes. It is actively expressed in unstable atherosclerotic plaques, suggesting its role in increasing plaque vulnerability.[33] Lp-PLA2 is both less variable than CRP and a more specific marker of vascular inflammation.[6] When adjusted for classic cardiovascular risk factors, Lp-PLA2 shows an attenuated but independent association with cardiovascular risk.[34]

In the serum, most (~80%) Lp-PLA is carried by LDL, whereas the remainder is carried by HDL and VLDL.[32] Lp-PLA2 can be measured by mass assay or by activity.[23] A recent meta-analysis of Lp-PLA2 studies showed associations between Lp-PLA2 and both CHD and stroke when assayed either by activity or mass.[35] Analyses of Lp-PLA2 in the JUPITER trial showed that Lp-PLA2 activity predicted new vascular events, but that Lp-PLA2 mass did not.[23] The association of Lp-PLA2 activity but not mass with cardiovascular events (myocardial infarction, stroke, and cardiovascular related mortality) was corroborated in a case-cohort sample from the Women's Health Initiative Observational study.[23]

The conflicting results of various Lp-PLA2 studies are not surprising given issues with assay calibration and reproducibility.[23] However, the Lp-PLA2 assays are in their infancy. As the assays become more standardized and the results more reproducible, it is likely that the role of Lp-PLA2 in the prediction of cardiovascular disease will be clarified. Until then, questions will remain as to whether Lp-PLA2 is an independent cardiovascular risk marker and, if so, what value it adds to risk assessment and decisions surrounding management.[34]

No major guidelines have been issued regarding Lp-PLA2 screening because clinical validation studies have not yet been completed.[6] However, given its specificity for vascular inflammation, Lp-PLA2 may be a useful assay to identify patients prone to cardiovascular risk masked by normal LDL in an early stage of atherosclerotic disease.[6] If a causal role between plaque stability and the presence of Lp-PLA2 can be established, Lp-PLA2 may additionally serve as a therapeutic target.

MYELOPEROXIDASE AND OXIDIZED LDL

Another promising class of biomarkers to emerge from the increased understanding of the role of inflammation in the pathogenesis of cardiovascular risk is based on the effects of oxidized LDL in the formation of atheromatous plaques and the involvement of the myeloperoxidase (MPO) pathway. Synthesized by macrophages in the arterial wall, MPO interacts with hydrogen peroxide (also produced by activated macrophages) to create hypochlorous acid. The MPO pathway functions as a barrier of innate immunity. However, in the presence of circulating LDL, oxidation results in increased uptake of LDL by macrophages, leading to the formation of foam cells.[36]

This process also inhibits the function of HDL. For ApoAI to properly associate with lipids and thereby facilitate effective efflux of cholesterol, it must undergo a conformational change. It has been hypothesized that MPO alters amino acid residues, preventing the conformational change, and thereby decreasing the rate of cholesterol reverse transport.[36] To investigate this phenomenon, one group recently developed a liquid chromatography mass spectrometry technique to quantify 2 known products of the MPO pathway: 3-chlorotyrosine and 3-nitrotyrosine. Using this technique, the group discovered that these MPO products were present at higher levels in atherosclerotic lesions than in circulating plasma in individuals with known CAD. In addition, circulating levels of the known MPO products were present at higher levels in patients with known disease than in normal, healthy controls. This finding suggests that chlorinated or nitrated products of the MPO pathway may be good markers of CAD, and possibly therapeutic targets as well.[36]

Another recently published technique for assessing the effects of MPO is based on the presence of MPO leading to the formation of an ApoAI-ApoAII heterodimer. An enzyme-linked immunosorbent assay (ELISA) sandwich assay was developed from goat antihuman AI and AII antibodies applied to HDL treated with MPO. Using immune blots, the group was able to show the presence of the ApoAI-ApoAII heterodimer. They went on to look for this heterodimer in patients with acute myocardial infarction and discovered modest but significant increases in the heterodimer level corresponding with the acute infarction.[37] This work is early but promising.

Another approach to the assessment of oxidation as a biomarker of cardiovascular risk has been to measure oxidized LDL directly. Direct measurement assays are based on the hypothesis that small, dense LDLs undergo oxidation that leads to conformational changes in the lipoprotein, facilitating uptake by macrophages, inducing platelet adhesion, and destabilizing the fibrous cap of arterial plaques. LDL that is heavily oxidized is quickly cleared from the circulation by Kupffer cells in the sinusoidal endothelial cells of the liver, making it difficult to measure. However, minimally oxidized LDL has a longer half-life in circulation and thus can be more easily measured.[19]

The development of assays to measure oxidized LDL directly has been met with numerous challenges. The first challenge is the development of antibodies directed against oxidized LDL that are sensitive enough to measure the multitude of heterogeneous oxidized epitopes but specific enough to target only oxidized particles. A second challenge is that many biological and lifestyle factors affect oxidized LDL levels. These factors include but are not limited to aging, male sex, obesity, inflammation, diabetes, impaired renal function, smoking, and physical inactivity.[19] If a sufficiently specific and sensitive assay can be developed, oxidized LDL could be an excellent marker for subclinical atherosclerosis. However, many challenges in terms of assay development and validation remain, as well as concerns about the influence of biologic factors.

LIPOPROTEIN (A)

Lipoprotein (a), also known as LP(a), is related to LDL, consisting of an LDL-like particle containing an ApoB100 covalently bound to an apolipoprotein (a) molecule by a disulfide bond.[38] Although the function of LP(a) is not known, it has been hypothesized, based on the ability of LP(a) to bind fibrin, that LP(a) may help to deliver cholesterol to healing tissues in the physiologic state and deliver cholesterol to plaques as a pathologic by-product.[39]

The association of high LP(a) levels with increased risk of CHD have long been proposed. However, early studies were underpowered to detect effects at any concentration lower than the highest levels. In addition, lack of assay standardization led to varied findings concerning the role of LP(a) and complicated early meta-analyses.[38,40] Recent mendelian randomization studies have helped to show the value of LP(a) as an independent predictor of CHD.[38,39] It has recently been shown that the association between LP(a) levels and CHD risk varies continuously and without a threshold effect.[38]

LP(a) levels in the population vary more than 1000-fold from less than 0.1 mg/dL to greater than 200 mg/dL, and are skewed toward low values with a long tail toward higher concentrations.[39] Although no significant variation exists between the sexes, mean and median values vary by as much as 4 times between ethnicities.[39] In addition, levels of LP(a) increase substantially in the setting of decreased glomerular filtration such as in chronic kidney disease.[39] Multiple platforms exist for measuring LP(a), including ELISA-based methods, as well as latex, immunonephelometric, immunoturbidimetric, and fluorescence assays.[38] These assays have become increasingly standardized in recent years.[40]

Consensus guidelines regarding LP(a) testing and treatment were proposed in 2010 in the *European Heart Journal*.[38] The proposed guidelines suggest single-time-point screening for patients with premature cardiovascular disease or a family history thereof, familial hypercholesterolemia, recurrent cardiovascular disease in the setting of statin treatment, greater than a 10% 10-year risk of cardiovascular disease event risk by US guidelines, or a greater than 3% 10-year fatal cardiovascular disease event risk by European guidelines. The group suggests treating patients with LP(a) levels greater than 80% of the population level (~50 mg/dL) with niacin and then rechecking LP(a) levels to monitor treatment goals.[38]

Although it is increasingly clear that LP(a) is an important independent predictor of cardiovascular disease, LP(a) faces a significant challenge as a biomarker because of a lack of effective treatments to reduce LP(a) concentrations.[39] Although recommended for use by the proposed European guidelines, extended-release niacin has not been shown to alter the course of CHD in patients treated with statins.[41] In addition, no prospective trials showing the effect of niacin on LP(a) levels have been published to date.[38] Phase 3 trials for cholesteryl ester transfer protein inhibitors targeting LP(a) levels are underway and may prove effective in modulating CHD risk caused by LP(a).[39] In the absence of an effective therapeutic targeting LP(a), routine screening is likely premature, despite the proposed guidelines.

GENETICS

Although the strong effect of genetics in the development of cardiovascular disease has long been known, only a small portion of the heritability of cardiovascular risk has been described to date.[42] The advent of genome-wide association studies (GWAS) has heralded the promise of a deeper understanding of the genetic contribution to cardiovascular risk and an unbiased approach for the discovery of new cardiovascular risk biomarkers.[18] Many loci were proposed during the early years of GWAS studies. However, because of the small effect of individual single-nucleotide polymorphisms (SNPs) to overall risk, few of the loci have been replicated in early studies.[42] Quantifying the effect of common SNPs, which typically correspond with odds ratios of cardiovascular disease risk of 0.7 to 1.3, requires large trials and was initially limited by the power of genetic technologies.[42] With the advancement of new genetic screening technology in recent years, new loci have been discovered and replicated, leading to new insight in the quantification of cardiac risk.

One such locus is a SNP on the p arm of chromosome 21. 9p21.3 is a promising target because it is found in a nonannotated region of the genome in which no genes conveying cardiovascular disease or risk have previously been identified.[42] A recent study has found that a single copy of the polymorphism confers a 15% to 20% increased risk of cardiovascular disease, whereas the homozygous state corresponds with an increased risk of 30% to 40%.[42,43] The biological correlate of the 9p21.3 locus has yet to be determined, but the magnitude of effect conferred by this polymorphism makes it an ideal target for risk prediction.

Another equally promising locus has been characterized on a highly conserved portion of chromosome 1. Locus 1p13.3 corresponds with the location of the sortillin gene, SORT1, which codes for a multiligand receptor associated with lipid and glucose metabolism. The gene product of SORT1 binds LDL-receptor (LDL-R) protein, increasing the uptake of LDL in the liver. This was shown in embryonic kidney cells, which, when transfected with the complementary DNA for SORT1, overexpressed the gene product of sortillin, and increased their uptake of LDL.[44] GWAS analyses have shown that each copy of the G-allele polymorphism leads to a 0.12-mmol/L decrease in LDL-C, thereby conferring a 9% decreased risk of CAD. The homozygous state confers an 18% decrease in CAD risk.[44]

APOLIPOPROTEIN E POLYMORPHISMS

Apolipoprotein E (APOE) is a structural component of many classes of lipoproteins and serves as a ligand to mediate the uptake and recycling of lipoprotein particles.[45] There are 3 major isoforms of APOE in the population: E2, E3, and E4, with E3 being the most common isoform.[45] Although the allele frequencies vary between ethnic groups, multiple studies have shown that LDL levels are higher in patients with the APOE4 genotype and lower in those with the APOE2 genotype.[45,46] Another study involving patients on dialysis found an increased risk of cardiovascular events and higher rates of cardiovascular mortality in patients with the APOE4 genotype.[47] As with polymorphisms in the sortillin gene, the APOE4 genotype may therefore be an important component of a multilocus approach to genetic risk factor profiling for cardiovascular disease.

APOLIPOPROTEIN (A) POLYMORPHISMS

In addition to the lipoprotein genetic variations discovered for apolipoprotein E, genetic variations in apolipoprotein (a) have also been described in recent years. The production of LP(a) by the liver is governed by the LPA locus on 6q27 and is significantly affected by copy number variation (CNV).[39] CNVs in the kringle IV domain 2 region of the LPA locus are present in numbers ranging from 2 to 40 per allele.[39] Increased copy numbers are associated with higher molecular weight isoforms, lower concentrations of LP(a), and thus a lower risk for cardiovascular disease.[39] Variations in copy numbers seem to explain between 30% and 70% of LP(a) variation.[39] An additional ~30% is explained by 2 SNPs that confer increased odds ratios of coronary disease of between 1.70 and 1.92.[48] As mentioned previously, although LP(a) levels are an increasingly important part of cardiovascular risk prediction, the current lack of effective LP(a)-directed therapy tempers the value of routine testing at a functional or genetic level.

PROPROTEIN CONVERTASE SUBTILISIN/KINEXIN TYPE 9

The most promising discovery to arise from genetic screening began in 2003 with the discovery of proprotein convertase subtilisin/kinexin type 9 (PCSK9).[49] Genetic analysis of patients with autosomal dominant familial hypercholesterolemia, but who were not adequately described by known mutations in ApoB, led to the discovery of a missense mutation in PCSK9.[49] Located on chromosome 1p32.3, PCSK9 is a serine protease that is produced in greatest concentrations by the liver and small intestine.[49] PCSK9 binds the LDL-R in circulation and facilitates low-density lipoprotein receptor (LDL-R) recycling.[49] In individuals with familial hypercholesterolemia, the missense mutation in PCSK9 leads to a gain of function and higher levels of circulating PCSK9. The net result is decreased density of LDL-R and higher circulating LDL.[49] Further genetic screening trials facilitated the discovery of a small number of patients with a loss-of-function mutation in PCSK9 with very low levels of circulating LDL.[49] This finding resulted in a race to develop pharmacologic therapies targeting the role of PCSK9.

Multiple monoclonal antibody–based therapies targeting PCSK9 have entered trials in recent years with promising results. The most thoroughly studied therapeutic to date is the monoclonal antibody REGN727, which binds PCSK9. In phase 1 trials, REGN727 significantly reduced LDL levels in healthy volunteers as well as in patients with both familial and nonfamilial forms of hypercholesterolemia.[49,50] Further studies have shown LDL reductions of up to 80% with REGN727 and reductions of at least 40% in all but 1 patient.[49] REGN727 has been well tolerated with no significant organ-specific side effects to date.[49] Eleven phase 3 clinical trials of REGN727, known as the ODYSSEY trials, and including 22,000 patients are ongoing and are equally promising.[49]

SUMMARY

Many advancements in the understanding of cardiovascular disease, risk assessment, and heritability have been made since the release of the ATP-III guidelines. Although important, LDL levels in isolation are not a sufficient predictor of cardiovascular risk or a means of assessing response to therapy. Atherosclerosis is a complex disease and it requires a model of prediction that acknowledges this complexity. The last decade has been an active time in lipid science, with many novel markers and risk prediction tools being proposed. Although only a small percentage of proposed markers have been validated successfully, those markers that have stood up to scientific scrutiny provide hope for more complete models of risk prediction. Even more importantly, some of these targets are serving as the inspiration for therapeutic targets. If successful, these novel therapies will change the landscape of disease, helping to control the immense burden of cardiovascular disease in developed countries. The clinical laboratories are in an excellent position to assist in the deployment of complex models and testing algorithms, including the standardization of assays and models of risk assessment, clinical consultation in the interpretation of risk scores, the evaluation of emerging risk factors, and the assurance of cost-effective strategies for screening.[6]

REFERENCES

1. Roger VL, Go AS, Lloyd-Jones DM, et al. Heart disease and stroke statistics–2012 update: a report from the American Heart Association. Circulation 2012; 125(1):e2–220.
2. Lloyd-Jones DM, Hong Y, Labarthe D, et al. Defining and setting national goals for cardiovascular health promotion and disease reduction: the American Heart Association's strategic impact goal through 2020 and beyond. Circulation 2010; 121(4):586–613.
3. Kumar V, Abbas A, Fausto N, et al. Robbins and Cotran pathologic basis of disease. 8th edition. Philadelphia: Saunders Elsevier; 2010.
4. Ross R. Atherosclerosis–an inflammatory disease. N Engl J Med 1999;340(2): 115–26.
5. Ábel G, Laposata M. Lipids, lipoproteins, and cardiovascular risk. In: Lewandrowski K, editor. Clinical chemistry: laboratory management and clinical correlations. Philadelphia: Lippincott Williams & Wilkins; 2002. p. 575–91.
6. Langlois MR. Laboratory approaches for predicting and managing the risk of cardiovascular disease: postanalytical opportunities of lipid and lipoprotein testing. Clin Chem Lab Med 2012;50(7):1169–81.
7. Ashen MD, Blumenthal RS. Clinical practice. Low HDL cholesterol levels. N Engl J Med 2005;353(12):1252–60.
8. Third report of the National Cholesterol Education Program (NCEP) Expert Panel on Detection, Evaluation, and Treatment of High Blood Cholesterol in Adults (Adult Treatment Panel III) final report. Circulation 2002;106(25):3143–421.
9. Brewer HB Jr. Increasing HDL cholesterol levels. N Engl J Med 2004;350(15): 1491–4.
10. Barter P, Gotto AM, LaRosa JC, et al. HDL cholesterol, very low levels of LDL cholesterol, and cardiovascular events. N Engl J Med 2007;357(13):1301–10.
11. Abudu N, Levinson SS. Calculated low-density lipoprotein cholesterol remains a viable and important test for screening and targeting therapy. Clin Chem Lab Med 2007;45(10):1319–25.
12. Mueller O, Chang E, Deng D, et al. PROCAM Study: risk prediction for myocardial infarction using microfluidic high-density lipoprotein (HDL) subfractionation is independent of HDL cholesterol. Clin Chem Lab Med 2008;46(4):490–8.
13. Rasouli M, Kiasari AM, Mokhberi V. The ratio of apoB/apoAI, apoB and lipoprotein(a) are the best predictors of stable coronary artery disease. Clin Chem Lab Med 2006;44(8):1015–21.
14. Genest J, Frohlich J, Fodor G, et al. Recommendations for the management of dyslipidemia and the prevention of cardiovascular disease: summary of the 2003 update. CMAJ 2003;169(9):921–4.
15. Anderson TJ, Gregoire J, Hegele RA, et al. 2012 update of the Canadian Cardiovascular Society guidelines for the diagnosis and treatment of dyslipidemia for

the prevention of cardiovascular disease in the adult. Can J Cardiol 2013;29(2): 151–67.

16. Master SR, Rader DJ. Beyond LDL cholesterol in assessing cardiovascular risk: apo B or LDL-P? Clin Chem 2013;59(5):723–5.

17. Cole TG, Contois JH, Csako G, et al. Association of apolipoprotein B and nuclear magnetic resonance spectroscopy-derived LDL particle number with outcomes in 25 clinical studies: assessment by the AACC Lipoprotein and Vascular Diseases Division Working Group on Best Practices. Clin Chem 2013;59(5):752–70.

18. Gilstrap LG, Wang TJ. Biomarkers and cardiovascular risk assessment for primary prevention: an update. Clin Chem 2012;58(1):72–82.

19. Verhoye E, Langlois MR, Asklepios I. Circulating oxidized low-density lipoprotein: a biomarker of atherosclerosis and cardiovascular risk? Clin Chem Lab Med 2009;47(2):128–37.

20. Morrow DA, de Lemos JA. Benchmarks for the assessment of novel cardiovascular biomarkers. Circulation 2007;115(8):949–52.

21. Devaraj S, Kumaresan PR, Jialal I. C-reactive protein induces release of both endothelial microparticles and circulating endothelial cells in vitro and in vivo: further evidence of endothelial dysfunction. Clin Chem 2011;57(12):1757–61.

22. Mora S, Musunuru K, Blumenthal RS. The clinical utility of high-sensitivity C-reactive protein in cardiovascular disease and the potential implication of JUPITER on current practice guidelines. Clin Chem 2009;55(2):219–28.

23. Cook NR, Paynter NP, Manson JE, et al. Clinical utility of lipoprotein-associated phospholipase A(2) for cardiovascular disease prediction in a multiethnic cohort of women. Clin Chem 2012;58(9):1352–63.

24. Ledue TB, Rifai N. Preanalytic and analytic sources of variations in C-reactive protein measurement: implications for cardiovascular disease risk assessment. Clin Chem 2003;49(8):1258–71.

25. Ridker PM, Cannon CP, Morrow D, et al. C-reactive protein levels and outcomes after statin therapy. N Engl J Med 2005;352(1):20–8.

26. Mora S, Ridker PM. Justification for the Use of Statins in Primary Prevention: an Intervention Trial Evaluating Rosuvastatin (JUPITER)–can C-reactive protein be used to target statin therapy in primary prevention? Am J Cardiol 2006; 97(2A):33A–41A.

27. Ridker PM, Danielson E, Fonseca FA, et al. Rosuvastatin to prevent vascular events in men and women with elevated C-reactive protein. N Engl J Med 2008;359(21):2195–207.

28. Biasucci LM, Biasillo G, Stefanelli A. Inflammatory markers, cholesterol and statins: pathophysiological role and clinical importance. Clin Chem Lab Med 2010; 48(12):1685–91.

29. Ridker PM, Rifai N, Rose L, et al. Comparison of C-reactive protein and low-density lipoprotein cholesterol levels in the prediction of first cardiovascular events. N Engl J Med 2002;347(20):1557–65.

30. Yousuf O, Mohanty BD, Martin SS, et al. High-sensitivity C-reactive protein and cardiovascular disease: a resolute belief or an elusive link? J Am Coll Cardiol 2013;62(5):397–408.

31. Ruckerl R, Peters A, Khuseyinova N, et al. Determinants of the acute-phase protein C-reactive protein in myocardial infarction survivors: the role of comorbidities and environmental factors. Clin Chem 2009;55(2):322–35.

32. Garza CA, Montori VM, McConnell JP, et al. Association between lipoprotein-associated phospholipase A2 and cardiovascular disease: a systematic review. Mayo Clin Proc 2007;82(2):159–65.

33. Kolasa-Trela R, Fil K, Bazanek M, et al. Lipoprotein-associated phospholipase A2 is elevated in patients with severe aortic valve stenosis without clinically overt atherosclerosis. Clin Chem Lab Med 2012;50(10):1825–31.
34. Stein EA. Lipoprotein-associated phospholipase A(2) measurements: mass, activity, but little productivity. Clin Chem 2012;58(5):814–7.
35. Thompson A, Gao P, Orfei L, et al. Lipoprotein-associated phospholipase A(2) and risk of coronary disease, stroke, and mortality: collaborative analysis of 32 prospective studies. Lancet 2010;375(9725):1536–44.
36. Shao B, Oda MN, Oram JF, et al. Myeloperoxidase: an oxidative pathway for generating dysfunctional high-density lipoprotein. Chem Res Toxicol 2010; 23(3):447–54.
37. Kameda T, Usami Y, Shimada S, et al. Determination of myeloperoxidase-induced apoAI-apoAII heterodimers in high-density lipoprotein. Ann Clin Lab Sci 2012;42(4):384–91.
38. Nordestgaard BG, Chapman MJ, Ray K, et al. Lipoprotein(a) as a cardiovascular risk factor: current status. Eur Heart J 2010;31(23):2844–53.
39. Kronenberg F, Utermann G. Lipoprotein(a): resurrected by genetics. J Intern Med 2013;273(1):6–30.
40. Erqou S, Kaptoge S, Perry PL, et al. Lipoprotein(a) concentration and the risk of coronary heart disease, stroke, and nonvascular mortality. JAMA 2009;302(4): 412–23.
41. Boden WE, Probstfield JL, Anderson T, et al. Niacin in patients with low HDL cholesterol levels receiving intensive statin therapy. N Engl J Med 2011; 365(24):2255–67.
42. Zeller T, Blankenberg S, Diemert P. Genomewide association studies in cardiovascular disease–an update 2011. Clin Chem 2012;58(1):92–103.
43. Samani NJ, Erdmann J, Hall AS, et al. Genomewide association analysis of coronary artery disease. N Engl J Med 2007;357(5):443–53.
44. Linsel-Nitschke P, Heeren J, Aherrahrou Z, et al. Genetic variation at chromosome 1p13.3 affects sortilin mRNA expression, cellular LDL-uptake and serum LDL levels which translates to the risk of coronary artery disease. Atherosclerosis 2010;208(1):183–9.
45. Burman D, Mente A, Hegele RA, et al. Relationship of the ApoE polymorphism to plasma lipid traits among South Asians, Chinese, and Europeans living in Canada. Atherosclerosis 2009;203(1):192–200.
46. Gronroos P, Raitakari OT, Kahonen M, et al. Association of high sensitive C-reactive protein with apolipoprotein E polymorphism in children and young adults: the Cardiovascular Risk in Young Finns Study. Clin Chem Lab Med 2008; 46(2):179–86.
47. Chmielewski M, Verduijn M, Dekker FW. ApoE genotype as risk factor in dialysis patients. Atherosclerosis 2010;212(2):695–6 [author reply: 697].
48. Clarke R, Peden JF, Hopewell JC, et al. Genetic variants associated with Lp(a) lipoprotein level and coronary disease. N Engl J Med 2009;361(26):2518–28.
49. Stein EA, Swergold GD. Potential of proprotein convertase subtilisin/kexin type 9 based therapeutics. Curr Atheroscler Rep 2013;15(3):310.
50. Stein EA, Mellis S, Yancopoulos GD, et al. Effect of a monoclonal antibody to PCSK9 on LDL cholesterol. N Engl J Med 2012;366(12):1108–18.

Lipoprotein(a)

An Important Cardiovascular Risk Factor and a Clinical Conundrum

Marlys L. Koschinsky, PhD*, Michael B. Boffa, PhD

KEYWORDS

- Lipoprotein(a) • Apolipoprotein(a) • Atherosclerosis • Thrombosis
- Oxidized phospholipids • Coronary heart disease • Genetics • Risk factors

KEY POINTS

- Concentrations of lipoprotein(a) (Lp[a]) are genetically determined predominantly at the level of *LPA*, the gene encoding apolipoprotein(a) (apo[a]); significant differences exist between ethnic groups in the genetic architecture of *LPA* and the distribution of Lp(a) concentrations.
- Although the role of the low-density lipoprotein (LDL) receptor in mediating clearance of Lp(a) from the circulation has been a point of controversy, it is becoming apparent that Lp(a) concentrations can be affected by therapies that influence this receptor, namely, statins and inhibitors of PCSK9.
- The true mechanism or mechanisms by which Lp(a) promotes coronary heart disease (CHD) remain elusive, although increasing evidence points to a key role for oxidized phospholipids that are possible covalently linked to apo(a).
- Although screening of the general population for elevated Lp(a) is not recommended, several types of patients could benefit from these measurements, possibly to target Lp(a) for lowering but more practically at this time to indicate those patients who would benefit most from rigorous attention to modifiable risk factors.
- A major unmet need in the field is a clinical trial in which the cardiovascular benefit of lowering plasma Lp(a) is assessed prospectively; such a trial would only be feasible with the advent of therapies to specifically lower Lp(a).

INTRODUCTION

A great deal of attention has recently focused on lipoprotein(a) (Lp[a]), an emerging risk factor for coronary heart disease (CHD) and possibly for other cardiovascular diseases. For decades, this lipoprotein particle has been an enigma: its true biological

This article originally appeared in Endocrinology and Metabolism Clinics, Volume 43, Issue 4, December 2014.

Department of Chemistry and Biochemistry, University of Windsor, 401 Sunset Avenue, Windsor, Ontario N9B 3P4, Canada

* Corresponding author. Office of the Dean, Faculty of Science, University of Windsor, Room 242 Essex Hall, 401 Sunset Avenue, Windsor, Ontario N9B 3P4, Canada.

E-mail address: mlk@uwindsor.ca

Clinics Collections 5 (2015) 63–76

http://dx.doi.org/10.1016/j.ccol.2015.05.005

function unknown; its status as a cardiovascular risk factor tenuous; and its clinical utility entirely unclear. Important advances have occurred over the last several years in the fields of genetics, epidemiology, biochemistry, and pharmacology to give new impetus to consider and manage Lp(a) in the clinical setting. After a brief introduction to Lp(a) structure and heterogeneity, this review focuses on the most recent findings in these spheres.

LIPOPROTEIN(a) STRUCTURE AND HETEROGENEITY

Lp(a) consists of a lipoprotein particle that is very similar to low-density lipoprotein (LDL), which is covalently linked to the unique glycoprotein apolipoprotein(a) (apo[a]) by a single disulfide bond (**Fig. 1**).[1,2] Apo(a) is homologous to the fibrinolytic proenzyme plasminogen.[3] Apo(a) lacks the amino-terminal tail region and first 3 kringle domains of plasminogen, but contains multiple copies of sequences homologous to plasminogen kringle IV (KIV) as well as a single copy of a kringle V–like domain and an inactive protease domain. Of the 10 different types of KIV-like sequences in apo(a), 9 are present in single copy in all isoforms, while one of them (KIV$_2$) is present in multiple repeats of between 3 and more than 30 copies.[4,5] This copy number variation is encoded at the level of the individual alleles of *LPA* (the gene encoding apo[a]) and accounts for the isoform size heterogeneity seen in the human population.[6]

Another level of significant heterogeneity in Lp(a) is in plasma levels of the lipoprotein. Plasma concentrations of Lp(a) are relatively stable within an individual, varying little in response to prandial status.[7] However, plasma concentrations of Lp(a) vary remarkably between individuals, with a range of greater than 1000-fold between the lowest and highest expressers.[8] Lp(a) concentrations are primarily genetically determined[8]: indeed, there is a general inverse correlation between apo(a) allele size and plasma Lp(a) levels[9] owing to the reduced secretion rate from hepatocytes of larger apo(a) isoforms.[10] Although the contributors to and magnitudes of genetic control of Lp(a) concentrations remain topics of debate, it is clear that the *LPA* gene itself is the major contributor to variation in plasma Lp(a) concentrations, with the size of the gene itself having the largest contribution.[9]

Compared with other lipoprotein classes, Lp(a) concentrations are relatively resistant to changes owing to dietary, exercise, or drug interventions.[11] However, evidence for lowering of plasma Lp(a) concentrations by several existing and investigational drugs has emerged, as in later discussion.

GENETICS OF *LPA*

Much of the recent interest in Lp(a) has emerged from genetic studies. Two landmark studies from 2009 showed that genetically elevated Lp(a) concentrations (from either small *LPA* allele sizes[12] or the presence of single nucleotide polymorphism (SNP) variants strongly associated with plasma concentrations[13]) are a risk factor for CHD. Indeed, the results of these studies indicate that elevated Lp(a) is causally related to the development of CHD.[12] Another recent study further reported that elevated Lp(a) is the strongest genetically determined risk factor for CHD.[14]

Significant questions remain as to the quantitative contribution of specific genetic variants to Lp(a) concentrations. Earlier data indicated that *LPA* genotype determined the vast majority (>90%) of variability in Lp(a) concentrations, with most of this, in turn, being accounted for by *LPA* allele size.[15] More recent estimates of the contribution of allele size or SNPs have furnished a much lower number (30%)[16]; it is possible that these later findings are, in part, a consequence of a real-time polymerase chain reaction (PCR)-based genotyping method that measures the total number of KIV$_2$

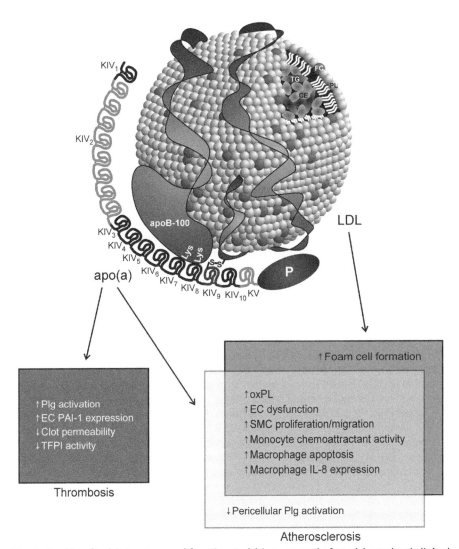

Fig. 1. Duality of Lp(a) structure and function. Lp(a) is composed of apo(a) covalently linked to the apoB-100 moiety of an LDL-like molecule. Apo(a) consists of multiple repeats of sequences related to plasminogen KIV and a single copy of kringle V (KV) and proteaselike (P) domains. The lipid content of the LDL-like moiety consists of a central core of triglycerides (TG) and cholesteryl esters (CE) surrounded by a shell of phospholipids (PL) and free cholesterol (FC). Lp(a) promotes both thrombosis and atherosclerosis: apo(a) promotes thrombosis because of its similarity to plasminogen (Plg), while LDL (and oxidized LDL) promotes atherosclerosis. Apo(a) also has several proatherosclerotic effects, shared with LDL/oxidized LDL, that are unrelated to it similarity to plasminogen. EC, endothelial cell; PAI-1, plasminogen activator inhibitor-1; SMC, smooth muscle cell; TFPI, tissue factor pathway inhibitor.

repeats in both alleles. Another complication of genetic studies is the differing genetic architecture of *LPA* in different ethnic groups, which likely underlies observed differences in the distribution of Lp(a) concentrations between different ethnic groups. In a multiethnic study, the same haplotype blocks were associated with Lp(a) concentrations in all 3 populations (South Asians, Chinese, and European Caucasians).[17]

However, the intronic variant (rs10455872) most strongly associated with allele size and Lp(a) concentrations in European Caucasians is not present in the other populations.[17] Another study in a Han Chinese population found that neither rs10455872 nor rs2798220 (encoding an Ile to Met substitution in the proteaselike domain and also strongly associated with elevated Lp[a] in Caucasians[18]) was associated with Lp(a) concentrations.[19]

It remains most likely that *LPA* allele size is the key driver of variation in plasma Lp(a) concentrations. Notably, there is no biochemical explanation for the association of any other polymorphism with Lp(a) concentrations, although this question has yet to be investigated directly. All *LPA* variants are in linkage disequilibrium with allele size, however.[17] Correlation of SNPs and haplotypes to allele size in a quantitative way will require allele-specific *LPA* genotyping for both SNPs and the length polymorphism.

LIPOPROTEIN(a) PRODUCTION AND METABOLISM

Variation in Lp(a) concentrations is primarily driven by differences in the rate of production, not catabolism,[20] which likely relates to the slower secretion of larger apo(a) isoforms.[10] It is notable, however, that very little is known about how Lp(a) is cleared from the circulation. Although the liver is the main organ responsible for Lp(a) catabolism,[21] the identity of the receptor or receptors that bind and internalize Lp(a) remains to be definitively established. In vitro studies point to a role for both the LDL receptor (LDLR) and the plasminogen receptors.[22] Studies conducted in mice or human subjects lacking the LDLR suggest against a major role for the LDLR in Lp(a) clearance, while still revealing a contribution of this receptor.[21,23] The effect of statins on Lp(a) concentrations has been controversial, again in keeping with the notion that LDLR levels are not a major driver of Lp(a) clearance. On the other hand, some studies in relatively large cohorts as well as a meta-analysis showed a measurable lowering effect of statins, albeit one that is dwarfed by the effect of these drugs on LDL-cholesterol (LDL-C).[24–26] Most recently, it has been demonstrated that inhibitory antibodies against proprotein convertase subtilisin/kexin type (PCSK9), a factor that diminishes LDLR numbers on the surface of hepatocytes, markedly decrease plasma Lp(a) concentrations.[27,28] Thus, it appears that the LDLR plays a role in Lp(a) catabolism that is most apparent when LDLR numbers are maximized while the concentration of LDL, a competitive ligand, is minimized.

A recent article has revealed a novel role for scavenger receptor-B1 (SR-B1) as an Lp(a) receptor.[29] SR-B1 mediates uptake of protein and, predominantly, neutral lipid from Lp(a). Knockout or overexpression of SR-B1 in mice clearly affects clearance of Lp(a), but the quantitative details clearly show that receptors other than SR-B1 play a role. The relative contribution of SR-B1 to Lp(a) catabolism remains to be clearly defined, and it will be interesting to determine if cholesteryl ester–depleted Lp(a) is targeted for preferential clearance and has any biological effects.

PATHOGENIC MECHANISMS OF LIPOPROTEIN(a)

The duality of Lp(a) structure that is readily apparent has given rise to the concept of a duality in the pathogenic effects of Lp(a), where the LDL-like moiety of Lp(a) serves to promote atherosclerosis, whereas the plasminogen-like apo(a) molecule promotes thrombosis by interfering with fibrinolysis (see **Fig. 1**). Although both of these effects have been documented for Lp(a),[30,31] extensive investigations have revealed many more facets than this simple model can account for. More specifically, several additional functions of apo(a) that do not necessarily arise from its similarity to plasminogen have emerged (see **Fig. 1**). These functions include initiation of signaling pathways in macrophages[32] and vascular endothelial cells,[33,34] resulting in proatherogenic changes in cell phenotype and gene expression.

Although a unifying mechanism underlying these unique proatherogenic effects of Lp(a) has yet to be conclusively demonstrated, a tantalizing possibility is that these effects may be attributable to modification of the particle by oxidized phospholipids (oxPL). In the EPIC-Norfolk study, oxidation modification of Lp(a) has been linked to CHD events and contributes additional predictive value to the suite of traditional CHD risk factors.[35] Moreover, the relationship of OxPL/apoB and Lp(a) to fatal and nonfatal CHD was accentuated in the highest tertiles of each, suggesting that they can provide independent information for risk prediction.[35]

Clinical studies have shown that Lp(a) is a preferential carrier of oxPL compared with LDL.[36] At least some of this is due to the ability of oxPL to become covalently linked to apo(a).[37] The oxPL, in turn, may act as ligands for cell-surface receptors, such as CD36, and Toll-like receptor 2 to initiate intracellular signaling cascades.[32] Interestingly, it has been reported recently that the addition of oxPL to apo(a) depends on an intact lysine-binding site in KIV_{10}.[38] Work in transgenic mice from almost 20 years ago showed that the lack of this site prevented the fatty-streak formation observed in mice overexpressing wild-type human apo(a).[39] More extensive structure-function studies will need to be undertaken to explore the importance of this lysine binding site and oxPL addition on the range of harmful effects of apo(a)/Lp(a).

Most recently, it has been reported that monocyte chemoattractant protein-1 (MCP-1), which is a proatherosclerotic molecule required for monocyte recruitment and migration across the vascular endothelium,[40] is carried by Lp(a) in human plasma.[41] In vitro, the binding interaction can be inhibited by E06, a monoclonal antibody against oxPL; this suggests that the oxPL modification of Lp(a) is essential for the binding of MCP-1. Overall, it is reasonable to speculate that the oxPL modification of Lp(a) contributes to its atherogenicity through the proinflammatory effects that are associated with oxPL; the association with Lp(a) allows these molecules to be targeted to the site of developing lesions.

ELEVATED PLASMA LIPOPROTEIN(a) CONCENTRATIONS AS A RISK FACTOR FOR VASCULAR DISEASE

It is well-established from retrospective case-control studies, prospective studies, and Mendelian randomization studies that elevated plasma Lp(a) is a risk factor for the development of CHD.[9] Most of the studies have focused on the influence of Lp(a) on a first occurrence of a coronary event. Some recent studies have sought to define whether elevated Lp(a) predicts the occurrence of events in patients with established disease. In a secondary prevention study that encompassed 18,979 subjects, Lp(a) in the highest quintile was associated with risk for subsequent events, although this relationship was lost for subjects with low LDL-C.[42] In the LIPID study, in which patients with a previous coronary event were randomized to statin or placebo, elevated Lp(a) (in the top quintile) was associated with risk for a variety of different cardiovascular endpoints.[43] In addition, in some patients, Lp(a) had increased after 1 year, and this was also associated with events.[43]

An important question is whether elevated Lp(a) remains a risk factor even in the face of aggressive lowering of LDL-C by statins. Analysis of data from the Justification for the Use of Statins in Prevention (JUPITER) trial did show a significant residual risk attributable to elevated Lp(a) in rosuvastatin-treated patients.[44] Thus, it appears reasonable at this time to consider the contribution of Lp(a) to a patient's risk even if the patient has existing disease and/or is receiving optimal lipid-lowering therapy.

Another longstanding question concerns whether small apo(a) isoforms are a risk factor independent of their association with elevated plasma concentrations of Lp(a). There are some biochemical data to suggest that small isoforms are more anti-fibrinolytic.[31] In the PROCARDIS study, adjustment for apo(a) isoform size did not alter the association of Lp(a) concentrations with CHD[13]; moreover, although small apo(a) isoforms were associated with increased risk, this association was abolished after adjustment for Lp(a) concentrations.

Two recent genetic studies have revealed that genetically elevated Lp(a) concentrations are associated with increased occurrence of aortic valve stenosis.[45,46] This disorder involves valvular calcification and is etiologically distinct from atherosclerosis, although it shares some common risk factors. Importantly, both studies demonstrated that elevated Lp(a) concentrations are in fact causal for aortic valve stenosis, as opposed to merely being a marker. The role of Lp(a) in the disease process is unknown, although Lp(a) appears to be deposited at sites of developing calcific valvular disease.

The ability of apo(a)/Lp(a) to inhibit fibrinolysis strongly suggests that elevated Lp(a) may pose a risk for pure thrombotic disorders such as venous thromboembolism. Although there have been discrepant results reported in the past, 3 recent, large, studies each also assessing *LPA* genotype at SNPs strongly associated with Lp(a) levels have concluded that no relationship between elevated Lp(a) and venous thromboembolism exists.[47–49] One study argued that this is evidence against a role for Lp(a) in the thrombotic complications of atherosclerosis.[47] There are, however, notable differences between the thrombi in arterial and venous compartments, with arterial thrombi being more platelet-rich, fibrin-poor, and initiated by the thrombogenic contents of the atherosclerotic core. Notably, a series of studies by Undas and coworkers[50] have shown that elevated Lp(a) is associated with reduced clot permeability and altered fibrin structure of plasma clots ex vivo.[51] In addition, Kardys and coworkers[52] found, in patients that had undergone percutaneous interventions, that elevated Lp(a) was associated with the incidence of major adverse coronary events within 1 year of the procedure, but not thereafter. One interpretation of these findings might be that they reflect the antifibrinolytic properties of Lp(a) because the early complications would be largely thrombotic in nature.

As surrogate markers of atherosclerosis become more specific and informative, the opportunity exists to more directly evaluate the role of Lp(a) in the atherosclerotic process itself. One such marker is coronary artery calcification (CAC), which is measured by computed tomography and is a sensitive indicator of preclinical atherosclerosis. The available data on the relationship between Lp(a) concentrations and CAC are conflicting. Studies have shown a positive correlation in large cohorts of European Caucasians or Asians,[53,54] although a smaller study found the Lp(a) was predictive of CAC only in Southeast Asians but not in European Caucasians.[55] Another study in a large cohort of European Caucasians found that although elevated Lp(a) correlated with increased CAC scores, Lp(a) was inferior to LDL-C or related measures,[56] the opposite of another study in a similar cohort.[53] Another study found that Lp(a) was only predictive of CAC in women with type 2 diabetes mellitus, but was not in women without diabetes or in men.[57] Clearly, additional studies are required to uncover the reasons for these discrepant findings and to determine the true relationship between elevated Lp(a) and subclinical atherosclerosis.

UTILITY OF LIPOPROTEIN(a) IN CLINICAL PRACTICE

Questions commonly posed by clinicians regarding the use of Lp(a) in clinical settings include the following: In which patients should Lp(a) levels be determined? How should Lp(a) concentrations be measured? What treatment strategy should be used for patients with elevated Lp(a) levels?

There is general agreement that measurement of Lp(a) in the general population is unnecessary.[58] However, there are specific clinical circumstances under which Lp(a) levels should be determined. These clinical circumstances are summarized in **Box 1**. Based on the current level of understanding, there is no additional benefit to the measurement of Lp(a) isoform size; this reflects the lack of evidence to suggest a role for apo(a) isoform size in CHD that is independent of the inverse relationship with Lp(a) levels.[59]

Because Lp(a) levels are genetically determined, it is suggested that a single measurement should be sufficient unless strategies are used that lower Lp(a) levels; in the latter case, response to treatment can be monitored through repeated measurement. An Lp(a) level above the 75th percentile has been taken as a decision point[58]; in Caucasian populations this corresponds to approximately 30 mg/dL. It is important to note that 30 mg/dL has been used in numerous epidemiologic studies to define elevated Lp(a) levels and is the most commonly used value used in clinical practice.[60] However, it must be recognized that this decision point might be expected to vary in different ethnic groups: in the Black population, for example, 30 mg/dL corresponds roughly to the 50th percentile,[58] although this cut-point still predicts risk for CHD in this population.[61] The Copenhagen Heart Study data reported greatly increased risk conferred by extreme Lp(a) concentrations greater than the 80th percentile of the study population (>approximately 50 mg/dL).[62] It has been suggested Lp(a) levels in excess of this value should be used to reclassify individuals into a higher risk category. This reclassification would include more aggressive LDL-lowering in this group, as well as the inclusion of niacin treatment as recommended by the European Atherosclerosis Society guidelines[63]; note that these recommendations are not universally accepted.[64]

As such, there is arguably no clearly defined cutoff point for the assessment of Lp(a) in CHD risk. The lack of this cutoff coupled with the lack of common reference materials for Lp(a) measurement and reporting of Lp(a) concentrations in different units, makes interlaboratory comparisons difficult. Although it is preferable to report Lp(a) measurements in molar concentrations (nmol/L) versus mass concentrations (mg/dL), many commercially available assays provide values in mass concentrations. A conversion factor of 3.17 (ie, 1 mg/mL of Lp[a] corresponds approximately to 3.17 nmol/L) has been suggested by the Lp(a) standardization group,[65] although a value of 2.4 has also been suggested[58]; using this latter value, 30 mg/dL converts to 72 nmol/L, which is a close approximation of the 75th percentile in Caucasian populations.[66] The ideal conversion factor will, of course, vary depending on the apo(a) isoform size present in the subject, so the suggested conversion factors are

---

Box 1
Patients in whom measurement of plasma lipoprotein(a) concentrations should be considered

- Patients with premature CHD in the absence of other risk factors

- Patients with a strong family history of premature CHD

- Patients who exhibit resistance to LDL lowering by statins

- Patients with recurrent restenosis or rapid disease progression with other risk factors controlled

- Patients with intermediate risk profiles[a]

[a] For example, 10-year Framingham risk score of 5%–19% or a CHD risk equivalent,[70] Lp(a) levels greater than 50 mg/dL would warrant reclassification into a higher risk category.[70]

necessarily average values. Another assay, the Vertical Auto Profile reports an Lp(a)-cholesterol value whereby 10 mg/dL (approximately the 75th percentile[67]) is the upper limit of normal.[68] Discrepant results have been reported for the relationship between Lp(a)-cholesterol and risk for cardiovascular disease,[67,69] and it has been suggested that measures of Lp(a)-cholesterol and Lp(a) particle concentration may be complementary.[68]

Based on the foregoing discussion, the authors' recommendations for Lp(a) concentrations above which intervention should be considered are as follows: 30 mg/dL (mass concentration); 75 nmol/L (particle concentration); and 10 mg/dL (Lp[a]-cholesterol).

Although there is no pharmacotherapy approved for use that specifically lowers Lp(a), in the subset of patients identified in **Box 1**, there remains a focus on aggressively reducing modifiable risk factors including elevated LDL-C; this would include the institution of statin therapy either alone or in combination with ezetimibe and/or bile acid sequestrants to achieve LDL-C levels less than 70 mg/dL, or a minimum of 50% reduction in LDL.[70] This recommendation is based on a study of 2769

Table 1
Current and future therapies to lower plasma lipoprotein(a) concentrations

Agent	Status[a]	Mechanism of Action	% ↓ in Lp(a)	Specific for Lp(a)?[b]
Niacin	Approved	Unknown (transcription of *LPA*?)	25	N
Simvastatin	Approved	↑ LDLR	19	N
Atorvastatin	Approved	↑ LDLR	22	N
Mipomersin	Approved (only for homozygous familial hypercholesterolemia)	↓ Translation of apoB mRNA	21–39	N
ASO 144367	Preclinical	↓ Translation of apo(a) mRNA	25 (in Lp[a] Tg mice)	Y
Anacetrapib	Phase III	Unknown	36	N
AMG145	Phase III	Unknown (↑ LDLR?)	30	N
REGN727/ SAR236553	Phase III	Unknown (↑ LDLR?)	30	N
Lomitapibe (AEGR-733)	Phase III	↓ Secretion of apoB-containing lipoproteins	16–19	N
Acetylsalicylic acid	Approved	↓ Transcription of apo(a) mRNA	20	Y
Lipoprotein-apheresis	Approved	Direct removal from plasma	69–73	N
Lp(a)-apheresis	Not available	Direct removal from plasma	73	Y
Tocilizumab	Approved	IL-6 receptor blockade, hence ↓ transcription of apo(a) mRNA	30	Y

[a] Refers to United States; note that no approval has been granted for the indication of elevated Lp(a), specifically.
[b] Refers to lipid profile.
Data from Refs.[25,27,28,42,73–93]

angiography patients wherein risk for major adverse coronary events attributable to Lp(a) was absent in patients with LDL-C less than 70 mg/dL.[71] Another study, in the setting of secondary prevention, found no significant contribution of Lp(a) to risk at LDL-C less than 120 mg/dL.[42] On the other hand, the large JUPITER trial found that a residual risk associated with elevated Lp(a) may persist in the background of low LDL levels resulting from aggressive statin therapy.[44]

It must be emphasized that there have been no randomized clinical trials to date that have specifically addressed the question of whether monitoring Lp(a) concentrations or lowering Lp(a) therapeutically has a clinical benefit. Nonetheless, it seems prudent, given the existing evidence for Lp(a) as a causal risk factor, to measure Lp(a) in specific groups of patients and to tailor their clinical management accordingly.

Some clinicians choose to treat patients with elevated Lp(a) levels using niacin (2 g/d); this may be useful in patients with elevated Lp(a) levels whose LDL concentrations cannot be aggressively lowered or in individuals with Lp(a) levels in excess of 50 mg/dL.[63] However, recent data from the AIM-HIGH trial indicate that niacin treatment did not significantly lower risk for cardiovascular events, despite being able to lower plasma Lp(a) concentrations.[72] Others may choose to include aspirin therapy given that aspirin has been shown to reduce Lp(a) levels and also may mitigate the potential prothrombotic role of Lp(a) in advanced lesions.[73] The latter approach may be of value in patients with existing prothrombotic disorders.[70] In addition to statins, niacin, and aspirin, several drugs in clinical trials or preclinical development have been shown to lower plasma Lp(a) concentrations (**Table 1**).Moreover, LDL-apheresis has been shown to reduce the risk of events attributable to Lp(a)[74,75] and specific Lp(a)-apheresis has been reported to reduce angiographically detectable CHD.[76] Therefore, the coming years may bring novel therapeutic approaches for the patient with elevated plasma Lp(a).

REFERENCES

1. Fless GM, ZumMallen ME, Scanu AM. Physicochemical properties of apolipoprotein(a) and lipoprotein(a−) derived from the dissociation of human plasma lipoprotein (a). J Biol Chem 1986;261:8712–8.
2. Koschinsky ML, Côté GP, Gabel BR, et al. Identification of the cysteine residue in apolipoprotein(a) that mediates extracellular coupling with apolipoprotein B-100. J Biol Chem 1993;268:19819–25.
3. McLean JW, Tomlinson JE, Kuang WJ, et al. cDNA sequence of human apolipoprotein(a) is homologous to plasminogen. Nature 1987;330:132–7.
4. van der Hoek YY, Wittekoek ME, Beisiegel U, et al. The apolipoprotein(a) kringle IV repeats which differ from the major repeat kringle are present in variably-sized isoforms. Hum Mol Genet 1993;2:361–6.
5. Marcovina SM, Albers JJ, Wijsman E, et al. Differences in Lp[a] concentrations and apo[a] polymorphs between black and white Americans. J Lipid Res 1996; 37:2569–85.
6. Lackner C, Cohen JC, Hobbs HH. Molecular definition of the extreme size polymorphism in apolipoprotein(a). Hum Mol Genet 1993;2:933–40.
7. Marcovina SM, Gaur VP, Albers JJ. Biological variability of cholesterol, triglyceride, low- and high-density lipoprotein cholesterol, lipoprotein(a), and apolipoproteins A-I and B. Clin Chem 1994;40:574–8.
8. Utermann G. Genetic architecture and evolution of the lipoprotein(a) trait. Curr Opin Lipidol 1999;10:133–41.

9. Kronenberg F, Utermann G. Lipoprotein(a): resurrected by genetics. J Intern Med 2013;273:6–30.

10. White AL, Guerra B, Lanford RE. Influence of allelic variation on apolipoprotein(a) folding in the endoplasmic reticulum. J Biol Chem 1997;272:5048–55.

11. Brewer HB Jr. Effectiveness of diet and drugs in the treatment of patients with elevated Lp(a) levels. In: Scanu AM, editor. Lipoprotein(a). New York: NY Academic Press, Inc; 1990. p. 211–20.

12. Kamstrup PR, Tybjaerg-Hansen A, Steffensen R, et al. Genetically elevated lipoprotein(a) and increased risk of myocardial infarction. JAMA 2009;301:2331–9.

13. Clarke R, Peden JF, Hopewell JC, et al. Genetic variants associated with Lp(a) lipoprotein level and coronary disease. N Engl J Med 2009;361:2518–28.

14. IBC 50K CAD Consortium. Large-scale gene-centric analysis identifies novel variants for coronary artery disease. PLoS Genet 2011;7:e1002260.

15. Boerwinkle E, Leffert CC, Lin J, et al. Apolipoprotein(a) gene accounts for greater than 90% of the variation in plasma lipoprotein(a) concentrations. J Clin Invest 1992;90:52–60.

16. Dubé JB, Boffa MB, Hegele RA, et al. Lipoprotein(a): more interesting than ever after 50 years. Curr Opin Lipidol 2012;23:133–40.

17. Lanktree MB, Anand SS, Yusuf S, et al. Comprehensive analysis of genomic variation in the LPA locus and its relationship to plasma lipoprotein(a) in South Asians, Chinese, and European Caucasians. Circ Cardiovasc Genet 2010;3:39–46.

18. Luke MM, Kane JP, Liu DM, et al. A polymorphism in the protease-like domain of apolipoprotein(a) is associated with severe coronary artery disease. Arterioscler Thromb Vasc Biol 2007;27:2030–6.

19. Li ZG, Li G, Zhou YL, et al. Lack of association between lipoprotein(a) genetic variants and subsequent cardiovascular events in Chinese Han patients with coronary artery disease after percutaneous coronary intervention. Lipids Health Dis 2013;12:127.

20. Rader DJ, Cain W, Ikewaki K, et al. The inverse association of plasma lipoprotein(a) concentrations with apolipoprotein(a) isoform size is not due to differences in Lp(a) catabolism but to differences in production rate. J Clin Invest 1994;93:2758–63.

21. Cain WJ, Millar JS, Himebauch AS, et al. Lipoprotein [a] is cleared from the plasma primarily by the liver in a process mediated by apolipoprotein [a]. J Lipid Res 2005;46:2681–91.

22. Tam SP, Zhang X, Koschinsky ML. Interaction of a recombinant form of apolipoprotein[a] with human fibroblasts and with the human hepatoma cell line HepG2. J Lipid Res 1996;37:518–33.

23. Rader DJ, Mann WA, Cain W, et al. The low density lipoprotein receptor is not required for normal catabolism of Lp(a) in humans. J Clin Invest 1995;95:1403–8.

24. Gonbert S, Malinsky S, Sposito AC, et al. Atorvastatin lowers lipoprotein(a) but not apolipoprotein(a) fragment levels in hypercholesterolemic subjects at high cardiovascular risk. Atherosclerosis 2002;164:305–11.

25. van Wissen S, Smilde TJ, Trip MD, et al. Long term statin treatment reduces lipoprotein(a) concentrations in heterozygous familial hypercholesterolaemia. Heart 2003;89:893–6.

26. Takagi H, Umemoto T. Atorvastatin decreases lipoprotein(a): a meta-analysis of randomized trials. Int J Cardiol 2012;154:183–6.

27. Desai NR, Kohli P, Giugliano RP, et al. AMG145, a monoclonal antibody against proprotein convertase subtilisin kexin type 9, significantly reduces lipoprotein(a)

in hypercholesterolemic patients receiving statin therapy: an analysis from the LDL-C assessment with proprotein convertase subtilisin kexin type 9 monoclonal antibody inhibition combined with statin therapy (LAPLACE)-thrombolysis in myocardial infarction (TIMI) 57 trial. Circulation 2013;128:962–9.

28. McKenney JM, Koren MJ, Kereiakes DJ, et al. Safety and efficacy of a monoclonal antibody to proprotein convertase subtilisin/kexin type 9 serine protease, SAR236553/REGN727, in patients with primary hypercholesterolemia receiving ongoing stable atorvastatin therapy. J Am Coll Cardiol 2012;59:2344–53.

29. Yang XP, Amar MJ, Vaisman B, et al. Scavenger receptor-BI is a receptor for lipoprotein(a). J Lipid Res 2013;54:2450–7.

30. Boffa MB, Koschinsky ML. Update on lipoprotein(a) as a cardiovascular risk factor and mediator. Curr Atheroscler Rep 2013;15:360.

31. Anglés-Cano E, de la Peña Díaz A, Loyau S. Inhibition of fibrinolysis by lipoprotein(a). Ann N Y Acad Sci 2001;936:261–75.

32. Seimon TA, Nadolski MJ, Liao X, et al. Atherogenic lipids and lipoproteins trigger CD36-TLR2-dependent apoptosis in macrophages undergoing endoplasmic reticulum stress. Cell Metab 2010;12:467–82.

33. Cho T, Jung Y, Koschinsky ML. Apolipoprotein(a), through its strong lysine-binding site in KIV(10'), mediates increased endothelial cell contraction and permeability via a Rho/Rho kinase/MYPT1-dependent pathway. J Biol Chem 2008;283:30503–12.

34. Cho T, Romagnuolo R, Scipione C, et al. Apolipoprotein(a) stimulates nuclear translocation of β-catenin: a novel pathogenic mechanism for lipoprotein(a). Mol Biol Cell 2013;24:210–21.

35. Tsimikas S, Mallat Z, Talmud PJ, et al. Oxidation-specific biomarkers, lipoprotein(a), and risk of fatal and nonfatal coronary events. J Am Coll Cardiol 2010; 56:946–55.

36. Tsimikas S, Bergmark C, Beyer RW, et al. Temporal increases in plasma markers of oxidized low-density lipoprotein strongly reflect the presence of acute coronary syndromes. J Am Coll Cardiol 2003;41:360–70.

37. Bergmark C, Dewan A, Orsoni A, et al. A novel function of lipoprotein [a] as a preferential carrier of oxidized phospholipids in human plasma. J Lipid Res 2008;49:2230–9.

38. Leibundgut G, Scipione C, Yin H, et al. Determinants of binding of oxidized phospholipids on apolipoprotein (a) and lipoprotein (a). J Lipid Res 2013;54: 2815–30.

39. Hughes SD, Lou XJ, Ighani S, et al. Lipoprotein(a) vascular accumulation in mice. In vivo analysis of the role of lysine binding sites using recombinant adenovirus. J Clin Invest 1997;100:1493–500.

40. Deshmane SL, Kremlev S, Amini S, et al. Monocyte chemoattractant protein-1 (MCP-1): an overview. J Interferon Cytokine Res 2009;29:313–26.

41. Wiesner P, Tafelmeier M, Chittka D, et al. MCP-1 binds to oxidized LDL and is carried by lipoprotein(a) in human plasma. J Lipid Res 2013;54:1877–83.

42. O'Donoghue ML, Morrow DA, Tsimikas S, et al. Lipoprotein(a) for risk assessment in patients with established coronary artery disease. J Am Coll Cardiol 2014;63:520–7.

43. Nestel PJ, Barnes EH, Tonkin AM, et al. Plasma lipoprotein(a) concentration predicts future coronary and cardiovascular events in patients with stable coronary heart disease. Arterioscler Thromb Vasc Biol 2013;33:2902–8.

44. Khera AV, Everett BM, Caulfield MP, et al. Lipoprotein(a) concentrations, rosuvastatin therapy, and residual vascular risk: an analysis from the JUPITER trial

(justification for the use of statins in prevention: an intervention trial evaluating rosuvastatin). Circulation 2014;129:635–42.

45. Thanassoulis G, Campbell CY, Owens DS, et al. Genetic associations with valvular calcification and aortic stenosis. N Engl J Med 2013;368:503–12.

46. Kamstrup PR, Tybjærg-Hansen A, Nordestgaard BG. Elevated lipoprotein(a) and risk of aortic valve stenosis in the general population. J Am Coll Cardiol 2014;63:470–7.

47. Kamstrup PR, Tybjærg-Hansen A, Nordestgaard BG. Genetic evidence that lipoprotein(a) associates with atherosclerotic stenosis rather than venous thrombosis. Arterioscler Thromb Vasc Biol 2012;32:1732–41.

48. Danik JS, Buring JE, Chasman DI, et al. Lipoprotein(a), polymorphisms in the LPA gene, and incident venous thromboembolism among 21483 women. J Thromb Haemost 2013;11:205–8.

49. Helgadottir A, Gretarsdottir S, Thorleifsson G, et al. Apolipoprotein(a) genetic sequence variants associated with systemic atherosclerosis and coronary atherosclerotic burden but not with venous thromboembolism. J Am Coll Cardiol 2012;60:722–9.

50. Undas A, Cieśla-Dul M, Drążkiewicz T, et al. Altered fibrin clot properties are associated with residual vein obstruction: effects of lipoprotein(a) and apolipoprotein(a) isoform. Thromb Res 2012;130:e184–7.

51. Rowland CM, Pullinger CR, Luke MM, et al. Lipoprotein (a), LPA Ile4399Met, and fibrin clot properties. Thromb Res 2014;133:863–7.

52. Kardys I, Oemrawsingh RM, Kay IP, et al. Lipoprotein(a), interleukin-10, C-reactive protein, and 8-year outcome after percutaneous coronary intervention. Clin Cardiol 2012;35:482–9.

53. Greif M, Arnoldt T, von Ziegler F, et al. Lipoprotein (a) is independently correlated with coronary artery calcification. Eur J Intern Med 2013;24:75–9.

54. Sung KC, Wild SH, Byrne CD. Lipoprotein (a), metabolic syndrome and coronary calcium score in a large occupational cohort. Nutr Metab Cardiovasc Dis 2013;23:1239–46.

55. Sharma A, Kasim M, Joshi PH, et al. Abnormal lipoprotein(a) levels predict coronary artery calcification in Southeast Asians but not in Caucasians: use of noninvasive imaging for evaluation of an emerging risk factor. J Cardiovasc Transl Res 2011;4:470–6.

56. Erbel R, Lehmann N, Churzidse S, et al. Gender-specific association of coronary artery calcium and lipoprotein parameters: the Heinz Nixdorf recall study. Atherosclerosis 2013;229:531–40.

57. Qasim AN, Martin SS, Mehta NN, et al. Lipoprotein(a) is strongly associated with coronary artery calcification in type-2 diabetic women. Int J Cardiol 2011;150:17–21.

58. Brown WV, Ballantyne CM, Jones PH, et al. Management of Lp(a). J Clin Lipidol 2010;4:240–7.

59. Hopewell JC, Seedorf U, Farrall M, et al. Impact of lipoprotein(a) levels and apolipoprotein(a) isoform size on risk of coronary heart disease. J Intern Med 2013;276(3):260–8. http://dx.doi.org/10.1111/joim.12187.

60. Anderson TJ, Grégoire J, Hegele RA, et al. 2012 update of the Canadian Cardiovascular Society guidelines for the diagnosis and treatment of dyslipidemia for the prevention of cardiovascular disease in the adult. Can J Cardiol 2013;29:151–67.

61. Virani SS, Brautbar A, Davis BC, et al. Associations between lipoprotein(a) levels and cardiovascular outcomes in black and white subjects: the atherosclerosis risk in communities (ARIC) study. Circulation 2012;125:241–9.

62. Kamstrup PR, Tybjærg-Hansen A, Nordestgaard BG. Extreme lipoprotein(a) levels and improved cardiovascular risk prediction. J Am Coll Cardiol 2013; 61:1146–56.
63. Nordestgaard BG, Chapman MJ, Ray K, et al. Lipoprotein(a) as a cardiovascular risk factor: current status. Eur Heart J 2010;31:2844–53.
64. Greenland P, Alpert JS, Beller GA, et al. American College of Cardiology Foundation; American Heart Association. 2010 ACCF/AHA guideline for assessment of cardiovascular risk in asymptomatic adults. J Am Coll Cardiol 2010;56:e50–103.
65. Kostner KM, März W, Kostner GM. When should we measure lipoprotein (a)? Eur Heart J 2013;34:3268–76.
66. Marcovina SM, Koschinsky ML, Albers JJ, et al. Report of the National Heart, Lung, and Blood Institute workshop on lipoprotein(a) and cardiovascular disease: recent advances and future directions. Clin Chem 2003;49:1785–96.
67. Seman LJ, DeLuca C, Jenner JL, et al. Lipoprotein(a)-cholesterol and coronary heart disease in the Framingham heart study. Clin Chem 1999;45:1039–46.
68. Konerman M, Kulkarni K, Toth PP, et al. Lipoprotein(a) particle concentration and lipoprotein(a) cholesterol assays yield discordant classification of patients into four physiologically discrete groups. J Clin Lipidol 2012;6:368–73.
69. Lamon-Fava S, Marcovina SM, Albers JJ, et al. Lipoprotein(a) levels, apo(a) isoform size, and coronary heart disease risk in the Framingham Offspring Study. J Lipid Res 2011;52:1181–7.
70. Jacobson TA. Lipoprotein(a), cardiovascular disease, and contemporary management. Mayo Clin Proc 2013;88:1294–311.
71. Nicholls SJ, Tang WH, Scoffone H, et al. Lipoprotein(a) levels and long-term cardiovascular risk in the contemporary era of statin therapy. J Lipid Res 2010;51: 3055–61.
72. Albers JJ, Slee A, O'Brien KD, et al. Relationship of apolipoproteins A-1 and B, and lipoprotein(a) to cardiovascular outcomes: the AIM-HIGH trial (atherothrombosis intervention in metabolic syndrome with low HDL/high triglyceride and impact on global health outcomes). J Am Coll Cardiol 2013;62:1575–9.
73. Chasman DI, Shiffman D, Zee RY, et al. Polymorphism in the apolipoprotein(a) gene, plasma lipoprotein(a), cardiovascular disease, and low-dose aspirin therapy. Atherosclerosis 2009;203:371–6.
74. Jaeger BR, Richter Y, Nagel D, et al. Longitudinal cohort study on the effectiveness of lipid apheresis treatment to reduce high lipoprotein(a) levels and prevent major adverse coronary events. Nat Clin Pract Cardiovasc Med 2009;6: 229–39.
75. Leebmann J, Roeseler E, Julius U, et al. Lipoprotein apheresis in patients with maximally tolerated lipid-lowering therapy, lipoprotein(a)-hyperlipoproteinemia, and progressive cardiovascular disease: prospective observational multicenter study. Circulation 2013;128:2567–76.
76. Safarova MS, Ezhov MV, Afanasieva OI, et al. Effect of specific lipoprotein(a) apheresis on coronary atherosclerosis regression assessed by quantitative coronary angiography. Atheroscler Suppl 2013;14:93–9.
77. Boden WE, Probstfield JL, Anderson T, et al. Niacin in patients with low HDL cholesterol levels receiving intensive statin therapy. N Engl J Med 2011;365: 2255–67.
78. Besseling J, Hovingh GK, Stroes ES. Antisense oligonucleotides in the treatment of lipid disorders: pitfalls and promises. Neth J Med 2013;71:118–22.
79. Raal FJ, Santos RD, Blom DJ, et al. Mipomersen, an apolipoprotein B synthesis inhibitor, for lowering of LDL cholesterol concentrations in patients with

homozygous familial hypercholesterolaemia: a randomised, double-blind, placebo-controlled trial. Lancet 2010;375:998–1006.

80. Stein EA, Dufour R, Gagne C, et al. Apolipoprotein B synthesis inhibition with mipomersen in heterozygous familial hypercholesterolemia: results of a randomized, double-blind, placebo-controlled trial to assess efficacy and safety as add-on therapy in patients with coronary artery disease. Circulation 2012;126: 2283–92.

81. McGowan MP, Tardif JC, Ceska R, et al. Randomized, placebo-controlled trial of mipomersen in patients with severe hypercholesterolemia receiving maximally tolerated lipid-lowering therapy. PLoS One 2012;7:e49006.

82. Thomas GS, Cromwell WC, Ali S, et al. Mipomersen, an apolipoprotein B synthesis inhibitor, reduces atherogenic lipoproteins in patients with severe hypercholesterolemia at high cardiovascular risk: a randomized, double-blind, placebo-controlled trial. J Am Coll Cardiol 2013;62:2178–84.

83. Visser ME, Wagener G, Baker BF, et al. Mipomersen, an apolipoprotein B synthesis inhibitor, lowers low-density lipoprotein cholesterol in high-risk statin-intolerant patients: a randomized, double-blind, placebo-controlled trial. Eur Heart J 2012;33:1142–9.

84. Merki E, Graham M, Taleb A, et al. Antisense oligonucleotide lowers plasma levels of apolipoprotein (a) and lipoprotein (a) in transgenic mice. J Am Coll Cardiol 2011;57:1611–21.

85. Cannon CP, Shah S, Dansky HM, et al. Safety of anacetrapib in patients with or at high risk for coronary heart disease. N Engl J Med 2010;363:2406–15.

86. Dias CS, Shaywitz AJ, Wasserman SM, et al. Effects of AMG 145 on low-density lipoprotein cholesterol levels: results from 2 randomized, double-blind, placebo-controlled, ascending-dose phase 1 studies in healthy volunteers and hypercholesterolemic subjects on statins. J Am Coll Cardiol 2012;60:1888–98.

87. Raal F, Scott R, Somaratne R, et al. Low-density lipoprotein cholesterol-lowering effects of AMG 145, a monoclonal antibody to proprotein convertase subtilisin/kexin type 9 serine protease in patients with heterozygous familial hypercholesterolemia: the reduction of LDL-C with PCSK9 Inhibition in heterozygous familial hypercholesterolemia disorder (RUTHERFORD) randomized trial. Circulation 2012;126:2408–17.

88. Sullivan D, Olsson AG, Scott R, et al. Effect of a monoclonal antibody to PCSK9 on low-density lipoprotein cholesterol levels in statin-intolerant patients: the GAUSS randomized trial. JAMA 2012;308:2497–506.

89. Roth EM, McKenney JM, Hanotin C, et al. Atorvastatin with or without an antibody to PCSK9 in primary hypercholesterolemia. N Engl J Med 2012;367: 1891–900.

90. Cuchel M, Bloedon LT, Szapary PO, et al. Inhibition of microsomal triglyceride transfer protein in familial hypercholesterolemia. N Engl J Med 2007;356:148–56.

91. Cuchel M, Meagher EA, du Toit Theron H, et al. Efficacy and safety of a microsomal triglyceride transfer protein inhibitor in patients with homozygous familial hypercholesterolaemia: a single-arm, open-label, phase 3 study. Lancet 2013; 381:40–6.

92. Samaha FF, McKenney J, Bloedon LT, et al. Inhibition of microsomal triglyceride transfer protein alone or with ezetimibe in patients with moderate hypercholesterolemia. Nat Clin Pract Cardiovasc Med 2008;5:497–505.

93. Schultz O, Oberhauser F, Saech J, et al. Effects of inhibition of interleukin-6 signalling on insulin sensitivity and lipoprotein (a) levels in human subjects with rheumatoid diseases. PLoS One 2010;5:e14328.

Genetic Testing in Hyperlipidemia

Ozlem Bilen, MD[a,1], Yashashwi Pokharel, MD, MSCR[b,c,1],
Christie M. Ballantyne, MD[c,d,e],*

KEYWORDS

- Dyslipidemia • Hereditary lipid disorder • Familial hypercholesterolemia
- Genetic testing

KEY POINTS

- Cascade screening of family members with lipid profile should be widely implemented for identification of familial hypercholesterolemia (FH) cases.
- Using cholesterol levels and other clinical information for FH diagnosis and screening can be specific but less sensitive.
- Some existing FH diagnostic criteria already incorporate genetic information for FH diagnosis. Identification of specific mutation or mutations in the affected individual with a focused screening of the mutation in family members can be quick and less expensive.
- Employment and insurance implications of genetic screening are important.
- Randomized clinical trials and cost-effectiveness analyses comparing the incremental benefit of genetic testing with clinical criteria are needed.

This article originally appeared in Cardiology Clinics, Volume 33, Issue 2, May 2015.
Disclosures: O. Bilen: Nothing to disclose. Y. Pokharel: Supported by American Heart Association SWA Summer 2014 Postdoctoral Fellowship Award. C.M. Ballantyne: Grant/Research support (All paid to institution, not individual): Abbott Diagnostic, Amarin, Amgen, Eli Lilly, Esperion, GlaxoSmithKline, Merck, Novartis, Pfizer, Regeneron, Roche Diagnostic, Sanofi-Synthelabo, National Institutes of Health, American Heart Association. Consultant: Abbott Diagnostics, Amarin, Amgen, Astra Zeneca, Cerenis, Esperion, Genentech, Genzyme, Kowa, Merck, Novartis, Pfizer, Regeneron, Sanofi-Synthelabo. Advisory panel: Merck, Pfizer.
[a] Department of Medicine, Baylor College of Medicine, 3131 Fannin Street, Houston, TX 77030, USA; [b] Section of Cardiovascular Research, Department of Medicine, Baylor College of Medicine, 6565 Fannin Street, Suite B157, Houston, TX 77030, USA; [c] Center for Cardiovascular Disease Prevention, Methodist DeBakey Heart and Vascular Center, 6565 Fannin Street, M.S. A-601, Houston, TX 77030, USA; [d] Section of Cardiovascular Research, Department of Medicine, Baylor College of Medicine, 6565 Fannin Street, M.S. A-601, Suite 656, Houston, TX 77030, USA; [e] Section of Cardiology, Department of Medicine, Baylor College of Medicine, 6565 Fannin Street, M.S. A-601, Suite 656, Houston, TX 77030, USA
[1] Both authors contributed equally.
* Corresponding author. 6565 Fannin Street, M.S. A-601, Suite 656, Houston, TX 77030.
E-mail address: cmb@bcm.edu

INTRODUCTION

Levels of certain plasma lipids and lipoproteins, such as low-density lipoprotein (LDL) cholesterol (LDL-C) and lipoprotein(a) (Lp[a]), are key risk factors for cardiovascular disease (CVD).[1,2] Although plasma lipids are determined largely by environmental and genetic factors, for some individuals levels are primarily determined by genotype. The Fredrickson classification of lipid disorders was based on common phenotypes (ie, abnormal lipid and lipoprotein subclasses) (**Table 1**).[3] Some of these phenotypes are frequently due to monogenic defects that directly affect lipoproteins and their function, and others are associated with polygenic abnormalities with multiple genetic variations.[3]

Familial hypercholesterolemia (FH), which most commonly has a Fredrickson IIa phenotype, is the most common hereditary lipid disorder, resulting in elevated blood cholesterol levels and premature atherosclerotic disease. FH has an autosomal-dominant inheritance with rare autosomal-recessive forms also described.[4] The most common cause of FH is mutation in the LDL receptor (LDL-R), with greater than 1600 different genetic mutations associated with FH.[5] Other causes include defects in apolipoprotein B (apoB), gain-of-function mutations in proprotein convertase subtilisin/kexin 9 (PCSK9), and other rare genetic abnormalities resulting in the FH phenotype.[6–8] FH can be heterozygous (HeFH), affecting only one allele; homozygous (HoFH), affecting 2 identical alleles; or compound heterozygous, affecting 2 different alleles. HeFH is among the most common metabolic disorders, affecting 1 in 300 to 1 in 500 individuals.[9] In founder populations such as French Canadians, Dutch, and Lebanese, HeFH is even more prevalent (1 in 50 to 1 in 100 individuals).[10–12] FH has a gene-dose effect such that in patients with HoFH, LDL-C level often exceeds 500 mg/dL. Patients with HeFH typically have LDL-C levels greater than 160 mg/dL as children and greater than 190 mg/dL as adults.[13] In addition to lifestyle changes, high-intensity statins are the pharmacotherapy of first choice, and if adequate response is not obtained, other lipid-lowering medications and LDL apheresis are available. In general, response to cholesterol-lowering medications that lead to increased LDL-R activity is determined by the degree of LDL-R function.[14]

In patients with HeFH, the risk of premature coronary heart disease increases by about 20-fold compared with individuals without FH.[15] Very often, a myocardial infarction is the first presenting sign in FH patients.[16] Approximately 20% of myocardial infarctions before the age of 45 years and 5% before the age of 60 years can be attributed to FH.[14] It is estimated that the risk of having CVD before age 50 is about 50% in men and 30% in women with FH. Despite the risk burden, most individuals with FH remain undiagnosed and either untreated or inadequately treated.[9,17] Furthermore, it has been shown that after FH patients attain optimal LDL-C levels by using lifestyle and pharmacologic therapies (such as high-intensity statins), the risk for ischemic events is reduced to that in non-FH populations.[18,19] Therefore, an improved screening and diagnostic tool for FH would be of immense public health value.

Lp(a) is another atherogenic lipoprotein, and higher levels increase the risk for ischemic cardiovascular events independent of other risk factors, including LDL-C.[20] Elevated Lp(a) is also one of the most commonly inherited dyslipidemias and is primarily genetically determined, but unfortunately, no approved therapies that lower Lp(a) also lower ischemic vascular events.[21] Currently, there is no clear role of genetic testing in routine practice in the management of individuals with elevated levels of Lp(a).

In this article genetic testing in the management of lipid disorders is reviewed, with a focus on FH.

Table 1
Genetics underlying Fredrickson phenotypes

ICD 10 Codes	Fredrickson Phenotype	↑ Lipid(s)	↑ Lipoprotein(s)	Genetic Mutations
E78.3 Hyperchylomicronemia	I	TG	CM	Monogenic; autosomal recessive: *LPL, APOC2*; other forms: *APOA5, LMF1, ?GPIHBP1*
E78.0 Pure hypercholesterolemia	IIa	Chol	LDL	~90% polygenic, ~10% monogenic; heterozygous: *LDLR, APOB, PCSK9*; homozygous: *LDLR, LDLRAP1*
E78.2 Mixed hyperlipidemia	IIb	Chol, TG	VLDL, LDL	Polygenic; some cases due to *USF1, APOB, LPL*; ~35% have *APOA5* S19W or −1131T>C
E78.2 Mixed hyperlipidemia	III	Chol, TG	IDL	Polygenic; *APOE* or homozygosity for E2 allele of *APOE* necessary but not sufficient; ~40% have *APOA5* S19W or −1131T>C
E78.1 Pure hypertriglyceridemia	IV	TG	VLDL	Polygenic; ~35% have *APOA5* S19W or −1131T>C
E78.3 Hyperchylomicronemia	V	Chol, TG	VLDL, CM	Polygenic; ~10%: *LPL, APOC2, APOA5*; ~55% have *APOA5* S19W or −1131T>C; small effects from *APOE, TRIB1, CHREBP, GALNT2, GCKR, ANGPTL3*

Abbreviations: 1131T>C, a T-to-C conversion at position −1131; *ANGPTL3*, angiopoietin-like 3; *APOA5*, apolipoprotein A-V; *APOB*, apolipoprotein B; *APOC2*, apolipoprotein C-II; *APOE*, apolipoprotein E; Chol, cholesterol; *CHREBP*, carbohydrate response element binding protein (also known as *MLXIPL*); CM, chylomicron; *GALNT2*, UDP-*N*-acetyl-α-*D*-galactosamine:polypeptide *N*-acetylgalactosaminyltransferase 2; *GCKR*, glucokinase regulator; HLP, hyperlipoproteinemia; IDL, intermediate-density lipoprotein; *LDLRAP1*, LDL receptor adaptor protein 1 (also known as *ARH*); *LPL*, lipoprotein lipase; *PCSK9*, proprotein convertase subtilisin/kexin type 9; S19W, serine to tryptophan conversion at amino acid 19; TG, triglyceride; *TRIB1*, tribbles homologue 1 (*Drosophila*); *USF1*, upstream transcription factor 1; VLDL, very low density lipoprotein.

GENETIC TESTING IN FAMILIAL HYPERCHOLESTEROLEMIA
Current Clinical Criteria for Diagnosis of Familial Hypercholesterolemia

It is currently estimated that only about 15% to 20% of patients with FH are actually diagnosed.[9] There are no internationally accepted criteria for FH diagnosis. However, the 3 commonly used criteria are the Dutch, Simon Broome, and US MedPed criteria (**Table 2**). Unlike the US criteria, which use total cholesterol levels and family history of FH, the Simon Broome and the Dutch criteria integrate personal and family lipid profiles, history of premature CVD (onset in men before age 55 years and in women before age 65 years), physical examination findings such as tendon xanthomas for the index person and family members, and genetic information.[22–24] The Simon Broome and the Dutch criteria classify definitive, probable, and possible FH. According to the Simon

Table 2
Clinical criteria in diagnosis of familial hypercholesterolemia

Simon Broome Familial Hypercholesterolemia Register Diagnostic Criteria for Familial Hypercholesterolemia: Criteria (Description)	
• TC >290 mg/dL in adults or >260 mg/dL in children aged <16 y, or LDL-C >190 mg/dL in adults or >155 mg/dL in children (A) • Tendinous xanthomata in the patient or a first-degree relative (B) • Positive DNA test (C) • Family history of premature CVD (D) • Family history of: TC >290 mg/dL in a first-degree or second-degree relative or >260 mg/dL in child or sibling aged <16 y (E)	Definitive FH: A and B or C Probable FH: A and D or A and E

Dutch Lipid Clinic Network Diagnostic Criteria for Familial Hypercholesterolemia: Criteria (Points)	
• First-degree relative with known premature (men <55 y; women <60 y) coronary and vascular disease, or first-degree relative with known LDL-C above the 95th percentile (1) • First-degree relative with tendinous xanthomata and/or arcus cornealis, or children aged <18 y with LDL-C above the 95th percentile (2) • Patient with premature CAD (2) • Patient with premature CVD or PVD (1) • Tendinous xanthoma (6) • Arcus cornealis before age 45 y (4) • LDL-C ≥329 (8), 251–329 (5), 193–251 (3), 155–193 (1) • Functional mutation in LDLR gene (8)	Definite FH: ≥8 points Probable FH: 6–8 points Possible FH: 3–5 points

US MedPed Program Diagnostic Criteria for Probable Heterozygous Familial Hypercholesterolemia				
	Total Cholesterol (mg/dL)			
Age (y)	First-Degree Relative with FH	Second-Degree Relative with FH	Third-Degree Relative with FH	General Population
<20	220	230	240	270
20–29	240	250	260	290
30–39	270	280	290	340
≥40	290	300	310	360

Broome criteria, to make a definitive FH diagnosis, either a positive genetic test or elevated cholesterol levels accompanied by tendon xanthomas in self or family are needed, whereas according to the Dutch criteria (which uses a scoring system), either a positive genetic test or a constellation of the aforementioned nongenetic criteria qualify for a definitive FH diagnosis (see **Table 2**).

The first steps in the assessment of a hereditary dyslipidemia in a clinic are to take a thorough history, including family history that covers at least 3 generations' history of CVD (including premature onset) and risk factors, family members' lipid profile (if available), performing a focused physical examination, and ordering a lipid profile. The presence of tendon xanthomas should be sought by careful inspection and palpation of the tendons commonly affected, such as the Achilles, finger extensor, and patellar tendons. Corneal arcus, if present in a patient under the age of 45 years, can indicate FH. Similarly, xanthelasma or tuberous xanthomas in a young patient should raise a concern for FH, although these are not FH specific.

Genetic Testing to Improve Diagnostic Accuracy

It is obvious that identification of the mutated gene or genes provides a definite diagnosis of FH, which is not always the case with a clinical diagnosis of FH. Clinical criteria are, in general, more specific than sensitive because they usually identify individuals with an extreme phenotype, such as those with very high LDL-C levels.[24] Although the clinical criteria are low cost and easy to assess, they lack sensitivity for several reasons. Some FH patients may not have severely elevated LDL-C levels and can be easily missed by using these clinical criteria.[25] The cholesterol levels used in these clinical criteria are off-treatment levels; however, most FH patients seen in a clinic are usually on cholesterol-lowering medications and therefore it is frequently difficult to obtain untreated total cholesterol and LDL-C levels in routine practice. Similarly, physical examination findings may not be as helpful in the modern era. Not only are findings such as corneal arcus and xanthelasma not specific to FH but common in the general aging population,[26] but more importantly, FH-specific findings such as tendon xanthoma, which results from lifelong cholesterol accumulation on tendons, are frequently not present when statins are used in FH patients since very early in life. Furthermore, family history may not be reliable in regard to premature CVD with improved medical therapy. Furthermore, women with FH usually manifest disease later than men. Therefore, it is possible that a male proband may present with premature onset of coronary heart disease, while his mother may have high levels of LDL-C but no history of an ischemic cardiac event. Genetic testing in the mother will be very helpful in this situation so that a proactive prevention strategy can be used to lower LDL-C for both the mother and her offspring, who may inherit the mutated genes. In all these situations, given its high sensitivity and specificity,[27,28] genetic testing can be of value in diagnosing FH.[24] Clearly, in both the Simon Broome and the Dutch criteria, a positive genetic test alone is sufficient to make the diagnosis of FH, whereas many individuals who would clinically have an autosomal-dominant pattern of high LDL-C and heart disease no longer meet these criteria.

Genetic Testing in Screening for Familial Hypercholesterolemia

Cascade screening involves stepwise diagnosis of all first-degree relatives of FH patients and it then extends to second-degree and third-degree relatives. Data from the United Kingdom suggest that cascade screening was associated with FH diagnosis at a younger age and led to higher rates of statin therapy in FH patients.[29] As mentioned previously, the institution of statin therapy in FH patients has been associated with a reduction in incident coronary heart disease.[18,30]

Cascade screening can be performed using clinical criteria, which rely mostly on cholesterol levels, or by using genetic testing. A mutation can be identified in up to 80% of the screened population depending on the clinical criteria used for FH diagnosis and sensitivity of the genetic test used. Once a mutation is found in the index case, genetic testing in first-degree relatives is quick, less expensive, and very sensitive and specific.[31] Although the cost of genetic testing may be of concern, cascade genetic testing has been shown to be the most effective strategy in screening for FH.[32,33]

The first successful model of a national genetic cascade screening program came from the Netherlands; since it started in 1994, more than 9000 FH patients have been identified.[32] Initially, without genetic testing, only 39% of these individuals were on cholesterol-lowering medications, and after 2 years of genetic screening, 85% were on medications. Other countries that followed similar strategies include Norway, Spain, Australia, New Zealand, and Wales. In general, mutation detection ranged from 36% to 59%, and the rates differed based on the original likelihood for having an FH diagnosis and on the methods used for genetic screening.[34–36] The National Institute for Health and Clinical Excellence in the United Kingdom recommends genetic cascade screening of close biological relatives of people with a clinical diagnosis of FH to identify additional FH patients effectively.[37,38] It should be noted that FH screening using a genetic approach has not been compared directly with using clinical FH criteria in a randomized controlled trial, and therefore, data are lacking on the potential benefit of a genetic approach compared with clinical criteria for FH diagnosis and screening. Furthermore, because FH remains underdiagnosed and cascade screening has been shown to be effective, it is very important to adopt wide implementation of cascade screening of family members (using cholesterol levels and clinical criteria) first.

In the United States as elsewhere, FH is underdiagnosed, indicating a need for better screening.[9] The American College of Cardiology/American Heart Association guidelines to treat cholesterol identified individuals with off-treatment LDL-C of 190 mg/dL or greater (individuals with FH usually have LDL-C >190 mg/dL) as a group that would benefit from statin therapy regardless of the underlying cause.[39] The National Lipid Association Expert Panel published clinical guidelines to address screening, diagnosis, and management of FH and recommended cascade screening with clinical criteria and using genetic testing in cases of diagnostic uncertainty.[40] The Familial Hypercholesterolemia Foundation recently established a multicenter registry in the United States, Cascade Screening for Awareness and Detection of Familial Hypercholesterolemia (CASCADE-FH), to improve awareness and eventually screening and outcomes in FH patients.[41] As cascade screening progresses in the United States, using genetic testing can be complementary to diagnosis and in certain situations may provide additional valuable information that may influence treatment decisions and outcomes.[40]

Genetic Testing in the Treatment of Familial Hypercholesterolemia

The presence of specific genetic mutations can be informative in FH treatment, especially given that currently there are numerous classes of approved and investigational therapies submitted for regulatory approval that work via different mechanisms.[40] Genetic sequencing may also identify new and unknown mutations, which may lead to novel therapeutic targets. Mutations in the PCSK9 gene were first identified in 2 French families who had phenotypic FH, and ultimately, led to the discovery that gain-of-function mutations in PCSK9 can cause FH.[7] Conversely, loss-of-function mutations were associated with lower LDL-C levels and lower risk of CVD.[42] These genetic data led to the development of a number of monoclonal antibodies against PCSK9 as a therapeutic target, which are currently under investigation in phase 3 trials, with 2 already submitted for regulatory approval.[43] In addition, response to lipid lowering, with some patients showing excellent response and others very resistant to treatment with statins,[44] may be predicted by genetic information in patients who are clinically thought to have HoFH, as shown in the Trial Evaluating PCSK9 Antibody in Subjects with LDL Receptor Abnormalities, in which the efficacy of evolocumab, a monoclonal antibody against PCSK9, for reducing LDL-C levels in clinically defined HoFH patients was dependent on LDL-R mutations without complete loss of function, suggesting that genetic data can provide incremental information to assess response to treatment.[45] Other studies have shown association of certain alleles with response to statins and CVD outcomes.[46–50]

Another use of genetic information is in pharmacogenomics. In addition to the usefulness in assessing response to certain medications as described previously, certain genetic variants may be associated with increased likelihood of having an adverse effect from a certain medication, such as SLCO1B1 with high-dose simvastatin,[51] although testing for such mutations has not been firmly established in lipid disorders.[13]

OTHER POTENTIAL USES OF GENETIC TESTING

Numerous biomarkers have been tested for CVD risk prediction,[52,53] and a growing area of interest is the identification of common genetic variants associated with the development of CVD.[54,55] Pilot studies have shown that single-nucleotide polymorphism data can assist in prediction of CVD risk.[55,56] Common variants at 9p21 exhibit the strongest and most reproducible associations with CVD in genome-wide association studies.[54,55,57] In the Atherosclerosis Risk in Communities study, the 9p21 allele was added to a base model with traditional risk factors to assess the incremental value of 9p21 variants to predict CVD and to assess potential reclassification of individuals among risk categories. The hazards ratio for incident CVD was 1.2 per allele ($P<.0003$), and 12.1% and 12.6% of the low-intermediate and high-intermediate groups were appropriately reclassified, respectively.[58] However, the addition of 9p21 variants to a conventional risk factor model in the Women's Health Study did not change the C statistic or improve calibration, and the net reclassification improvement was modest (2.7%, $P<.02$).[59] Therefore, these data suggest that the 9p21 variation is associated with modestly increased risk for CVD; however, the net reclassification improvement was less than that provided by imaging tests or assessment of biomarkers.

GENETIC TESTING IN HYPERTRIGLYCERIDEMIA

Another important plasma lipid is triglyceride. Mild-to-moderate hypertriglyceridemia, as commonly encountered in clinical practice, is typically lifestyle related, but can also be polygenic and result from the cumulative burden of common and rare variants in several genes.[60] Familial chylomicronemia syndrome is a monogenic autosomal-recessive disorder caused by 2 mutant alleles of the genes encoding lipoprotein lipase, apoC-II, apoA-V, lipase maturation factor 1, glycosylphosphatidylinositol-anchored high-density lipoprotein binding protein 1, or glycerol-3-phosphate dehydrogenase 1.[60] Because of clustering of susceptibility alleles and lifestyle-related factors in families, biochemical screening and counseling for family members are essential, but routine genetic testing is not warranted.[60]

DISADVANTAGES OF GENETIC TESTING

The yield of genetic testing varies by referral criteria used and the population studied. Up to 10% to 30% of individuals may lack a mutation, especially in populations without founder effects and with significant ancestral heterogeneity such as the US population.[61] Most of these individuals are thought to have polygenic disease. Mutation detection rates are also lower in individuals classified as having possible or probable FH than in those with definite FH. Although the specificity for genetic testing is very high, false-positive cases may be seen with nonpathogenic sequences.

Cost of genetic testing can be a potential problem, although the price of genetic testing for patients with severe hypercholesterolemia has substantially decreased over time (**Table 3**). The psychological or emotional impact of "labeling" on patients and family members should also be considered. Legal ramifications regarding insurance or employment can be important and are covered in the United States by the Genetic Information Nondiscrimination Act (GINA), which prohibits the use of genetic information in health insurance and employment.[62] However, it should be noted that GINA does not apply to employers with less than 15 employees. The protection in employment does not extend to the US military, nor does it apply to health insurance through the Tricare Military Health System, the Indian Health Service, the Veterans Health Administration, or the Federal Employees Health Benefits Program. Finally, the law does not cover long-term care insurance, life insurance, and disability insurance.[63]

Interpretation of genetic test results may appear confusing to physicians and can require specialized expertise unless presented in simplified form. In addition, "incidentally found mutations" without known phenotypic associations can be confusing to both patients and health care providers.

CURRENT TESTS AVAILABLE

Currently available tests and testing centers can be identified from the Gene Tests Web site (see **Table 3**).[64] **Table 3** summarizes currently available US laboratories that offer specific genetic tests.

Table 3
Laboratories offering genetic testing in the United States and costs of the tests

Gene	% of FH	No. of Mutations/Cost	US Laboratories
LDLR	60%–80%	• >1000 mutations ○ Whole gene analysis ■ ~$1400 ○ Deletion/duplication test ■ ~$2030	• 7 in USA: (20 International) ○ Ambry Genetics (CA) ○ Correlagen Diagnostics (MA) ○ Athena Diagnostics (MA) ○ Mayo Clinic (MN) ○ Baylor College of Medicine (TX) ○ Progenika (MA) ○ Prevention Genetics (WI)
ApoB	1%–10%	• 1 common mutation ○ Targeted mutation analysis ■ ~$400	• 2 in USA: (6 International) ○ Ambry Genetics (CA) ○ ARUP Laboratories (UT)
PCSK9	<5%	• 1 common mutation ○ Targeted mutation analysis ■ ~$1400	• 1 in USA: (2 International) ○ Ambry Genetics (CA)

NOTE: Subsequent testing in family members is inexpensive once causal variant is already identified (~$250–$400). The costs for genetic tests may or may not be covered by health insurance.

SUMMARY

FH is a common disorder in which early diagnosis and treatment can prevent the development of CVD in most individuals. Unfortunately, this common disorder is underdiagnosed and undertreated. Using clinical screening and diagnostic tools, such as CASCADE-FH, screening can be very effective and should be widely adopted. As advances in human genome sequencing are being made, there is increasing evidence that genetic information can be helpful in screening, diagnosis, and treatment of FH. However, randomized trials and cost-effectiveness studies to assess the incremental benefit of genetic testing over clinical criteria for screening and diagnosis of FH are needed to provide definitive answers for wider implementation of genetic testing in clinical practice.

ACKNOWLEDGMENTS

We thank Kerrie Jara for her editorial assistance.

REFERENCES

1. Lusis AJ. Atherosclerosis. Nature 2000;407:233–41.
2. Rader DJ, Daugherty A. Translating molecular discoveries into new therapies for atherosclerosis. Nature 2008;451:904–13.
3. Hegele RA. Plasma lipoproteins: genetic influences and clinical implications. Nat Rev Genet 2009;10:109–21.
4. Tada H, Kawashiri MA, Nohara A, et al. Autosomal recessive hypercholesterolemia: a mild phenotype of familial hypercholesterolemia: insight from the kinetic study using stable isotope and animal studies. J Atheroscler Thromb 2014. [Epub ahead of print].
5. Brown MS, Goldstein JL. A receptor-mediated pathway for cholesterol homeostasis. Science 1986;232:34–47.
6. Innerarity TL, Weisgraber KH, Arnold KS, et al. Familial defective apolipoprotein B-100: low density lipoproteins with abnormal receptor binding. Proc Natl Acad Sci U S A 1987;84:6919–23.
7. Abifadel M, Varret M, Rabes JP, et al. Mutations in PCSK9 cause autosomal dominant hypercholesterolemia. Nat Genet 2003;34:154–6.
8. Garcia CK, Wilund K, Arca M, et al. Autosomal recessive hypercholesterolemia caused by mutations in a putative LDL receptor adaptor protein. Science 2001; 292:1394–8.
9. Nordestgaard BG, Chapman MJ, Humphries SE, et al. Familial hypercholesterolaemia is underdiagnosed and undertreated in the general population: guidance for clinicians to prevent coronary heart disease: consensus statement of the European Atherosclerosis Society. Eur Heart J 2013;34:3478–3490a.
10. Moorjani S, Roy M, Gagne C, et al. Homozygous familial hypercholesterolemia among French Canadians in Quebec Province. Arteriosclerosis 1989;9:211–6.
11. Seftel HC, Baker SG, Jenkins T, et al. Prevalence of familial hypercholesterolemia in Johannesburg Jews. Am J Med Genet 1989;34:545–7.
12. Fahed AC, Nemer GM. Familial hypercholesterolemia: the lipids or the genes? Nutr Metab (Lond) 2011;8:23.
13. Bays HE, Jones PH, Brown WV, et al. National Lipid Association annual summary of clinical lipidology 2015. J Clin Lipidol 2014;8:S1–36.
14. Hopkins PN, Toth PP, Ballantyne CM, et al. Familial hypercholesterolemias: prevalence, genetics, diagnosis and screening recommendations from the National

Lipid Association Expert Panel on Familial Hypercholesterolemia. J Clin Lipidol 2011;5:S9–17.

15. Watts GF, Lewis B, Sullivan DR. Familial hypercholesterolemia: a missed opportunity in preventive medicine. Nat Clin Pract Cardiovasc Med 2007;4:404–5.

16. Wu NQ, Guo YL, Xu RX, et al. Acute myocardial infarction in an 8-year old male child with homozygous familiar hypercholesterolemia: laboratory findings and response to lipid-lowering drugs. Clin Lab 2013;59:901–7.

17. Neil HA, Hammond T, Huxley R, et al. Extent of underdiagnosis of familial hypercholesterolaemia in routine practice: prospective registry study. BMJ 2000;321:148.

18. Versmissen J, Oosterveer DM, Yazdanpanah M, et al. Efficacy of statins in familial hypercholesterolaemia: a long term cohort study. BMJ 2008;337:a2423.

19. Rees A. Familial hypercholesterolaemia: underdiagnosed and undertreated. Eur Heart J 2008;29:2583–4.

20. Emerging Risk Factors. Lipoprotein(a) concentration and the risk of coronary heart disease, stroke, and nonvascular mortality. JAMA 2009;302:412–23.

21. Koschinsky ML, Boffa MB. Lipoprotein(a): an important cardiovascular risk factor and a clinical conundrum. Endocrinol Metab Clin North Am 2014;43:949–62.

22. Civeira F. International Panel on Management of Familial Hypercholesterolemia. Guidelines for the diagnosis and management of heterozygous familial hypercholesterolemia. Atherosclerosis 2004;173:55–68.

23. Scientific Steering Committee on behalf of the Simon Broome Register Group. Risk of fatal coronary heart disease in familial hypercholesterolaemia. BMJ 1991;303:893–6.

24. Williams RR, Hunt SC, Schumacher MC, et al. Diagnosing heterozygous familial hypercholesterolemia using new practical criteria validated by molecular genetics. Am J Cardiol 1993;72:171–6.

25. Graadt van Roggen JF, van der Westhuyzen DR, Coetzee GA, et al. FH Afrikaner-3 LDL receptor mutation results in defective LDL receptors and causes a mild form of familial hypercholesterolemia. Arterioscler Thromb Vasc Biol 1995;15:765–72.

26. Kotulak JC, Brungardt T. Age-related changes in the cornea. J Am Optom Assoc 1980;51:761–5.

27. National Institute for Health and Care Excellence. Identification and Management of Familial Hypercholesterolaemia (NICE clinical guideline 71). London; 2008. Available at: http://www.guidance.nice.org.uk/cg71. Accessed February 23, 2015.

28. Humphries SE, Norbury G, Leigh S, et al. What is the clinical utility of DNA testing in patients with familial hypercholesterolaemia? Curr Opin Lipidol 2008;19:362–8.

29. Ballantyne CM, Pazzucconi F, Pintó X, et al. Efficacy and tolerability of fluvastatin extended-release delivery system: a pooled analysis. Clin Ther 2001;23:177–92.

30. Neil A, Cooper J, Betteridge J, et al. Reductions in all-cause, cancer, and coronary mortality in statin-treated patients with heterozygous familial hypercholesterolaemia: a prospective registry study. Eur Heart J 2008;29:2625–33.

31. The Task Force for the management of dyslipidaemias of the European Society of Cardiology (ESC) and the European Atherosclerosis Society (EAS). ESC/EAS Guidelines for the management of dyslipidaemias. Eur Heart J 2011;32:1769–818.

32. Leren TP. Cascade genetic screening for familial hypercholesterolemia. Clin Genet 2004;66:483–7.

33. Marks D, Wonderling D, Thorogood M, et al. Screening for hypercholesterolaemia versus case finding for familial hypercholesterolaemia: a systematic review and cost-effectiveness analysis. Health Technol Assess 2000;4:1–123.

34. Austin MA, Breslow JL, Hennekens CH, et al. Low-density lipoprotein subclass patterns and risk of myocardial infarction. JAMA 1988;260:1917–21.
35. Muir LA, George PM, Laurie AD, et al. Preventing cardiovascular disease: a review of the effectiveness of identifying the people with familial hypercholesterolaemia in New Zealand. N Z Med J 2010;123:97–102.
36. Aviram M, Lund-Katz S, Phillips MC, et al. The influence of the triglyceride content of low density lipoprotein on the interaction of apolipoprotein B-100 with cells. J Biol Chem 1988;263:16842–8.
37. Ned RM, Sijbrands EJ. Cascade screening for familial hypercholesterolemia (FH). PLoS Curr 2011;3:RRN1238.
38. Austin MA. Plasma triglyceride as a risk factor for coronary heart disease: the epidemiologic evidence and beyond. Am J Epidemiol 1989;129:249–59.
39. Stone NJ, Robinson JG, Lichtenstein AH, et al. 2013 ACC/AHA guideline on the treatment of blood cholesterol to reduce atherosclerotic cardiovascular risk in adults: a report of the American College of Cardiology/American Heart Association Task Force on Practice Guidelines. J Am Coll Cardiol 2014;63:2889–934.
40. Goldberg AC, Hopkins PN, Toth PP, et al. Familial hypercholesterolemia: screening, diagnosis and management of pediatric and adult patients: clinical guidance from the National Lipid Association Expert Panel on Familial Hypercholesterolemia. J Clin Lipidol 2011;5:133–40.
41. O'Brien EC, Roe MT, Fraulo ES, et al. Rationale and design of the familial hypercholesterolemia foundation Cascade screening for awareness and detection of familial hypercholesterolemia registry. Am Heart J 2014;167:342–9.e17.
42. Cohen JC, Boerwinkle E, Mosley TH Jr, et al. Sequence variations in PCSK9, low LDL, and protection against coronary heart disease. N Engl J Med 2006;354:1264–72.
43. Dadu RT, Ballantyne CM. Lipid lowering with PCSK9 inhibitors. Nat Rev Cardiol 2014;11:563–75.
44. Choumerianou DM, Dedoussis GV. Familial hypercholesterolemia and response to statin therapy according to LDLR genetic background. Clin Chem Lab Med 2005;43:793–801.
45. Raal FJ, Honarpour N, Blom DJ, et al. Inhibition of PCSK9 with evolocumab in homozygous familial hypercholesterolaemia (TESLA Part B): a randomised, double-blind, placebo-controlled trial. Lancet 2014. [Epub ahead of print].
46. Shiffman D, Chasman DI, Zee RY, et al. A kinesin family member 6 variant is associated with coronary heart disease in the Women's Health Study. J Am Coll Cardiol 2008;51:444–8.
47. Morrison AC, Bare LA, Chambless LE, et al. Prediction of coronary heart disease risk using a genetic risk score: the Atherosclerosis Risk in Communities study. Am J Epidemiol 2007;166:28–35.
48. Iakoubova OA, Tong CH, Rowland CM, et al. Association of the Trp719Arg polymorphism in kinesin-like protein 6 with myocardial infarction and coronary heart disease in 2 prospective trials: the CARE and WOSCOPS trials. J Am Coll Cardiol 2008;51:435–43.
49. Ridker PM, MacFadyen JG, Glynn RJ, et al. Kinesin-like protein 6 (KIF6) polymorphism and the efficacy of rosuvastatin in primary prevention. Circ Cardiovasc Genet 2011;4:312–7.
50. Arsenault BJ, Boekholdt SM, Hovingh GK, et al. The 719Arg variant of KIF6 and cardiovascular outcomes in statin-treated, stable coronary patients of the Treating to New Targets and Incremental Decrease in End Points through Aggressive Lipid-lowering prospective studies. Circ Cardiovasc Genet 2012;5:51–7.

51. Search Collaborative Group. SLCO1B1 variants and statin-induced myopathy–a genomewide study. N Engl J Med 2008;359:789–99.
52. Ridker PM, Danielson E, Fonseca FA, et al. Rosuvastatin to prevent vascular events in men and women with elevated C-reactive protein. N Engl J Med 2008;359:2195–207.
53. Vasan RS. Biomarkers of cardiovascular disease: molecular basis and practical considerations. Circulation 2006;113:2335–62.
54. Samani NJ, Erdmann J, Hall AS, et al. Genomewide association analysis of coronary artery disease. N Engl J Med 2007;357:443–53.
55. McPherson R, Pertsemlidis A, Kavaslar N, et al. A common allele on chromosome 9 associated with coronary heart disease. Science 2007;316:1488–91.
56. Schunkert H, Gotz A, Braund P, et al. Repeated replication and a prospective meta-analysis of the association between chromosome 9p21.3 and coronary artery disease. Circulation 2008;117:1675–84.
57. Myocardial Infarction Genetics Consortium. Genome-wide association of early-onset myocardial infarction with single nucleotide polymorphisms and copy number variants. Nat Genet 2009;41:334–41.
58. Brautbar A, Ballantyne CM. Pharmacological strategies for lowering LDL cholesterol: statins and beyond. Nat Rev Cardiol 2011;8:253–65.
59. Paynter NP, Chasman DI, Buring JE, et al. Cardiovascular disease risk prediction with and without knowledge of genetic variation at chromosome 9p21.3. Ann Intern Med 2009;150:65–72.
60. Hegele RA, Ginsberg HN, Chapman MJ, et al. The polygenic nature of hypertriglyceridaemia: implications for definition, diagnosis, and management. Lancet Diabetes Endocrinol 2014;2:655–66.
61. Palacios L, Grandoso L, Cuevas N, et al. Molecular characterization of familial hypercholesterolemia in Spain. Atherosclerosis 2012;221:137–42.
62. Avogaro P, Bittolo Bon G, Cazzolato G. Presence of a modified low density lipoprotein in humans. Arteriosclerosis 1988;8:79–87.
63. Ballantyne CM, Houri J, Notarbartolo A, et al. Effect of ezetimibe coadministered with atorvastatin in 628 patients with primary hypercholesterolemia: a prospective, randomized, double-blind trial. Circulation 2003;107:2409–15.
64. Berry EM, Eisenberg S, Haratz D, et al. Effects of diets rich in monounsaturated fatty acids on plasma lipoproteins—the Jerusalem Nutrition Study: high MUFAs vs high PUFAs. Am J Clin Nutr 1991;53:899–907.

Familial Hypercholesterolemia

Victoria Enchia Bouhairie, MD, Anne Carol Goldberg, MD*

KEYWORDS

- Familial hypercholesterolemia • Statins • Ezetimibe • Bile acid sequestrants
- LDL apheresis • Lomitapide • Mipomersen

KEY POINTS

- Familial hypercholesterolemia (FH) is a common genetic disorder leading to high cholesterol levels from birth and increased risk of atherosclerotic cardiovascular disease.
- Heterozygous FH occurs in approximately 1 in 250 people in many populations.
- Homozygous FH can lead to coronary artery disease in childhood and adolescence.
- Early treatment can decrease the risk of premature atherosclerotic cardiovascular disease in FH patients.

INTRODUCTION

Familial hypercholesterolemia (FH) is an inherited condition resulting in high levels of low-density lipoprotein cholesterol (LDL-C) and increased risk of premature cardiovascular disease in men and women. FH causes lifetime exposure to high LDL-C levels. It is not rare, but it is underdiagnosed. Although therapies for FH are available, it is commonly undertreated. Early diagnosis and treatment mitigate the excess risk of premature atherosclerotic cardiovascular disease that occurs with FH.[1-3]

Pathophysiology

The pathophysiology of FH is due to decreased function of LDL receptors (LDLRs) (**Box 1**).

This article originally appeared in Cardiology Clinics, Volume 33, Issue 2, May 2015.
Conflict of Interest Statement: Dr V.E. Bouhairie receives support from Award Number T32DK007120 from the National Institute of Diabetes and Digestive and Kidney Diseases. The content is solely the responsibility of the authors and does not necessarily represent the official views of the National Institute of Diabetes and Digestive and Kidney Diseases or the National Institutes of Health; Dr A.C. Goldberg: Research Support: Research contracts to institution— Merck, Genzyme/ISIS/Sanofi-Aventis, GlaxoSmithKline, Amgen, Amarin, Regeneron/Sanofi-Aventis, Roche/Genentech, Pfizer; Consulting: Tekmira, Astra-Zeneca, uniQure; Editorial: Merck Manual. Division of Endocrinology, Metabolism, and Lipid Research, Department of Medicine, Washington University School of Medicine, Campus Box 8127, 660 South Euclid, St Louis, MO 63110, USA
* Corresponding author.
E-mail address: agoldber@dom.wustl.edu

Box 1
Pathophysiology of familial hypercholesterolemia

- Decreased LDLR function due to a genetic defect, typically one of the following classes[1]:
  - LDLR is not synthesized
  - LDLR is not properly transported from the endoplasmic reticulum to the Golgi apparatus for expression on the cell surface
  - LDLR does not properly bind LDL on the cell surface
  - LDLR does not properly cluster in clathrin-coated pits for receptor endocytosis
  - LDLR is not recycled back to the cell surface
- Therefore, LDLR-mediated endocytosis is decreased
- Leading to markedly elevated LDL levels
- Premature development of atherosclerotic plaque

Genetics of Familial Hypercholesterolemia

FH is an autosomal-dominant disorder with a gene dosage effect. Patients who are homozygotes (or compound heterozygotes) have much higher LDL-C levels and earlier coronary artery disease (CAD) onset than heterozygous patients.[1–4] The underlying defect in FH was initially thought to be due to increased synthesis of cholesterol, but it is now known that the fractional catabolic rate of LDL is decreased in heterozygous FH individuals compared with normal subjects.[5] The LDLR pathway was characterized by Brown and Goldstein and revealed receptor-mediated endocytosis.[6]

The most common form of FH is a monogenic, autosomal-dominant disorder, which causes defects in the gene that encodes the LDLR.[1–3]

More than 900 mutations of this gene have been identified,[1] most pathogenic, leading to the LDLR having decreased capacity to clear LDL from the circulation.

There are also defects in the LDLR binding region of apolipoprotein B (apoB)[1] and rare gain-of-function proprotein convertase subtilisin/kexin type 9 (PCSK9) gene mutations.[7] A rare autosomal-recessive form of FH caused by loss-of-function mutations in the LDL receptor adaptor protein 1 (LDLRAP1), which encodes a protein required for clathrin-mediated internalization of the LDLR, has also been described (**Table 1**).[3]

Table 1
Types of mutations causing familial hypercholesterolemia

Mutation	Gene	Mechanism	Numbers of Mutations (% of FH Cases)
LDLR	LDLR	LDLR is absent or has decreased capacity to clear LDL from circulation	>900 (85%–90%)
ApoB (also known as familial defective apoB)	ApoB	Impaired LDLR binding—mutation at binding site on LDL particle	Mutations around the 3500 residues–most common is Arg3500Gln (5%–10%)
PCSK9 gain of function	PCSK9	Increased PCSK9 level leads to increased degradation of LDLRs	Rare
LDLR adaptor protein	LDLRAP1	Protein needed for clathrin-mediated internalization of LDLR	Rare; autosomal-recessive hypercholesterolemia

Prevalence of Familial Hypercholesterolemia

Historically, the prevalence of heterozygous FH was 1 in 500 persons. Recent genetic studies suggest a prevalence of 1 in 200 to 250.[8,9] In populations such as French Canadians, Ashkenazi Jews, Lebanese, and several South African populations, the prevalence may be as high as 1 in 100.[10] Based on a prevalence of 1 in 500, there are an estimated 620,000 FH patients in the United States,[11] but this number may be as high as 1,500,000 based on a prevalence of 1 in 250. The historical prevalence estimate of homozygous (or compound heterozygous) patients is 1 in 1 million, and this would also change based on current studies. Recent data from the Netherlands suggest that the prevalence could be as low as 1 in 160,000 and is likely to be about 1 in 250,000.[9] Most patients with homozygous FH have extreme hypercholesterolemia with rapidly accelerated atherosclerosis when left untreated.[3,10]

Although single-gene disorders play a crucial role in the cause of FH, linkage studies suggest that some cases are caused by the presence of multiple single-nucleotide polymorphisms.[12] Heterozygotes arise when a mutation is inherited from one parent only, whereas homozygotes develop when the same mutated gene is inherited from both parents. Compound heterozygotes are due to inheritance of a different mutation from each parent. Untreated heterozygotes have LDL-C in the range of 155 to 500 mg/dL, whereas untreated homozygotes (or compound heterozygotes) typically have LDL-C greater than 500 mg/dL. Recent data suggest wide variation in LDL-C levels.[1–3,10]

PATIENT EVALUATION
Screening Strategies

Although the atherosclerotic manifestations of FH usually occur in adulthood, the clinical effects of the disease can start in the first decade of life in homozygous patients.[3] Unfortunately, FH is often diagnosed late and after the occurrence of a major coronary event. A combination of screening methods to identify at-risk individuals is needed[11,13,14] to prevent premature atherosclerosis.

There are many barriers to the diagnosis and treatment of FH. Many individuals and family members with FH who have CAD have other common CAD risk factors; thus, genetic hypercholesterolemia is not suspected and ultimately not diagnosed. Primary care physicians manage most patients with hypercholesterolemia, and there is often a lack of awareness of FH among physicians and the general public with only very severe cases being referred to specialists.[2,13]

Cascade screening, in which health care providers actively screen for disease among the first-degree and second-degree relatives of patients diagnosed with FH,[13] can increase detection rates but risks missing affected individuals. Several national and international guidelines recommend universal screening for elevated serum cholesterol by age 20 and cascade testing of first-degree relatives of all individuals with FH.[2,11,13,15,16] For children, cholesterol screening should be done at age 9 to 11 and considered beginning at age 2 in those with a family history of premature cardiovascular disease or elevated cholesterol.[11,17,18]

Diagnosis

Diagnosis of FH is based on lipid levels, family history, physical findings (if present), and, if available, genetic analysis (**Box 2**). Physical examination findings of tendon xanthomas, arcus corneae (under the age of 45), and tuberous xanthomas or xanthelasma (under the age of 25) when present at an early age should also prompt suspicion for FH. However, physical findings are not present in all patients with FH.[1]

Box 2
Clinical approach to diagnosis of familial hypercholesterolemia

Consider FH in the following

- Presence of premature atherosclerotic cardiovascular disease
- Fasting LDL-C levels greater than 190 mg/dL in adults after exclusion of secondary causes of elevated LDL-C (hypothyroidism, nephrotic syndrome)
- Fasting untreated LDL-C levels that have an 80% probability of FH in the general population:
  - ≥250 mg/dL in adults ≥30 years
  - ≥220 mg/dL in adults aged 20 to 29
  - ≥190 mg/dL in patients under the age of 20
- Presence of full corneal arcus under the age of 40
- Presence of tendon xanthomas
- Family history of premature atherosclerotic cardiovascular disease
- Family history of high cholesterol levels

There are 3 well-defined clinical diagnostic tools that are used to diagnose FH:

- The US Make Early Diagnoses Prevent Early Deaths Program Diagnostic Criteria,[19]
  - Uses total and LDL-C measurements and family history
- The Dutch Lipid Clinic Network Diagnostic Criteria[20]
  - Uses a point system of LDL-C levels, physical examination findings, and family and personal history of CAD; presence of genetic mutations
- The Simon Broome Register Diagnostic Criteria[15]
  - Uses LDL-C levels, family history, tendon xanthomas, presence of genetic mutations

The Dutch Lipid Clinic criteria are generally not useful in children. These sets of criteria are typically used to diagnose heterozygous FH.

The diagnosis of homozygous (or compound heterozygous) FH has been defined in several ways,[3,10] with one possible definition shown in **Box 3**. However, recent data on the heterogeneity and prevalence of genetically defined homozygous FH suggest that older criteria may not always apply.[9]

Genetic Testing

Clinical criteria may not identify all patients with FH, and genetic testing is part of the screening strategies in many countries, with the costs covered by national health services.[2,3,13,15,16] In the United States, it is done infrequently, partly because of cost and lack of insurance coverage. Genetic testing in certain populations has changed the understanding of the frequency of both heterozygous and homozygous FH. However, a mutation is not always found in patients with clinical FH, and lack of a mutation should not change treatment.[1]

Prognosis

Patients with heterozygous FH are generally asymptomatic in childhood and early adulthood. About 5% of heart attacks in patients under the age of 60 and as many as 20% under the age of 45 are due to FH.[1,2]

Box 3
Diagnosis of homozygous familial hypercholesterolemia

Genetic analysis showing mutations in 2 alleles at gene locus for *LDLR, APOB, PCKS9, LDLRAP1*

OR

Presence of untreated LDL greater than 500 mg/dL or treated LDL greater than 300 mg/dL plus:

Presence of cutaneous or tendon xanthomas before the age of 10 years

OR

Both parents with evidence of heterozygous FH (except for the rare LDLRAP1 mutations)

Note that the range of untreated LDL-C levels in homozygous FH can be lower, especially in children.

Data from Cuchel M, Bruckert E, Ginsberg H. Homozygous familial hypercholesterolaemia: new insights and guidance for clinicians to improve detection and clinical management. A position paper from the Consensus Panel on Familial Hypercholesterolaemia of the European Atherosclerosis Society. Eur Heart J 2014;35(32):2146–57; and Raal FJ, Santos RD. Homozygous familial hypercholesterolemia: current perspectives on diagnosis and treatment. Atherosclerosis 2012;223:262–8.

Homozygous or compound heterozygous FH has a severe and variable clinical presentation usually within the first decade of life. Most of these individuals have extreme hypercholesterolemia with rapidly accelerated atherosclerosis when left untreated. The variation depends on the amount of LDLR activity.[3,10] CAD is the most common cause of premature death in these patients, but other cardiovascular diseases, including aortic and supravalvular aortic stenosis and aortic root disease, are also common.[3,10]

Risk assessment tools

Risk assessment tools do not adequately predict 10-year coronary heart disease (CHD) risk in FH patients, and the Framingham Risk Score is not recommended in FH patients.[4] Risk calculators underestimate risk in patients with FH because of the significant effect of exposure to high cholesterol levels from birth.

TREATMENT

The lifetime risk of CHD and premature onset CHD is very high in individuals with FH. Early treatment is beneficial and long-term drug therapy can substantially reduce or eliminate the added lifetime risk of CHD from having FH and can lower the CHD event rate in heterozygous FH patients to levels similar to those of the general population.[2,21,22] The 2013 American College of Cardiology/American Heart Association (ACC/AHA) cholesterol treatment guideline recommends potent statin use in adult patients with LDL-C levels of 190 mg/dL or higher.[23] The National Lipid Association recommends that both children and adults with LDL-C of 190 mg/dL or higher (or non-high-density lipoprotein [HDL] cholesterol $\geq$220 mg/dL) after lifestyle changes be started on drug therapy.[17,24]

Lifestyle and Noncholesterol Risk Factor Modification

Lifestyle and noncholesterol risk factor modification is an important part of treatment (**Box 4**).[13,24]

Box 4
Lifestyle and noncholesterol risk factor modification

- Dietary modification contributes to improvement in lipid profiles
  - A heart-healthy diet including vegetables, fruit, nonfat dairy, beans, tree nuts, fish, and lean meats should be encouraged
  - Restrict intake of saturated fat to less than 7% of calories
  - Avoid trans fats
  - If alcohol is used, amount should be moderate
  - Addition of plant stanols (2 g/d) and insoluble fiber (10–20 g/d) can provide some LDL-C lowering
  - Dietitian counseling is beneficial
- Physical activity
- Avoidance of weight gain
- Avoidance and cessation of smoking is mandatory
  - Discourage exposure to passive smoking
- Treat diabetes and hypertension
- Consider low-dose aspirin

Homozygous patients require treatment as soon as the diagnosis is made and need lifestyle, medication, and additional modalities. Treatment of homozygous FH patients can delay major cardiovascular events and early death.[3,25]

Pharmacologic Therapy

Statins should be the initial drug for all adults with FH and in children with heterozygous FH starting at 8 to 10 years of age.[4,13,15–17,24] Patients with homozygous FH should be treated as soon as the diagnosis is made.[3,10,13] The US Food and Drug Administration (FDA) has approved lovastatin, atorvastatin, simvastatin, and rosuvastatin in children over the age of 10 years and pravastatin in those over 8 years of age.[26] Statins increase the expression of LDLRs by reducing HMG-CoA reductase, the rate-limiting step in cholesterol synthesis. Moderate-potency to high-potency statins should be used as first-line treatment (atorvastatin, rosuvastatin, simvastatin, pitavastatin) (**Table 2**). Low-potency statins are usually inadequate for FH patients.[13,24] Adult FH patients should have a treatment goal of 50% LDL-C reduction or better from baseline. Statin therapy is effective in heterozygous FH patients and may also benefit homozygous patients who have some LDLR activity (see **Table 2**).[3,10]

Long-term safety of statins in the pediatric population is still unknown, but the current benefits of therapy outweigh the risk of untreated pediatric populations.[17,26–28] Children and adolescents being treated with statins should have regular follow-up with close monitoring of creatinine kinase, aspartate aminotransferase (AST), and alanine aminotransferase levels (ALT). Baseline levels, then repeat testing, should be done at 1 to 3 months after drug initiation and then yearly. If **creatine kinase** levels reach 5 times the upper limit of normal and AST or ALT levels reach 3 times the upper limit of normal, a 3-month drug-free holiday should be initiated with reintroduction of the same drug at a lower dose or a different statin if levels return to baseline.[29]

Patients with FH who have a higher risk of CHD require more intensive drug therapy.[4,13]

Table 2
Lipid-lowering medications for use in familial hypercholesterolemia: statins

Statin	Dose Range (mg)	Mean Reduction LDL-C (%)	Pharmacologic and Safety Issues
Rosuvastatin	5–40	46–55	Dose reduction in renal insufficiency, Asian, and elderly patients
Atorvastatin	10–80	37–51	Minimal renal excretion CYP3A4 substrate
Simvastatin	5–80[a]	26–47	CYP3A4 substrate, dose reduction in severe renal insufficiency
Lovastatin	10–80	21–40	CYP3A4 substrate
Pravastatin	10–80	20–36	Dose reduction in severe renal insufficiency
Fluvastatin	20–80	22–35	Minimal renal excretion
Pitavastatin	1–4	32–43	Dose reduction in severe renal insufficiency

[a] Simvastatin 80-mg dosage should only be used in patients previously taking this dose for greater than 1 year and no other contraindications.

High-risk patients include those with the following:

- Clinically evident CHD or other atherosclerotic cardiovascular disease
- Diabetes
- Family history of very early CHD (<45 years in men and <55 years in women)
- Current smoking
- Two or more CHD risk factors
- High lipoprotein (a) (≥50 mg/dL)

In these patients, the LDL goal is less than 100 mg/dL and non-HDL goal is less than 130 mg/dL.

Combination Therapy

Many patients with FH will require more than one medication to obtain optimal LDL-C lowering. Patients may require multiple medications depending on their baseline LDL-C levels and their responsiveness to therapy. Drugs that can be added to statins for LDL-C reduction include ezetimibe, bile-acid sequestrants, and niacin (**Table 3**).

The addition of ezetimibe to a statin is the preferred approach in the treatment of patients with FH.[2,3,13,16] Some patients may require 3 or more medications to lower LDL-C adequately.

Fibrates are most useful for triglyceride lowering but may have some LDL-C lowering effect.

Ezetimibe, niacin, and bile acid sequestrants are also treatment options for drug intensification or for those intolerant of a statin; this should also be considered in FH patients who are not at very high risk when LDL-C does not decrease by 50% with statin monotherapy. It is important to note that doubling the dose of statin only achieves an additional LDL reduction by 6% to 7%.[30] Therefore, if additional reduction is needed, other medications should be added. Other options for those intolerant of statins include every-other-day statin therapy or lowering the dose while adding other treatment medications.

Table 3
Low-density lipoprotein–lowering drugs for familial hypercholesterolemia: nonstatins

Medication	Dose Range	Mean Reduction LDL-C (%)	Pharmacologic and Safety Issues
Ezetimibe	10 mg daily	15–20	Diarrhea, abdominal pain, myalgias
Bile acid sequestrants			
Colesevelam	3.75–4.375 g/d	15–18	Should be given with meals.
Colestipol	4–15 g bid	12–30	Side effects: constipation, abdominal
Cholestyramine	4–12 g bid	7–30	pain, bloating, nausea, flatulence
			Interference with absorption of other medications: warfarin, digoxin, thyroid hormone, thiazide diuretics, amiodarone, glipizide, statins (less with colesevelam)
Niacin	500–2000 mg daily	5–20	Side effects: flushing, pruritus, nausea, bloating, elevation of liver transaminases, hyperuricemia, and hyperglycemia
Fenofibrate (multiple preparations)	30–200 mg daily	0–20	Reduced dosage in renal insufficiency Side effects: abdominal pain, gastrointestinal, elevation of liver enzymes, myalgias, risk of rhabdomyolysis, increased creatinine

Drug interactions with statins are primarily due to cytochrome P450 metabolism, drug transporters, and glucuronidation; thus, caution should be used with medications metabolized by cytochrome P450 isoenzyme CYP 3A4.[31]

Ezetimibe is localized to the brush border of the small intestine and inhibits the absorption of cholesterol. It reduces LDL-C by about 15% to 20% when used alone and provides 20% additional reduction in combination with a statin.[32]

Bile acid sequestrants inhibit the enterohepatic reuptake and increase fecal loss of bile salts. They decrease LDL-C by preventing the reabsorption of bile acids in the terminal ileum. Because they are not absorbed systemically, they are considered safer to use than other cholesterol-lowering medications.[33] Like ezetimibe, the effect on LDL-C reduction can be additive with statins and even ezetimibe.[34] The need for suspensions or large numbers of pills, gastrointestinal side effects, and multiple drug-drug interactions limits patient adherence and use. Colesevelam, as compared with other bile acid sequestrants, has fewer gastrointestinal side effects and drug-drug interactions. Colesevelam is also approved for treatment of diabetes and may help patients achieve both glycemic and lipid goals.[35] Colesevelam is the recommended bile acid sequestrant for FH patients.[24]

Niacin, a water-soluble B vitamin, lowers LDL-C and raises HDL. It comes in crystalline and extended release forms. Because of concerns for liver toxicity, most nonprescription sustained release forms are not recommended.[24] The maximum dose of 2 g daily of niacin when added to statin is effective in lowering LDL-C.[24]

Fibrates lower triglycerides and raise HDL-C. Because of the increased risk of fibrate-induced myositis (particularly with gemfibrozil) with statins, they need to be used with caution.[31]

Women with FH who are of child-bearing age should be advised to use contraception while on therapy and to stop any statin (category X), niacin (category C), or ezetimibe (category C) therapy at least 4 weeks before stopping contraception.[24]

Those who become pregnant on therapy or are breastfeeding should be advised to discontinue therapy immediately. colesevelam is a category B drug and can used when clinically indicated.[24] For pregnant women with homozygous FH, or heterozygous FH and atherosclerotic disease, LDL apheresis should be considered.[13,24]

Low-Density Lipoprotein Apheresis

LDL apheresis is an important treatment modality for homozygous FH patients and for heterozygous patients who have not met treatment goals despite optimal tolerated medical therapy (**Box 5**).[24,36] It is an extracorporeal treatment that uses various methods to remove LDL from the circulation. LDL apheresis is currently FDA approved and has been shown in clinical trials to prevent and slow the progression of CHD.[13,37,38]

Apheresis is generally done every 1 to 2 weeks, with each session taking about 3 hours and removing greater than 60% of Apo-B-containing lipoproteins.[38] The LDL reduction with LDL apheresis is temporary and associated with a rebound elevation in lipid levels after the procedure. The efficacy of LDL apheresis can be enhanced by the addition of statin therapy. LDL apheresis treatment in homozygous FH patients has improved their life expectancy to more than 50 years.[38] Cost and limited availability decrease widespread use of LDL apheresis.

Homozygous Familial Hypercholesterolemia: Treatment Considerations

Treatment starts at the time of diagnosis and involves age-appropriate diet, statin, ezetimibe, and often apheresis.[3,13] The FDA has approved 2 novel treatments for

---

Box 5
Low-density lipoprotein apheresis recommendations (National Lipid Association and American College of Cardiology/American Heart Association cholesterol guideline)

LDL apheresis is recommended for the following patients

- LDL goal reduction has not been achieved despite diet and maximum drug therapy (after 6 months)
- Adequate drug therapy is not tolerated or contraindicated
- Functional homozygous FH patients with LDL-C 300 mg/DL or higher (or non-HDL cholesterol ≥330 mg/dL)
- Functional heterozygous FH patients with LDL-C 300 mg/dL or higher (or non-HDL ≥330 mg/dL) and 0–1 risk factors
- Functional heterozygous FH patients with LDL-C 200 mg/dL or higher (or non-HDL cholesterol ≥230 mg/dL) and with risk characteristics such as 2 or more risk factors or high lipoprotein (a) 50 mg/dL or higher
- Functional heterozygotes with LDL-C 160 mg/dL or higher (or non-HDL cholesterol ≥190 mg/dL) and very high-risk characteristics (established CHD, other cardiovascular disease, or diabetes).

Data from Ito M, McGowan M, Moriarty P. National Lipid Association Expert Panel on Familial Hypercholesterolemia. Management of familial hypercholesterolemias in adult patients: recommendations from the National Lipid Association Expert Panel on Familial Hypercholesterolemia. J Clin Lipidol 2011;5:S38–45; and Stone NJ, Robinson JG, Lichtenstein AH, et al. Report on the treatment of blood cholesterol to reduce atherosclerotic cardiovascular disease in adults: full panel report supplement. 2013. Available at: http://circ.ahajournals.org/content/suppl/2013/11/07/01.cir.0000437738.63853.7a.DC1/Blood_Cholesterol_Full_Panel_Report.docx. Accessed January 21, 2015.

homozygous FH individuals older than 18 years of age: lomitapide and mipomersen (**Table 4**).[39] Lomitapide also has European approval. Lomitapide is a microsomal triglyceride transfer (MTP) protein inhibitor available as a capsule and used as an adjunct to other cholesterol-lowering medications, lifestyle changes, and LDL apheresis if needed. The function of MTP, which resides in the lumen of endoplasmic reticulum of enterocytes and hepatocytes, is to assist in the transfer of triglycerides to apolipoprotein B to form very-low-density lipoprotein particles.[40] Lomitapide enabled some homozygous FH patients to discontinue or decrease the frequency of apheresis in some in a clinical trial.[41] Because of concerns about hepatotoxicity, prescription of lomitapide requires an FDA-approved Risk Evaluation and Mitigation Strategy (REMS) program.

Mipomersen is delivered by subcutaneous injection with weekly dosing. It is an antisense oligonucleotide that causes a reduction in LDL by binding to messenger RNA and inhibiting apolipoprotein B-100 synthesis.[42] LDL, apo B, and lipoprotein (a) concentrations are reduced.[43,44] Reported side effects include injection site reactions, flulike symptoms, increased ALT, and steatosis.[42–44] Thus, this medication also requires frequent monitoring of liver function tests and prescription approval via REMS.

SURGICAL THERAPY

For patients who do not achieve sufficient lipid reduction by the above-mentioned modalities, other potential treatment options include partial ileal bypass and liver transplantation. Liver transplantation produces a significant lowering of LDL-C by providing normal LDLRs. Liver transplantation is now used primarily in children with homozygous FH when apheresis is not an option or with concurrent heart transplantation.[13,45] Its use, however, is limited due to the risk of transplant surgery and the limited number of donor livers.[13,24,29] Partial ileal bypass is rarely used and works by interrupting enterohepatic bile acid circulation.[13,24]

Table 4					
Pharmacologic agents approved for homozygous familial hypercholesterolemia					
Treatment	Dosage	Mean Reduction LDL-C (%)	Drug Interactions	Safety Issues	Side Effects
Mipomersen	200 mg subcutaneously once per week	24–28	None	Increased hepatic transaminases Increased hepatic fat	Injection site reactions, pyrexia, malaise, fatigue, headache, nausea
Lomitapide	5 to 60 mg orally per day	38–50	Cytochrome p450 3A4 (atorvastatin)	Increased hepatic enzymes Increased hepatic fat Cytochrome p450 3A4 interactions	Diarrhea, gastrointestinal side effects Requires low-fat diet and supplemental fat-soluble vitamins

TREATMENT RESISTANCE/COMPLICATIONS
Side Effects of Medications

Statins and muscle problems

Statin side effects, particularly muscle complaints, are the limiting factors in their optimal usage. Muscle symptoms are the most common cause of statin discontinuation. They are typically dose dependent and can vary with the statin used. Statin-induced myopathy appears to be positively associated with the dose and potency of the statin.[23,46] Symptoms tend to occur more often with increasing age and number of medications, and decreasing renal function and body size. Management of statin-related myopathy can be difficult (**Box 6**).[23,46]

Statins and liver issues

Although liver toxicity from statins is often a concern for patients and physicians, it is not common, and serious hepatotoxicity is extremely rare. Hepatic aminotransferase elevation is usually mild and does not require discontinuation of the statin. It may be dose dependent.

Only about 1% of patients have aminotransferase increases to greater than 3 times the upper limit of normal, and the elevation often decreases even if patients continue on the statin. A common cause is hepatic steatosis, which responds to weight loss. Statins can be used cautiously in the presence of liver disease as long as it is not decompensated.[47] In particular, nonalcoholic fatty liver disease is not a contraindication. Hepatic transaminases should be obtained at baseline and during treatment if there is a clinical indication for their measurement.[23] Routine monitoring of hepatic transaminases was removed from product labeling by the FDA in 2012. If aminotransferases remain greater than 3 times the upper limit of normal, change to a different statin and identifying other contributing conditions or drugs should be considered.[48] Irreversible liver damage resulting from statins is extremely rare, with a rate of liver failure of 1 case per 1 million person-years of use.[49]

Clinical trials and meta-analyses have shown a small increase in the risk of diabetes with statin use. In most cases of FH, the benefits of statin treatment far outweigh this risk.[23]

Box 6
Approach to statin-related muscle problems

- Discontinue statin in patients who develop muscle symptoms until they can be evaluated. For severe symptoms, evaluate for rhabdomyolysis.

- For mild to moderate symptoms, evaluate for conditions increasing the risk of muscle symptoms, including renal or hepatic impairment, hypothyroidism, vitamin D deficiency, rheumatologic disorders, and primary muscle disorders

- Statin-induced myalgias are likely to resolve within 2 months of discontinuing the drug.

- If symptoms resolve, the same or lower dose of the statin can be reintroduced.

- If symptoms recur, use a low dose of a different statin and increase as tolerated.

- If the cause of symptoms is determined to be unrelated, restart the original statin.

Data from Stone NJ, Robinson J, Lichtenstein AH, et al. 2013 ACC/AHA guideline on the treatment of blood cholesterol to reduce atherosclerotic cardiovascular risk in adults: a report of the American College of Cardiology/American Heart Association Task Force on Practice Guidelines. J Am Coll Cardiol 2014;63(25 Pt B):2889–934; and Rosenson RS, Baker SK, Jacobson TA. An assessment by the Statin Muscle Safety Task Force: 2014 update. J Clin Lipidol 2014;8:S58–71.

DRUGS IN DEVELOPMENT

Drugs in development have the potential for additive effects with statins or other lipid-lowering medications to achieve further reduction of LDL-C.

The most promising new therapeutic approach for FH involves monoclonal antibodies to PCSK9. PCSK9 increases LDL-C by binding to the epidermal growth factor-like repeat A domain of the LDLR, causing LDL-receptor degradation, thus reducing the amount of LDL cleared from the plasma.[7] Gain-of-function mutations of PCSK9 result in elevation of LDL, whereas loss-of-function mutations lead to life-long low LDL levels and are associated with decreased risk of cardiovascular disease.[50] Given by subcutaneous injection once every 2 to 4 weeks, monoclonal antibodies that inhibit the binding of PCSK9 to LDLRs have produced 40% to 70% reductions of LDL-C in a variety of clinical situations, including FH.[51–55] Cardiovascular outcomes trials with several of these antibodies are in progress.

SUMMARY

FH is a serious and treatable condition with a significantly increased risk of cardiovascular disease. Its onset is in early childhood with resultant premature death if not treated adequately. FH is underdiagnosed and undertreated, and more effort needs to be made to effectively screen and diagnose these patients because early treatment is necessary to decrease morbidity and mortality to the same level as in the general population. Lifestyle and diet changes are necessary but generally insufficient, and patients should be started on moderate-potency and high-potency statin therapy as initial treatment. Combination therapy is required in many patients. LDL apheresis should be considered in heterozygous and homozygous FH patients who have insufficient response to medical therapy. Recent medications for treatment of homozygous FH patients have been approved with other new treatment options currently undergoing clinical trials.

REFERENCES

1. Hopkins P, Toth P, Ballantyne CM, et al. Familial hypercholesterolemias: prevalence, genetics, diagnosis and screening recommendations from the National Lipid Association Expert Panel on Familial Hypercholesterolemia. J Clin Lipidol 2011;5(3 Suppl):S9–17.
2. Nordestgaard B, Chapman M, Humphries S, et al. Familial hypercholesterolaemia is underdiagnosed and undertreated in the general population: guidance for clinicians to prevent coronary heart disease: consensus statement of the European Atherosclerosis Society. Eur Heart J 2013;34(45):3478–3490a.
3. Cuchel M, Bruckert E, Ginsberg H, et al. Homozygous familial hypercholesterolaemia: new insights and guidance for clinicians to improve detection and clinical management. A position paper from the Consensus Panel on Familial Hypercholesterolaemia of the European Atherosclerosis Society. Eur Heart J 2014;35(32):2146–57.
4. Robinson JG, Goldberg AC, National Lipid Association Expert Panel on Familial Hypercholesterolemia. Treatment of adults with familial hypercholesterolemia and evidence for treatment: recommendations from the National Lipid Association Expert Panel on Familial Hypercholesterolemia. J Clin Lipidol 2011;5(3 Suppl):S18–29.
5. Langer T, Strober W, Levy RI. The metabolism of low density lipoprotein in familial type II hyperlipoproteinemia. J Clin Invest 1972;51(6):1528–36.

6. Brown M, Goldstein J. A receptor-mediated pathway for cholesterol homeostasis. Science 1986;232(4746):34–47.
7. Abifadel M, Elbitar S, El Khoury P, et al. Living the PCSK9 adventure: from the identification of a new gene in familial hypercholesterolemia towards a potential new class of anticholesterol drugs. Curr Atheroscler Rep 2014;16(9):439.
8. Benn M, Watts GF, Tybjaerg-Hansen A, et al. Familial hypercholesterolemia in the Danish general population: prevalence, coronary artery disease, and cholesterol-lowering medication. J Clin Endocrinol Metab 2012;97(11):3956–64.
9. Sjouke B, Kusters D, Kindt I, et al. Homozygous autosomal dominant hypercholesterolaemia in the Netherlands: prevalence, genotype–phenotype relationship, and clinical outcome. Eur Heart J 2014. http://dx.doi.org/10.1093/eurheartj/ehu058.
10. Raal FJ, Santos RD. Homozygous familial hypercholesterolemia: current perspectives on diagnosis and treatment. Atherosclerosis 2012;223:262–8.
11. Goldberg A, Hopkins P, Toth P, et al, National Lipid Association Expert Panel on Familial Hypercholesterolemia. Familial hypercholesterolemia: screening, diagnosis and management of pediatric and adult patients: clinical guidance from the National Lipid Association Expert Panel on Familial Hypercholesterolemia. J Clin Lipidol 2011;5:S1–8.
12. Talmud PJ, Shah S, Whittall R, et al. Use of low-density lipoprotein cholesterol gene score to distinguish patients with polygenic and monogenic familial hypercholesterolaemia: a case-control study. Lancet 2013;381(9874):1293–301.
13. Watts GF, Gidding S, Wierzbicki AS, et al. Integrated guidance on the care of familial hypercholesterolemia from the International FH Foundation. J Clin Lipidol 2014;8:148–72.
14. Haase A, Goldberg A. Identification of people with heterozygous familial hypercholesterolemia. Curr Opin Lipidol 2012;23(4):282–9.
15. DeMott K, Nherera L, Shaw EJ, et al. Clinical guidelines and evidence review for familial hypercholesterolaemia: the identification and management of adults and children with familial hypercholesterolaemia. London: National Collaborating Centre for Primary Care and Royal College of General Practitioners; 2008.
16. Watts GF, Sullivan DR, Poplawski N, et al. Familial hypercholesterolaemia: a model of care for Australasia. Atheroscler Suppl 2011;12(2):221–63.
17. Daniels SR, Gidding SS, de Ferranti SD, National Lipid Association Expert Panel on Familial Hypercholesterolemia. Pediatric aspects of familial hypercholesterolemias: recommendations from the National Lipid Association Expert Panel on Familial Hypercholesterolemia. J Clin Lipidol 2011;5:S30–7.
18. Expert Panel on Integrated Guidelines for Cardiovascular Health and Risk Reduction in Children and Adolescents, National Heart, Lung, and Blood Institute. Expert panel on integrated guidelines for cardiovascular health and risk reduction in children and adolescents: summary report. Pediatrics 2011;128(Suppl 5):S213–56.
19. Williams RR, Hunt SC, Schumacher MC. Diagnosing heterozygous familial hypercholesterolemia using new practical criteria validated by molecular genetics. Am J Cardiol 1993;72(2):171–6.
20. World Health organization. Familial hypercholesterolaemia. Report of a second WHO consultation. Geneva (Switzerland): World Health Organization; 1999.
21. Neil A, Cooper J, Betteridge J, et al. Reductions in all-cause, cancer, and coronary mortality in statin-treated patients with heterozygous familial hypercholesterolaemia: a prospective registry study. Eur Heart J 2008;29:2625–33.

22. Versmissen J, Oosterveer DM, Yazdanpanah M, et al. Efficacy of statins in familial hypercholesterolaemia: a long term cohort study. BMJ 2008;337:a2423.

23. Stone NJ, Robinson J, Lichtenstein AH, et al. 2013 ACC/AHA guideline on the treatment of blood cholesterol to reduce atherosclerotic cardiovascular risk in adults: a report of the American College of Cardiology/American Heart Association Task Force on Practice Guidelines. J Am Coll Cardiol 2014;63(25 Pt B): 2889–934.

24. Ito M, McGowan M, Moriarty P, National Lipid Association Expert Panel on Familial Hypercholesterolemia. Management of familial hypercholesterolemias in adult patients: recommendations from the National Lipid Association Expert Panel on Familial Hypercholesterolemia. J Clin Lipidol 2011;5:S38–45.

25. Raal FJ, Pilcher GJ, Panz VR, et al. Reduction in mortality in subjects with homozygous familial hypercholesterolemia associated with advances in lipid-lowering therapy. Circulation 2011;124:2202–7.

26. Forrester J. Redefining normal low-density lipoprotein cholesterol: a strategy to unseat coronary disease as the nation's leading killer. J Am Coll Cardiol 2010; 56(8):630–6.

27. Wiegman A, Hutten BA, de Groot EE. Efficacy and safety of statin therapy in children with familial hypercholesterolemia: a randomized controlled trial. JAMA 2004;292(3):331–7.

28. McCrindle BW, Urbina EM, Dennison BA, et al. Drug therapy of high-risk lipid abnormalities in children and adolescents: a scientific statement from the American Heart Association Atherosclerosis, Hypertension, and Obesity in Youth Committee, Council of Cardiovascular Disease in the Young, with the Council on Cardiovascular Nursing. Circulation 2007;115:1948–67.

29. Varghese M. Familial hypercholesterolemia. A review. Ann Pediatr Cardiol 2014; 7(2):107–17.

30. Jones P, Davidson M, Stein E, et al. Comparison of the efficacy and safety of rosuvastatin versus atorvastatin, simvastatin, and pravastatin across doses (STELLAR* Trial). Am J Cardiol 2003;92(2):152–60.

31. Kellick KA, Bottorff M, Toth PP. A clinician's guide to statin drug-drug interactions. J Clin Lipidol 2014;8:S30–46.

32. Gagne C, Gaudet D, Bruckert E, et al. Efficacy and safety of ezetimibe coadministered with atorvastatin or simvastatin in patients with homozygous familial hypercholesterolemia. Circulation 2002;105(21):2469–75.

33. Insull W Jr. Clinical utility of bile acid sequestrants in the treatment of dyslipidemia: a scientific review. South Med J 2006;99:257–73.

34. Huijgen R, Abbink E, Bruckert E, et al. Colesevelam added to combination therapy with a statin and ezetimibe in patients with familial hypercholesterolemia: a 12-week, multicenter, randomized, double-blind, controlled trial. Clin Ther 2010; 32(4):615–25.

35. Zieve F, Kalin M, Schwartz S, et al. Results of the glucose-lowering effect of WelChol study (GLOWS): a randomized, double-blind, placebo-controlled pilot study evaluating the effect of colesevelam hydrochloride on glycemic control in subjects with type 2 diabetes. Clin Ther 2007;29(1):74–83.

36. Stone, NJ, Robinson JG, Lichtenstein AH, et al. Report on the Treatment of blood cholesterol to reduce atherosclerotic cardiovascular disease in adults: full panel report supplement. 2013. Available at: http://circ.ahajournals.org/content/suppl/2013/11/07/01.cir.0000437738.63853.7a.DC1/Blood_Cholesterol_Full_Panel_Report.docx. Accessed January 21, 2015.

37. Thompson G. LDL apheresis. Atherosclerosis 2003;167(1):1–13.

38. Thompson GR, Catapano A, Saheb S, et al. Severe hypercholesterolaemia: therapeutic goals and eligibility criteria for LDL apheresis in Europe. Curr Opin Lipidol 2010;21(6):492–8.

39. Rader D, Kastelein J. Lomitapide and mipomersen: two first-in-class drugs for reducing low-density lipoprotein cholesterol in patients with homozygous familial hypercholesterolemia. Circulation 2014;129(9):1022–32.

40. Cuchel M, Bloedon L, Szapary P, et al. Inhibition of microsomal triglyceride transfer protein in familial hypercholesterolemia. N Engl J Med 2007;356:148–56.

41. Cuchel M, Meagher EA, du Toit Theron H, et al. Efficacy and safety of a microsomal triglyceride transfer protein inhibitor in patients with homozygous familial hypercholesterolaemia: a single-arm, open-label, phase 3 study. Lancet 2013; 381:40–6.

42. Stein E, Dufour R, Gagne C, et al. Apolipoprotein B synthesis inhibition with mipomersen in heterozygous familial hypercholesterolemia: results of a randomized, double-blind, placebo-controlled trial to assess efficacy and safety as add-on therapy in patients with coronary artery disease. Circulation 2012; 126(19):2283–92.

43. Raal FJ, Santos RD, Blom DJ, et al. Mipomersen, an apolipoprotein B synthesis inhibitor, for lowering of LDL cholesterol concentrations in patients with homozygous familial hypercholesterolaemia: a randomized, double-blind, placebo-controlled trial. Lancet 2010;375(9719):998–1006.

44. McGowan M, Tardif J, Ceska R, et al. Randomized, placebo-controlled trial of mipomersen in patients with severe hypercholesterolemia receiving maximally tolerated lipid-lowering therapy. PloS ONE 2012;7:e49006.

45. Palacio CH, Harring TR, Nguyen NT, et al. Homozygous familial hypercholesterolemia: case series and review of the literature. Case Rep Transplant 2011; 2011:154908.

46. Rosenson RS, Baker SK, Jacobson TA. An assessment by the statin muscle safety task force: 2014 update. J Clin Lipidol 2014;8:S58–71.

47. Herrick C, Litvin M, Goldberg AC. Lipid lowering in liver and chronic kidney disease. Best Pract Res Clin Endocrinol Metab 2014;28:339–52.

48. Bays H, Cohen DE, Chalasani N, et al. An assessment by the statin liver safety task force: 2014 update. J Clin Lipidol 2014;8:S47–57.

49. Cohen DE, Anania FA, Chalasani N. An assessment of statin safety by hepatologists. Am J Cardiol 2006;97:77C–81C.

50. Cohen JC, Boerwinkle E, Mosley TH Jr, et al. Sequence variations in PCSK9, low LDL, and protection against coronary heart disease. N Engl J Med 2006;354: 1264–72.

51. Stein EA, Raal F. Reduction of low-density lipoprotein cholesterol by monoclonal antibody inhibition of PCSK9. Annu Rev Med 2014;65:417–31.

52. Stein EA, Honarpour N, Wasserman SM, et al. Effect of the proprotein convertase subtilisin/kexin 9 monoclonal antibody, AMG 145, in homozygous familial hypercholesterolemia. Circulation 2013;128(19):2113–20.

53. Stein E, Mellis S, Yancopoulos G, et al. Effect of a monoclonal antibody to PCSK9 on LDL cholesterol. N Engl J Med 2012;366:1108–18.

54. Raal F, Scott R, Somaratne R, et al. Low-density lipoprotein cholesterol-lowering effects of AMG 145, a monoclonal antibody to proprotein convertase subtilisin/ kexin type 9 serine protease in patients with heterozygous familial hypercholesterolemia: the Reduction of LDL-C with PCSK9 Inhibition in Heterozygous Familial Hypercholesterolemia Disorder (RUTHERFORD) randomized trial. Circulation 2012;126(20):2408–17.

55. Stein EA, Gipe D, Bergeron J, et al. Effect of a monoclonal antibody to PCSK9, REGN727/SAR236553, to reduce low-density lipoprotein cholesterol in patients with heterozygous familial hypercholesterolaemia on stable statin dose with or without ezetimibe therapy: a phase 2 randomised controlled trial. Lancet 2012; 380(9836):29–36.

New Therapies for Reducing Low-Density Lipoprotein Cholesterol

Evan A. Stein, MD, PhD[a],*, Frederick J. Raal, MBBCh, MMED, PhD[b]

KEYWORDS

- LDL cholesterol • Apo B antisense • MTP inhibitors • PCSK9 inhibitors

KEY POINTS

- Although the past 4 decades have probably been the most fruitful and productive in transitioning from a low-density lipoprotein (LDL) cholesterol hypothesis to demonstration of clinical benefit, cardiovascular disease still remains the major cause of mortality and morbidity in industrialized societies.
- Cardiovascular disease is rapidly becoming the major cause of morbidity and mortality in recently industrializing countries, like India and China, that together constitute nearly half the world's population.
- It is fortunate that most of the most effective lipid-lowering drugs, the statins, have become, or will soon become, generic and inexpensive.
- There remains a large unmet medical need for new and effective agents that are also well tolerated and safe, especially for patients unable to either tolerate statins or achieve optimal LDL-C on current therapies.

INTRODUCTION

It is now nearly 3 decades since the first HMG CoA reductase inhibitor ("statin") was approved for general use on September 1, 1987, to lower low-density lipoprotein cholesterol (LDL-C).[1] Since that time, the statins have become the cornerstone and mainstay of guidelines in every country to reduce cardiovascular disease.[2–5] Large placebo or comparator trials have clearly demonstrated that statins significantly and substantially reduce morbidity and mortality of all forms of atherosclerotic disease, especially coronary heart disease (CHD) and stroke, no matter what the starting levels of LDL-C and the underlying absolute risk of CHD in the population in the trial.[6] As more effective statins have been developed and approved, with the most effective

This article originally appeared in Endocrinology and Metabolism Clinics, Volume 43, Issue 4, December 2014.

[a] Metabolic and Atherosclerosis Research Center, 5355 Medpace Way, Cincinnati, OH 45227, USA; [b] Department of Medicine, Faculty of Health Sciences, University of the Witwatersrand, 7 York Road, Parktown, Johannesburg 2193, South Africa
* Corresponding author.
E-mail address: esteinmrl@aol.com

of these agents at its highest dose reducing LDL-C by 55% on average, associated CHD outcome trials also have been carried out to show that the lower LDL-C levels attained are associated with lower CHD events.[7,8] The initial statins started becoming available as generic formulations in late 2001, with the major selling agents, simvastatin becoming generic in 2006 and atorvastatin in 2011.[9,10] The last remaining major and most effective statin, rosuvastatin, became generic in a number of countries, such as Canada and Brazil in 2012, and will do so in the United States in 2016 and in Europe a year later.[11] Thus, with generic atorvastatin even at its highest dose now costing less than a cup of coffee a week, even without insurance coverage,[12] and being able to achieve LDL-C reductions on average of 50%, new LDL-C–lowering agents are, and will in the future, be confined to specific situations in which statins are either not tolerated, are contraindicated, or cannot on their own achieve optimal LDL-C reductions.

Patients unable to tolerate statins, effective doses of statins, or achieve optimal control despite statins, currently have limited options that achieve LDL-C–lowering efficacy even in the range of the less effective statins of 2 decades ago. Among the alternative agents are the cholesterol absorption transport inhibitor, ezetimibe, extended release (ER) niacin, bile acid sequestrants, and fibrates. However, these agents reduce LDL-C only by 12% to 18%, may be associated with significant adverse events, and in recent outcome trials have not been shown to further reduce CHD events when added to statins.[13–16]

Therefore, the need for new or additional LDL-C–lowering agents can be summarized as follows (**Box 1**):

1. The largest need is in the large and growing number of statin-adverse patients,[17] in whom there are limited alternatives to achieving significant LDL-C reductions if even low-dose or intermittent-dose statin can be tolerated.[18] During the first 2 decades of statin development and use, the concern for statin toxicity was the severe and life-threatening, although rare, rhabdomyolysis. However, as statin use has grown to tens of millions of the population and extended to primary prevention in high-risk individuals, there has been more attention paid to milder nonspecific myalgias, and other muscle-related side effects (MRSE), as these symptoms are an impediment to maintaining successful long-term lipid-lowering therapy in everyday medical practice. The magnitude of the problem has recently been more fully addressed[19] and estimated to be 5% to 10% of statin-treated patients. With more

---

Box 1
Unmet medical needs for new effective, well-tolerated, and safe low-density lipoprotein-cholesterol (LDL-C)–lowering agents

1. Severe hypercholesterolemia: Despite reduction of 50%–60% with high-dose efficacious stains and ezetimibe, many of the millions of patients with autosomal dominant forms of elevated LDL-C still do not reach optimal levels.

2. Statin intolerance: Although only approximately 5%–10% of patients requiring statins cannot tolerate them, or high enough doses, this constitutes many millions of actual patients.

3. Lower is better: Based on evidence-based clinical trials involving more than 170,000 patients, greater LDL-C reduction results in greater cardiovascular disease (CVD) risk reduction.

4. Treatment guidelines: The overwhelming majority of countries recommend LDL-C treatment goals in patients with high-risk and very high risk CVD, which are often not attainable with current therapies.

than 20 million patients in the United States alone requiring statin therapy or more than a 35% reduction in LDL-C, there are a projected 1 to 2 million patients who will complain of statin side effects and therefore need effective nonstatin LDL-C lowering.

2. There are populations with more severe elevations of LDL-C, such as autosomal dominant hypercholesterolemia (ADH), where most do not achieve optimal levels of LDL-C, despite reductions of 50% to 65% achievable by combining the highest dose of the most effective statins and ezetimibe.[20,21] Recent revisions from 1 in 500 to 1 in 250, based on genetic screening, to the previously thought prevalence of ADH has also further highlighted the unmet need in this population.[22]

3. Pooled analysis by the Cholesterol Treatment Trialists' Collaborators (CTTC) from 27 trials of statin versus placebo or more versus less statin, with 174,149 randomized patients, showed a reduction in the 5-year incidence of major coronary events, coronary revascularizations, and ischemic strokes by approximately 20% for every 40-mg/dL reduction in LDL-C. In addition, greater reductions in LDL-C obtained with more intensive statin regimens further reduced the incidence of major vascular events.[6] Based on this large body of evidence, clinical practice guidelines, with the recent exception of those from the American Heart Association/American College of Cardiology have recommended lower LDL-C goals, currently less than 70 mg/dL, in high-risk patients with CHD.[2–5]

This review describes a number of agents either recently approved or currently in advanced large-scale trials that produce sufficient LDL-C reduction to potentially meet the current unmet needs outlined previously.

LOW-DENSITY LIPOPROTEIN CHOLESTEROL LOWERING AGENTS RECENTLY APPROVED

Although statins increase removal of LDL-C from the circulation, depending to a significant extent on the LDL receptor, an alternative approach is to decrease apolipoprotein (Apo) B containing lipoprotein formation and/or release from the liver and/or the intestines (**Fig. 1**). If inhibition is selective for hepatic Apo B (B_{100}) lipoprotein formation, then very low density lipoprotein (VLDL), intermediate density lipoprotein (IDL), and LDL will be prevented from entering the circulation. If inhibition is nonspecific, then in addition to reduction in B_{100} lipoprotein formation, there will be reductions in Apo B_{48} containing lipoproteins, chylomicrons, and remnants. The 2 current approaches are selective inhibition of hepatic Apo B_{100} synthesis with gene silencing antisense technology and nonselective inhibition of lipidation of Apo B_{100} and B_{48} lipoproteins by the enzyme microsomal triglyceride transport protein (MTP).[23] Mipomersen, an Apo B antisense drug, and lomitapide, an MTP inhibitor, have both recently been approved in the United States by the Food and Drug Administration (FDA) solely for the treatment of homozygous familial hypercholesterolemia (HoFH), although they carry black box warnings about significant side effects (**Table 1**) and are prescribed only under a risk evaluation and mitigation strategy (REMS) program (**Table 2**).[24,25]

Apolipoprotein B Antisense (Mipomersen)

The principle for inhibiting hepatic Apo B_{100} production is shown in **Fig. 2**. Briefly, as for all protein synthesis the process is initiated from deoxyribonucleic acid (DNA), which consists of 2 strands, one representing the "sense" genetic code sequence, and the other strand, containing complementary base pairs, is the "antisense" coding. During transcription, the "sense" and "antisense" strands separate, and the "antisense" strand serves as a template for the next step, which is to produce a single-stranded messenger ribonucleic acid (mRNA). The mRNA also has a base-pairing

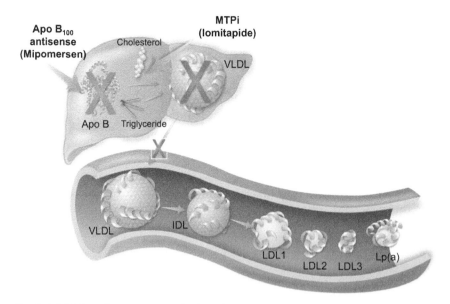

Fig. 1. Inhibition of Apo B100 synthesis and MTP activity. Apo B-100 is an important structural and functional component of lipoproteins. Inhibiting Apo B100 production reduces VLDL, IDL, LDL, and Lp(a) production. MTP is an enzyme required for lipidation of Apo B100 and B48 for formation of VLDL in liver and chylomicrons in gut. Inhibiting MTP reduces hepatic VLDL, IDL, LDL, and intestinal chylomicron formation and remnant production. (*Adapted from* Brautbar A, Ballantyne CM. Pharmacological strategies for lowering LDL cholesterol: statins and beyond. Nat Rev Cardiol 2011;8:253–265; and Parhofer KG. Mipomersen: evidence-based review of its potential in the treatment of homozygous and severe heterozygous familial hypercholesterolemia. Core Evid 2012;7:29–38.)

matching the DNA antisense and is also termed "sense." On reaching the cytosol, ribosomes translate the mRNA to produce proteins, in this case Apo B. By developing agents with RNase activity that will degrade a specific mRNA, it has been possible to impair translation of the downstream protein (see **Fig. 2**). Mipomersen thus binds by Watson and Crick base-pairing and is complementary to a 20-nucleotide segment of the coding region for the mRNA for Apo B. This selective hybridization/binding to its cognate mRNA results in the RNase H-mediated degradation of the Apo B message and inhibits Apo B protein synthesis.[23]

A potential advantage of antisense drugs is their increased specificity for the liver and thus they are best used to inhibit proteins that are predominantly made in the liver, such as Apo B and a number of other proteins important in lipid metabolism, such as Apo CIII, the "small a" component of lipoprotein (a) (Lp(a)), and proprotein convertase subtilisin/kexin type 9 (PCSK9).

All antisense drugs developed to date have been of single-strand antisense nucleotide sequences that are complementary to mRNA, called antisense oligonucleotides or ASOs. The tissue levels are predictable from plasma concentrations, where they are 90% protein bound, and correlate well with the pharmacology of ASOs. They disappear from the bloodstream rapidly but remain in tissue for prolonged periods, often months.

ASOs are generally 20 base-pairs long and behave stably and predictably irrespective of sequence. Mipomersen (ISIS 301012) is the nonadecasodium salt of a 20-base (20-mer) phosphorothioate oligonucleotide. Each of the 19 internucleotide

Table 1
Food and Drug Administration required "boxed warning" for lomitapide and mipomersen regarding risk of hepatotoxicity

Concern	Lomitapide	Mipomersen
Hepatic transaminases	Can cause elevations; 34% of patients in the phase 3 trial had at least one elevation in ALT or AST $\geq$3 times ULN.	Can cause elevations; 12% of patients in the phase 3 trial treated compared with 0% of the placebo-treated group had at least one elevation in ALT $\geq$3 times ULN.
Bilirubin, INR, and alkaline phosphatase	No concomitant clinically meaningful elevations.	No concomitant clinically meaningful elevations.
Hepatic fat	Increases hepatic fat, with or without concomitant increases in transaminases. The median absolute increase in hepatic fat was 6% after both 26 and 78 wk of treatment, from 1% at baseline, measured by magnetic resonance spectroscopy.	Increases hepatic fat, with or without concomitant increases in transaminases. In trials with heterozygous FH, the median absolute increase in hepatic fat was 10% after 26 wk of treatment, from 0% at baseline, measured by magnetic resonance imaging.
Hepatic steatosis	Treatment may be a risk factor for progressive liver disease, including steatohepatitis and cirrhosis.	Hepatic steatosis is a risk factor for advanced liver disease, including steatohepatitis and cirrhosis.
Monitoring recommendations	Measure ALT, AST, alkaline phosphatase, and total bilirubin before initiating treatment and then ALT and AST regularly as recommended. During treatment, adjust the dose if the ALT or AST are $\geq$3 times ULN. Discontinue the drug for clinically significant liver toxicity.	Measure ALT, AST, alkaline phosphatase, and total bilirubin before initiating treatment and then ALT and AST regularly as recommended. During treatment, withhold the dose if the ALT or AST are $\geq$3 times ULN. Discontinue the drug for clinically significant liver toxicity.

Abbreviations: ALT, alanine aminotransferase; AST, aspartate aminotransferase; FH, familial hyper-cholesterolemia; INR, international normalized ratio; ULN, upper limit of normal.

linkages is a $3'$-O to $5'$-O phosphorothioate diester. Ten of the 20 sugar residues are 2-deoxy-D-ribose; the remaining 10 are 2-O-(2-methoxyethyl)-D-ribose (MOE). The residues are arranged such that 5 MOE nucleosides at the $5'$ and $3'$ ends of the molecule flank a gap of ten $2'$-deoxynucleosides.[23] Each of the 9 cytosine bases is methylated at the 5-position (MeC). The $2'$-methoxyethyl-5-methyluridine ($2'$-MOE MeU) nucleosides are also designated as $2'$-methoxyethylribothymidine ($2'$-MOE T) and are also termed "second-generation" ASOs. The molecular formula of mipomersen is $C_{230}H_{305}N_{67}O_{122}P_{19}S_{19}Na_{19}$, and the molecular weight is 7594.9 amu.

Mipomersen is the only Apo B antisense drug to have entered clinical development and progressed to approval for any clinical use. Mipomersen is metabolized by nucleases, both endonucleases and exonucleases, and the fragments are excreted in the urine.

Drug-drug interaction is minimal, as there is no CYP 450 metabolism and studies have shown essentially no interaction with statins or ezetimibe.[26] Mipomersen is poorly

Table 2
Risk evaluation and mitigation strategy (REMS) requirements for lomitapide and mipomersen: common features

I. Goals

To educate prescribers about the following:	a. The risk of hepatotoxicity associated with the drugs.
	b. The need to monitor patients as per product labeling.
	c. Restricting access to patients with a clinical or laboratory diagnosis consistent with homozygous familial hypercholesterolemia (HoFH).

II. REMS elements

A. Elements to ensure safe use

1. Health care providers (HCPs) who prescribe are specially certified	a. To become specially certified, prescribers must enroll in the drug's REMS program and complete the following:
	i. Review the prescribing information.
	ii. Reviewing the materials or module in the REMS Prescriber Education and Enrollment Kit.
	iii. Complete, sign and submit the prescriber enrollment form.
	b. The drug company will
	i. Ensure REMS Prescriber Education and Enrollment Kit or Training Module and prescriber enrollment form are on REMS Web site or a coordinating center.
	ii. Ensure that HCPs complete training and enrollment form before activating prescribers' certification.
	iii. Inform prescribers of substantive changes to REMS program.
	iv. Communicate information to HCPs and specific professional associations through their REMS program Web site and *Dear Healthcare Provider* and *Dear Professional Association* letters.
2. The drug will be dispensed only by specially certified pharmacies.	a. The company will ensure that the drug will be dispensed only by certified pharmacies.
	b. To be certified, the pharmacy representative must agree to the following:
	i. To educate all pharmacy staff involved on the drug's REMS program requirements.
	ii. Put processes and procedures in place to verify that
	1. The prescriber is certified in REMS program.
	2. The drug's REMS prescription authorization form is received for each NEW prescription.
	iii. To be audited to ensure that all processes and procedures are in place and are being followed for the REMS Program.
	iv. To provide prescription data to the REMS program.
3. The drug will be dispensed only with evidence or documentation of safe-use conditions.	a. To patients whose prescribers are certified in the REMS Program and *attest* on the REMS prescription authorization form that
	i. They understand that the drug is indicated as an adjunct to lipid-lowering medications and diet to reduce LDL-C and Apo B in patients with *HoFH*;
	ii. Affirm that their patient has a clinical or laboratory diagnosis consistent with *HoFH*;
	iii. They understand that the drug has not, or has not been adequately, studied in patients <18 y of age; and
	iv. Liver function tests have been obtained as directed in the prescribing information.

(continued on next page)

Table 2 (continued)	

B. Implementation system	a. The companies will ensure that their drug is distributed to and dispensed only by certified pharmacies.
	b. The companies will maintain, monitor, and evaluate the implementation of their REMS program.
	  i. Develop and follow written procedures and scripts to implement the REMS.
	  ii. Maintain a secure, validated database of all certified prescribers and pharmacies that is in compliance with 21 CFR Part 11 regulations.
	  iii. Send confirmation of certification to each certified pharmacy.
	  iv. Maintain a REMS program coordinating center with a call center to support patients, prescribers, and pharmacies.
	  v. Ensure materials listed in their REMS program will be available on a Web site or from a REMS program coordinating center.
	  vi. Update all affected materials and notify enrolled prescribers and certified pharmacies if there are substantive changes to the REMS or REMS program.
	  vii. Monitor and audit the certified pharmacies and institute corrective action if noncompliance is found.

C. Timetable for submission of assessments	Companies will submit REMS assessments to the Food and Drug Administration at 6 mo, 12 mo, and annually thereafter from the date of initial approval.

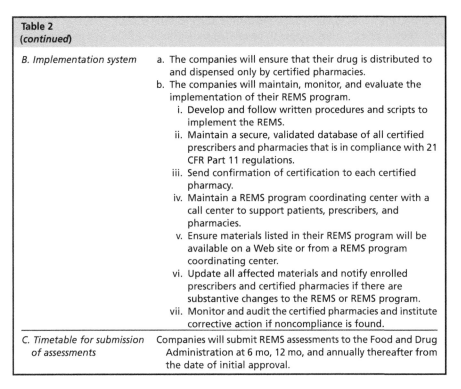

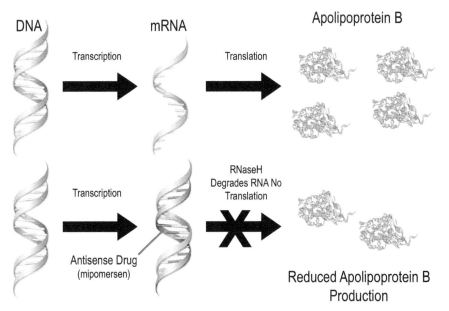

Fig. 2. Mechanism of action: antisense oligonucleotide to reduce hepatic Apo B100 synthesis. (*Adapted from* Goldberg AC. Novel therapies and new targets of treatment for familial hypercholesterolemia. J Clin Lipidol 2010;4(5):353; with permission.)

absorbed from the intestinal tract and is thus administered subcutaneously.[23] Side effects seen in clinical trials appear to be related mostly to the ASOs, and to the mechanism of action: predominantly injection site reactions and liver enzyme elevation.[23]

Mipomersen, and the resultant LDL-C reduction, take up to 6 months to achieve steady state. In early dose-ranging studies[26] carried out in patients with moderately elevated LDL-C on diet alone, mipomersen at dosages of 50, 100, 200, 300, and 400 mg were administered weekly and demonstrated a progressive dose-response–related reduction in LDL-C and Apo B reaching nearly 70% at the 400-mg per week dosage after 12 weeks.[26] Consistent with the long period required to achieve maximal and stable LDL-C reductions, these reductions were sustained even 90 days after cessation of treatment.

Phase 1 and 2 studies performed in patients with heterozygous (He) FH[27] and HoFH[23] in which mipomersen was added to current and maximal lipid therapy showed robust dose-related and time-related reductions in Apo B, triglycerides, non–high-density lipoprotein (HDL)-C and Lp(a) with no significant changes seen in HDL-C or Apo A1. Based on the phase 2 trials, a mipomersen dosage of 200 mg per week was selected for longer and larger phase 3 trials in HeFH[28] and HoFH.[29]

The phase 3 HeFH trial was double-blind, placebo-controlled, and randomized 124 adult patients with coronary artery disease (CAD) on maximally tolerated statin and LDL-C $\geq$100 mg/dL to mipomersen 200 mg subcutaneously (SC) weekly or placebo (2:1) for 26 weeks. A total of 114 patients, 41/41 on placebo and 73/81 on mipomersen, completed treatment. LDL-C, the primary end point, reduced by a mean (95% confidence interval [CI]) of 28.0% (–34.0% to –22.1%) with mipomersen and increased by 5.2% (–0.5%–10.9%) with placebo, $P<.001$. Mipomersen similarly and significantly reduced Apo B and Apo B containing lipoproteins including Lp(a).[28]

The definitive trial in 51 patients with HoFH, which resulted in the FDA granting marketing approval as an orphan drug for HoFH, was the largest randomized, double-blind, and placebo-controlled trial in this patient population.[29] Seventeen patients were randomized to placebo and 34 to mipomersen 200 mg SC weekly for 26 weeks. Baseline LDL-C concentrations were 400 mg/dL and 439 mg/dL, respectively. Mipomersen treatment resulted in mean (95% CI) LDL-C reductions of 24.7% (–31.6 to –17.7%) compared with a decrease of 3.3% (–12.1%–5.5%) with placebo ($P<.001$), as shown in **Table 3**. Significant ($P<.001$) reductions also were observed

---

Table 3
Comparative[a] efficacy on LDL-C and other lipoproteins in homozygous FH between microsomal triglyceride transport protein inhibitor (lomitapide), Apo B_{100} antisense inhibitor (mipomersen), and PCSK9 inhibitor (evolocumab)

Parameter	Lomitapide (%)[23,93]	Mipomersen (%)[29]	Evolocumab (%)[80]
LDL-C[b]	−40.1	−21.3	−30.9
Apo B[b]	−39	−24.3	−23.1
Lp(a)[c]	−13.4	−23.2	−11.8
HDL-C[b]	−6.9	+11.2	0
Apo A1[b]	−6.5	+3.9	Not done

Abbreviations: Apo, apolipoprotein; FH, familial hypercholesterolemia; HDL-C, high-density lipoprotein cholesterol; LDL-C, low-density lipoprotein cholesterol; PCSK9, proprotein convertase subtilisin/kexin type 9.
[a] Based on ITT (intent to treat) analysis and primary/secondary end points from 26-week trials.
[b] Mean % change (vs placebo for mipomersen and evolocumab, from baseline for lomitapide).
[c] Median % change.
Data from Refs.[23,29,80,93]

for Apo B (–27%) and Lp(a) (–31%) and HDL-C increased 15% in the mipomersen group (P = .035).[29]

Safety and tolerability
The most common adverse events in all trials were injection site reactions, being twice as frequent with mipomersen than placebo in the HeFH trial and 3 times as frequent in patients with HoFH.[28,29] Additional clinically important side effects included flulike symptoms.[23] The most common laboratory findings related to liver function tests: in the HoFH trial, increases of 3 or more times upper limit of normal (ULN) in hepatic transaminases, occurred in 12% of mipomersen-treated patients versus none in the placebo group. In the HeFH trial, hepatic transaminase elevations of 3 or more times ULN occurred in 14.5% mipomersen patients compared with 2.4% on placebo, and in 6.0% of those treated with mipomersen these elevations were confirmed 1 week or more later, whereas none were sustained in placebo patients. One mipomersen-treated patient had maximal alanine aminotransferase of 10 or more times ULN.[28] No patient met Hy's law. A small study had previously demonstrated minimal increases in hepatic triglyceride content as measured by magnetic resonance spectroscopy over 15 weeks of treatment[30]; however, in the phase 3 HeFH trial of 26 weeks, more marked and more frequent hepatitis steatosis was seen with mipomersen.[28] In none of the trials was mipomersen observed to have adverse effects on blood pressure, renal function (serum creatinine, estimated glomerular filtration rate), muscle (myalgia, CK elevation), glucose homeostasis, or platelet count. In the HeFH study, serious adverse events were reported in 4.9% of placebo (CAD and supraventricular tachycardia) and 7.2% of mipomersen-treated patients (basal cell carcinoma, angina pectoris, acute myocardial infarction, chest pain, pulmonary embolism, and noncardiac chest pain). In the HoFH study, serious adverse events were reported in 5.9% in both the placebo and mipomersen groups.

Longer-term and larger studies are needed to determine whether hepatic steatosis will become self-limiting or clinically significant and result in hepatic damage. To address this, "A Study of the Safety and Efficacy of Two Different Regimens of Mipomersen in Patients With Familial Hypercholesterolemia and Inadequately Controlled Low-Density Lipoprotein Cholesterol (FOCUS FH)" commenced in 2011.[31]

Summary
Treatment with mipomersen has been approved only in the United States and is confined to use in HoFH under a strict REMS program (see **Table 2**). The marketing application for HoFH has been submitted in Europe but in December 2012, the Europe Medicines Agency's Committee for Medicinal Products for Human Use (CHMP) rejected the application out of concern that for a drug intended for lifelong use, a high percentage of even homozygous FH patients stopped taking the medicine within 2 years. The CHMP also expressed reservations as to the potential long-term consequences of elevated hepatic transaminases associated with hepatic steatosis and the risk of irreversible liver damage. Along with slightly more cardiovascular events in the mipomersen-treated arms compared with placebo, the agency, at that point in time, felt the benefits of mipomersen did not outweigh its risks and recommended that it be refused marketing authorization.[32] Mipomersen was resubmitted in early 2013 but was again rejected, as the CHMP stated their concerns remained unresolved.[33]

Even though the elevated hepatic transaminases do not appear to reflect drug toxicity and are likely mechanism related from hepatic triglyceride accumulation, this does present a concern for long-term, usually lifelong, therapy. The larger and longer FOCUS FH trial, currently in progress, should provide additional safety information along with information on clinical events.[31] Presumably this will also allow reevaluation by the European agency for homozygous FH. However, even with this information, it is highly unlikely that the use of mipomersen will ever extend to patients without HoFH.

Microsomal Triglyceride Transfer Protein Inhibitors

Microsomal triglyceride transport protein (MTP) is a heterodimeric lipid transfer protein that is localized in the endoplasmic reticulum of hepatocytes and enterocytes and plays a critical role in lipidation of both hepatic Apo B_{100} and intestinal Apo B_{48} (see **Fig. 1**) to form lipoproteins that are then released into the circulation. Without MTP, the formation of chylomicrons, VLDL and their downstream lipoproteins including remnants, IDL, and LDL does not occur.

Inhibition of MTP became a potential therapeutic target following the discovery in 1992 by Wetterau and others[34] of MTP deficiency as the cause of a rare inherited disorder associated with very low levels of LDL-C, called abetalipoproteinemia. Abetalipoproteinemia is also characterized by fat malabsorption, steatorrhea, hepatic steatosis,[35] and neurologic disorders due to the very low levels of Apo B_{48}-containing lipoproteins that transport vitamin E and other lipid-soluble vitamins.[36]

The first MTP inhibitor studied in humans, implitapide (BAY 13-9952), demonstrated significant effects on both hepatic and intestinal lipoproteins within 10 days of exposure.[37] By the early 2000s there were 2 systemic compounds in development: implitapide from Bayer and lomitapide (BMS-201038) from Bristol-Myers Squibb.[38]

Following a large phase 2 trial in Europe with implitapide, the gastrointestinal side effects and hepatic transaminase elevations resulted in Bayer abandoning further development of their compound.[39]

BMS-201038 (lomitapide) was reported in a 7-day multiple ascending-dose, phase-1 study to produce large reductions in LDL-C, ranging from 54% to 86% with doses of 25 to 100 mg per day.[40] A similar effect was seen with implitapide, but a high rate of hepatosteatosis and gastrointestinal adverse experiences were encountered, even with the 25-mg dose in a longer phase 2 trial, the results of which were never published. Subsequently, Bristol-Myers Squibb halted further development.

After being abandoned by major pharmaceutical companies, both implitapide and lomitapide were given to individual academic investigators or academic institutions and small studies to develop them in HoFH and severe HeFH were continued.[40,41] In 2005, lomitapide was licensed by the University of Pennsylvania to Aegerion, and in 2006 the same company obtained implitapide.[42] Lomitapide entered a new phase 2 trial in patients with mildly elevated LDL-C levels at significantly lower starting doses of 5.0 mg daily and after 4 weeks the dose was escalated to 7.5 mg and then to 10.0 mg daily. The reductions in Apo B and LDL-C were dose related and robust. Mean LDL-C decreased 19%, 26%, and 30% at 5.0, 7.5, and 10.0 mg per day respectively (all $P<.01$). As seen for implitapide, statistically significant reductions ranging from 6.5% to 9.2% in HDL-C and 9% to 11% for Apo A1 were reported with all doses over the 12-week trial.[43] The side-effect profile was not favorable, with 32% of patients in the lomitapide monotherapy group discontinuing the trial, mainly for gastrointestinal side effects, which were experienced by 64% of subjects on the drug. Transaminase elevations greater than 3 times ULN occurred in nearly 20% of the patients treated with lomitapide alone or in combination with ezetimibe, resulting in their stopping the drug in the 12-week trial.[43]

Thus, while development of lomitapide was apparently halted for the broad population, a small dose-escalating pilot trial had been done in patients with HoFH.[41] Significant reductions in LDL-C were seen at the higher doses, reaching approximately 50%

at the 55-mg to 80-mg dose. Significant elevations of the hepatic transaminase, alanine aminotransferase, were seen in more than half of the subjects and hepatic magnetic resonance imaging showed hepatic fat accumulation in nearly all patients, with substantial increases seen in some, starting before administration of the highest and most-effective dose.

Following on the results of this proof-of-concept study, and partially funded by the FDA orphan drug program, a larger, open-label phase 3 study of lomitapide in HoFH was undertaken.[44] The study enrolled 29 adult patients, on maximally tolerated lipid-lowering drug therapy, including 16 on LDL apheresis, which remained unchanged during the initial 26 weeks of the trial. Lomitapide was started at a dose of 5 mg per day and titrated at approximately 4-week intervals to a maximum of 60 mg daily. The primary efficacy end point was the LDL-C change at week 26, after which time changes in lipid-lowering therapy were permitted. Six patients terminated with 23 patients completing the 26-week efficacy phase. Based on an intention-to-treat analysis of all 29 patients, the mean LDL-C reduction was 40% from baseline ($P<.001$) with a median dosage of 40 mg per day of lomitapide (see **Table 3**). Individual responses varied even at the same daily dose, similar to the variability seen in HoFH with statins and mipomersen. Parallel reductions in Apo B of 39% and lipoprotein(a) of 13% were seen. Although all the patients were genotyped, the effect of genotype on response was not reported. The result of this open-label trial was the basis for FDA approval in December 2012 of lomitapide solely for the treatment of adults. Similar approval by the European Medicines Agency was obtained in early 2013. The FDA approval carried a black-box warning (see **Table 1**), identical to that for mipomersen, regarding the potential for hepatic toxicity as well as the REMS program, similar to that of mipomersen (see **Table 2**).[24] The FDA also required additional trials in pediatric patients with HoFH, which are ongoing.[24] In addition, as required by the Japanese authorities, a phase 3, open-label trial in Japan of similar design to the trial discussed previously is being performed. This trial is estimated to enroll 5 to 10 adult patients with HoFH receiving concomitant lipid-lowering therapies, including apheresis. Patients will receive lomitapide for 26 weeks, again starting at 5 mg daily and escalating to a maximum dose of 60 mg based on tolerability and hepatic transaminases. Patients will continue into an additional 30-week safety phase with changes in hepatic fat being assessed from baseline to week 56.[45]

Although use of both lomitapide and mipomersen are likely to find a limited role in the treatment of HoFH, it is extremely unlikely, due to their poor tolerability and associated potential for hepatic toxicity, that they will ever become a therapeutic option in less-severe patient populations.

LOW-DENSITY LIPOPROTEIN CHOLESTEROL–LOWERING AGENTS IN ADVANCED CLINICAL DEVELOPMENT

Two therapeutic classes of drugs with LDL-C–lowering potential are currently in phase 3 development. The most exciting are agents inhibiting PCSK9, which, based on supporting genetics, mechanism of action, and larger and predictable reductions in LDL-C, promise to be as revolutionary as the statins were a generation ago, as outlined in detail in the next section.[46] The other class consists of agents that reduce or prevent the exchange of cholesterol between HDL and Apo B containing lipoproteins by inhibiting the enzyme cholesterol ester transfer protein (CETP).[47] The original development concept of CETP inhibitors was to increase HDL-C based on the hypothesis that raising this "anti-atherogenic" lipoprotein would in itself reduce cardiovascular morbidity and mortality. In early trials with the first CETP inhibitor to enter development, torcetrapib, it was noted that LDL-C was concomitantly reduced along with an increase in HDL-C.[48] Minimal, or no reduction in LDL-C was found with a second agent, dalcetrapib, which also raised HDL-C more modestly.[49] These first CETP inhibitors were terminated from clinical development, as outlined later in this article, but 2 additional agents, anacetrapib and evacetrapib, which also produce larger reductions in LDL-C, continue in development.[50,51]

Proprotein Convertase Subtilisin/Kexin Type 9 Inhibitors

In 2003, Abifadel and colleagues[52] described a new form of autosomal dominant hypercholesterolemia (ADH), which was not associated with mutations in the genes coding for the low-density lipoprotein receptor (LDLr) or its ligand, Apo B, but mutations in the gene encoding PCSK9. The role of PCSK9, at that time a recently described member of a nuclear protease family, was unknown and the mechanism by which it impacted LDL-C a complete mystery. By studying transgenic mice that overexpressed PCSK9, Maxwell and Breslow[53] discovered that their LDL receptor (LDLr) function, but not synthesis, was reduced, leading to elevated LDL-C levels. Thus the PCSK9 mutation causing the new form of FH appeared to be due to "gain-of-function" (GOF) in PCSK9, which somehow impacted LDLr function but not production. Additional GOF mutations in PCSK9 leading to elevated LDL-C have since been identified (**Fig. 3**). However, how PCSK9 decreased LDLr activity was not clear, but it did not appear to be due to reduced receptor synthesis, as LDLr mRNA production was unchanged.[54] These observations were soon followed by studies by Rashid and colleagues,[55] in which PCSK9 production was eliminated using a knockout mouse model and LDLr activity was substantially increased with resultant LDL-C reduction. Further studies in humans by Cohen and colleagues[56] confirmed that participants in a large longitudinal epidemiologic cardiovascular study with low plasma levels of LDL-C had "loss-of-function" (LOF) mutations in PCSK9. These families were reported to have a significant reduction in lifetime risk of coronary heart disease, and no adverse health effects. A number of LOF mutations have now been described associated with both reduced LDL-C and risk of cardiovascular disease (CVD) (see **Fig. 3, Table 4**). These observations of no adverse health

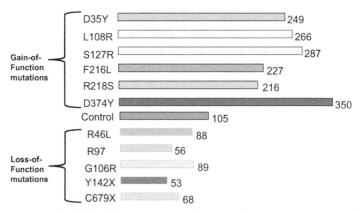

Fig. 3. Mean LDL-C levels (mg/dL) in patients with GOF and LOF PCSK9 mutations. (*Adapted from* Poirier S, Mayer G. The biology of PCSK9 from the endoplasmic reticulum to lysosomes: new and emerging therapeutics to control low-density lipoprotein cholesterol. Drug Des Devel Ther 2013;7:1136.)

Table 4
Risk of early myocardial infarction in subjects with PCSK9 loss-of-function, missense mutation R46L in different populations

Country	Study	Odds Ratio (95% CI)	P Value
Finland	FINRISK	0.30 (0.11–0.81)	.02
Sweden	Malmo: Cardiovascular cohort	0.32 (0.07–1.61)	.17
Spain	REGICOR	0.35 (0.15–0.82)	.02
USA (Seattle)	Puget Sound: heart attack risk	0.45 (0.21–0.98)	.049
USA (Boston)	Massachusetts General: study premature CAD	0.59 (0.21–1.69)	.46
Combined		0.40 (0.26–0.61)	.00002

Abbreviations: CI, confidence interval; PCSK9, proprotein convertase subtilisin/kexin type 9.

Adapted from Kathiresan S, the Myocardial Infarction Genetics Consortium. A PCSK9 missense variant associated with a reduced risk of early-onset myocardial infarction. N Engl J Med 2008;358:2299; with permission.

effects with LOF have been further supported by reports in now a number of healthy unrelated subjects with homozygous or compound heterozygous LOF mutations in PCSK9 and extremely low LDL-C levels, lower than 20 mg/dL, and undetectable PCSK9, essentially equivalent to the mouse PCSK9 model.[57] The mechanism by which PCSK9 reduced LDLr activity was elucidated by Lagace and coworkers in 2006,[58] when they demonstrated that circulating or plasma PCSK9 bound to the LDLr was internalized along with the receptor and LDL-C and targeted the LDLr for degradation (**Fig. 4**), thus preventing the LDLr from recycling back to the cell surface. This provided the critical information needed to design possible methods to inhibit PCSK9 and rapidly lead to development of a monoclonal antibody (mAb) targeted to PCSK9 knowing that preventing PCSK9 in the plasma from binding to the LDLr could restore or increase LDLr activity (see **Fig. 4C**). Proof-of-concept studies in mice and nonhuman primates showed the approach to be effective in binding PCSK9 and reducing LDL-C.[59] As total and free PCSK9 plasma levels can be measured and monitored in plasma it also provided a unique ability to monitor the effect of mAb on both the "target" and LDL-C. Over the past decade, much has been learned about the production and metabolism of PCSK9 before it enters the circulation. PCSK9 is produced mainly by hepatocytes as proPCSK9 in the endoplasmic reticulum and synthesis appears to be mediated via the same transcription factor, sterol receptor element binding protein-2 (SREBP2), which leads to increased synthesis of the LDLr. As plasma PCSK9 ultimately results in degradation of LDLr, this action is mostly likely a counter-regulatory mechanism designed to prevent excessive uptake of cholesterol into liver cells, as the adrenal and other organs in need of LDL-C delivery do not appear to be affected by PCSK9. However, as SREBP2 is upregulated by inhibition of intracellular cholesterol synthesis, for example by HMG CoA reductase inhibitors or "statins," leading to simultaneous increased production of LDLr and PCSK9, it has been postulated that the log linear dose response seen with statins may be due, at least in part, to concomitant reduction in LDLr recycling.[60] In 2009, 2 fully human mAbs, alirocumab and evolocumab, targeted to PCSK9, were being tested in humans.[61,62] The results of the single and multiple ascending dose, phase 1, trials were published in early 2012 demonstrating that administration of a PCSK9 mAb led to dramatic reductions in LDL-C in a broad range of patient phenotypes, whether added to diet alone or to background statin therapy.[61,62] Over the past 2 years, clinical development has progressed very rapidly with 3 mAbs already

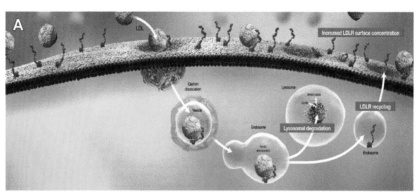

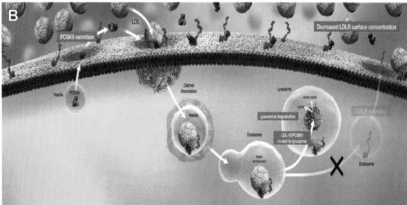

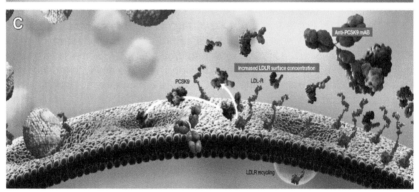

Fig. 4. LDLr, PCSK9, and mAbs to PCSK9 role in receptor function and recycling. (*A*) Normal LDLr recycling. (*B*) Effect of PCSK9 on LDLr recycling. (*C*) Impact of monoclonal antibody to PCSK9 on LDLr recycling. (*From* Stein EA, Wasserman SM, Dias C, et al. AMG-145. Drugs Future 2013;38:453; with permission.)

in phase 3 clinical development.[63–65] The most advanced of these are Amgen's evolocumab (AMG 145) followed by alirocumab (REGN 727/SAR 236553), originally produced by Regeneron and being codeveloped with Sanofi. Comprehensive data have been published on the phase 1 and 2 trials of both drugs,[61,62,66–72] as well as a number of trials from the evolocumab phase 3 program.[73–76] The phase 1b, multiple ascending dose (MAD) program of alirocumab incorporated a number of novel elements that accelerated the knowledge and future clinical development by including patients on stable statin therapy, which is known to increase plasma PCSK9, subjects on diet alone, and patients with HeFH and non-FH.[61] Three different doses, 50, 100, and 150 mg, were administered subcutaneously at differing intervals of 2 and 4 weeks. Using standardized "biomarker" measurements allowed a unique opportunity for direct measurement during these early trials, making it possible to assess the pharmacokinetics and pharmacodynamics by monitoring the mAb, the level of free/unbound PCSK9, and the biomarker of clinical importance, namely LDL-C (**Fig. 5**), in the bloodstream. Even in this fairly small phase 1 trial, it was clear that there was no difference in LDL-C reduction between patients with FH and non-FH, or between those on background statin therapy and those on modified diet alone. By pooling the different patient phenotypes it was also feasible to assess dose response and dose scheduling (ie, dosing at 2-week or 4-week intervals). Although there was a large difference in LDL-C reduction between the 50-mg and 100-mg doses, there was virtually no difference in maximal LDL-C reduction between the 100-mg and 150-mg doses.[61] This indicated, and subsequent studies later confirmed, that nearly all the plasma PCSK9 was bound by the mAb at the 100-mg dose. The effect on LDL-C was rapid, reaching maximum effect within approximately 5 to 7 days after the dose and the reduced LDL-C levels were stable for approximately 2 weeks before free PCSK9 levels started increasing followed quickly by LDL-C. It was also apparent from this limited study that the higher the dose of mAb, the longer the duration of effect, consistent with excess mAb not initially bound to PCSK9 remaining available to bind newly synthesized PCSK9, preventing PCSK9 binding to the LDLr and maintaining lower LDL-C. A similar MAD study with the Amgen monoclonal antibody to PCSK9, evolocumab (AMG 145), in terms of patient phenotypes and background treatments, but with higher doses, and dosing intervals ranging from 1 to 4 weeks, produced almost identical results.[62] Both drugs were well tolerated and had no significant or unexpected clinical or laboratory side effects, and the drugs moved rapidly into larger phase 2 trials in 2011. The results of 3 alirocumab and 4 evolocumab phase 2 trials were published in 2012. The trials can be best summarized by the questions they answered. McKenney and colleagues[66] highlighted 2 issues, whether even higher doses than tested in phase 1 would result in greater LDL-C reduction, prolonged duration of reduction, or both. The study assessed the

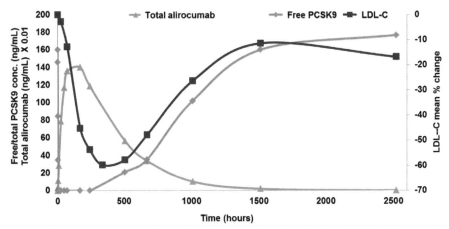

Fig. 5. Pharmacokinetics and dynamics of a monoclonal antibody to PCSK9 (alirocumab), free PCSK9, and LDL-C.

same 100-mg and 150-mg alirocumab doses administered every 2 weeks and compared them with 200 and 300 mg given every 4 weeks. It clearly demonstrated that despite the very large increase of mAb administered, there was no further reduction in LDL-C at any time after dosing. Although the duration of effect with the higher doses of even 300 mg was still not sufficient to maintain for 4 weeks the reductions in LDL-C seen at 2 weeks, there still remained the potential that even larger doses, if practical and cost-effective, could provide a long enough duration of effect to merit 4-week dosing. This was in fact assessed with evolocumab in 2 large studies that used doses up to 420 mg administered every 4 weeks and compared them with lower doses given every 2 weeks.[68,69] As shown in **Fig. 6**, from a pooled and very robust analysis of these trials, when evolocumab was given at a dosage of 420 mg every 4 weeks, the approximate 60% reductions in LDL-C were sustained, with minimal increase between weeks 2 and 4.[77] These data indicated that with high enough dosing there is potential to achieve excellent reductions with monthly therapy with a rough 3-to-1 "rule of thumb" in that 420 mg every 4 weeks would achieve the same stable LDL-C reductions as 140 mg every 2 weeks.

To assess (1) if the "rule of 6s," dose response with statins was due to upregulation of PCSK9 and (2) if there was a maximum to which LDLr activity could be upregulated with statin/PCSK9 mAb combination, Roth and colleagues[67] compared patients on stable doses of atorvastatin 10 mg daily, who were randomized to receive 80 mg of atorvastatin plus alirocumab or placebo or to remain on atorvastatin 10 mg plus alirocumab. The eightfold increase of atorvastatin from 10 to 80 mg alone followed the "rule of 6s" and resulted in the anticipated roughly 18% further reduction in LDL-C. The addition of 150 mg of alirocumab every 2 weeks to the group that maintained atorvastatin 10 mg daily resulted in a 66% decrease in LDL-C from baseline, or a 49% difference from the 80-mg dose of atorvastatin. The group that increased atorvastatin to 80 mg combined with the 150 mg of alirocumab experienced a decrease in LDL-C of 73%, a 55% additional decrease compared with atorvastatin 80 mg alone. The net reduction between 10 and 80 mg atorvastatin combined with the same dose of alirocumab was therefore only 6%.[67] Thus, although inhibiting PCSK9 in patients on maximal-dose atorvastatin was still very effective, the effect was definitely not synergistic, and not even additive, and ruled out the role of PCSK9 as the reason for the log-linear dose response seen with statin dosing. The trial also suggested that there may well be a point at which further upregulation of the LDLr is not possible.

Two trials in HeFH patients, 1 with alirocumab and 1 with evolocumab, assessed if the response seen in the small phase 1 trials in HeFH would be consistent in a global population with FH and more diverse LDLr defects.[68,71] In both trials, the mAb was added to stable treatment of high-dose effective statins and ezetimibe. The trials differed in that the alirocumab study used lower dose, 100 and 150 mg, dosed at 2 weeks, and 200 and 300 mg at 4-week intervals, whereas the evolocumab trial assessed 2 larger doses, 350 mg and 420 mg, given every 4 weeks. Both trials showed excellent mean LDL-C reductions of 60% to 70%, with responses fairly uniform in all FH patients.[68,71]

The final question to be assessed in the phase 2 program was to determine if patients unable to tolerate statins or high doses of statins would tolerate a PCSK9 mAb. The trial of evolocumab used ezetimibe as a nonstatin control group, and enrolled patients with documented muscle-related side effects on at least 1 statin.[72] The study also confirmed the need for additional effective lipid-lowering agents, as baseline LDL-C was close to 200 mg/dL with most patients having CHD or at high risk. The reductions in LDL-C seen across the various doses of evolocumab were consistent with those seen in previous populations, with reductions approaching

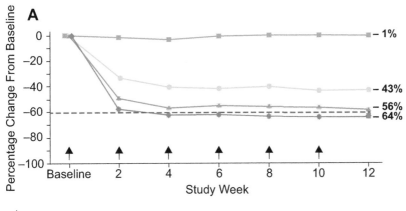

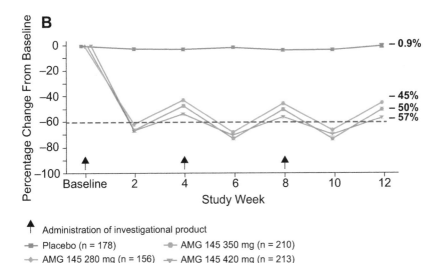

Fig. 6. (*A*) Evolocumab (AMG 145) every 2 weeks: LDL-C percentage change from baseline. (*B*) Evolocumab (AMG 145) every 4 weeks: LDL-C percentage change from baseline. (*From* Stein EA, Giugliano RP, Koren MJ, et al. Efficacy and safety of evolocumab (AMG 145), a fully human monoclonal antibody to PCSK9, in hyperlipidaemic patients on various background lipid therapies: pooled analysis of 1359 patients in 4 phase 2 trials. Eur Heart J 2014;35:2253; with permission.)

55% with evolocumab 420 mg every 4 weeks. Few patients stopped the study, evolocumab was well tolerated, and minimal elevations in the muscle enzyme creatine kinase were seen.[72]

Reductions in LDL-C have been accompanied by parallel large reductions in Apo B, although the decrease in Apo B is approximately 6% lower than that for LDL-C at any given dose, similar to what is seen with statins.[77] A novel and unexpected finding, consistent in all trials, is an as-yet-unexplained reduction in Lp(a), in the 25% to 30% range (**Fig. 7**).[78]

Consistent with upregulation of LDLr and removal of Apo B–containing lipoproteins, including triglyceride-rich, small, very-low-density and intermediate-density lipoproteins, has been the finding of modest reductions in triglycerides. As anticipated, with improved clearance of LDL-C there have been modest increases in HDL-C and its major constituent apolipoprotein A1.[77]

The last question addressed in phase 2 was to determine if patients with HoFH would respond to PCSK9 inhibition. This was assessed in a small open-label pilot trial of 8 patients: 6 LDLr defective status and 2 with negative LDLr function.[79] Somewhat counter to expectations, a moderate approximate 20% reduction in LDL-C was seen with the response confined to those patients with some residual LDLr activity. The study achieved sufficient response to warrant a large definitive phase 3 trial in patients with HoFH.[80]

More than 1600 patients were randomized between the Sanofi/Regeneron and Amgen programs, with more than 1200 patients treated with active drug, most for 12 weeks. To view this in the context of statin development, the phase 2 trials were

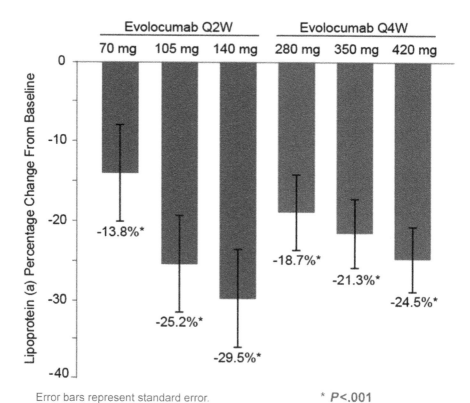

Error bars represent standard error.   * P<.001

Fig. 7. Reduction in lipoprotein (a) with PCSK9 monoclonal antibody evolocumab (AMG 145): a pooled analysis of more than 1300 patients in 4 phase II trials. (*From* Raal FJ, Giugliano RP, Sabatine MS, et al. Reduction in lipoprotein (a) with the PCSK9 monoclonal antibody evolocumab (AMG 145): a pooled analysis of over 1300 patients in 4 phase 2 trials. J Am Coll Cardiol 2014;63(13):1284; with permission.)

generally 4 or 6 weeks long and fairly small, usually fewer than 100 patients. Thus, by the end of the phase 2 PCSK9 program for these 2 agents, the patient exposure likely exceeds that of all statins combined at the same stage of development. Even though the drugs are administered by SC injection, tolerability has been good, and patients terminating trials no higher than that of statin or other oral lipid-lowering drugs. Elevations of liver function and muscle enzymes seen with statins and some other lipid-lowering drugs have been minimal with PCSK9 mAbs.[77] Nonspecific adverse effects have been reported, although the frequency in the trials has not been noticeably different from placebo or control therapy. Both alirocumab and evolocumab monoclonal antibodies are fully humanized, which minimizes the potential for immune reactions and the development of consistent or high titers of neutralizing antibodies to the agents has not been seen in phase 2 trials.

Concern has been raised regarding very low levels of LDL-C that are achieved in some patients. Although it is reassuring from the epidemiologic studies and the few patients with genetic abnormalities leading to lifelong very low LDL-C, this question will be answered only by the long-term clinical outcome trials currently ongoing in phase 3.[63–65] Alirocumab and evolocumab are now well into large phase 3 programs, with 6 evolocumab trials already published or publically presented.[73–76,78] The major purpose of phase 3 is to assess long-term safety in a larger population so as to provide sufficient information for regulatory agencies to determine the risk to benefit in approving an LDL-C–lowering agent for general use. Thus, little additional information is anticipated with regard to efficacy, which is solidly established and robust in terms of LDL-C reduction and in itself an approvable end point, as recently reiterated by the FDA. However, unlike the long hiatus between development and marketing approval of statins where CHD and clinical outcome trials were only started many years after release general use, evolocumab, alirocumab, and the Pfizer humanized PCSK9 mAb, bococizumab, have already entered large CVD outcome trials as part of their phase 3 programs (**Table 5**).[63–65,81] The first of these trials is anticipated to conclude in late 2016 or early 2017.

To summarize the highlights from the phase 3 trials of evolocumab results available to date, the following can be stated. (1) LDL-C efficacy after 52 weeks was consistent with that seen in the 12-week phase 2.[73] (2) LDL-C efficacy was consistent across a wide spectrum of background therapies including diet alone, various statin doses, to statin plus ezetimibe.[73,76] (3) Trials comparing 140 mg every 2 weeks to 420 mg monthly with assessments at both 2 and 4 weeks after dosing confirmed equivalent LDL-C reductions consistent with the "rule of 3" regarding the 2-week dose needed to achieve stability for 4 weeks.[74,76] (4) Patients intolerant to at least 2 statins still tolerated evolocumab and had the same 60% reductions in LDL-C seen in the phase 2 statin intolerant trial.[75] (5) the definitive double-blind randomized trial in HoFH involving 49 patients showed an overall 31% mean reduction in LDL-C with evolocumab compared with placebo (see **Table 3**), and 40% in those patients with at least 1 LDLr defective allele.[81] (6) Perhaps most important, tolerability and safety continues to be good with no additional findings from the phase 2 studies.

In summary, PCSK9 mAb therapy appears to be the most promising therapeutic class since statins and is able to fill the current medical need outlined in the introduction. Despite the mode of administration by SC injection, and the likely high cost associated with biological agents, the substantial reduction in LDL-C and self-administration of these drugs either every 2 or 4 weeks will likely result in PCSK9 mAbs being widely accepted and used by patients. It is anticipated that the addition of PCSK9 mAbs to current therapy in the CHD outcome trials currently in progress will augment the reductions in CVD that have been achieved by statins.

Table 5
PCSK9 monoclonal antibody cardiovascular outcome trials currently in progress

	Evolocumab (AMG 145)	Alirocumab (SAR236553/REGN727)	Bococizumab (RN 316)	
Sponsor	Amgen	Sanofi/Regeneron	Pfizer	
Trial	FOURIER	ODYSSEY Outcomes	SPIRE I	SPIRE II
Sample size	22,500	18,000	12,000	6300
Patients	MI, stroke, or PAD	4–52 wk post-ACS	High risk of CV event	
Statin	Atorva ≥20 mg or equiv	Evidence-based medicine Rx	Lipid-lowering Rx	
LDL-C mg/dL (mmol/L)	≥70 (≥1.8)	≥70 (≥1.8)	70–99 (1.8–2.6)	≥100 (≥2.6)
PCSK9i Dosing	Q2W or Q4W	Q2W	Q2W	
End point	1. CV death, MI, stroke, revasc or hosp for UA 2. CV death, MI, or stroke	CHD death, MI, ischemic stroke, or hosp for UA	CV death, MI, stroke, or urgent revasc	
Completion	12/2017	1/2018	8/2017	

Abbreviations: ACS, acute coronary syndrome; CHD, coronary heart disease; CV, cardiovascular; hosp, hospitalization; MI, myocardial infarction; PAD, peripheral arterial disease; PCSK9, proprotein convertase subtilisin/kexin type 9; revasc, revascularization; Rx, prescription; UA, unstable angina.

An alternative therapeutic approach to mAbs using the similar antisense technology described previously for Apo B was demonstrated in an animal model,[82] in which a second-generation antisense ASO directed at murine PCKS9 reduced PCSK9 expression and decreased LDLc by 38% in 6 weeks. Despite the promise shown in these animal experiments, combined with the human experience with the Apo B ASO, mipomersen, and a partnership announced in 2007 between ISIS Pharmaceuticals and Bristol-Myers Squibb,[83] this approach has not entered human trials. An alternative method for gene "silencing" by using short interfering RNA has been developed by Alnylam. In a proof-of-concept single ascending dose study, both plasma PCSK9 and LDL-C reductions were reported.[84]

Cholesterol Ester Transfer Protein Inhibitors

CETP, a plasma protein that catalyzes the exchange of cholesteryl esters and triglyceride between HDL and Apo B containing lipoproteins, was identified as a potential therapeutic target from populations with elevated HDL-C and apparent reduction in CVD risk.[85] Subsequently, genetic mutations in CETP were found to be related to elevations in HDL-C and pharmacologic inhibition was able to reproduce a similar elevation.[48,85] Along with the increase in HDL-C, it was noted that there was a reduction in LDL-C, which mechanistically was consistent with the prevention of cholesterol transfer from HDL to LDL.[48] The magnitude of LDL-C reduction has varied with different CETP inhibitors, as well as with the dose of specific inhibitors.[86,87] For example, minimal or no LDL-C reduction was seen with dalcetrapib, to moderate reductions of approximately 20% with torcetrapib.[48,49] Both of these agents were terminated after large CVD outcome trials were stopped, for toxicity in the case of torcetrapib and futility in the case of dalcetrapib.[50,51] However 2 CETP inhibitors, evacetrapib and anacetrapib, continue in development, both now in large CVD outcome trials.[88,89]

Anacetrapib, a potent and selective CETP inhibitor at 150 and 300 mg daily, increased HDL-C and Apo A-I of 39% and 47%, respectively. At dosages of 10, 40, 150, and 300 mg daily, LDL-C reductions ranged from 15% to approximately 40%.[90] A dose of 100 mg was selected for the CVD outcome trial, which in a large trial lowered LDL-C by 25% to 35%.[91,92] This dose is also being used in the large 30,624-patient CVD outcome trial, REVEAL (Randomized EValuation of the Effects of Anacetrapib Through Lipid-modification), currently in progress with results anticipated in 2017.[89]

Evacetrapib, also a potent inhibitor of CETP, showed a dose response in both HDL-C and LDL-C in a dose ranging trial with increases of HDL-C of 54%, 95%, and 129%, and reductions in LDL-C of 14%, 22%, and 36% with doses of 30, 100, and 500 mg per day.[87] A dose of 130 mg was selected for the 12,000-patient ACCELERATE CVD outcome trial currently in progress, with results expected in late 2016.[88]

Depending on the results, it may be that these agents would be used to reduce LDL-C, although their primary action is to increase HDL-C and their effect on LDL-C is relatively small compared with PCSK9 inhibitors.

SUMMARY

Although the past 4 decades have probably been the most fruitful and productive in transitioning from an LDL-C hypothesis to demonstration of clinical benefit, CVD still remains the major cause of mortality and morbidity in industrialized societies. It is rapidly becoming the major cause of morbidity and mortality in recently industrializing countries, such as India and China, that together constitute nearly half of the world's population. It is fortunate that most of the most-effective lipid-lowering drugs, the statins, have become, or will soon become, generic and very inexpensive. However, there remains a large unmet medical need for new and effective agents that are also well tolerated and safe, especially for patients unable to either tolerate statins or achieve optimal LDL-C on current therapies. It is likely that the agents discussed in this review will fill that need.

REFERENCES

1. Statins: a success story involving FDA, academia and industry. Available at: http://www.fda.gov/AboutFDA/WhatWeDo/History/ProductRegulation/Selections FromFDLIUpdateSeriesonFDAHistory/ucm082054.htm. Accessed July 25, 2014.
2. Stone N, Robinson J, Lichtenstein AH, et al. 2013 ACC/AHA guideline on the treatment of blood cholesterol to reduce atherosclerotic cardiovascular risk in adults: a report of the American College of Cardiology/American Heart Association Task Force on Practice Guidelines. Circulation 2014;129:S1–45.
3. European Association for Cardiovascular Prevention & Rehabilitation, Reiner Z, Catapano AL, et al, ESC Committee for Practice Guidelines (CPG) 2008-2010 and 2010-2012 Committees. ESC/EAS Guidelines for the management of dyslipidaemias: the Task Force for the management of dyslipidaemias of the European Society of Cardiology (ESC) and the European Atherosclerosis Society (EAS). Eur Heart J 2011;32:1769–818.
4. Anderson TJ, Grégoire J, Hegele RA, et al. 2012 Update of the Canadian Cardiovascular Society guidelines for the diagnosis and treatment of dyslipidemia for the prevention of cardiovascular disease in the adult. Can J Cardiol 2013; 29:151–67.

5. National Heart Foundation of Australia and the Cardiac Society of Australia and New Zealand. Reducing risk in heart disease: an expert guide to clinical practice for secondary prevention of coronary heart disease. Melbourne (Australia): National Heart Foundation of Australia; 2012. Available at: http://www.heartfoundation.org.au/SiteCollectionDocuments/Reducing-risk-inheart-disease.pdf. Accessed July 10, 2014.

6. Cholesterol Treatment Trialists' (CTT) Collaboration, Baigent C, Blackwell L, et al. Efficacy and safety of more intensive lowering of LDL cholesterol: a meta-analysis of data from 170,000 participants in 26 randomised trials. Lancet 2010;376:1670–81.

7. Jones PH, Davidson MH, Stein EA, et al, STELLAR Study Group. Comparison of efficacy and safety of rosuvastatin versus atorvastatin, simvastatin, and pravastatin across doses (STELLAR Trial). Am J Cardiol 2003;92:152–60.

8. LaRosa JC, Grundy SM, Waters DD, et al, Treating to New Targets (TNT) Investigators. Intensive lipid lowering with atorvastatin in patients with stable coronary disease. N Engl J Med 2005;352(14):1425–35.

9. Billups SJ, Plushner SL, Olson KL, et al. Clinical and economic outcomes of conversion of simvastatin to lovastatin in a group-model health maintenance organization. J Manag Care Pharm 2005;11(8):681–6.

10. Jackevicius CA, Chou MM, Ross JS, et al. Generic atorvastatin and health care costs. N Engl J Med 2012;366(3):201–4.

11. Howard L. Drug in focus: rosuvastatin. Available at: http://www.genericsweb.com/index.php?object_id=680. Accessed July 12, 2014.

12. Available at: http://www2.costco.com/Pharmacy/DrugInfo.aspx?p=1&SearchTerm=atorvastatin&Drug=ATORVASTATIN. Accessed July 12, 2014.

13. Ezzet F, Wexler D, Statkevich P, et al. The plasma concentration and LDL-C relationship in patients receiving ezetimibe. J Clin Pharmacol 2001;41(9):943–9.

14. Davidson MH, Dillon MA, Gordon B, et al. Colesevelam hydrochloride (cholestagel): a new, potent bile acid sequestrant associated with a low incidence of gastrointestinal side effects. Arch Intern Med 1999;159(16):1893–900.

15. Capuzzi DM, Guyton JR, Morgan JM, et al. Efficacy and safety of an extended-release niacin (Niaspan): a long-term study. Am J Cardiol 1998;82(12A):74U–81U.

16. Knopp RH, Brown WV, Dujovne CA, et al. Effects of fenofibrate on plasma lipoproteins in hypercholesterolemia and combined hyperlipidemia. Am J Med 1987;83(5B):50–9.

17. Maningat P, Gordon BR, Breslow JL. How do we improve patient compliance and adherence to long-term statin therapy? Curr Atheroscler Rep 2013;15(1):291.

18. Stein EA, Ballantyne CM, Windler E, et al. Efficacy and tolerability of Fluvastatin XL 80 mg alone, ezetimibe alone and the combination of Fluvastatin XL 80 mg with ezetimibe in patients with a history of muscle-related side effects with other statins: a randomized, double-blind, double-dummy trial. Am J Cardiol 2008;101:490–6.

19. Bruckert E, Hayem G, Dejager S, et al. Mild to moderate muscular symptoms with high-dosage statin therapy in hyperlipidemic patients—the PRIMO study. Cardiovasc Drugs Ther 2005;19:403–14.

20. Stein E, Stender S, Mata P, et al, Ezetimibe Study Group. Achieving lipoprotein goals in patients at high risk with severe hypercholesterolemia: efficacy and safety of ezetimibe co-administered with atorvastatin. Am Heart J 2004;148(3):447–55.

21. Stein EA, Ose L, Retterstol K, et al. Further reductions in low-density lipoprotein cholesterol and C-reactive protein with the addition of ezetimibe to maximum dose rosuvastatin in patients with severe hypercholesterolemia. J Clin Lipidol 2007;1:280–6.
22. Nordestgaard BG, Chapman MJ, Humphries SE, et al. Familial hypercholesterolaemia is underdiagnosed and undertreated in the general population: guidance for clinicians to prevent coronary heart disease. Eur Heart J 2013;34:3478–90.
23. Rader DJ, Kastelein JJ. Lomitapide and mipomersen: two first-in-class drugs for reducing low-density lipoprotein cholesterol in patients with homozygous familial hypercholesterolemia. Circulation 2014;129:1022–32.
24. FDA approves new orphan drug for rare cholesterol disorder. US Food and Drug Administration Web site. 2012. Available at: http://www.fda.gov/NewsEvents/Newsroom/PressAnnouncements/ucm333285.htm. Accessed May 28, 2014.
25. FDA approves new orphan drug Kynamro to treat inherited cholesterol disorder. US Food and Drug Administration Web site. 2013. Available at: http://www.fda.gov/NewsEvents/Newsroom/PressAnnouncements/ucm337195.htm. Accessed May 28, 2014.
26. Kastelein JJ, Wedel MK, Baker BF, et al. Potent reduction of apolipoprotein B and low-density lipoprotein cholesterol by short-term administration of an antisense inhibitor of apolipoprotein B. Circulation 2006;114:1729–35.
27. Akdim F, Visser ME, Tribble DL, et al. Effect of mipomersen, an apolipoprotein B synthesis inhibitor, on low-density lipoprotein cholesterol in patients with familial hypercholesterolemia. Am J Cardiol 2010;105:1413–9.
28. Stein EA, Dufour R, Gagne C, et al. Apolipoprotein B synthesis inhibition with mipomersen in heterozygous familial hypercholesterolemia: results of a randomized, double-blind, placebo-controlled trial to assess efficacy and safety as add-on therapy in patients with coronary artery disease. Circulation 2012;126:2283–92.
29. Raal FJ, Santos RD, Blom DJ, et al. Mipomersen, an apolipoprotein B synthesis inhibitor, for lowering of LDL cholesterol concentrations in patients with homozygous familial hypercholesterolaemia: a randomised, double-blind, placebo-controlled trial. Lancet 2010;375:998–1006.
30. Visser ME, Akdim F, Tribble DL, et al. Effect of apolipoprotein-B synthesis inhibition on liver triglyceride content in patients with familial hypercholesterolemia. J Lipid Res 2010;51(5):1057–62.
31. A Study of the safety and efficacy of two different regimens of mipomersen in patients with familial hypercholesterolemia and inadequately controlled low-density lipoprotein cholesterol (FOCUS FH). Available at: http://clinicaltrials.gov/show/NCT01475825. Accessed July 12, 2014.
32. Available at: http://www.ema.europa.eu/docs/en_GB/document_library/Summary_of_opinion_-_Initial_authorisation/human/002429/WC500140678.pdf. Accessed July 12, 2014.
33. Available at: http://www.forbes.com/sites/larryhusten/2013/03/22/europe-and-us-diverge-on-two-new-drugs/. Accessed July 12, 2014.
34. Wetterau JR, Aggerbeck LP, Bouma ME, et al. Absence of microsomal triglyceride transfer protein in individuals with abetalipoproteinemia. Science 1992;258:999–1001.
35. Scriver CR, Sly WS, Childs B, et al, editors. The metabolic and molecular bases of inherited disease. 8th edition. McGraw-Hill Professional; 2000.
36. Rader DJ, Brewer HB Jr. Abetalipoproteinemia: new insights into lipoprotein assembly and vitamin E metabolism from a rare genetic disease. JAMA 1993;270:865–9.

37. Stein EA, Isaacsohn JL, Mazzu A, et al. Effect of BAY 13-9952, a microsomal triglyceride transfer protein inhibitor on lipids and lipoproteins in dyslipoproteinemic patients. Circulation 1999;100(18 Suppl 1) [abstract: 1342].

38. Wetterau JR, Gregg RE, Harrity TW, et al. An MTP inhibitor that normalizes atherogenic lipoprotein levels in WHHL rabbits. Science 1999;282:751–4.

39. Farnier M, Stein E, Megnien S, et al. Efficacy and safety of implitapide, a microsomal triglyceride transfer protein inhibitor in patients with primary hypercholesterolemia. Abstract Book of the XIV International Symposium on Drugs Affecting Lipid Metabolism. New York, September 9–12, 2001. p. 4.

40. Available at: http://www.clinicaltrials.gov/ct/show/NCT00079859. Accessed June 10, 2008.

41. Cuchel M, Bloedon LT, Szapary PO, et al. Inhibition of microsomal triglyceride transfer protein in familial hypercholesterolemia. N Engl J Med 2007;356:148–56.

42. Available at: http://www.sec.gov/Archives/edgar/data/1338042/000119312 507123502/ds1a.htm. Aegerion Pharmaceuticals, Inc. Common Stock Registration Statement. AMENDMENT NO. 3 to FORM S-1; May 25, 2007. United States Securities and Exchange Commission. Washington, DC. 20549. 2007. Accessed July 12, 2014.

43. Samaha FF, McKenney J, Bloedon LT, et al. Inhibition of microsomal triglyceride transfer protein alone or with ezetimibe in patients with moderate hypercholesterolemia. Nat Clin Pract Cardiovasc Med 2008;5:497–505.

44. Cuchel M, Meagher EA, du Toit Theron H, et al. Efficacy and safety of a microsomal triglyceride transfer protein inhibitor in patients with homozygous familial hypercholesterolaemia: a single-arm, open-label, phase 3 study. Lancet 2013; 381:40–6.

45. Efficacy and safety of lomitapide in Japanese patients with HoFH on concurrent lipid-lowering therapy. Available at: http://clinicaltrials.gov/ct2/show/record/ NCT02173158?term=lomitapide&rank=8. Accessed July 12, 2014.

46. Stein EA, Raal FJ. Reduction of low density lipoprotein cholesterol by monoclonal antibody inhibition of PCSK9. Annu Rev Med 2014;65:417–31.

47. Tall AR, Jiang X, Luo Y, et al. 1999 George Lyman Duff memorial lecture: lipid transfer proteins, HDL metabolism, and atherogenesis. Arterioscler Thromb Vasc Biol 2000;20:1185–8.

48. Clark RW, Sutfin TA, Ruggeri RB, et al. Raising high-density lipoprotein in humans through inhibition of cholesteryl ester transfer protein: an initial multidose study of torcetrapib. Arterioscler Thromb Vasc Biol 2004;24:490–7.

49. de Grooth GJ, Kuivenhoven JA, Stalenhoef AF, et al. Efficacy and safety of a novel cholesteryl ester transfer protein inhibitor, JTT-705, in humans: a randomized phase II dose-response study. Circulation 2002;105:2159–65.

50. Barter PJ, Caulfield M, Eriksson M, et al. Effects of torcetrapib in patients at high risk for coronary events. N Engl J Med 2007;357:2109–22.

51. Schwartz GG, Olsson AG, Abt M, et al. Effects of dalcetrapib in patients with a recent acute coronary syndrome. N Engl J Med 2012;367(22):2089–99.

52. Abifadel M, Varret M, Rabès JP, et al. Mutations in PCSK9 cause autosomal dominant hypercholesterolemia. Nat Genet 2003;34:154–6.

53. Maxwell KN, Breslow JL. Adenoviral-mediated expression of PCSK9 in mice results in a low-density lipoprotein receptor knockout phenotype. Proc Natl Acad Sci U S A 2004;101:7100–5.

54. Maxwell KN, Fisher EA, Breslow JL. Overexpression of PCSK9 accelerates the degradation of the LDLR in a post–endoplasmic reticulum compartment. Proc Natl Acad Sci U S A 2005;102(6):2069–74.

55. Rashid S, Curtis DE, Garuti R, et al. Horton decreased plasma cholesterol and hypersensitivity to statins in mice lacking PCSK9. Proc Natl Acad Sci U S A 2005;102:5374–9.
56. Cohen JC, Boerwinkle E, Mosley TH Jr, et al. Sequence variations in PCSK9, low LDL, and protection against coronary heart disease. N Engl J Med 2006;354:1264–72.
57. Zhao Z, Tuakli-Wosornu Y, Lagace TA, et al. Molecular characterization of loss-of-function mutations in PCSK9 and identification of a compound heterozygote. Am J Hum Genet 2006;79(3):514–23.
58. Lagace TA, Curtis DE, Garuti R, et al. Secreted PCSK9 decreases the number of LDL receptors in hepatocytes and in livers of parabiotic mice. J Clin Invest 2006; 116:2995–3005.
59. Chan JC, Piper DE, Cao Q, et al. A proprotein convertase subtilisin/kexin type 9 neutralizing antibody reduces serum cholesterol in mice and nonhuman primates. Proc Natl Acad Sci U S A 2009;106:9820–5.
60. Berthold HK, Seidah NG, Benjannet S, et al. Evidence from a randomized trial that simvastatin, but not ezetimibe, upregulates circulating PCSK9 levels. PLoS One 2013;8(3):e60095. http://dx.doi.org/10.1371/journal.pone.0060095.
61. Stein EA, Mellis S, Yancopoulos GD, et al. Effect of a monoclonal antibody to PCSK9 on LDL cholesterol. N Engl J Med 2012;366:1108–83.
62. Dias CS, Shaywitz AJ, Wasserman SM, et al. Effects of AMG 145 on low-density lipoprotein cholesterol levels: results from 2 randomized, double-blind, placebo controlled, ascending-dose phase 1 studies in healthy volunteers and hyper-cholesterolemic subjects on statins. J Am Coll Cardiol 2012;60:1888–98.
63. Further Cardiovascular Outcomes Research With PCSK9 Inhibition in Subjects With Elevated Risk (FOURIER). Available at: http://clinicaltrials.gov/show/ NCT01764633. Accessed July 12, 2014.
64. ODYSSEY outcomes: evaluation of cardiovascular outcomes after an acute coronary syndrome during treatment with Alirocumab SAR236553 (REGN727). Available at: http://clinicaltrials.gov/ct2/show/NCT01663402? term=odyssey&rank=6. Accessed July 12, 2014.
65. The evaluation of PF-04950615 (RN316), in reducing the occurrence of major cardiovascular events in high risk subjects (SPIRE-1). Available at: http:// clinicaltrials.gov/ct2/show/NCT01975376?term=PF-04950615&rank=13.   Accessed July 12, 2014.
66. McKenney JM, Koren MJ, Kereiakes DJ, et al. Safety and efficacy of a mono-clonal antibody to proprotein convertase subtilisin/kexin type 9 serine prote-ase, SAR236553/REGN727, in patients with primary hypercholesterolemia receiving ongoing stable atorvastatin therapy. J Am Coll Cardiol 2012;59: 2344–53.
67. Roth EM, McKenney JM, Hanotin C, et al. Atorvastatin with or without an antibody to PCSK9 in primary hypercholesterolemia. N Engl J Med 2012;367:1891–900.
68. Stein EA, Gipe D, Bergeron J, et al. Effect of a monoclonal antibody to PCSK9, REGN727/SAR236553, to reduce low-density lipoprotein cholesterol in patients with heterozygous familial hypercholesterolaemia on stable statin dose with or without ezetimibe therapy: a phase 2 randomised controlled trial. Lancet 2012;380:29–36.
69. Giugliano RP, Desai NR, Kohli P, et al. Efficacy, safety, and tolerability of a mono-clonal antibody to proprotein convertase subtilisin/kexin type 9 in combination with a statin in patients with hypercholesterolaemia (LAPLACE-TIMI 57): a rand-omised, placebo-controlled, dose-ranging, phase 2 study. Lancet 2012;380: 2007–17.

70. Koren MJ, Scott R, Kim JB, et al. Efficacy, safety, and tolerability of a monoclonal antibody to proprotein convertase subtilisin/kexin type 9 as monotherapy in patients with hypercholesterolaemia (MENDEL): a randomised, double-blind, placebo-controlled, phase 2 study. Lancet 2012;380:1995–2006.

71. Raal F, Scott R, Somaratne R, et al. Low-density lipoprotein cholesterol-lowering effects of AMG 145, a monoclonal antibody to proprotein convertase subtilisin/kexin type 9 serine protease in patients with heterozygous familial hypercholesterolemia: the Reduction of LDL-C with PCSK9 Inhibition in Heterozygous Familial Hypercholesterolemia Disorder (RUTHERFORD) randomized trial. Circulation 2012;126:2408–17.

72. Sullivan D, Olsson AG, Scott R, et al. Effect of a monoclonal antibody to PCSK9 on low-density lipoprotein cholesterol levels in statin-intolerant patients: the GAUSS randomized trial. JAMA 2012;308:2497–506.

73. Blom DJ, Hala T, Bolognese M, et al, for the DESCARTES Investigators. A 52-week placebo-controlled trial of evolocumab in hyperlipidemia. N Engl J Med 2014;370:1809–19.

74. Koren MJ, Lundqvist P, Bolognese M, et al, MENDEL-2 Investigators. Anti-PCSK9 monotherapy for hypercholesterolemia: the MENDEL-2 randomized, controlled phase III clinical trial of evolocumab. J Am Coll Cardiol 2014; 63(23):2531–40.

75. Stroes E, Colquhoun D, Sullivan D, et al, GAUSS-2 Investigators. Anti-PCSK9 antibody effectively lowers cholesterol in patients with statin intolerance: the GAUSS-2 randomized, placebo-controlled phase 3 clinical trial of evolocumab. J Am Coll Cardiol 2014;63(23):2541–8.

76. Robinson JG, Nedergaard BS, Rogers WJ, et al, LAPLACE-2 Investigators. Effect of evolocumab or ezetimibe added to moderate- or high-intensity statin therapy on LDL-C lowering in patients with hypercholesterolemia: the LAPLACE-2 randomized clinical trial. JAMA 2014;311(18):1870–82.

77. Stein EA, Giugliano RP, Koren MJ, et al. Efficacy and safety of evolocumab (AMG 145), a fully human monoclonal antibody to PCSK9, in hyperlipidaemic patients on various background lipid therapies: pooled analysis of 1359 patients in 4 phase 2 trials. Eur Heart J 2014. http://dx.doi.org/10.1093/eurheartj/ehu085.

78. Raal FJ, Giugliano RP, Sabatine MS, et al. Reduction in lipoprotein (a) with the PCSK9 monoclonal antibody evolocumab (AMG 145): a pooled analysis of over 1300 patients in 4 phase 2 trials. J Am Coll Cardiol 2014;63:1278–88.

79. Stein EA, Honarpour N, Wasserman SM, et al. Effect of the proprotein convertase Subtilisin/Kexin 9 monoclonal antibody, AMG 145, in homozygous familial hypercholesterolemia. Circulation 2013;128:2113–20.

80. Raal FJ, Honarpour N, Blom DJ, et al. Inhibition of PCSK9 with evolocumab in homozygous familial hypercholesterolaemia (TESLA Part B): a randomised, double-blind, placebo-controlled trial. Lancet 2014.

81. The evaluation of PF-04950615 (RN316) in reducing the occurrence of major cardiovascular events in high risk subjects (SPIRE-2). Available at: http://clinicaltrials.gov/ct2/show/NCT01975389?term=PF-04950615&rank=14. Accessed July 12, 2014.

82. Graham MJ, Lemonidis KM, Whipple CP, et al. Antisense inhibition of proprotein convertase subtilisin/kexin type 9 reduces serum LDL in hyperlipidemic mice. J Lipid Res 2007;48:763–7.

83. ISIS Press Release. Bristol-Myers SQUIBB selects ISIS drug targeting PCSK9 as development candidate for prevention and treatment of cardiovascular disease. Carlsbad (CA): PRNewswire-FirstCall; 2008. Available at: http://ir.isispharm.

com/phoenix.zhtml?c=222170&p=irol-newsArticle&ID=1289499.   Accessed September 23, 2014.

84. Fitzgerald K, Frank-Kamenetsky M, Shulga-Morskaya S, et al. Effect of an RNA interference drug on the synthesis of proprotein convertase subtilisin/kexin type 9 (PCSK9) and the concentration of serum LDL cholesterol in healthy volunteers: a randomised, single-blind, placebo-controlled, phase 1 trial. Lancet 2014; 383(9911):60–8.

85. Thompson A, Di Angelantonio E, Sarwar N, et al. Association of cholesteryl ester transfer protein genotypes with CETP mass and activity, lipid levels, and coronary risk. JAMA 2008;299:2777–88.

86. Krishna R, Anderson MS, Bergman AJ, et al. Effect of the cholesteryl ester transfer protein inhibitor, anacetrapib, on lipoproteins in patients with dyslipidaemia and on 24-h ambulatory blood pressure in healthy individuals: two double-blind, randomised placebo-controlled phase I studies. Lancet 2007;370: 1907–14.

87. Nicholls SJ, Brewer HB, Kastelein JJ, et al. Effects of the CETP inhibitor evacetrapib administered as monotherapy or in combination with statins on HDL and LDL cholesterol: a randomized controlled trial. JAMA 2011;306(19):2099–109.

88. A study of evacetrapib in high-risk vascular disease (ACCELERATE). Available at: http://clinicaltrials.gov/show/NCT01687998. Accessed July 12, 2014.

89. REVEAL: randomized evaluation of the effects of anacetrapib through lipid-modification. Available at: http://clinicaltrials.gov/show/NCT01252953. Accessed July 15, 2014.

90. Bloomfield D, Carlson GL, Sapre A, et al. Efficacy and safety of the cholesteryl ester transfer protein inhibitor anacetrapib as monotherapy and coadministered with atorvastatin in dyslipidemic patients. Am Heart J 2009;157(2):352–60.

91. Cannon CP, Shah S, Dansky HM, et al. Safety of anacetrapib in patients with or at high risk for coronary heart disease. N Engl J Med 2010;363:2406–15.

92. Anacetrapib: Merck provides information about a different method to measure LDL cholesterol and progress on REVEAL study. Available at: http://www.mercknewsroom.com/press-release/research-and-developmentnews/merck-provides-update-cardiovascular-development-program. Accessed July 12, 2014.

93. FDA briefing document NDA 203858. Available at: http://www.fda.gov/downloads/AdvisoryCommittees/CommitteesMeetingMaterials/Drugs/Endocrinologicand MetabolicDrugsAdvisoryCommittee/UCM323841.pdf. Accessed July 16, 2014.

Combination Therapy with Statins: Who Benefits?

Amita Singh, MD, Michael Davidson, MD*

KEYWORDS

- Lipids • Cholesterol • Statin • Niacin • Fibrates • Ezetimibe • Omega-3 fatty acids
- Cardiovascular risk

KEY POINTS

- When therapies have been studied in addition to statins, which remain the standard of treatment, it has been challenging to consistently show an additional clinical benefit in terms of cardiovascular (CV) event reduction, although overall safety seems acceptable.
- Combination therapy is a viable and often used strategy, which allows more patients to successfully reach their ideal lipid targets.
- There may be particular benefit with fenofibrate and niacin in patients with more severe atherogenic dyslipidemias who are unable to achieve intensive low-density lipoprotein (LDL) reduction with statins alone.
- Patients with very high CV risk because of recurrent events on therapy, or those with statin intolerance, are potential candidates for combination strategies.
- Further testing of novel therapies, particularly the PCSK9 class of medications, may introduce an era of potent LDL lowering without dependence on statins, but until then, they remain the mainstay of therapy.

INTRODUCTION

Cardiovascular (CV) disease (CVD) has been the leading cause of death in the United States since the early twentieth century, with worldwide rates similarly on the increase.[1] Increased low-density lipoprotein cholesterol (LDL-C) and, to a lesser extent, low high-density lipoprotein cholesterol (HDL-C) and increased triglyceride (TG) levels are all independent risk factors for CVD. Since the introduction of lovastatin in 1987, statins (hemoglobin [HMG]-coenzyme A [CoA] reductase inhibitors) have been repeatedly shown to decrease LDL-C, thereby reducing the risk for CVD events for patients with or without established vascular disease, and have long comprised the foundation of lipid-lowering therapy.

The importance of decreasing LDL levels in modification of CV risk has driven interest in and development of several novel cholesterol-modifying drugs, many of

This article originally appeared in Endocrinology and Metabolism Clinics, Volume 43, Issue 4, December 2014.
Section of Cardiology, University of Chicago, Chicago, IL, USA
* Corresponding author. 140 Belle Avenue, Highland Park, IL 60035.
E-mail address: mdavidsonmd@gmail.com

which are under investigation in ongoing clinical trials. However, until these pharmacotherapies are widely available, the established cholesterol-modifying drugs remain the cornerstone of therapy; among these are statins, niacin, fibrates, ezetimibe, bile acid sequestrants (BASs), and omega-3 fatty acids (OM3FAs). In the last 10 years, clinical trials of combination therapy, primarily used as add-on therapies to statins, have yielded inconsistent results with regards to CV-related morbidity and mortality outcomes. Further complicating the picture are the release of the 2013 American College of Cardiology (ACC)/American Heart Association (AHA) Guidelines on the Treatment of Blood Cholesterol, which shifted the focus of therapy away from LDL-C targets.[2] The juxtaposition of these guidelines with previous algorithms has invoked questions regarding the safety and efficacy of combination lipid-lowering therapies as part of an optimal medical regimen for CV risk reduction. Although combination therapy may not be broadly recommended for all patients, closer examination of the available data suggests that combination therapy is largely safe and that careful selection provides tailored lipid-lowering strategies, which may benefit specific populations.

QUESTIONING THE PARADIGM: UPDATED BLOOD CHOLESTEROL GUIDELINES

Until recently, the aim of lipid-lowering therapy had focused on an established LDL-C target, which was calculated based on the presence of CV risk factors or equivalent disease states. In turn, this risk estimate and target LDL-C mandated how medication therapies were initiated and further titrated, typically beginning with statins.[3] The National Cholesterol Education Panel delineated LDL-C as the primary target of statin therapy, with a secondary non–HDL-C goal (designated as 30 mg/dL more than the LDL-C target). Intensive therapy was geared toward patients with higher risk, as assessed by the 10-year risk estimates using the Framingham scoring system, with consideration for use of add-on therapies for achievement of LDL-C or non–HDL-C targets. Commonly cited weaknesses of the 2001 guidelines and 2004 update were the limited generalizability of the Framingham risk score in women and nonwhite populations, and the monolithic emphasis on LDL-C targets, which could possibly lead to underuse of statin therapy. Efforts to expound on these guidelines emerged from consensus statements and guidelines from the American Diabetes Association and AHA/ACC, which further elaborated on the identification of high-risk patients (so-called cardiometabolic patients and those with established CVD), for whom intensive lipid-lowering therapy would provide incremental benefit in residual CV risk reduction.[4–6]

In a hotly debated turn, the 2013 ACC/AHA Guidelines on the Treatment of Blood Cholesterol abandoned the prespecified LDL-C and non–HDL-C targets in favor of the identification of 4 risk groups for whom statin therapy is most likely to be beneficial in reducing the risk of atherosclerotic CVD.[2] Furthermore, in lieu of designated on-treatment LDL-C targets, the guidelines suggested an empirical statin potency (low, mid, or high potency) without clear targets. It can be surmised that assessing a response to therapy (ie, percent LDL reduction) could be obtained from measuring on-treatment lipid values, although the panel did not recommend routine pursuit of LDL-C targets. The 2013 guidelines do not discuss details of combination therapy, although it is implied that there may be a role for add-on strategies in individuals with statin intolerance or those with a suboptimal response to therapy. Thus, the guideline-driven use of combination therapy in the era of statin therapy remains open ended, with answers likely to be clarified by the results of future clinical trials.

STATINS AS FIRST-LINE THERAPY

The largest and most convincing body of clinical trial–based evidence supporting reduction in CV outcomes with lipid-lowering therapies is ascribed to the statin class of drugs. Statins act as competitive inhibitors with HMG-CoA reductase, an enzyme critical to the rate-limiting step in the biosynthesis of cholesterol, because it catalyzes the conversion of HMG-CoA to mevalonic acid. The downstream effects of reduced cholesterol synthesis lead to upregulation of LDL receptors and increased plasma clearance of LDL-C. Lipid-independent pleiotropic effects of statins include improved endothelial function via activation of eNOS, reduction of circulating oxidized lipoproteins, and antiinflammatory effects via suppressed production of proinflammatory cytokines.[7] Imaging studies including intravascular ultrasonography and magnetic resonance imaging modalities have suggested the stabilizing effects of statin therapy on plaque composition by showing plaque lipid depletion and even regression in limited studies.[8–10]

Primary prevention studies of statin therapy have shown benefits through reduction of LDL-C levels along with subsequent decreases in the incidence of coronary disease events in numerous populations, including diabetics (CARDS [Collaborative Atorvastatin Diabetes Study]), the elderly (PROSPER), hypertensive patients (ASCOT-BPLA), and those with high LDL-C levels (WOSCOPS, AFCAPS/Tex-CAPS [Air Force/Texas Coronary Atherosclerosis Prevention Study]).[11–17] Furthermore, an increasing body of evidence suggests that individuals with baseline evidence of increased inflammation, manifest as increases in high-sensitivity C-reactive protein, may experience an even greater benefit of statins mediated through both LDL-lowering and antiinflammatory effects.[18–21] Secondary prevention studies have not only shown a reduction in recurrent CV events with statin therapy for patients with established vascular disease but also a reduction in mortality.[22–27] Data from more recent clinical trials and meta-analyses[22,27,28] have underscored the observation that further LDL-C lowering may be of additional benefit in a very high-risk secondary prevention population. Furthermore, the benefits gleaned from statin use may be continuous over decreasing levels of LDL. An estimated 10% to 12% reduction in all-cause mortality, driven by CV-related mortality, accompanies each 1-mmol/L reduction of LDL-C, which supported the pursuit of more intensive LDL-C goals for certain high-risk populations.[23,29]

LIMITATIONS OF STATIN MONOTHERAPY

Ideally, combining another drug with a statin would improve on CV risk reduction and lessen the likelihood of adverse side effects. Although statins are clearly beneficial, they can be associated with clinically significant adverse reactions and side effects, which may impair adherence or prevent optimal titration. The incidence of musculoskeletal-related issues, most commonly myalgias, was reported in only 1.5% to 5% of patients in clinical trials, whereas observational studies in general statin-treated populations have reported significantly higher rates of up to 10%.[30,31] More serious side effects include myopathy, defined as increased creatine phosphokinase level 10 times the upper limit of normal, and rhabdomyolysis (myopathy with concomitant renal injury), although both entities are less common. Predisposing patient factors associated with a greater incidence of myopathy include elderly age, female gender, renal impairment, hypothyroidism, and the use of interacting drugs (eg, CYP3A4 or CYP2C9 substrates).[32] Statins have also been shown to potentially increase aminotransferase levels, although this may be dose related and also associated with underlying nonalcoholic hepatic steatosis, which improves with therapy.

Overt hepatotoxicity is rare, but caution should be advised for patients with a history of liver dysfunction.[33] Recent attention has been drawn to the potential unmasking of incident diabetes with statin use. This situation seems to be more pronounced with intensive-dose compared with moderate-dose statins, although the risk is outweighed by the magnitude of CV risk reduction seen with their use.[34]

Although statin therapy results in significant reductions in LDL-C levels, it does not affect all components of the lipid profile equally. In cardiometabolic patients with atherogenic dyslipidemia, manifest as increased TG and low HDL-C levels, there may be a role for combination therapy. Post hoc analyses of intensive statin therapy have suggested that persistently increases apolipoprotein B (ApoB) and TG levels are associated with recurrent CV events, reinforcing the concept that although statins are part of optimal medical therapy, they do not entirely mitigate residual risk.[35,36] Therefore, add-on therapies may be appropriate for patients with increased TG or ApoB levels, in addition to those who experience recurrent events on statin therapy.

Strategies for Combination Therapy: Safety and Efficacy

Niacin and statin combination therapy

Niacin is one of the oldest lipid-lowering drugs in active use, and acts to lower LDL-C levels through several mechanisms, including limiting peripheral mobilization of free fatty acids, thereby limiting hepatic very low-density lipoprotein (VLDL) synthesis, as well as interfering with the conversion of VLDL to LDL-C. It results in dose-dependent reductions in LDL-C of up to 15%, and at lower doses, can improve HDL-C by 15% to 40%, and lower TG levels by 25% to 50%. Some of the earliest data using niacin monotherapy in men with previous myocardial infarction (MI) showed a durable CV morbidity and mortality benefit gained with administration of niacin at 3 g per day.[37,38] Additional data gleaned from combination niacin-statin trials using surrogate measures of atherosclerosis, as in the HATS (HDL Atherosclerosis Treatment Study) and ARBITER-3 studies, suggested a possible regression in coronary stenosis and carotid intima-medial thickness, respectively, with combination therapy.[39,40] There are concerns related to its number of side effects, which include flushing, hepatotoxicity, worsening of impaired glucose tolerance, and hyperuricemia.

Recent larger-scale clinical trials of niacin as add-on therapy to statins have yielded less convincing results in altering CVD events. Results from AIM-HIGH (Atherothrombosis Intervention in Metabolic Syndrome with Low HDL/High Triglycerides: Impact on Global Health Outcomes) were released in 2011, because the trial ended earlier than anticipated because of an interim analysis suggesting futility in proving its hypothesis.[41] The study population, comprising patients with atherogenic dyslipidemia and previous CVD, had achieved intensive LDL-C control with combination simvastatin-ezetimibe, with a mean of 71 mg/dL at the start of the trial. Thus, many of these high-risk patients embarked on the trial having already achieved their lipid goals. During the truncated 3-year follow-up period, there was no difference in the composite event of coronary heart disease, nonfatal MI, ischemic stroke, hospitalization for an acute coronary syndrome, or symptom-driven coronary or cerebral revascularization (hazard ratio [HR] 1.02, 95% confidence interval [CI] 0.87–1.21, $P = .79$). Recently published subgroup data posited that there was a trend toward benefit with niacin therapy for patients with the highest tertile of TG (>198 mg/dL) and lowest tertile of HDL-C (<33 mg/dL), although it did not meet significance (HR 0.74, $P = .073$).[42]

Although formal publications are forthcoming, data are available from the HPS2-THRIVE (Treatment of HDL to Reduce the Incidence of Vascular Events) trial, in which niacin-laropiprant versus placebo was tested against a background therapy for simvastatin-ezetimibe and failed to prove benefit in rates of major vascular events (relative risk [RR] 0.96, 95% CI 0.90–1.03, $P = .29$) over 4 years of follow-up.[43] Furthermore, safety end points from the trial raised concerns because of a signal for increased hemorrhagic stroke rates associated with treatment, although the trend toward risk with niacin-laropiprant therapy was not significant (RR 1.28, 95% CI 0.97–1.69, $P = .08$). The well-publicized increased rates of myopathy (RR 4.4, $P<.0001$), particularly in patients of Chinese descent, were not accompanied by a significant increase in rhabdomyolysis (7 cases in treatment vs 5 in placebo, RR 1.4, $= 0.54$), they still suggested a common reason for drug discontinuation.[44] Subgroup data are yet to be made available from this trial, although there was a hint toward possible benefit for a small subgroup of patients with LDL-C levels more than 77 mg/dL (12% for niacin-laropiprant vs 13.5% for placebo, $P = .02$). Both trials aimed to assess the CV benefits gleaned from primarily HDL increasing, although niacin was shown to lower LDL-C levels in both trials (−12.5% reduction in AIM-HIGH, −10% LDL-C reduction in HPS2-THRIVE) without conferring clear and additional CV risk benefit. A flaw in study design that may have contributed to the failure of either AIM-HIGH or HPS2-THRIVE to prove a significant difference in outcomes relates to the small differences in non–HDL-C between treatment groups at the conclusion of the study. In AIM-HIGH, the non-HDL difference was 101 mg/dL, whereas in HPS2-THRIVE, the non-HDL difference was a mere 17 mg/dL. These small differences may have made it difficult to detect a treatment effect between groups, and helps underscore why there was no improvement in risk detected for these populations who were already on intensive lipid-lowering therapy with statins.

The 2013 ACC/AHA guidelines cite that based on the results of AIM-HIGH, there is no apparent CVD benefit for patients who are at their LDL-C goal (between 40 and 80 mg/dL).[2] Although the 2 trials discussed have weakened the strength of evidence supporting the use of niacin, it remains an effective LDL-lowering agent and should be considered as a combination strategy, particularly for patients who have combined increased TG and LDL-C levels without contraindications for its use.

Statins and fibrate combination therapy

Fibric acid derivatives exert a primarily TG-lowering effect via activation of the α subtype of the peroxisome proliferator-activated receptor (PPAR-α), a nuclear hormone receptor. Stimulation of PPAR-α increases lipolysis through simultaneous upregulation of LPL, thereby increasing VLDL catabolism and TG clearance from plasma, but can also lead to small increases in LDL in patients with baseline increased TG levels.

Although fibrates are used in conjunction with statin therapy, their lipid-lowering effects extend beyond reductions in LDL-C ($\leq$10%–20%, again primarily in patients without increased TG levels), because they have also been shown to lower TG levels up to 20% to 50% and increase HDL-C by 5% to 15%.[45] Gemfibrozil is a first-generation fibric acid derivative, and was shown in VA-HIT (Veterans Affairs HDL Intervention Trial)[46] to reduce nonfatal MI and CV death by 4.4% (RR reduction [RRR] of 22%, $P = .006$) when used in dyslipidemic men with previous coronary artery disease compared with the placebo group, despite similarly achieved LDL-C levels. There was an even greater benefit seen for patients with diabetes mellitus or those with increasing plasma insulin levels without overt diabetes.[47] However, gemfibrozil acts by inhibiting hepatic glucuronidation and may potentiate circulating levels of statin, potentially leading to greater risk of toxicity in combination therapy.

Newer formulations, particularly fenofibrate, have been shown to have a lower toxicity profile. This finding was verified in a pooled analysis of 6 clinical trials[48] evaluating coadministration of fenofibrate with statins, in which there were no significant differences in overall adverse events compared with statin monotherapy, including no reports of myopathy or rhabdomyolysis in the 1628 subjects studied. Although the fenofibrate-statin combination fares better in safety data, there is inconsistent evidence for their use to modify CV outcomes. The well-publicized results from the ACCORD (Lipid-lowering Action to Control Cardiovascular Risk in Diabetes) trial,[49] which pitted combination simvastatin-fenofibrate versus simvastatin alone in a diabetic population, failed to show any reduction in the primary composite end point over 4.7 years of follow-up, despite improvements in TG and HDL-C levels in the combination arm. However, an important subgroup emerged, in whom the combination of fenofibrate-simvastatin did confer benefit; although the overall cohort had a nonsignificant RRR in the primary outcome of 8%, patients with TG levels greater than 204 mg/dL and HDL-C levels less than 34 mg/dL had a trend toward a greater RRR (–31%, P = .057). Review of data from older fibrate monotherapy studies (FIELD, HHS, BIP)[50] similarly seem to point to this low–HDL-C/high-TG group as one that experiences the greatest degree of benefit with the use of fibrate therapy.

Furthermore, the safety of this combination seems to have been borne out in trials using fenofibrate. In ACCORD, there was no significant difference in rates of myopathy or increases in creatine phosphokinase levels, again suggesting that the combination of fenofibrate with simvastatin was well tolerated. Although the FIELD trial was intended to analyze the benefit of fibrate monotherapy, nearly one-third of patients in the fibrate arm were initiated on statin therapy, and of those nearly 1000 patients, there were no reported cases of rhabdomyolysis.[51]

A meta-analysis of 18 trials[52] including more than 45,000 patients found that there was no significant mortality benefit with fibrate therapy, but a 10% RRR (P = .048) for overall CV events and 13% RRR for coronary events (P<.001). Taken together, these data suggest that fibrates are not routinely indicated second-line therapy for LDL lowering, nor do they alter mortality outcomes, but their use may result in CV and coronary event reduction for patients with diabetes and an atherogenic dyslipidemic lipid profile.

Bile acid sequestrant and statin combination therapy

Before the advent of statins, BAS therapy with either cholestyramine or colestipol was proved to be an effective LDL-C–lowering strategy, with early data showing associated reductions in coronary heart disease (CHD) event rates compared with placebo.[53–55] In conjunction with statin therapy, BAS can provide an additive reduction in LDL-C levels by 10% to 25%. A caveat for their use relates to a potential increase in TG level for patients with baseline hypertriglyceridemia, which may be related to a compensatory increase in VLDL production. In addition, the use of BAS as part of a combination therapy is limited by their interference with statin absorption, potentially leading to decreased efficacy of therapy.[56]

The emergence of a second-generation BAS, colesevelam, has largely circumvented the drug-drug interactions that marred the use of older-generation BAS. Colesevelam is further appealing among the BAS class because of added improvements in HDL-C and ApoB in combination with atorvastatin.[57] An intriguing glucose-lowering effect of colesevelam was shown in the GLOWS (Glucose Lowering Effect of WelChol Study), in which a small population of diabetic patients were randomized to colesevelam 3.65 g/d versus placebo for 12 weeks, at which time there was a significant reduction in A1c by –0.5% (up to –1.0% for those with baseline HbA1c >8.0%) and reductions in LDL-C (–11.7% treatment difference), as well as ApoB and LDL particle number.[58] Thus, there may be a role for add-on BAS therapy to statins, namely colesevelam, in patients with type 2 diabetes mellitus, although caution must be exercised to avoid its use in patients with hypertriglyceridemia.

Ezetimibe and statin combination therapy

Ezetimibe is a cholesterol absorption inhibitor that works at the level of the Niemann-Pick C1-like 1 protein in the small bowel, capable of decreasing LDL-C levels by up to 20% when used in conjunction with statins.[59–61] Use of ezetimibe as add-on therapy reduces circulating levels of proinflammatory oxidized LDL-C and LDL particle number.[62,63]

Despite the contemporary use of ezetimibe, there are only a few clinical trials that have examined its use within specific patient populations. A secondary analysis from SANDS (Stop Atherosclerosis in Native Diabetics Study)[64] showed regression in carotid intima-medial thickness in diabetics treated to aggressive LDL-C targets regardless of treatment (statin monotherapy vs combination with ezetimibe), indicating that although it was an effective strategy to achieve LDL lowering, there was no treatment-independent benefit gained from its use. The SHARP (Study of Heart and Renal Protection) trial[60] randomized 9270 patients with renal disease to simvastatin-ezetimibe versus placebo, with a significant reduction seen in the primary end point of coronary death, nonfatal MI, stroke, or revascularization (13.4% vs 11.3%, $P = .002$). Evidence of a reduction in CV events within the population with renal disease is particularly notable, because previous statin trials had not been able to replicate a magnitude of benefit. Another study comparing simvastatin-ezetimibe with placebo in patients with mild to moderate aortic stenosis (SEAS [Simvastatin and Ezetimibe in Aortic Stenosis])[59] did not show a reduction in the primary outcome of valvular and ischemic events, but there was a significant reduction in ischemic events by 22%, which was a prespecified secondary outcome. The most common side effects of combination statin-ezetimibe related to transaminase abnormalities, with 1 pooled analysis of safety outcomes[65] estimating an overall incidence less than 1%, consistent with what is reported in the prescribing information.

Benefits of ezetimibe use are extrapolated from the limited series of studies as outlined earlier. IMPROVE-IT (Improved Reduction of Outcomes: Vytorin Efficacy International Trial), which is assessing the use of simvastatin-ezetimibe versus simvastatin in a post-ACS population, should be completed soon and will no doubt enrich the current body of evidence on add-on ezetimibe use.[66]

Omega-3 fatty acids and statin combination therapy

OM3FAs, namely docosahexaenoic acid (DHA) and eicosapentanoic acid (EPA), have been shown to reduce TG levels in a dose-dependent fashion, with largely neutral effects on LDL-C. Earlier secondary prevention studies[67,68] suggested that supplementation with low-dose daily OM3FAs resulted in 15% to 20% reduction in composite CV events for patients with and without a history of coronary artery disease. Subsequent prospective studies[69–71] performed in the era of high-potency statins have failed to replicate these findings. This finding is well illustrated by results from the Alpha Omega trial,[72] which examined the outcomes of low-dose supplementation EPA+DHA in a secondary prevention setting in conjunction with modern medical therapy, with 86% of patients enrolled receiving statin therapy. The negative results for the overall study population suggested that there was a significant interaction in treatment effect seen in patients who were treated with statins, although post hoc analyses did suggest significant benefit for diabetic patients with history of an MI and for patients who were not on statin therapy. The doses of omega-3s used in these trials were ineffective in lowering TGs and therefore may have been inadequate to provide a lipid benefit necessary to reduce CHD events.

Newer formulations of OM3FA (Vascepa, Epanova), highly refined to allow for higher potency of EPA or EPA+DHA, have been shown to effectively treat hypertriglyceridemia and seem to have non–HDL-C–lowering effects, which may be augmented by concomitant high-potency statin use.[73–76] In addition, the combination of statins and OM3FAs seem to be safe and well tolerated, with the most frequent side effect of gastrointestinal intolerance. However, there are no definitive data to suggest a further reduction of CV events with the use of these newer OM3FA formulations. Ongoing clinical trials (REDUCE-IT, STRENGTH) will aim to answer whether the benefits of OM3FA with statin therapy extend beyond TG level lowering to confer any primary or secondary CV RR in patients with hypertriglyceridemia on statin therapy.

Novel Add-On Therapies

Mipomersen and lomitapide are both therapies approved by the US Food and Drug Administration for use as adjunctive to maximally tolerated lipid-lowering medications and diet, specifically for the treatment of homozygous familial hypercholesterolemia (FH). Mipomersen is an apoB-100 antisense oligonucleotide, administered as a subcutaneous injection, which binds to ApoB messenger RNA and curtails hepatic synthesis of ApoB-containing lipoproteins.[77] Main side effects relate to increased liver transaminase levels, injection site reactions, and systemic symptoms of fatigue and pyrexia. Lomitapide is an inhibitor of microsomal TG transfer protein and decreases LDL as well as TG levels.[77] The primary side effect relates to gastrointestinal side effects, and more serious complications related to hepatotoxicity and fatty liver, and have led to limiting prescribing under terms of Risk Evaluation and Mitigation Strategy in the United States.

The promise of PCSK-9 inhibitors, which targets the enzyme that regulates LDL-receptor degradation to promote receptor-mediated clearance of LDL from plasma, only continues to grow with accumulating phase 2 and phase 3 clinical trials. Various antibody formulations have been shown to result in marked LDL-C reductions in FH and the statin-intolerant population, and preliminary data suggest safety and sustained efficacy when used in conjunction with statin therapy with up to 1 year of treatment. Reductions have been dramatic, with 49% to 76% decreases in LDL-C levels as part of monotherapy or used alongside either high-potency statins or daily ezetimibe.[78–83] This striking potency in lipid lowering has allowed greater numbers of at-risk patients to achieve ideal LDL-C targets, which may be difficult for patients with FH or intensive goals of less than 70 mg/dL.[84,85] Concurrent reductions in ApoB, Lp(a), TG, VLDL, and modest increases in HDL-C levels have all been reported, further reinforcing their appeal for clinical use. However, when and for whom this class of medications will be approved and adopted for widespread use will depend on the ease of their required subcutaneous administration routes and durable safety data, which are still undergoing longer-term investigation.

SUMMARY

Individually, many of the lipid-lowering drugs in use have been shown to improve CV outcomes. However, when therapies have been studied in addition to statins, which remain the standard of treatment, it has been challenging to consistently show an additional clinical benefit in terms of CV event reduction, although overall safety seems acceptable. This debate has been further complicated by the advent of recent guidelines, which emphasize treatment with high-potency statin monotherapy over achievement of discrete LDL-C and non–HDL-C targets. Combination therapy is a viable and often used strategy that allows more patients to successfully reach their ideal lipid targets. There may be particular benefit with fenofibrate and niacin in patients with more severe atherogenic dyslipidemias who are unable to achieve intensive LDL reduction with statins alone. In addition, patients with very high CV risk because of recurrent events on therapy, or those with statin intolerance, are potential candidates for combination strategies. Further testing of novel therapies, particularly the PCSK-9 class of medications, may introduce an era of potent LDL lowering without dependence on statins, but until then, they remain the mainstay of therapy.

REFERENCES

1. Fuster V, Kelly BB, editors. Promoting cardiovascular health in the developing world: a critical challenge to achieve global health. Washington, DC: 2010.
2. Stone NJ. 2013 ACC/AHA guideline on the treatment of blood cholesterol to reduce atherosclerotic cardiovascular risk in adults: a report of the American College of Cardiology/American Heart Association Task Force on Practice Guidelines. J Am Coll Cardiol 2013;63(25 Pt B):2889–934.
3. National Cholesterol Education Program (NCEP) Expert Panel on Detection, Evaluation, and Treatment of High Blood Cholesterol in Adults (Adult Treatment Panel III). Third Report of the National Cholesterol Education Program (NCEP) Expert Panel on Detection, Evaluation, and Treatment of High Blood Cholesterol in Adults (Adult Treatment Panel III) final report. Circulation 2002;106(25): 3143–421.
4. American Diabetes Association. Standards of medical care in diabetes–2013. Diabetes Care 2013;36(Suppl 1):S11–66.
5. Brunzell JD. Lipoprotein management in patients with cardiometabolic risk: consensus statement from the American Diabetes Association and the American College of Cardiology Foundation. Diabetes Care 2008;31(4):811–22.
6. AHA. AHA/ACC guidelines for secondary prevention for patients with coronary and other atherosclerotic vascular disease: 2006 update endorsed by the National Heart, Lung, and Blood Institute. J Am Coll Cardiol 2006;47(10):2130–9.
7. Bonetti PO. Statin effects beyond lipid lowering–are they clinically relevant? Eur Heart J 2003;24(3):225–48.
8. Nicholls SJ. Effect of two intensive statin regimens on progression of coronary disease. N Engl J Med 2011;365(22):2078–87.
9. Nissen SE. Effect of very high-intensity statin therapy on regression of coronary atherosclerosis: the ASTEROID trial. JAMA 2006;295(13):1556–65.
10. Zhao XQ. MR imaging of carotid plaque composition during lipid-lowering therapy a prospective assessment of effect and time course. JACC Cardiovasc Imaging 2011;4(9):977–86.
11. Downs JR. Primary prevention of acute coronary events with lovastatin in men and women with average cholesterol levels: results of AFCAPS/TexCAPS. Air Force/Texas Coronary Atherosclerosis Prevention Study. JAMA 1998;279(20): 1615–22.
12. Heart Protection Study Collaborative Group. MRC/BHF Heart Protection Study of cholesterol lowering with simvastatin in 20,536 high-risk individuals: a randomised placebo-controlled trial. Lancet 2002;360(9326):7–22.
13. ALLHAT Officers and Coordinators for the ALLHAT Collaborative Research Group, The Antihypertensive and Lipid-Lowering Treatment to Prevent Heart Attack Trial. Major outcomes in moderately hypercholesterolemic, hypertensive

patients randomized to pravastatin vs usual care: The Antihypertensive and Lipid-Lowering Treatment to Prevent Heart Attack Trial (ALLHAT-LLT). JAMA 2002;288(23):2998–3007.

14. Shepherd J. Prevention of coronary heart disease with pravastatin in men with hypercholesterolemia. West of Scotland Coronary Prevention Study Group. N Engl J Med 1995;333(20):1301–7.

15. Shepherd J. Pravastatin in elderly individuals at risk of vascular disease (PROSPER): a randomised controlled trial. Lancet 2002;360(9346):1623–30.

16. Colhoun HM. Primary prevention of cardiovascular disease with atorvastatin in type 2 diabetes in the Collaborative Atorvastatin Diabetes Study (CARDS): multicentre randomised placebo-controlled trial. Lancet 2004;364(9435): 685–96.

17. Sever PS. Prevention of coronary and stroke events with atorvastatin in hypertensive patients who have average or lower-than-average cholesterol concentrations, in the Anglo-Scandinavian Cardiac Outcomes Trial–Lipid Lowering Arm (ASCOT-LLA): a multicentre randomised controlled trial. Lancet 2003; 361(9364):1149–58.

18. Ridker PM. C-reactive protein levels and outcomes after statin therapy. N Engl J Med 2005;352(1):20–8.

19. Ridker PM. Relative efficacy of atorvastatin 80 mg and pravastatin 40 mg in achieving the dual goals of low-density lipoprotein cholesterol <70 mg/dl and C-reactive protein <2 mg/l: an analysis of the PROVE-IT TIMI-22 trial. J Am Coll Cardiol 2005;45(10):1644–8.

20. Morrow DA. Clinical relevance of C-reactive protein during follow-up of patients with acute coronary syndromes in the Aggrastat-to-Zocor Trial. Circulation 2006; 114(4):281–8.

21. Ridker PM. Rosuvastatin to prevent vascular events in men and women with elevated C-reactive protein. N Engl J Med 2008;359(21):2195–207.

22. LaRosa JC. Intensive lipid lowering with atorvastatin in patients with stable coronary disease. N Engl J Med 2005;352(14):1425–35.

23. Cholesterol Treatment Trialists' (CTT) Collaboration, et al. Efficacy and safety of more intensive lowering of LDL cholesterol: a meta-analysis of data from 170,000 participants in 26 randomised trials. Lancet 2010;376(9753):1670–81.

24. Prevention of cardiovascular events and death with pravastatin in patients with coronary heart disease and a broad range of initial cholesterol levels. The Long-Term Intervention with Pravastatin in Ischaemic Disease (LIPID) Study Group. N Engl J Med 1998;339(19):1349–57.

25. Sacks FM. The effect of pravastatin on coronary events after myocardial infarction in patients with average cholesterol levels. Cholesterol and Recurrent Events Trial investigators. N Engl J Med 1996;335(14):1001–9.

26. Randomised trial of cholesterol lowering in 4444 patients with coronary heart disease: the Scandinavian Simvastatin Survival Study (4S). Lancet 1994; 344(8934):1383–9.

27. Cannon CP. Intensive versus moderate lipid lowering with statins after acute coronary syndromes. N Engl J Med 2004;350(15):1495–504.

28. Pedersen TR. High-dose atorvastatin vs usual-dose simvastatin for secondary prevention after myocardial infarction: the IDEAL study: a randomized controlled trial. JAMA 2005;294(19):2437–45.

29. Baigent C. Efficacy and safety of cholesterol-lowering treatment: prospective meta-analysis of data from 90,056 participants in 14 randomised trials of statins. Lancet 2005;366(9493):1267–78.

30. Bays H. Statin safety: an overview and assessment of the data–2005. Am J Cardiol 2006;97(8A):6C–26C.
31. Bruckert E. Mild to moderate muscular symptoms with high-dosage statin therapy in hyperlipidemic patients–the PRIMO study. Cardiovasc Drugs Ther 2005; 19(6):403–14.
32. Bitzur R. Intolerance to statins: mechanisms and management. Diabetes Care 2013;36(Suppl 2):S325–30.
33. Tandra S, Vuppalanchi R. Use of statins in patients with liver disease. Curr Treat Options Cardiovasc Med 2009;11(4):272–8.
34. Preiss D. Risk of incident diabetes with intensive-dose compared with moderate-dose statin therapy: a meta-analysis. JAMA 2011;305(24):2556–64.
35. Mora S. Determinants of residual risk in secondary prevention patients treated with high- versus low-dose statin therapy: the Treating to New Targets (TNT) study. Circulation 2012;125(16):1979–87.
36. Faergeman O. Plasma triglycerides and cardiovascular events in the Treating to New Targets and Incremental Decrease in End-Points through Aggressive Lipid Lowering trials of statins in patients with coronary artery disease. Am J Cardiol 2009;104(4):459–63.
37. Canner PL. Fifteen year mortality in Coronary Drug Project patients: long-term benefit with niacin. J Am Coll Cardiol 1986;8(6):1245–55.
38. Clofibrate and niacin in coronary heart disease. JAMA 1975;231(4):360–81.
39. Taylor AJ, Lee HJ, Sullenberger LE. The effect of 24 months of combination statin and extended-release niacin on carotid intima-media thickness: ARBITER 3. Curr Med Res Opin 2006;22(11):2243–50.
40. Brown BG. Simvastatin and niacin, antioxidant vitamins, or the combination for the prevention of coronary disease. N Engl J Med 2001;345(22):1583–92.
41. AIM-HIGH Investigators, et al. Niacin in patients with low HDL cholesterol levels receiving intensive statin therapy. N Engl J Med 2011;365(24):2255–67.
42. Guyton JR. Relationship of lipoproteins to cardiovascular events: the AIM-HIGH Trial (Atherothrombosis Intervention in Metabolic Syndrome With Low HDL/High Triglycerides and Impact on Global Health Outcomes). J Am Coll Cardiol 2013; 62(17):1580–4.
43. HPS2-THRIVE: Randomized placebo-controlled trial of ER niacin and laropiprant in 25,673 patients with pre-existing cardiovascular disease. American College of Cardiology Scientific Sessions.
44. HPS2-THRIVE Collaborative Group. HPS2-THRIVE randomized placebo-controlled trial in 25 673 high-risk patients of ER niacin/laropiprant: trial design, pre-specified muscle and liver outcomes, and reasons for stopping study treatment. Eur Heart J 2013;34(17):1279–91.
45. Staels B. Mechanism of action of fibrates on lipid and lipoprotein metabolism. Circulation 1998;98(19):2088–93.
46. Rubins HB. Gemfibrozil for the secondary prevention of coronary heart disease in men with low levels of high-density lipoprotein cholesterol. Veterans Affairs High-Density Lipoprotein Cholesterol Intervention Trial Study Group. N Engl J Med 1999;341(6):410–8.
47. Rubins HB. Diabetes, plasma insulin, and cardiovascular disease: subgroup analysis from the Department of Veterans Affairs high-density lipoprotein intervention trial (VA-HIT). Arch Intern Med 2002;162(22):2597–604.
48. Guo J. Meta-analysis of safety of the coadministration of statin with fenofibrate in patients with combined hyperlipidemia. Am J Cardiol 2012;110(9): 1296–301.

49. ACCORD Study Group. Effects of combination lipid therapy in type 2 diabetes mellitus. N Engl J Med 2010;362(17):1563–74.
50. Singh A. What should we do about hypertriglyceridemia in coronary artery disease patients? Curr Treat Options Cardiovasc Med 2013;15(1):104–17.
51. Keech A, Simes RJ, Barter P. Effects of long-term fenofibrate therapy on cardiovascular events in 9795 people with type 2 diabetes mellitus (the FIELD study): randomised controlled trial. Lancet 2005;366(9500):1849–61.
52. Jun M. Effects of fibrates on cardiovascular outcomes: a systematic review and meta-analysis. Lancet 2010;375(9729):1875–84.
53. Glueck CJ. Colestipol and cholestyramine resin. Comparative effects in familial type II hyperlipoproteinemia. JAMA 1972;222(6):676–81.
54. Hashim SA, Vanitallie TB. Cholestyramine resin therapy for hypercholesteremia: clinical and metabolic studies. JAMA 1965;192:289–93.
55. The Lipid Research Clinics Coronary Primary Prevention Trial results. I. Reduction in incidence of coronary heart disease. JAMA 1984;251(3):351–64.
56. Bellosta S, Paoletti R, Corsini A. Safety of statins: focus on clinical pharmacokinetics and drug interactions. Circulation 2004;109(23 Suppl 1):III50–7.
57. Hunninghake D. Coadministration of colesevelam hydrochloride with atorvastatin lowers LDL cholesterol additively. Atherosclerosis 2001;158(2):407–16.
58. Zieve FJ. Results of the glucose-lowering effect of WelChol study (GLOWS): a randomized, double-blind, placebo-controlled pilot study evaluating the effect of colesevelam hydrochloride on glycemic control in subjects with type 2 diabetes. Clin Ther 2007;29(1):74–83.
59. Rossebo AB. Intensive lipid lowering with simvastatin and ezetimibe in aortic stenosis. N Engl J Med 2008;359(13):1343–56.
60. Baigent C. The effects of lowering LDL cholesterol with simvastatin plus ezetimibe in patients with chronic kidney disease (Study of Heart and Renal Protection): a randomised placebo-controlled trial. Lancet 2011;377(9784):2181–92.
61. Morrone D. Lipid-altering efficacy of ezetimibe plus statin and statin monotherapy and identification of factors associated with treatment response: a pooled analysis of over 21,000 subjects from 27 clinical trials. Atherosclerosis 2012; 223(2):251–61.
62. Moutzouri E. Comparison of the effect of simvastatin versus simvastatin/ezetimibe versus rosuvastatin on markers of inflammation and oxidative stress in subjects with hypercholesterolemia. Atherosclerosis 2013;231(1):8–14.
63. Le NA. Changes in lipoprotein particle number with ezetimibe/simvastatin coadministered with extended-release niacin in hyperlipidemic patients. J Am Heart Assoc 2013;2(4):e000037.
64. Fleg JL. Effect of statins alone versus statins plus ezetimibe on carotid atherosclerosis in type 2 diabetes: the SANDS (Stop Atherosclerosis in Native Diabetics Study) trial. J Am Coll Cardiol 2008;52(25):2198–205.
65. Toth PP. Safety profile of statins alone or combined with ezetimibe: a pooled analysis of 27 studies including over 22,000 patients treated for 6-24 weeks. Int J Clin Pract 2012;66(8):800–12.
66. Cannon CP. Rationale and design of IMPROVE-IT (IMProved Reduction of Outcomes: Vytorin Efficacy International Trial): comparison of ezetimbe/simvastatin versus simvastatin monotherapy on cardiovascular outcomes in patients with acute coronary syndromes. Am Heart J 2008;156(5):826–32.
67. Yokoyama M. Effects of eicosapentaenoic acid on major coronary events in hypercholesterolaemic patients (JELIS): a randomised open-label, blinded endpoint analysis. Lancet 2007;369(9567):1090–8.

68. Dietary supplementation with n-3 polyunsaturated fatty acids and vitamin E after myocardial infarction: results of the GISSI-Prevenzione trial. Gruppo Italiano per lo Studio della Sopravvivenza nell'Infarto miocardico. Lancet 1999;354(9177): 447–55.
69. ORIGIN Trial Investigators. n-3 fatty acids and cardiovascular outcomes in patients with dysglycemia. N Engl J Med 2012;367(4):309–18.
70. Risk and Prevention Study Collaborative Group, et al. n-3 fatty acids in patients with multiple cardiovascular risk factors. N Engl J Med 2013;368(19):1800–8.
71. Kromhout D. n-3 fatty acids and cardiovascular events after myocardial infarction. N Engl J Med 2010;363(21):2015–26.
72. Eussen SR. Effects of n-3 fatty acids on major cardiovascular events in statin users and non-users with a history of myocardial infarction. Eur Heart J 2012; 33(13):1582–8.
73. Ballantyne CM. Efficacy and safety of eicosapentaenoic acid ethyl ester (AMR101) therapy in statin-treated patients with persistent high triglycerides (from the ANCHOR study). Am J Cardiol 2012;110(7):984–92.
74. Bays HE. Eicosapentaenoic acid ethyl ester (AMR101) therapy in patients with very high triglyceride levels (from the Multi-center, plAcebo-controlled, Randomized, double-blINd, 12-week study with an open-label Extension [MARINE] trial). Am J Cardiol 2011;108(5):682–90.
75. Kastelein JJ. Omega-3 free fatty acids for the treatment of severe hypertriglyceridemia: the EpanoVa fOr Lowering Very high triglyceridEs (EVOLVE) trial. J Clin Lipidol 2014;8(1):94–106.
76. Maki KC. A highly bioavailable omega-3 free fatty acid formulation improves the cardiovascular risk profile in high-risk, statin-treated patients with residual hypertriglyceridemia (the ESPRIT trial). Clin Ther 2013;35(9):1400–11.e1–3.
77. Rader DJ, Kastelein JJ. Lomitapide and mipomersen: two first-in-class drugs for reducing low-density lipoprotein cholesterol in patients with homozygous familial hypercholesterolemia. Circulation 2014;129(9):1022–32.
78. Blom DJ. A 52-week placebo-controlled trial of evolocumab in hyperlipidemia. N Engl J Med 2014;370(19):1809–19.
79. Raal F. Low-density lipoprotein cholesterol-lowering effects of AMG 145, a monoclonal antibody to proprotein convertase subtilisin/kexin type 9 serine protease in patients with heterozygous familial hypercholesterolemia: the Reduction of LDL-C with PCSK9 Inhibition in Heterozygous Familial Hypercholesterolemia Disorder (RUTHERFORD) randomized trial. Circulation 2012;126(20):2408–17.
80. Roth EM. Atorvastatin with or without an antibody to PCSK9 in primary hypercholesterolemia. N Engl J Med 2012;367(20):1891–900.
81. Stein EA. Effect of a monoclonal antibody to PCSK9, REGN727/SAR236553, to reduce low-density lipoprotein cholesterol in patients with heterozygous familial hypercholesterolaemia on stable statin dose with or without ezetimibe therapy: a phase 2 randomised controlled trial. Lancet 2012;380(9836):29–36.
82. Stroes E. Anti-PCSK9 antibody effectively lowers cholesterol in patients with statin intolerance: the GAUSS-2 randomized, placebo-controlled phase 3 clinical trial of evolocumab. J Am Coll Cardiol 2014;63(23):2541–8.
83. Sullivan D. Effect of a monoclonal antibody to PCSK9 on low-density lipoprotein cholesterol levels in statin-intolerant patients: the GAUSS randomized trial. JAMA 2012;308(23):2497–506.
84. Desai NR. AMG 145, a monoclonal antibody against PCSK9, facilitates achievement of national cholesterol education program-adult treatment panel III low-density lipoprotein cholesterol goals among high-risk patients: an analysis

from the LAPLACE-TIMI 57 trial (LDL-C assessment with PCSK9 monoclonal antibody inhibition combined with statin thErapy-thrombolysis in myocardial infarction 57). J Am Coll Cardiol 2014;63(5):430–3.

85. RUTHERFORD-2: The addition of evolocumab (AMG 145) allows the majority of heterozygous familial hypercholesterolemic patients to achieve low-density lipoprotein cholesterol goals - results from the phase 3 randomized, double-blind, placebo-controlled study. Presented at ACC Scientific Sessions. 2014.

Lipid-Lowering Agents and Hepatotoxicity

Michael Demyen, MD[a], Kawtar Alkhalloufi, MD[b],
Nikolaos T. Pyrsopoulos, MD, PhD, MBA[a],*

KEYWORDS

- Lipid-lowering agents • Hepatotoxicity • Statins • Drug-induced liver injury

KEY POINTS

- Lipid-lowering therapy is increasingly being used in patients for a variety of diseases, the most important being the secondary prevention of cardiovascular disease.
- Many lipid-lowering drugs carry side effects that include elevations in hepatic function tests and liver toxicity.
- In many cases, these drugs are not prescribed or they are underprescribed because of fears of injury to the liver.
- This article attempts to review key trials with respect to the hepatotoxicity of these drugs.
- Recommendations are also provided with respect to the selection of low-risk patients and strategies to lower the risk of hepatotoxicity when prescribing these medications.

INTRODUCTION

One of the main causes of death in industrialized countries is ischemic heart disease, accounting for approximately 1 out of every 6 deaths in the United States according to 2007 data.[1] Aggressive lipid management strategies have been successful in reducing risk of events in patients with coronary heart disease. Lowering low-density lipoprotein cholesterol (LDL-C) has shown to decrease cardiovascular morbidity and mortality in patients with coronary artery disease and at risk groups for ischemic heart disease. In addition, lowering of non HDL cholesterol is advocated in some circles for primary prevention of heart disease as well.[2]

Concern among primary care physicians and specialists for liver injury due to lipid lowering agents (**Table 1**) may prevent many patients from benefiting from these medications.[3] This article attempts to present the data regarding the risk of hepatotoxicity of these agents and provide strategies and patient selection criteria that will reduce the risk of these side effects.

This article originally appeared in Clinics in Liver Disease, Volume 17, Issue 4, November 2013.
Conflict of Interest: The authors have nothing to disclose.
[a] Rutgers New Jersey Medical School, Newark, New Jersey 07103, USA; [b] Howard University College of Medicine, Washington, DC 20059, USA
* Corresponding author.
E-mail address: npyrsopoulos@yahoo.com

Clinics Collections 5 (2015) 147–162
http://dx.doi.org/10.1016/j.ccol.2015.05.010
2352-7986/15/$ – see front matter © 2015 Elsevier Inc. All rights reserved.

Table 1
Lipid-lowering drug therapies, usual starting doses and dose ranges

Agent	Recommended Starting Daily Dose	Dose Range
Statins		
Lovastatin	20 mg	10–80 mg
Pravastatin	40 mg	10–80 mg
Simvastatin	20–40 mg	5–80 mg
Fluvastatin	40 mg	20–80 mg
Atorvastatin	10–20 mg	10–80 mg
Rosuvastatin	10 mg	5–40 mg
Pitavastatin	2 mg	2–4 mg
Fibrates		
Fenofibrate	48–145 mg	48–145 mg
Gemfibrozil	1200 mg	1200 mg
Fenofibric acid	45–135 mg	45–135 mg
Niacin		
Immediate release	250 mg	250–3000 mg
Extended release	500 mg	50 mg 0–2000 mg
Bile acid sequestrants		
Cholestyramine	8–16 g	4–24 g
Colestipol	2 g	2–16 g
Colesevelam	3.8 g	3.8–4.5 g
Cholesterol absorption inhibitors		
Ezetimibe	10 mg	10 mg
Combination therapies (single pill)		
Ezetimibe/simvastatin	10/20 mg	10/10–10/80 mg
Extended release		
Niacin/simvastatin	500/20 mg	500/20–1000/20 mg

Data from Jellinger PS, Smith DA, Mehta AE, et al. American Association of Clinical Endocrinologists' guidelines for management of dyslipidemia and prevention of atherosclerosis. Endocr Pract 2012;18(Suppl 1):18.

STATINS

Statins are competitive inhibitors of the 3-hydroxy-3-methylglutarylcoenzyme A (HMG-CoA) reductase enzyme and are efficient agents in reducing plasma cholesterol and LDL. The effects of the HMG-CoA reductase inhibitors are related to their capacity to reduce endogenous cholesterol synthesis by inhibiting the enzyme that converts HMG-CoA into mevalonic acid, a cholesterol precursor. Statins also increase plasma LDL uptake of hepatocytes by upregulation of these receptors because of the reduction in plasma concentrations (**Table 2**).[4]

The initial safety trials and postmarketing surveillance studies of statins consistently show that although a significant portion of patients may have elevated aminotransferases, these are usually mild. One of the most convincing articles to demonstrate this was the Greek Atorvastatin and Coronary Heart Disease Evaluation (GREACE) study, by Law and colleagues,[5] which attempted to assess the severity of these abnormalities in hepatic function tests in patients who are prescribed statin medication. The

Table 2
Primary lipid-lowering drug classes and their metabolic effect

Drug Class	Metabolic Effect
HMG-CoA reductase inhibitors (statins: lovastatin, pravastatin, fluvastatin, simvastatin, atorvastatin, rosuvastatin, pitavastatin)	Primarily ↓ LDL-C 21%–55% by competitively inhibiting rate-limiting step of cholesterol synthesis in the liver Effect on HDL-C is less pronounced (↑ 2%–10%) ↓ TG 6%–30%
Fibric acid derivatives (gemfibrozil, fenofibrate, fenofibric acid)	Primarily ↓ TG 20%–35%, ↑ HDL-C 6%–18% by stimulating lipoprotein lipase activity Fenofibrate may ↓ TC and LDL-C 20%–25% Lower VLDL-C and LDL-C; reciprocal increase in LDL-C transforms the profile into a less atherogenic form by shifting fewer LDL particles to larger size Fenofibrate ↓ fibrinogen level
Niacin (nicotinic acid)	↓ LDL-C 10%–25%, ↓ TG 20%–30%, ↑HDL-C 10%–35% by decreasing hepatic synthesis of LDL-C and VLDL-C ↓ Lipoprotein (a) Transforms LDL-C to less atherogenic form by increasing particle size and thus decreasing particle number
Bile acid sequestrants (cholestyramine, colestipol, colesevelam hydrochloride)	Primarily ↓ LDL-C 15%–25% by binding bile acids at the intestinal level Colesevelam ↓ glucose and hemoglobin A1c (~0.5%)
Cholesterol absorption inhibitors (ezetimibe)	Primarily ↓ LDL-C 10%–18% by inhibiting intestinal absorption of cholesterol and decreasing delivery to the liver, ↓ Apo B 11%–16%

Abbreviations: Apo B, apolipoprotein B; HDL-C, HDL cholesterol; TC, total cholesterol; TG, triglyceride; VLDL-C, very low-density lipoprotein cholesterol.
Data from Jellinger PS, Smith DA, Mehta AE, et al. American Association of Clinical Endocrinologists' guidelines for management of dyslipidemia and prevention of atherosclerosis. Endocr Pract 2012;18(Suppl 1):16–17.

study used Hy's law, which used serum bilirubin twice the upper limit of normal (ULN) or alanine aminotransferase (ALT) more than 3 times the ULN in patients without other liver dysfunction as a definition of serious drug-induced toxicity. In a placebo-matched control trial, 10- to 40-mg doses of simvastatin, lovastatin, fluvastatin, atorvastatin, and pravastatin were given to patients; hepatic function tests were compared. The incidence of an ALT elevation more than 3 times the ULN was 1.3% with the tested drugs and 1.1% to placebo, statistically insignificant (**Table 3**).[5]

Data from other trials seem to confirm this data. In one meta-analysis, 4 large trials, involving more than 48,000 patients, compared statins with placebo in patients and showed no difference in the frequency or degree of abnormal Hepatic Function Tests between the treatment and placebo groups. Moreover, if abnormal hepatic function tests were seen, these values tended to normalize, even with continuation of the same dose of statin.[6] Other studies have reported only an insignificant increase in ALT after statin administration.[7]

Perhaps the most striking endorsement for the safety of statins comes from the American Journal of Cardiology in 2006, which stated that after systematically

Table 3
Incidence rate of liver enzyme increase in participants of randomized controlled trials of statins

Trials	Participants (N)		Type of Statins	Duration (y)	Single Measure (%)		2 Consecutive Measures (%)	
	Statin	Placebo			Statin	Placebo	Statin	Placebo
HPS	10,269	10,267	Simvastatin	5.3	0.4	0.3	0.1	0.0
EXCEL	6582	1663	Lovastatin	0.9	1.4	0.9	0.7	0.1
ASCOT	5168	5137	Atorvastatin	3.3	—	—	—	—
LIPID	4512	4502	Pravastatin	6.1	2.1	1.9	—	—
AFCAPS/TexCAPS	3304	3301	Lovastatin	5.2	—	—	0.5	0.3
WOSCOPS	3302	3293	Pravastatin	4.9	0.5	0.4	—	—
PROSPER	2891	2913	Pravastatin	3.2	0.0	0.0	—	—
4S	2221	2223	Simvastatin	5.4	2.1	1.4	0.6	0.5
CARE	2081	2078	Pravastatin	5.0	3.2	3.5	—	—
MIRACL	1538	1548	Atorvastatin	0.3	2.5	0.6	—	—
LIPS	844	833	Fluvastatin	3.9	—	—	1.2	0.4

Study								
GREACE	800	800	Atorvastatin	3.0	—	—	—	—
PMSG	530	535	Pravastatin	0.5	1.1	0.2	0.0	0.0
ACAPS	460	459	Lovastatin	3.0	1.3	1.3	—	—
REGRESS	450	434	Pravastatin	2.0	0.0	0.2	0.0	0.0
FLARE	409	425	Fluvastatin	0.8	1.7	0.7	0.0	0.0
KAPS	224	223	Pravastatin	3.0	1.8	1.3	—	—
LRT	203	201	Lovastatin	0.5	1.5	0.5	—	—
MAAS	193	188	Simvastatin	4.0	0.0	0.0	—	—
Riegger et al[55]	187	178	Fluvastatin	2.5	0.0	0.0	—	—
LCAS	157	164	Fluvastatin	0.9	—	—	1.3	0.1
Total	46,355	41,362	—	—	—	—	—	—
Incidence per 1000 per person-year	82,411	72,457	—	—	3.0	2.0	1.1	0.4

The liver enzyme increase is defined as more than 3 times the ULN or more than 120 U/L.

Abbreviations: 4S, The Scandinavian Simvastatin Survival Study; ACAPS, Asymptomatic Carotid Artery Progression Study; AFCAPS/TexCAPS, Air Force/Texas Coronary Atherosclerosis Prevention Study; ASCOT, Anglo-Scandinavian Cardiac Outcomes Trial; CARE, Cholesterol and Recurrent Events; EXCEL, Expanded Clinical Evaluation of Lovastatin; FLARE, Fluvastatin Angioplasty Restenosis; GREACE, GREek Atorvastatin and Coronary-heart-disease Evaluation; HPS, Heart Protection Study; KAPS, Kuopio Atherosclerosis Prevention Study; LCAS, Lipoprotein and Coronary Atherosclerosis Study; LIPID, The Long-Term Intervention with Pravastatin in Ischaemic Disease; LIPS, Lescol Intervention Prevention Study; LRT, Lovastatin Restenosis; MAAS, Multicentre Anti-Atheroma Study; MIRACL, Myocardial Ischemia Reduction with Acute Cholesterol Lowering; PMSG, Pravastatin Multinational Study Group; PROSPER, The Prospective Study of Pravastatin in the Elderly at Risk; REGRESS, Regression growth evaluation statin study; WOSCOPS, West of Scotland Coronary Prevention Study.

Adapted from Law M, Rudnicka AR. Statin safety: a systematic review. Am J Cardiol 2006;97(8A):52C–60C; with permission.

reviewing cohort studies, randomized trials, voluntary notifications to national regulatory authorities, and published case reports, fewer hepatobiliary disorders were found in statin patients than in placebo patients.[8]

Hepatotoxicity of Different Statins

The safety of statins with regard to hepatotoxicity seems to be a class-wide phenomenon, as evidenced by multiple trials. In the Expanded Clinical Evaluation of Lovastatin Study (EXCEL), a double-blinded, diet- and placebo-controlled trial, 6500 patients were randomized and followed for a median of 5 years. The number of patients who developed ALT elevations greater than 3 times the ULN did not differ between the lovastatin and the placebo group (18 [0.6%] vs 11 [0.3%]).[9]

In the Scandinavian Simvastatin Survival Study (4S), involving over 4000 subjects, the number of patients developing an ALT level greater than 3 times the ULN did not differ between the simvastatin and placebo groups (14 [0.7%]) vs 12 [0.6%]).[10] In the Heart Protection Study, another simvastatin-placebo controlled trial with more than 20,000 patients monitored over 5 years, no evidence of hepatitis (defined as ALT of more than 4 ULN) was found in either group.[11]

Pravastatin also shows robust safety data. Pooled data from 3 large trials involving more than 19,000 patients that were randomized into drug versus placebo showed that marked ALT or aspartate aminotransferase (AST) elevations occurred with similarly low frequency in the pravastatin or placebo group (1.2%).[12–14]

Rosuvastatin was also shown to have a low incidence of hepatoxicity because a 2.5-year database survey of more than 10,000 patients did not show any cases of acute hepatitis.[15]

With atorvastatin, a review article looked at randomized trials, postmarketing analysis, and case reports and concluded that the drug is safe with respect to hepatotoxicity, especially if the dosage is kept less than 80 mg/d.[16]

In a meta-analysis of all statins, fluvastatin was the only statin found to have a significant difference versus placebo in liver test abnormalities (1.13% vs 0.29% with placebo [$P = .04$]). However, this was in a relatively small group of just more than 2000 patients in 2 small trials (**Box 1**).[7]

Hydrophilicity

There was a suggestion in a meta-analysis that higher-intensity hydrophilic statin therapy (ie, rosuvastatin and pravastatin) may increase the risk of elevated

---

Box 1
Percentages of aminotransferase increases in patients treated with placebo and different doses of statins

Stain	Placebo (%)	STATIN Dose (%)			
		10 mg	20 mg	40 mg	80 mg
Lovastatin	0.1	—	0.1	0.9	2.3
Simvastatin	—	—	0.7	0.9	2.3
Pravastatin	1.3	—	—	1.4	—
Fluvastatin	0.3	—	0.2	1.5	2.7
Atorvastatin	—	0.2	0.2	0.6	2.3

Data from De Denus S, Spinler SA, Miller K, et al. Statins and liver toxicity: a meta-analysis. Pharmacotherapy 2004;24:584–91; and *Adapted from* Bellosta S, Paoletti R, Corsini A. Safety of statins: focus on clinical pharmacokinetics and drug interactions. Circulation 2004;109(23 Suppl 1):III50–7, with permission.

aminotransferases (risk ratio [RR] 3.54 [95% confidence interval (CI), 1.83–6.85]) over higher-intensity lipophilic therapy (RR 1.58 [95% CI, 0.81–3.08]). However, this meta-analysis included only 9 trials, and pravastatin was the only hydrophilic statin evaluated. More data are needed before this relationship can be proven.[17]

Statins Dose

There are many studies that demonstrate a dose-dependence risk of aminotransferase elevation in statins. In a 2007 meta-analysis of 9 trials involving multiple statin drugs, there was an increased risk of elevated aminotransferases in patients on high statin therapy when compared with low statin therapy (RR 3.1 [95% CI, 1.72–5.58]).[17] An article by Law and Rudnicka[8] further attempted to quantify the risk as approximately 2 per 1000 patient-years with high doses and 1 per 1000 patient-years with a low-dose regimen. Perhaps the most well-known dose-related risk of hepatic enzyme abnormalities is found in atorvastatin. In a retrospective analysis of data reported in 49 clinical trials, no differences were identified between low-dose atorvastatin (10 mg) versus placebo; however, elevated aminotransferases were significantly elevated in a higher (80 mg) dose of atorvastatin.[18]

It is important to note that the effectiveness of the statin on LDL does not relate in any meaningful way to the risk of liver toxicity. In a large prospective randomized trial of 23 treatment arms, the dose of therapy rather than the effectiveness in lowering LDL was a more important determinant of liver toxicity.[19] The results were similar to a pooled analysis of all statin new drug application data.[20]

Hepatic Function Testing in Patients Taking Statins

There is no evidence that monitoring hepatic function tests while on treatment with statins reduces the rate of hepatotoxicity.[21] According to the US Food and Drug Administration (FDA), a baseline hepatic function tests should be done before starting statins except lovastatin, for which liver-function monitoring is no longer requested for asymptomatic patients without a history of liver disease. Although these warnings and considerations are required on package inserts, the clinical utility may not be warranted.

As so eloquently calculated in Bader's article in the *American Journal of Gastroenterology*, the estimated cost of routine liver function tests on patients prescribed statins in 2005 might approach $3 billion a year.[3] The number has almost certainly increased in the years after this as more patients are found to benefit from this class of drug.

The lack of data supporting routine testing does not imply, however, that patients on statins should not be monitored for liver damage. As pointed out in the article by Björnsson and colleagues,[22] most of the safety studies of statin drugs were severely

---

Risk factors for adverse hepatotoxic effects of statins

- High dose
- Recent addition of statin (within 3 months)
- Drug-drug interactions
- Advanced age and chronic illness
- Concomitant use of other lipid-lowering agents

Adapted from Bellosta S, Paoletti R, Corsini A. Safety of statins: focus on clinical pharmacokinetics and drug interactions. Circulation 2004;109(23 Suppl 1):III50–7.

underpowered to detect such a rare side effect as clinically significant statin hepato-toxicity. Although rare, the side effects, including liver failure, have been reported and should be investigated aggressively in symptomatic patients starting statins for the first time.

Drug Interaction

Hepatotoxicity in statins is more common among patients receiving drugs that are metabolized by the cytochrome P450 enzyme systems (**Table 4**).[23] All statins undergo metabolism by cytochrome P450, with the exception of pravastatin, which is trans-formed enzymatically inside hepatocytes, and rosuvastatin, which is only minimally metabolized by cytochrome P450 2C9. In studies comparing the interaction profiles of pravastatin, simvastatin, and atorvastatin alone versus coadministration with cyto-chrome P450 3A4 inhibitors in healthy subjects, variable effects were reported with different statin preparations. The coadministration of pravastatin with verapamil or itraconazole does not seem to change its pharmacokinetics. However, verapamil increased simvastatin concentrations; itraconazole increased atorvastatin concentra-tions; and clarithromycin enhanced all 3 statin concentrations.[24] Additionally, there has been evidence that cyclosporine may interact with statins via mechanisms that are not exclusively CYP450 3A4 inhibitor related because increases in pravastatin bioavailability have been reported in the literature.[23] This interaction does not seem to affect the overall safety of administration, as was shown in the renal transplant patients receiving cyclosporine in the Assessment of Lescol in Renal Transplantation (ALERT) trial.[25]

Statins in Patients with Chronic Liver Disease

Statin and chronic hepatitis C
Several large trials have shown the administration of statins is safe in patients with hepatitis C.[26] In a study by Khorashadi and colleagues,[27] 830 patients matched for body mass index were randomized into 3 groups: 166 patients who were hepatitis C positive on statin therapy, 332 patients who were hepatitis C negative on statin ther-apy, and 332 patients who were hepatitis C positive who did not receive statin treat-ment. Liver function tests were evaluated 1 year before therapy as well as 1 year after starting the trial. The results showed that all patients receiving statins had a higher inci-dence of mild to moderate increases in liver biochemistry values, but no difference in the frequency or severity of these increases existed between hepatitis C positive and

Table 4		
Summary of important drug-drug interactions with statin use		
May Interact with Statins	**Potentiated by Statin Therapy**	**Similar Side Effects to Statins**
Macrolides	Digoxin	Fibrates
HIV protease inhibitors	Coumarin anticoagulants	Niacin
Azole antifungals	Oral contraceptives	
Diclofenac		
Nefazodone		
Calcium antagonists		
Cyclosporine, tacrolimus		

Abbreviation: HIV, human immunodeficiency virus.
Adapted from Bellosta S, Paoletti R, Corsini A. Safety of statins: focus on clinical pharmacoki-netics and drug interactions. Circulation 2004;109(23 Suppl 1):III50–7.

negative patients on statin therapy. It was the nontreated group who had the highest incidence of severe increases in laboratory values. There were no significant differences in the discontinuation rates of patients taking statins, regardless of hepatitis C status. There is even evidence that the statins may possess antiviral properties, as a fluvastatin trial suggested in hepatitis C interferon treatment failures.[28]

Statins in nonalcoholic steatohepatitis

Statins cannot only be used safely in patients with nonalcoholic fatty liver disease or nonalcoholic steatohepatitis (NASH), there are several trials that suggest statin use may improve or normalize aminotransferases in these patients.[29] Post hoc data from the GREACE trial sought to report the safety of statins in patients with NASH and ALT values that were more than 3 times the ULN versus a control. Serious increases of ALT were no different in each group, and ALT values in the statin group were improved in contrast to the control group. More strikingly, this resulted in an overall 68% risk reduction in cardiovascular events (including all-cause mortality and coronary heart disease mortality and morbidity) in patients taking statins over the control group.[30,31]

Statins in cirrhosis and transplant

Low doses of statins can be used with careful monitoring in compensated cirrhosis, chronic liver disease, and partially obstructed liver disease. One of the best studies was performed by Lewis and colleagues,[32] which was a placebo-controlled trial with 80 mg of pravastatin in more than 300 well-compensated patients with chronic liver disease of all types. Some patients in the group had up to 5 times the normal limit of aminotransferase levels before the study started. Nevertheless, no significant ALT elevations were observed between the two groups, prompting the Liver Expert Panel to recommend that statin therapy not be contraindicated in patients with well-compensated liver disease.[33]

In patients with decompensated cirrhosis, the data support extreme caution with the use of statins because these patients may have severely impaired metabolic pathways. This finding was revealed in a study by Simonson and colleagues[34] in which concentrations of rosuvastatin were increased significantly in a Child-Pugh B cohort when compared with a Child-Pugh A patient population. Uncertainties in plasma concentration might increase the risk of severe hepatotoxicity in these patients.

After a liver transplant, patients must be monitored carefully when they are placed on statins mostly because of the effects of immunosuppressive agents. As noted earlier, these drugs are metabolized by the cytochrome P450 system and increase the risk of statin toxicity. Using pravastatin, which is not metabolized through this pathway, might mitigate these risks. In a controlled crossover study, 6 weeks of pravastatin or cerivastatin did not show significant effects in liver function and immunosuppression. However, the study was small and short-term, so more clinical evidence is likely needed.[35] As noted earlier though, care must be taken when combining pravastatin and cyclosporine because increased bioavailability was seen in these patients.[23]

In the future, statins may play a role in the treatment of patients with cirrhosis as one study suggests. In this trial, simvastatin decreased the hepatic venous pressure gradient and improved liver perfusion in patients with cirrhosis as compared with placebo.[36]

Acute liver failure associated with statin use

The rate of statin-induced hepatic failure is exceedingly rare. Only 30 cases were reported to the FDA between 1987 and 2000. The rate of liver failure with statins use is estimated at about one case per million person-years of use.[5,33] The incidence is very similar to the rate of idiopathic acute liver failure in the general public, which in the United States ranges from 0.5 to 1.0 cases per million.[21]

In an article by Bjornsson and colleagues,[22] all 3 patients who suffered acute liver failure related to statin therapy experienced similar toxicity when rechallenged with the medication.

This finding reinforces the consensus opinion among hepatologists that "if a causal relationship between significant liver injury and statins therapy cannot be excluded, then re-initiation of statin therapy is not recommended."[33]

Summary of the hepatotoxic effects of statins

Mild elevations of ALT (less than 3 times the ULN value) commonly occur in patients who are started on statin therapy; however, this rarely reflects true hepatotoxicity. Such elevations are usually transient, asymptomatic, and do not require interruption of therapy.

Lower doses of statins and lipophilic statin preparations might further reduce that risk. Care should be taken in reducing drug-drug interactions, especially in medications that use the cytochrome P450 3A4 pathway. Many patients with chronic liver disease, such as patients with chronic hepatitis C and patients with NASH, can safely take statins with little risk and possible hepatoprotective benefits. Patients with well-compensated NASH should be strongly considered for statin therapy because of their high cardiovascular risk.[33] On the other hand, statin hepatotoxicity should be monitored more carefully in patients with cirrhosis and in posttransplant patients, especially with patients on significant doses of immunosuppressive medication.

Routine monitoring of hepatic function tests in average-risk patients taking statins, although recommended in several package inserts, is not helpful in discovering serious hepatic events. Björnsson and colleagues[22] suggested a reasonable monitoring strategy whereby patients are counseled on the rare, serious risk of idiosyncratic statin-induced hepatitis; patients with signs and symptoms of this reaction are vigilantly monitored and treated.

Statins should be discontinued in patients having unexplained, persistent elevations of more than 3 times the ULN. Statins should not be restarted in these patients who have hepatotoxic reactions unless another cause for the laboratory abnormality is found. Acute liver failure associated with statins is rare but has been reported.

EZETIMIBE

Ezetimibe was the first member of the lipid-lowering drugs that inhibit the uptake of dietary and biliary cholesterol. The FDA approved it in 2002 for hypercholesterolemia alone or in combination with statins. Ezetimibe inhibits the absorption of dietary and biliary cholesterol by blocking transport proteins, specifically the Niemann-Pick C1-Like 1 protein found in jejunal enterocytes.[37] Ezetimibe reduces the LDL level by 15% to 20%,[38] triglyceride (TG) levels by 5%, and increases the HDL level by 1% to 2% (see **Table 2**).[39] Ezetimibe is commonly combined with a statin and is marketed with simvastatin under the trade name Zetia.

Clinical safety trials of ezetimibe report the incidence of asymptomatic, reversible elevations in aminotransferase levels 3 or more times the ULN at 0.7%, which were similar to placebo.[40] There has been a single case report of a woman who developed a serious hepatocellular drug-induced liver disease after 4 months of therapy with 10 mg daily of ezetimibe, with withdrawal of the drug resulting in slow recovery.[41] To date, no cases of liver failure, liver transplantation, or death have been reported with ezetimibe.

Aminotransferase levels may be slightly higher with combination ezetimibe-simvastatin therapy compared with simvastatin alone,[42] although another trial involving atorvastatin monotherapy versus an atorvastatin-ezetimibe combination showed no significant difference in aminotransferase elevations.[43] In conclusion, ezetimibe monotherapy seems to be extremely safe with regard to aminotransferase elevations, and the value of monitoring liver function among patients receiving a statin-ezetimibe regimen (as stated on the package insert of Zetia [Merck & Co., Inc., Whitehouse Station, NJ, 2001]) should be similar to that of statin therapy alone.

BILE ACID SEQUESTRANTS

As a class, bile acid sequestrants, by the nature of their mechanism, are poorly absorbed and so theoretically have little potential for hepatotoxicity. However, hepatic abnormalities are seen in patients that are administered these drugs.[44] Typical preparations (cholestyramine, colestipol, and colesevelam) bind bile acids in the intestine, preventing enterohepatic recirculation of cholesterol. As a result, the hepatic cholesterol content declines, stimulating the production of LDL receptors, which leads to increased LDL clearance and, thus, low LDL levels. In the Coronary Primary Prevention Trial, cholestyramine reduced the total cholesterol by 13%, LDL by 20%, and Coronary Heart Disease (CHD) events (fatal and nonfatal) by 19% (see **Table 2**). Higher AST levels were seen, on average, in patients on cholestyramine versus placebo in this trial, although this was only seen in the first year of therapy and no episodes of acute liver injury or serious adverse hepatic events were seen.[45] Similarly, in the Lovastatin Study Group III, ALT levels more than 2 times the ULN occurred in 9% of patients in the study.[46]

Colestipol has been shown to have a similar excellent safety record with regard to hepatic derangement; however, there is a case report of a patient with type IIa dyslipidemia who developed asymptomatic elevation of his liver enzymes 10 times the ULN after a 3-month treatment period. One week after discontinuing colestipol, serum aminotransferases decreased dramatically. Four weeks after colestipol was discontinued, all liver function tests were normal.[47]

Colesevelam has greater specificity for bile acids and, thus, has less drug interactions and gastrointestinal adverse effects as compared with cholestyramine and colestipol. In the best study looking at hepatic effects of colesevelam, 509 patients with type 2 diabetes were followed for a year in an open-label study. Only one patient had ALT of more than 3 times the ULN and 2 patients had AST of more than 3 times the ULN. These abnormalities resolved despite the fact that the drug was not stopped during the trial.[48]

In summary, these drugs seem to be extremely safe with regard to serious hepatotoxic events, although they do seem, in some cases, to raise aminotransferase levels. In nearly all cases, these elevations are mild and self-limited and, in cases of severe insult, resolve with the discontinuation of the drug.

NIACIN

Niacin inhibits the lipolysis of TG by hormone-sensitive lipase, thereby decreasing hepatic TG synthesis. Niacin also reduces TG synthesis by inhibiting both the synthesis and esterification of fatty acids in the liver. Niacin reduces TG by 35% to 50% and LDL by 25% and increases the HDL level by 15% to 30% (see **Table 2**).

There are 3 different formulations of niacin: immediate release (IR) or crystalline, extended release (ER), and sustained released (SR), with absorption rates of 1 hour,

8 hours, and 12 hours, respectively. ER and SR preparations are given to reduce the rate of unwanted physical side effects, such as flushing.

IR niacin has been shown to have the least risk of hepatotoxicity, whereas ER and SR preparations seem to be more commonly associated with dose-dependent amino-transferase elevations.[49]

A comparative study indicated that approximately 50% of those receiving SR niacin experienced hepatotoxicity, especially with dosages of more than 2000 mg/d, compared with none in the IR niacin group.[50] The differences in hepatotoxicity among formulations are likely explained by 2 different metabolic pathways. Conjugation of niacin with glycine to form nicotinic acid is a low-affinity, high-capacity system, which leads to flushing. The second nonconjugative pathway involves multiple reactions that convert niacin to nicotinamide and is a high-affinity, low-capacity system with greater potential for hepatotoxicity. IR products will quickly saturate the nonconjugative pathway, with most of the drug being metabolized by conjugation, resulting in increased flushing and a low incidence of hepatotoxicity. Slowly absorbed preparations (SR niacin) are metabolized primarily by the high-affinity nonconjugative pathway, resulting in less flushing but increased hepatotoxicity.[49]

Thus, as is so often the case with niacin, the benefits of this drug must be weighed against the physical and metabolic side effects of the drug. Preparations of SR niacin less than 2 g/d might reduce the risk of hepatic events in these patients.

FIBRATES

Currently, 5 fibrates are used clinically; 3 are available in the United States, 2 of which are found in generic formulations: gemfibrozil and fenofibrate. The FDA has not approved bezafibrate and ciprofibrate, which are available in Europe and elsewhere. The FDA has approved a new fenofibrate formulation known as fenofibric acid (Trilipix) with a specific indication for use with a statin in patients with mixed dyslipidemia.[51]

The pharmacologic actions of fibrates are mediated by their interaction with peroxisome proliferator-activated receptor alpha. Fibrates decrease TG levels by up to 50% and LDL by 15% to 20% and increases HDL by 15%. Most of the fibrates have potential antithrombotic effects, including the inhibition of coagulation and enhancement of fibrinolysis (see **Table 2**).

The effects of fibrate monotherapy on the liver have been discussed and succinctly summarized in Dr Zimmerman's[44] textbook on hepatotoxicity. Clofibrate is associated with several different adverse liver effects. The first is a 10% incidence of AST elevations, which may be partly caused by muscle injury. There have also been case reports of granulomatous cholestatic jaundice and anicteric hepatitis. Also, care should be taken in patients who are at risk for gallbladder disease because this may enhance the formation of stones or in patients with primary biliary cirrhosis in whom clofibrate may increase plasma cholesterol. As far as fenofibrate, elevated aminotransferases have been seen in up to 20% of patients, and several cases of cholestatic and chronic hepatitis have been reported. Gemfibrozil seems to have the least hepatic effects, although a low incidence of elevated aminotransferases have been reported as well as possible evidence of microvesicular steatosis.[44]

The most common use of fibrates today is in combination with other lipid-lowering agents, such as statins; in these preparations, an increased risk of myopathy and elevated aminotransferase levels have been observed, especially when a high dose of statin is used.[52] However, if the concomitant statin dose remains low to moderate, adverse events, including hepatotoxicity, generally remain low.[53] In case of transaminase elevations, levels normalized within weeks after the discontinuation of the drug treatment.[54]

SUMMARY

In patients with hypercholesterolemia and heart disease, lipid-lowering agents have been shown to decrease cardiovascular events and extend lifespans. Nearly all lipid-lowering agents may cause an elevation in aminotransferases in patients. The risk of hepatotoxicity from lipid-lowering agents, however, is generally very low; this risk can be minimized using careful patient selection, attention to the type of drugs used, and knowledge of the potential for drug-drug interactions. Statins, in particular, seem to be extremely safe in most patients, including patients with chronic compensated liver disease. Special care must be taken in patients with evidence of decompensated disease and in patients who are on immunosuppressive medications after undergoing a transplant. Physicians must be vigilant for the signs and symptoms of serious statin-related idiosyncratic drug reaction; statins should never be restarted in these patients.

Ezetimibe seems to be extremely safe with regard to liver toxicity, but physicians should be aware that this drug might be combined with other lipid-lowering agents that may increase the risk of hepatic derangement.

Bile acid sequestrants are also considered very safe with respect to liver toxicity, although mild elevated aminotransferases may be experienced in a significant proportion of patients, which is almost always completely reversible.

Niacin doses of 2 g or more in the ER or higher doses in the SR are associated with higher rates of hepatotoxicity events and should be avoided if possible.

Fibrates, as a class, also have a low risk of elevated aminotransferases; however, this risk is increased when the medication is used in combination with statin therapy.

It seems that hepatic function testing does not need to be routinely performed except in patients that are at risk for hepatic injury, although clinicians should be wary of the small but serious risk of severe liver injury that has been reported with these medications. In general, mild elevations in aminotransferases less than 3 times the ULN should not merit discontinuation of therapy. In elevations greater than 3 times the ULN or in more ominous signs of liver damage, such as hepatomegaly, clinical evidence of jaundice, elevated direct bilirubin, or increased prothrombin time, the discontinuation of statin therapy should be seriously considered.[33]

As always, with any therapy, the overall benefit to patients must be considered when therapy is considered. Indeed, as originally stated in Ted Bader's editorial in the *Journal of Hepatology*, the benefits of lipid-lowering drugs, such as statin therapy, in patients with liver disease and cardiac risk factors may increase the overall lifespan more than any other therapy. In addition, this mortality benefit is accomplished with only minimal risk, especially when compared with the extremely risky therapies offered to many patients with liver disease, such as liver transplantation for patients with NASH or peg interferon–based triple therapy for hepatitis C.[51]

REFERENCES

1. Jellinger PS, Smith DA, Mehta AE, et al. American Association of Clinical Endocrinologists' guidelines for management of dyslipidemia and prevention of atherosclerosis. Endocr Pract 2012;18(Suppl 1):1–78.
2. Smith SC Jr, Benjamin EJ, Bonow RO, et al. AHA/ACCF secondary prevention and risk reduction therapy for patients with coronary and other atherosclerotic vascular disease: 2011 update: a guideline from the American Heart Association and American College of Cardiology Foundation endorsed by the World Heart

Federation and the Preventive Cardiovascular Nurses Association. J Am Coll Cardiol 2011;58(23):2432–46.

3. Bader T. The myth of statin-induced hepatotoxicity. Am J Gastroenterol 2010; 105:978–80. http://dx.doi.org/10.1038/ajg.2010.102.

4. Hunninghake DB. HMG-CoA reductase inhibitors. Curr Opin Lipidol 1992;3: 22–8.

5. Law MR, Wald NJ, Rudnicka AR. Quantifying effect of statins on low density lipoprotein cholesterol, ischaemic heart disease, and stroke: systematic review and meta-analysis. BMJ 2003;326:1423.

6. Rzouq FS, Volk ML, Hatoum HH, et al. Hepatotoxicity fears contribute to under-utilization of statin medications by primary care physicians. Am J Med Sci 2010; 340:89–93.

7. De Denus S, Spinler SA, Miller K, et al. Statins and liver toxicity: a meta-analysis. Pharmacotherapy 2004;24:584–91.

8. Law M, Rudnicka AR. Statin safety: a systematic review. Am J Cardiol 2006; 97(8A):52C–60C.

9. Bradford RH, Shear CL, Chremos AN, et al. Expanded Clinical Evaluation of Lovastatin (EXCEL) study results. I. Efficacy in modifying plasma lipoproteins and adverse event profile in 8245 patients with moderate hypercholesterolemia. Arch Intern Med 1991;151(1):43–9.

10. Randomised trial of cholesterol lowering in 4444 patients with coronary heart disease: the Scandinavian Simvastatin Survival Study (4S). Lancet 1994; 344(8934):1383–9.

11. MRC/BHF Heart Protection Study Collaborative Group, Armitage J, Bowman L, Collins R, et al. Effects of simvastatin 40 mg daily on muscle and liver adverse effects in a 5-year randomized placebo-controlled trial in 20,536 high-risk people. BMC Clin Pharmacol 2009;9:6.

12. Shepherd J, Cobbe SM, Ford I, et al, for the West of Scotland Coronary Prevention Study Group (WOS). Prevention of coronary heart disease with pravastatin in men with hypercholesterolemia. N Engl J Med 1995;333:1301–7.

13. The Long-term Intervention with Pravastatin in Ischemic Disease Group (LIPID). Prevention of cardiovascular events and death with pravastatin in patients with coronary heart disease and a broad range of initial cholesterol levels. N Engl J Med 1998;339:1349–57.

14. Sacks FM, Pfeffer MA, Moye LA, et al, for the Cholesterol and Recurrent Events Trial Investigators (CARE). The effect of pravastatin on coronary events after myocardial infarction in patients with average cholesterol levels. N Engl J Med 1996;335:1001–9.

15. Garcia-Rodriguez LA, Masso-Gonzalez EL, Wallander MA, et al. The safety of rosuvastatin in comparison with other statins in over 100,000 statin users in UK primary care. Pharmacoepidemiol Drug Saf 2008;17:943–52.

16. Arca M. Atorvastatin: a safety and tolerability profile. Drugs 2007;67(Suppl 1): 63–9.

17. Dale KM, White CM, Henyan NN, et al. Impact of statin dosing intensity on transaminase and creatine kinase. Am J Med 2007;120(8):706–12.

18. Newman C, Tsai J, Szarek M, et al. Comparative safety of atorvastatin 80 mg versus 10 mg derived from analysis of 49 completed trials in 14,236 patients. Am J Cardiol 2006;97(1):61–7.

19. Alsheikh-Ali AA, Maddukuri PV, Han H, et al. Effect of the magnitude of lipid lowering on risk of elevated liver enzymes, rhabdomyolysis, and cancer: insights from large randomized statin trials. J Am Coll Cardiol 2007;50:409–18.

20. Jacobson TA. Statin safety: lessons from new drug applications for marketed statins. Am J Cardiol 2006;97(8A):44C–51C.
21. Tolman KG. Defining patient risks from expanded preventive therapies. Am J Cardiol 2000;85:15E–9E.
22. Björnsson E, Jacobsen EI, Kalaitzakis E. Hepatotoxicity associated with statins: reports of idiosyncratic liver injury post-marketing. J Hepatol 2012;56(2):374–80. http://dx.doi.org/10.1016/j.jhep.2011.07.023.
23. Bellosta S, Paoletti R, Corsini A. Safety of statins: focus on clinical pharmacokinetics and drug interactions. Circulation 2004;109(23 Suppl 1):III50–7.
24. Jacobson TA. Comparative pharmacokinetic interaction profiles of pravastatin, simvastatin, and atorvastatin when coadministered with cytochrome P450 inhibitors. Am J Cardiol 2004;94(9):1140–6.
25. Holdaas H, Fellström B, Jardine AG, et al. Effect of fluvastatin on cardiac outcomes in renal transplant recipients: a multicentre, randomised, placebo-controlled trial. Lancet 2003;361(9374):2024–31.
26. Madhoun MF, Bader T. Statins improve ALT values in chronic hepatitis C patients with abnormal values. Dig Dis Sci 2010;55:870–1.
27. Khorashadi S, Hasson NK, Cheung RC. Incidence of statin hepatotoxicity in patients with hepatitis C. Clin Gastroenterol Hepatol 2006;4(7):902–7 [quiz: 806].
28. Bader T, Fazili J, Madhoun M, et al. Fluvastatin inhibits hepatitis C replication in humans. Am J Gastroenterol 2008;103:1383–9.
29. Matalka MS, Ravnan MC, Deedwania PC. Is alternate daily dose of atorvastatin effective in treating patients with hyperlipidemia? The Alternate Day versus Daily Dosing of Atorvastatin Study (ADDAS). Am Heart J 2002;144:674–7.
30. Athyros VG, Tziomalos K, Gossios TD, et al. Safety and efficacy of long-term statin treatment for cardiovascular events in patients with coronary heart disease and abnormal liver tests in the Greek Atorvastatin and Coronary Heart Disease Evaluation (GREACE) study: a post hoc analysis. Lancet 2010;376:1916–22.
31. Bader T. Liver tests are irrelevant when prescribing statins. Lancet 2010;376:1882–3.
32. Lewis JH, Mortensen ME, Zweig S, et al. Efficacy and safety of high-dose pravastatin in hypercholesterolemic patients with well-compensated chronic liver disease: Results of a prospective, randomized, double-blind, placebo-controlled, multicenter trial. Hepatology 2007;46(5):1453–63.
33. Cohen D, Anania F, Chalasani N. An assessment of statin safety by hepatologists. Am J Cardiol 2006;97:C77–81.
34. Simonson SG, Martin PD, Mitchell P, et al. Pharmacokinetics and pharmacodynamics of rosuvastatin in subjects with hepatic impairment. Eur J Clin Pharmacol 2003;58(10):669–75.
35. Onofrei MD, Butler KL, Fuke DC, et al. Safety of statin therapy in patients with preexisting liver disease. Pharmacotherapy 2008;28(4):522–9.
36. Abraldes JG, Albillos A, Bañares R, et al. Simvastatin lowers portal pressure in patients with cirrhosis and portal hypertension: a randomized controlled trial. Gastroenterology 2009;136:1651–8.
37. Garcia-Calvo M, Lisnock J, Bull HG, et al. The target of ezetimibe is Niemann-Pick C1-Like 1 (NPC1L1). Proc Natl Acad Sci U S A 2005;102:8132–7.
38. Gagné C, Bays HE, Weiss SR, et al. Efficacy and safety of ezetimibe added to ongoing statin therapy for treatment of patients with primary hypercholesterolemia. Am J Cardiol 2002;90:1084–91.

39. Knopp RH, Dujovne CA, Le Beaut A, et al. Evaluation of the efficacy, safety, and tolerability of ezetimibe in primary hypercholesterolaemia: a pooled analysis from two controlled phase III clinical studies. Int J Clin Pract 2003;57:363–8.

40. Dujovne CA, Suresh R, McCrary Sisk C, et al. Safety and efficacy of ezetimibe monotherapy in 1624 primary hypercholesterolaemic patients for up to 2 years. Int J Clin Pract 2008;62:1332–6.

41. Castellote J, Ariza J, Rota R, et al. Xavier Xiol Serious drug-induced liver disease secondary to ezetimibe. World J Gastroenterol 2008;14(32):5098–9.

42. Goldman-Levine JD, Bohlman LG. Ezetimibe/simvastatin (Vytorin) for hypercholesterolemia. Am Fam Physician 2005;72:2081–2.

43. Conard S, Bays H, Leiter LA, et al. Ezetimibe added to atorvastatin compared with doubling the atorvastatin dose in patients at high risk for coronary heart disease with diabetes mellitus, metabolic syndrome or neither. Diabetes Obes Metab 2010;12:210–8.

44. Zimmerman HJ. Hepatotoxicity: the adverse effects of drugs and other chemicals on the liver. 2nd edition. Philadelphia: Lippincott; 1999. p. 660, 662.

45. The Lipid Research Clinics Coronary Primary Prevention Trial results. I. Reduction in incidence of coronary heart disease. JAMA 1984;251(3):351–64.

46. The Lovastatin Study Group III. A multicenter comparison of lovastatin and cholestyramine therapy for severe primary hypercholesterolemia. JAMA 1988; 260:359–66.

47. Sirmans SM, Beck JK, Banh HL, et al. Colestipol-induced hepatotoxicity. Pharmacotherapy 2001;21(4):513–6.

48. Goldfine AB, Fonseca VA, Jones MR, et al. Long-term safety and tolerability of colesevelam HCl in subjects with type 2 diabetes. Horm Metab Res 2010;42: 23–30.

49. Backes JM, Padley RJ, Moriarty PM. Important considerations for treatment with dietary supplement versus prescription niacin products. Postgrad Med 2011; 123:70–83.

50. Mckenney JM, Proctor JD, Harris S, et al. A comparison of the efficacy and toxic effects of sustained versus immediate release niacin in hypercholesterolemic patients. JAMA 1994;271:672–7.

51. Mohiuddin SM, Pepine CJ, Kelly MT, et al. Efficacy and safety of ABT-335 (fenofibric acid) in combination with simvastatin in patients with mixed dyslipidemia: a phase 3, randomized, controlled study. Am Heart J 2009;157(1):195–203.

52. Backes JM, Howard PA, Ruisinger JF, et al. Does simvastatin cause more myotoxicity compared with other statins? Ann Pharmacother 2009;43:2012–20.

53. Murdock DK, Murdock AK, Murdock RW, et al. Long-term safety and efficacy of combination gemfibrozil and HMG-CoA reductase inhibitors for the treatment of mixed lipid disorders. Am Heart J 1999;138:151–5.

54. Athyros VG, Papageorgiou AA, Hatzikonstandinou HA, et al. Safety and efficacy of long-term statin-fibrate combinations in patients with refractory familial combined hyperlipidemia. Am J Cardiol 1997;80:608–13.

55. Riegger G, Abletshauser C, Ludwig M, et al. The effect of fluvastatin on cardiac events in patients with symptomatic coronary artery disease during one year of treatment. Atherosclerosis 1999;144(1):263–70.

Screening Strategies for Cardiovascular Disease in Asymptomatic Adults

Margaret L. Wallace, PharmD, BCACP*, Jason A. Ricco, MD, MPH,
Bruce Barrett, MD, PhD

KEYWORDS

- Cardiovascular disease screening • Primary care • Evidence-based
- General-risk adult population

KEY POINTS

- Assessment of risk factors (eg, age, smoking, hypertension, family history) is key in determining the need for additional screening.
- Use of risk assessment tools, such as the Pooled Cohort Equations or Framingham in a United States population or Systematic Coronary Risk Evaluation or Prospective Cardiovascular Münster in a European population, improves the estimation of individual risk; however, these tools do not perform as well in Latinos or Asian Americans.
- Guidelines recommend assessment of risk factors, including lipid levels, every 4 to 6 years in adults 20 to 79 years of age without evidence of atherosclerotic cardiovascular disease (ASCVD), including the estimation of 10-year risk for ASCVD in those individuals aged 40 to 79 years.
- Abdominal aortic ultrasound is recommended one time in men aged 65 to 75 years who have ever smoked.
- There is insufficient evidence to recommend the use of lipoprotein (a), homocysteine, carotid intima-media thickness, or electrocardiography in a general-risk, asymptomatic, adult population.
- If risk-based decisions are uncertain after quantitative risk assessment, some guidelines suggest that family history, high-sensitivity C-reactive protein, or a coronary artery calcium score may be considered to further inform decision making.
- Cardiovascular disease results from a complex interplay of multiple genetic, environmental, and behavioral factors. Genetic screening is not recommended.

This article originally appeared in Primary Care: Clinics in Office Practice, Volume 41, Issue 2, June 2014.
Conflict of Interest: None.
Drs M.L. Wallace and J.A. Ricco are supported by a National Research Service Award (T32HP10010) from the Health Resources and Services Administration to the University of Wisconsin Department of Family Medicine. Dr B. Barrett is supported by a Midcareer Investigator Award in Patient-Oriented Research and Mentoring (K24AT006543) from NIH NCCAM.
Department of Family Medicine, University of Wisconsin, 1100 Delaplaine Court, Madison, WI 53715, USA
* Corresponding author.
E-mail address: Margaret.Wallace@fammed.wisc.edu

EPIDEMIOLOGY AND RISK FACTORS

Heart disease is the leading cause of death in the United States,[1] with heart attack and stroke accounting for about a third of all US deaths.[2] Cardiovascular diseases (CVDs) are also a leading cause of disability, with more than 4 million reporting a related disability in the United States.[2] The total cost of CVDs in the United States was estimated at $444 billion in 2010.[2] This number is expected to increase significantly as the US population ages.[2] Abdominal aortic aneurisms (AAA) affect 5% to 10% of men aged 65 to 79 years, and mortality following rupture of an abdominal aneurism is very high.[3]

Risk factors for CVD include family history, hypertension (HTN), dyslipidemia, smoking history, and diabetes mellitus. Smoking is associated with a 3- to 5-fold increase in the risk of AAA and AAA mortality.[4] Although most people with CVD have at least one conventional risk factor, it is important to know that almost 15% of men and 10% of women with CVD do not have any of the conventional risk factors.[5]

The risk for CVD varies across different populations, including race/ethnicity, age, and sex. Although a leading cause of death in the United States as a whole, heart disease has a higher prevalence, morbidity, and mortality in African Americans.[6,7] The reasons for these disparities have been debated. Risk factors, such as smoking, HTN, diabetes mellitus, and physical inactivity, are more common in African Americans; however, nondisease factors, such as genetic differences, health behaviors, and social factors, also play a role.[6] Race and ethnicity often correlate with social conditions or a person's environment, including education level, access to health care, and socioeconomic status. Lower socioeconomic status is linked to calorie-rich and nutrient-poor diets, which increases the risk of developing CVD.[8]

As the main point of contact within the health care system for most individuals, primary care providers play a critical role in the detection and management of risk factors for the primary prevention of CVD.

GLOBAL RISK ASSESSMENT TOOLS

Although evaluating cardiac risk is crucial for both determining the need for preventive treatment as well as specifying treatment intensity,[9–11] research suggests that health care providers tend to be poor estimators of patients' CVD risk.[12] The relative risk reduction from a given treatment tends to be constant across populations.[13] For example, if a treatment produces a relative risk reduction of approximately 30%, an individual with a baseline risk of 10% would have an absolute risk reduction of 3%. However, an individual with a baseline risk of 20% would have an absolute risk reduction of 6%. Thus, risk assessment is critical because the absolute risk reduction observed from treatment is a function of an individual's baseline risk, and treatment benefits may not outweigh treatment harms (which are likely constant) in low-risk individuals.

A variety of screening tools exist to help providers estimate the risk of a first cardiovascular event in adult patients,[12] including the Pooled Cohort Equations,[14] Framingham Risk Score (FRS), QRISK2 (version 2 of the QRISK CVD risk algorithm), Assessing Cardiovascular Risk using Scottish Intercollegiate Guidelines Network, Systematic Coronary Risk Evaluation (SCORE), Prospective Cardiovascular Münster (PROCAM), and United Kingdom Prospective Diabetes Study (UKPDS). Each tool is derived from a different sample and has associated advantages and disadvantages. As delineated in **Table 1**, consideration of unique characteristics and the source population is useful in guiding the selection of an appropriate risk assessment tool for a particular patient.

Table 1
Commonly used externally validated risk prediction models

Model	Outcome	Number of External Evaluations	Source Populations	Online Tool
Pooled Cohort Equations[33]	Nonfatal MI, CHD death, fatal and nonfatal stroke	—	Atherosclerosis Risk in Communities Study • United States • Aged 45–64 y • Men and women • Whites and African American[34] Cardiovascular Health Study • United States • Aged 65 y and older • Men and women[35] Coronary Artery Risk Development in Young Adults Study • United States • Aged 18–30 y • Men and women • White and African American[36] Framingham Heart Study • United States • Aged 30–62 y • 55% women • Primarily white Framingham Offspring Study • United States • Aged <10–70 y • 52% female • Primarily white[37]	http://my.americanheart.org/professional/StatementsGuidelines/PreventionGuidelines/Prevention-Guidelines_UCM_457698_SubHomePage.jsp

(continued on next page)

Table 1
(continued)

Model	Outcome	Number of External Evaluations	Source Populations	Online Tool
1991 Framingham Risk Score Model	CVD	26	Framingham Heart Study • United States • Aged 30–62 y • 55% women • Primarily white Framingham Offspring Study • United States • Aged <10–70 y • 52% female • Primarily white[37]	http://reference.medscape.com/calculator/framingham-coronary-risk-ldl
1998 Framingham Risk Score Model	Total CHD (ie, angina, MI, sudden CHD death, cardiac procedure)	24	Framingham Heart Study, Framingham Offspring Study[38] • United States • Aged 30–74 y • 53% women • Primarily white[37]	
Framingham Risk Score Adult Treatment Panel III	Hard CHD (ie, sudden CHD death or MI)	16	Framingham Heart Study • United States • Aged 30–62 y • 55% women • Primarily white Framingham Offspring Study • United States • Aged <10–70 y • 52% female • Primarily white[37] *Excludes people with diabetes*	http://cvdrisk.nhlbi.nih.gov/calculator.asp

PROCAM	Hard CHD (ie, sudden CHD death or MI)	11	PROCAM[39] • Germany • Aged 35–65 y • White *Excludes women*	http://www.chd-taskforce.de/procam_interactive.html
SCORE	CVD mortality	11	SCORE[40] • Finland, Russia, Norway, United Kingdom, Denmark, Sweden, Belgium, Germany, Italy, France, Spain • Aged 19–80 y • Pooled dataset from cohort studies in 12 European countries; most of the cohorts were population-based; some occupational cohorts were included to increase representation from lower-risk areas	Access from the European Society of Cardiology

Abbreviations: CHD, coronary heart disease; MI, myocardial infarction.

Data from Matheny M, McPheeters M, Glasser A, et al. Systematic review of cardiovascular disease risk assessment tools. Evidence Synthesis No. 85. Rockville (MD): AHRQ Publication; 2011.

DESCRIPTION OF COMMONLY USED SCREENING METHODS
Blood Pressure Measurement

HTN is a common, preventable risk factor for the development of CVD and death.[15] Individuals with HTN have a much higher risk of stroke, myocardial infarction, heart failure, peripheral vascular disease, and AAA than those without HTN.[16] Office blood pressure measurement with an appropriately sized upper arm cuff is the standard screening test for HTN. In practice, errors may occur in measuring blood pressure as a result of instrument, observer, or patient factors. Factors leading to error include issues with the manometer, stethoscope, poorly fitting cuffs for the patient's arm size, trouble hearing Korotkoff sounds, inattention on the part of the observer, rapid release of air from the blood pressure cuff, and many more.[16] Precision in identifying those with HTN improves with the number of blood pressure measurements taken.[16]

When performed properly, office blood pressure measurement is highly correlated with the intra-arterial measurement and is predictive of cardiovascular risk.[16] The relationship between blood pressure and cardiovascular risk is continuous.[17] Individual blood pressure measurements tend to be variable; thus, HTN diagnosis should be made after at least 2 elevated readings taken on at least 2 visits.[17]

Blood Tests

Dyslipidemia is considered a major risk factor for the development of CVD. Lipid-lowering therapies, especially statins, are widely used in the primary and secondary prevention of CVD.[9] There are known associations between elevations in total cholesterol, low-density lipoproteins (LDL), and triglycerides as well as reductions in high-density lipoproteins (HDL) and CVD. Fasting lipid profiles including these 4 lipid biomarkers are widely used in screening and decision making in contemporary medicine. In recent years, some have also advocated for measuring elevations in lipoprotein (a).[18]

Inflammation seems to play an important role in the development of atherosclerosis. C-reactive protein (CRP) is a biomarker that increases in response to inflammation in the body. An elevated CRP level has been suggested as a potential nontraditional risk factor to use in estimating risk for those without known CVD.[19]

Homocysteine first became of interest in the prediction of CVD after observing that most children with genetic homocystinuria die of premature vascular disease. Severe homocysteine elevations can be the result of genetic mutations causing enzyme abnormalities. Insufficient consumption of folate, vitamin B_6, and vitamin B_{12}—vitamins that play a large role in homocysteine metabolism—accounts for most homocysteine elevations in the United States.[20]

Imaging

A variety of imaging tools have been studied and are increasingly used in practice to screen for CVD, including coronary artery calcium (CAC) obtained by computed tomography (CT), carotid artery ultrasound, and abdominal aorta ultrasound. CAC and carotid artery imaging are both used as markers of atherosclerosis,[21,22] although the interpretation of the 2 modalities differs in prediction of specific cardiovascular risk.[23]

Carotid intima-media thickness (cIMT) reflects primarily hypertensive medial hypertrophy, which is more predictive of stroke than myocardial infarction and is weakly associated with traditional cardiovascular risk factors.[23] Alternatively, carotid plaque area is more predictive of myocardial infarction than stroke and is often associated with traditional risk factors.[23] CAC scores predict cardiovascular events in asymptomatic adults[24] as well as both cardiovascular events and all-cause mortality in people with type 2 diabetes.[25] Screening for abdominal aneurism is conducted using ultrasonography to detect asymptomatic aneurisms for which surgery may reduce the risk of future rupture.[3]

Electrocardiography

Electrocardiography (ECG) has been used since the late 1800s in the diagnosis of CVD. ECG is frequently used to detect cardiac irregularities such as ventricular hypertrophy or conduction system delays. ECG abnormalities are associated with an increased risk of coronary heart disease (CHD) events[26] and mortality.[27]

Genetic Screening

Family history plays an important role in assessing the risk of CVD. In most cases, multiple genetic changes, which individually do not result in disease, are working together with environment and behavior to cause disease. Genetic screening is not yet sophisticated enough to detect this complex interplay between genes. However, some less common inherited heart diseases are caused by one or a few genetic changes that work to cause disease. Examples of these include familial hyperlipidemia, some forms of hypertrophic and dilated cardiomyopathy, arrhythmogenic right ventricular cardiomyopathy, long-QT syndrome, and Brugada syndrome. Genetic testing can help determine which relatives are at risk for developing a condition but cannot predict whether it will develop or its severity.[28]

EVIDENCE FOR RISK ASSESSMENT AND SCREENING
Global Risk Assessment

An impressive body of research demonstrates that the treatment of some cardiovascular risk factors reduces the rate of cardiovascular events. Numerous risk prediction models have been developed, but relatively few have been externally validated. An evidence review from the US Preventive Services Task Force (USPSTF) identified 17 risk prediction models that were validated in a population other than the one in which the model was developed. Risk prediction models are considered general population first-outcome incidence calculators, meaning they are intended to assess the individual risk of a first CVD event in a general-risk population.[12]

US models (ie, Framingham) validated in nationally representative US cohorts performed well in white and black populations but performed poorly among Hispanics and people of Asian descent living in the United States.[12,29,30] Social, cultural, and ethnic differences seem to influence CHD risk; thus, models are more likely to perform well in populations resembling the source population.[12,30] Models that excluded diabetes mellitus performed well in a general population. There are currently no externally validated models for use in a diabetic population in the United States.[12] US models had mixed performance when tested in European cohorts: US models underpredicted risk in European cohorts from high-risk populations (eg, people with diabetes) and overpredicted risk in the general population.[12]

More recently, the American College of Cardiology and the American Heart Association (ACC/AHA) have jointly developed new Pooled Cohort Equations in 2013 to estimate both the 10-year and lifetime risks for developing a first atherosclerotic cardiovascular disease (ASCVD) event, defined as CHD death, nonfatal myocardial infarction, and fatal or nonfatal stroke.[14] Participants from several large cohort studies were ultimately included for analysis and equation development, including participants in the ARIC (Atherosclerosis Risk in Communities) study,[22] Cardiovascular

Health Study,[21] and the CARDIA (Coronary Artery Risk Development in Young Adults) study,[31] in combination with data from the Framingham Study cohorts. The Pooled Cohort Equations include age, total and HDL cholesterol, systolic blood pressure (treated or untreated), diabetes, and current smoking status as statistically warranted variables and are only validated for use in African American and non-Hispanic white men and women because of insufficient data from the pooled cohorts for other racial/ethnic groups.[14]

In general, US models, such as the Pooled Cohorts Equations or FRS, should be used for screening in the United States, whereas European models, such as SCORE or PRO-CAM, should be used in European patients. Recognize that these models have significant limitations when used in populations that do not resemble the source population with regard to social, cultural, and ethnic characteristics. A major concern of the new Pooled Cohort Equations is that it systematically overestimated risks by roughly 75% to 150% based on its performance in 5 external validation cohorts. It is thought that this is caused by the use of cohort data from studies conducted more than 2 decades ago that do not necessarily reflect current levels of morbidity or improvements in overall health and health care since that time.[32] This conclusion suggests the need for routinely performing new external validation studies for any of these risk assessment models in contemporary cohorts to maintain model predictive value. Outcomes and cohort characteristics of several validated risk prediction models are described in **Table 1**.

Blood Pressure

Although there have been no randomized controlled trials (RCTs) evaluating the direct effect of screening for HTN on CVD event rates, trials evaluating HTN treatment demonstrated improved outcomes in the treatment of patients who were enrolled as a result of elevated blood pressures detected in screening.[16] Additionally, no studies have evaluated the relative effectiveness of selective versus universal blood pressure screening or the optimal frequency for blood pressure screening.[16] Although no direct evidence for HTN screening exists, indirect evidence supports screening adults for HTN because it is an important risk factor for CVD events and is reliably detected through office blood pressure screening. Additionally, treatment with lifestyle and pharmacologic therapy can effectively reduce blood pressure and CVD events.[16]

Lipids

Lipid screening in individuals with known CHD has been widely supported for some time. The benefits of lipid screening in a general risk population are relatively unknown because there have been no RCTs evaluating the direct effect of screening on CVD event rates. Because there is growing evidence demonstrating that statins reduce rates of CVD events in both intermediate- and high-risk individuals, dyslipidemia is considered a modifiable risk factor and lipids have become a target for CVD screening.[41] Nevertheless, there has not been clear consensus on whom, how, and when to screen for dyslipidemia for primary prevention of CHD.[42,43]

Because the absolute benefit of treating dyslipidemia is a function of baseline risk, a 10% baseline risk of events has been commonly used as a threshold for producing a meaningful difference in CVD outcomes given the significant drop-off in effectiveness for reducing CVD events in individuals with lower than a 10-year risk.[41,44] A 2008 USPSTF evidence review demonstrated that no combination of FRS ATP-III (Adult Treatment Panel III) risk factors in men aged 18 to 35 years or women younger than 40 years would result in a 10-year risk of cardiovascular events greater than 10% in nonsmokers or those without a history of HTN or diabetes mellitus. This finding means that limiting screening in men aged 18 to 35 years or women younger than 40 years to those with a smoking, HTN, or diabetes history will sufficiently identify those most likely to benefit from treating dyslipidemia.[43]

In 2013, the ACC/AHA released new guidelines for both cardiovascular risk assessment and treatment of cholesterol with statins that defined the threshold for 10-year risk at 7.5% rather than 10.0% as previously defined by ATP-III.[14,45] This risk threshold was based on data from both primary prevention statin RCTs and meta-analyses of statin RCTs included in the 2013 Cochrane review on statins for primary prevention of CVD that suggested that the ASCVD risk reduction benefit clearly outweighed the risks of statin therapy at a 7.5% or more 10-year risk threshold.[41,45,46] However, this redefinition of low ASCVD risk was met with controversy based on conflicting evidence for statin benefits in low-risk individuals as well as the methodology for setting the new threshold.[47–50] Indeed, the meta-analysis performed by the Cholesterol Treatment Trialists' (CTT) collaborators showed a 20% decrease in major vascular events for roughly every 40 mg/dL reduction in LDL cholesterol with statin treatment in low-risk individuals (the most significant finding for the meta-analysis of the 27 RCTs). However, 35% of the major vascular events were actually coronary revascularization procedures and not hard cardiovascular end points.[46,49]

Additionally, data from the CTT meta-analyses do not demonstrate that statins have a significant effect on overall mortality among low-risk individuals; the CTT collaborators did not consider the effect of statins on serious adverse effects despite having access to patient-level data.[49] Regardless of whether the threshold for low ASCVD 10-year risk is less than 7.5% or less than 10.0%, more research is currently needed to determine whether statin treatment in low-risk individuals actually provides a net benefit when taking into account the potential risks and harms of treatment. Future studies addressing this may very well influence the 10-year risk cutoff for risk assessment and more accurately determine whom and when to screen for dyslipidemia.

Screening for lipid disorders is recommended by both the ATP-III's and the USPSTF's guidelines. There are no trials that evaluate the effect of screening for triglycerides on clinical end points in individuals who would not otherwise qualify for lipid-lowering therapy. Although triglycerides seem to be a significant predictor when used as the sole predictor of CHD events, this association is reduced or eliminated when adjusting for other variables, such as those included in the FRS.[43] According to a 2001 evidence synthesis from the USPSTF, a Framingham-based algorithm that incorporates total cholesterol and HDL is the most accurate approach for predicting CHD events.[42] The updated 2013 risk assessment guidelines from the ACC/AHA retain both total and HDL cholesterol as statistically significant variables in the new Pooled Cohort Equations.[14] **Table 2** displays the reliability and accuracy, patient acceptance, and provider feasibility of different lipid screening strategies.

Evidence from epidemiologic studies and RCTs supports the use of CHD risk equivalents (ie, peripheral artery disease, AAA, carotid artery disease, and diabetes)[9] in targeting individuals who may benefit from lipid-lowering therapy.[43] There is not sufficient evidence to inform the recommended frequency of lipid screening in asymptomatic adults, although ATP-III suggests once every 5 years and the ACC/AHA's 2013 guidelines recommend risk factor assessment (including total and HDL cholesterol) every 4 to 6 years among adults.[14,42,43]

Lipoprotein (a)

There is insufficient evidence that using lipoprotein (a) improves risk stratification in asymptomatic adults compared with traditional risk factors alone.[51,52] A plasma lipoprotein (a) level of 30 mg/dL or greater is associated with an increased risk of CVD. There is little correlation between lipoprotein (a) and traditional CHD risk factors,

Table 2
Features of different lipid screening strategies for adults

Test	Reliability	Accuracy	Patient Acceptability	Feasibility for Providers
Nonfasting TC	Intermediate	Lower	Higher	Higher
Nonfasting TC/HDL	Lower	Intermediate	Higher	Intermediate
LDL/HDL ratio requires fasting TC, HDL, triglycerides	Higher	Intermediate	Lower	Intermediate
Nonfasting TC + HDL and NCEP guidelines	Intermediate	Intermediate	Intermediate	Lower
Nonfasting TC + HDL with calculation of Framingham risk	Intermediate	Higher	Intermediate	Lower

Abbreviations: NCEP, National Cholesterol Education Program; TC, total cholesterol.
From Helfand M, Carson S. Screening for lipid disorders in adults: selective update of 2001 US Preventive Services Task Force Review. Evidence synthesis no. 49. Rockville (MD): AHRQ Publication; 2008.

and studies have not evaluated the additive value of lipoprotein (a) with traditional risk factors in predicting CHD.[52]

CRP

Several studies have reported associations of CRP with CVD event rates; nevertheless, there is insufficient evidence that using CRP to stratify risk in asymptomatic adults leads to a reduction in CHD.[52] Adjusting for all Framingham risk factors in the evaluation of CRP, a meta-analysis of 10 studies of good quality from the USPSTF's 2009 evidence review found an increased relative risk (1.58; confidence interval [CI] 1.37–1.83) for those with high CRP (>3.0 mg/L) compared with those with low CRP (<1.0 mg/L). The included studies did not directly assess the impact of adding CRP to the assessment of FRS to reclassify individuals at intermediate risk. Several studies have evaluated the impact of CRP in reclassifying intermediate-risk individuals as high risk; however, the results of these studies are imprecise and conflicting and are not able to quantify how many people would be reclassified.[53]

Homocysteine

Homocysteine levels are positively associated with CVD and can be lowered by folic acid and other nutrients[54]; however, there is no evidence that screening with a homocysteine level in asymptomatic adults leads to a reduction in the prevalence of CHD events. An increase in homocysteine by 5 μmol/L was associated with a small increase in relative risk for total CHD (1.18; CI 1.10–1.26) when those with known CHD were excluded from the cohort. Administering folic acid can result in a reduction in homocysteine, though 2 large randomized trials, Health Outcomes Prevention (HOPE) trial and the Norwegian Vitamin Trial (NORVIT), testing whether folic acid can result in a decrease in myocardial infarction or recurrent CVD events were both negative.[55,56] The HOPE trial demonstrated a decreased relative risk of stroke from decreasing homocysteine with folic acid[56]; however, this was not confirmed in the NORVIT trial.[55] The Swiss Heart Study, which included 553 individuals following successful angioplasty of at least one coronary stenosis, demonstrated decreased relative risk of myocardial infarction or repeat revascularization after percutaneous coronary intervention with the use of homocysteine-lowering therapy.[57] These effects have not been confirmed in other studies.[52]

CAC Score

There is insufficient evidence that screening using a CAC score in asymptomatic adults leads to a reduction in the rate of CHD events.[51,52] A meta-analysis of 3 good-quality population-based cohort studies demonstrated increased relative risk for coronary events as the CAC score increased. Adjusted for other Framingham risk factors, the CAC score demonstrated the ability to better predict individuals at an increased risk over the estimated 10-year risk using FRS alone. Nevertheless, it is important to know that older studies overestimated the independent effect of CAC scores and that no studies have shown that CAC screening leads to better outcomes.[52]

A population-based cohort study from Rotterdam, Netherlands evaluated the utility of using 12 newer risk factors with standard risk factors. This study found that relative to the other emerging risk factors, the CAC score contributed significantly to the standard risk factors to predict CHD risk. However, these results are from a primarily white, European population and did not assess whether CAC screening results in better clinical outcomes.[58]

A cost-effectiveness modeling analysis of CAC score screening in an intermediate-risk population was conducted based on the Rotterdam study. In this analysis, CAC score screening in men just met a commonly used threshold for cost-effectiveness. Because of its retrospective nature, however, many assumptions were made. Sensitivity analysis demonstrated that by altering these assumptions, CAC screening was no longer cost-effective. In women, CAC screening was not cost-effective, even when using assumptions that generally favor CAC screening.[59]

cIMT

A USPSTF's 2009 evidence synthesis evaluating emerging risk factors for CHD found 3 cohort studies evaluating the potential utility of cIMT in screenings. However, these studies had serious limitations, such as including patients with known CAD, symptomatic peripheral vascular disease, or not reporting CHD events as end points. Although cIMT is predictive of some CVD events after adjusting for traditional risk factors, there is not consensus on examination technique or standards for interpreting the cIMT measures. The studies included in the analysis had differing methods for evaluating cIMT, making the synthesis of results unreliable.[51,52] A cohort study published following the USPSTF's 2009 report demonstrated similarly modest improvements in CHD risk prediction.[58]

Ultrasound of Abdominal Aorta

A Cochrane review evaluating ultrasound screening of asymptomatic adults for AAA identified 4 studies with 127891 men and 9342 women randomly assigned to receive ultrasound screening or no screening.[3] Only one trial included women. None of the trials were conducted in the United States (2 were in the United Kingdom, one in Denmark, and one in Australia). In 3 of these trials, screening was associated with a reduction in death from AAA in men aged 65 to 83 years (odds ratio [OR] 0.60; range 0.47–0.78). There was no reduction in mortality among women. Three to 5 years following the screening, all-cause mortality was not significantly different between the screened and unscreened groups. Screened men were more likely to have undergone surgery for AAA than men who were not screened (OR 2.03; range 1.59–2.59).

Screening among men aged 65 to 74 years seems to be cost-effective, but there is no evidence related to life expectancy, complications from surgery, or quality of life.[3]

In 2005, the USPSTF also completed an evidence synthesis. This synthesis included the same 4 trials identified in the Cochrane review; however, the USPSTF's review focused on answering questions related to screening in a high-risk population, repeat screening in individuals without AAA on initial screening, harms associated with AAA screening, and harms associated with repairing AAAs 5.5 cm or greater in diameter.[4] Age, smoking, family history, coronary artery disease, hypercholesterolemia, and cerebrovascular disease are risk factors for AAA. Only one trial evaluated mortality from AAA in different age groups. Invitation to screen was associated with significantly reduced mortality in men aged 65 to 75 years (OR 0.19, CI 0.04–0.89) and increased mortality in older men.[4] The researchers of the USPSTF's evidence syntheses developed a model to evaluate the impact of selectively screening those with a history of smoking. This model demonstrated that invitation to screen men aged 65 to 74 years with a lifetime history of smoking 100 or more cigarettes accounts for 89% of the expected reduction in mortality from screening all men aged 65 to 74 years.[4] However, limiting screening to current smokers was too restrictive and resulted in many missed AAAs. Population screening strategies based on coronary artery disease, hypercholesterolemia, and cerebrovascular disease do not perform better than approaches using age, sex, and smoking history in identifying high-risk populations for screening.[4]

Repeat screening in men with a negative AAA ultrasound at 65 years of age does not seem to be advantageous. In men with negative AAA screening at 65 years of age, the incidence of new AAA was low in 10 years of periodic AAA screening. When AAAs were found in follow-up screening, they were most commonly less than 4.0 cm and did not have a significant risk of rupture.[4] Ultrasonography is not associated with any physical harm in adults. Participants with positive ultrasonography compared with negative ultrasonography had slightly more anxiety and lower mental and physical health scores initially but soon returned to normal within 6 weeks of screening. Elective AAA repair has risks and is associated with significant morbidity and mortality. Outcomes are improved in hospitals conducting more AAA repairs and when repairs are done by experienced vascular surgeons.[4]

ECG

The USPSTF published an evidence synthesis evaluating the use of ECG in screening asymptomatic adults in 2011.[60] There were no RCTs or prospective cohort studies evaluating clinical outcomes following screening versus no screening in asymptomatic adults. No studies assessed the improved accuracy of stratifying cardiovascular risk by using traditional risk factors plus resting or stress ECG compared with traditional risk factors alone. A pooled analysis including 63 prospective cohort studies demonstrated that ST-segment or T-wave abnormalities, left ventricular hypertrophy, bundle branch block, or left-axis deviation on resting ECG or ST-segment depression with exercise, failure to reach maximum target heart rate, or low exercise capacity on exercise ECG are associated with an increased risk of a cardiovascular event after adjusting for traditional risk factors.[60]

Genetic Screening

Although most CVD results from a complex interaction of genetic and environmental influence, thereby precluding effective genetic screening, familial hypercholesterolemia (FH) is a monogenic disease that can be identified with genetic testing. The rate of FH varies greatly by region and ethnicity and responds well to treatment.[61] Genetic screening in family members of people with known FH demonstrated cost-effectiveness in analysis from the Netherlands. This type of screening allows detection of FH before it is symptomatic.[62] A second cost-effectiveness analysis in the United Kingdom demonstrated superiority of DNA testing in family members of people with known or probable FH followed by LDL testing in individuals in which a genetic mutation was not identified.[63] Importantly, these studies used a cascade design, meaning all first-degree relatives of those with known or probable FH are tested rather than general population-based genetic screening, which is not recommended.

CVD PREVENTION AND SCREENING RECOMMENDATIONS

Evidence-based research has allowed for the development of clinical practice guidelines as professional recommendations to guide clinical and health policy decision making. The USPSTF, the ACC/AHA, and other organizations have provided assessments of the current evidence for CVD prevention and screening through professional recommendations. The USPSTF is an independent group of 16 US experts in prevention and evidence-based medicine from the fields of preventive medicine and primary care assembled to provide recommendations based on scientific evidence reviews on a variety of clinical preventive medicine services.[64] The USPSTF provides recommendations for services when benefits clearly outweigh the harms, with a focus on health and quality of life. The USPSTF assigns a grade definition (A, B, C, D, or I) based on the strength of evidence and net benefit, and grade A and B services have clear benefit and should be offered to patients.[65]

The ACC and AHA have jointly produced guidelines for CVD since 1980, with experts in the subjects under consideration providing recommendations based on a thorough evidence review. The experts rank supporting evidence for recommendations according to previously established methodology, with level A evidence coming from multiple randomized clinical trials, level B evidence derived from a single randomized trial or nonrandomized studies, and level C evidence largely based on consensus opinion, case studies, or standard of care. In 2010, the ACC/AHA published a clinical guideline for assessing CVD risk in asymptomatic adults, addressing many of the screening strategies discussed in this article.[66] The ACC/AHA's updated 2013 guideline for assessing cardiovascular risk focuses mainly on the new model for global risk assessment, the Pooled Cohort Equations.[14]

The Joint National Committee on Prevention, Detection, Evaluation, and Treatment of High Blood Pressure (JNC) was established to provide an evidence-based approach to the prevention and management of HTN.[67] JNC is made up of a panel of experts; the most recent set of guidelines, JNC8, was published in 2013 focusing on the treatment of HTN in adults.[15] The National Heart, Lung, and Blood Institute established the National Cholesterol Education Program (NCEP) in 1985 with the goal of reducing CVD morbidity and mortality by lowering the percent of Americans with high cholesterol. As part of its educational efforts, NCEP has published a series of 3 clinical practice guidelines for cholesterol management beginning in 1988.[68] The most recent version, published in 2002 and updated in 2004, The Third Report of the Expert Panel on Detection, Evaluation, and Treatment of High Blood Cholesterol in Adults (ATP-III) was drafted by expert panel members, including representative experts from both ACC and AHA.[44,68] **Table 3** provides a summary of guidelines and recommendations for various screening strategies from these organizations.

CURRENT PRACTICE PATTERNS

Data documenting the current practice patterns for CVD screening using the newest testing modalities are limited. Health system reports and observational data provide

Table 3
Summary of guidelines

Screening	USPSTF's Guideline (Evidence Grade)[a]	ACC Foundation/AHA's Guideline (Evidence Grade)[b]	Other Guidelines
Global Risk Assessment	—	The race- and sex-specific Pooled Cohort Equations should be used in non-Hispanic African Americans and non-Hispanic whites 40–79 y of age (B) Use of the sex-specific Pooled Cohort Equations for non-Hispanic whites may be considered when estimating risk in patients from populations other than African Americans and non-Hispanic whites (C) It is reasonable to assess traditional ASCVD risk factors (age, sex, total and HDL cholesterol, systolic blood pressure, use of antihypertensive therapy, diabetes, and current smoking) every 4–6 y in adults 20–79 y of age who are free from ASCVD (B) Assessing 30-y or lifetime ASCVD risk based on traditional risk factors may be considered in adults 20–59 y of age without ASCVD and who are not at high short-term risk (C)[33]	—
Genetic Screening	—	Genotype testing for CHD risk assessment in asymptomatic adults is not recommended (B)[66]	National Institute for Health and Clinical Excellence: Recommends cascade screening with both cholesterol and DNA testing for the diagnosis of FH[69]
Blood Pressure	Recommends screening for high blood pressure in adults aged 18 y and older (A)[70]	Blood pressure screening is not specifically addressed; however, blood pressure is included in the Pooled Cohort Equation recommended for estimating risk[33]	Joint National Committee on Prevention, Detection, Evaluation, and Treatment of High Blood Pressure: Blood pressure screening is not specifically addressed[15]

Blood Tests

Lipids	Strongly recommends FLP screening men aged 35 y and older for lipid disorders (A) Recommends FLP screening men aged 20 to 35 y for lipid disorders if they have additional risks, such as smoking, HTN, or diabetes (B) Strongly recommends FLP screening women aged 45 y and older (A) Recommends FLP screening women aged 20 to 45 y for lipid disorders if they are at increased risk for coronary heart disease, such as smoking, HTN, or diabetes (B) No recommendation for or against routine screening for lipid disorders in men aged 20 to 35 y or in women aged 20 y and older who are not at increased risk for CHD (C)[71]	Measurement of lipid parameters beyond a standard FLP (total cholesterol, HDL, LDL, triglycerides) are not recommended in asymptomatic adults (C)[66]	NCEP ATP-III: Recommends a complete FLP (total cholesterol, LDL, HDL, and triglycerides) as the preferred initial test, rather than screening for total cholesterol and HDL alone Recommends screening all adults aged 20 y and older every 5 y or more frequently with a borderline result[44]
High-Sensitivity CRP	Current evidence is insufficient to the balance of benefits and harms of using nontraditional risk factors to screen asymptomatic men and women with no history of CHD to prevent CHD events (I)[72]	If, after quantitative risk assessment, a risk-based treatment decision is uncertain, assessment of high-sensitivity CRP may be considered to inform treatment decision making (B)[33]	ACPM: Does not recommend routine screening of the general adult population using high-sensitivity CRP[73] NCEP ATP-III: Does not recommend routine measurement of inflammatory markers for the purpose of modifying LDL cholesterol goals in primary prevention[44]
Homocysteine	Current evidence is insufficient to the balance of benefits and harms of using nontraditional risk factors to screen asymptomatic men and women with no history of CHD to prevent CHD events (I)[72]	Not addressed	NCEP ATP-III: Does not recommend routine measurement of homocysteine as part of risk assessment to modify LDL-cholesterol goals for primary prevention[44]

(continued on next page)

Table 3
(continued)

Screening	USPSTF's Guideline (Evidence Grade)[a]	ACC Foundation/AHA's Guideline (Evidence Grade)[b]	Other Guidelines
Imaging			
CAC Score	Current evidence is insufficient to the balance of benefits and harms of using nontraditional risk factors to screen asymptomatic men and women with no history of CHD to prevent CHD events (I)[72]	If, after quantitative risk assessment, a risk-based treatment decision is uncertain, assessment of CAC score may be considered to inform treatment decision making (B)[33]	NCEP ATP-III: Does not recommend indiscriminate screening for CAC in asymptomatic persons, particularly in persons without multiple risk factors Measurement of CAC is an option for advanced risk assessment in appropriately selected persons[44] ACPM: Does not recommend routine screening of the general adult population using CT scanning[73]
cIMT	Current evidence is insufficient to the balance of benefits and harms of using nontraditional risk factors to screen asymptomatic men and women with no history of CHD to prevent CHD events (I)[72]	cIMT is not recommended for routine measurement in clinical practice for risk assessment for first ASCVD event (B)[33]	ACPM: Does not recommend routine screening of the general adult population using cIMT[73]
Ultrasound of Abdominal Aorta	Recommends one-time screening for AAA by ultrasonography in men aged 65–75 y who have ever smoked (B) No recommendation for or against screening for AAA in men aged 65–75 y who have never smoked (C) Recommends against routine screening for AAA in women (D)[74]	Not addressed	ACPM: Recommends one-time AAA screening in men aged 65–75 y who have ever smoked Routine AAA screening in women is not recommended[73]

ECG			
Stress	Recommends against routine screening with exercise treadmill test in adults with low risk for CHD events (D)[75]	An exercise ECG may be considered for cardiovascular risk assessment in intermediate-risk asymptomatic adults (including sedentary adults considering starting a vigorous exercise program), predominantly when attention is paid to non-ECG markers, such as exercise capacity (B)[66]	ACPM: Does not recommend routine screening of the general adult population using exercise stress testing[73]
Resting	Insufficient evidence to recommend for or against routine ECG in adults at increased risk for CHD events (I)[75]	A resting ECG is reasonable for cardiovascular risk assessment in asymptomatic adults with HTN or diabetes (C) / A resting ECG may be considered for cardiovascular risk assessment in asymptomatic adults without HTN or diabetes (C)[66]	ACPM: Does not recommend routine screening of the general adult population using ECG[73]

Abbreviations: ACPM, American College of Preventive Medicine; FLP, fasting lipid panel.

[a] Strength of recommendation. Grade A: The USPSTF recommends the service. There is high certainty that the net benefit is substantial. Grade B: The USPSTF recommends the service. There is high certainty that the net benefit is moderate or there is moderate certainty that the net benefit is moderate to substantial. Grade C: The USPSTF recommends selectively offering or providing this service to individual patients based on professional judgment and patient preferences. There is at least moderate certainty that the net benefit is small. Grade D: The USPSTF recommends against the service. There is moderate or high certainty that the service has no net benefit or that the harms outweigh the benefits. Grade I: The USPSTF concludes that the current evidence is insufficient to assess the balance of benefits and harms of the service. Evidence is lacking, of poor quality, or conflicting; the balance of benefits and harms cannot be determined.[65]

[b] Evidence based on certainty of treatment effect. Level A: Multiple populations evaluated; data derived from multiple randomized clinical trials or meta-analyses. Level B: Limited populations evaluated; data derived from a single randomized trial or nonrandomized study. Level C: Very limited populations evaluated; only consensus opinion of experts, case studies, or standards of care.[66]

a source for information on blood pressure measurement, lipid screening, and use of ECGs in the primary care setting.

Studies report variable rates of blood pressure screening in the United States. One study of women in central Pennsylvania reported blood pressure measurement as the most commonly received preventive service, with 94.1% receiving screening in a 2-year period.[76] Another study demonstrated that blood pressure was measured in 56% of all adult visits and 93% of visits with hypertensive patients in office visits conducted in 2003 to 2004.[77] Seeing a specialist other than a cardiologist, older than 75 years, lack of insurance, absence of HTN-related comorbidities, and visits other than general medical examination visits were all associated with decreased odds of being screened for HTN.[77] Because blood pressure is one of the most important modifiable risk factors for CVD, this variability in blood pressure screening indicates that efforts are needed to improve the consistency of blood pressure screening in clinical practice.

Lipid screening is currently performed at highly variable rates throughout the United States. Among 6830 patients from 44 primary care practices in the Midwest, the rate of cholesterol screening every 5 years varied from 45% to 88%.[78] Similarly, cholesterol screening rates varied widely among 5071 patients at 60 non–university-based primary care practices in North Carolina. Although the median clinic screening rate of 40% every 2 years met the frequency recommended by the ATP-III's guidelines (once every 5 years), the rate of screening varied broadly from 26% to 54% among the different clinics.[79] Additionally, the 2-year screening rate differed significantly by specialty, with internal medicine providers screening at higher rates than family medicine providers (54% vs 38%) across the clinics.[79]

Lipid screening rates differ based on both patient and contextual factors. Patient factors associated with higher rates of lipid screening include older age, a diagnosis of diabetes, and higher body mass index.[76,79,80] Additionally, having a regular provider, having continuous health insurance coverage for the past year, and the presence of at least one chronic medical condition are associated with higher lipid screening rates.[76] At the contextual level, primary care provider density by county is positively associated with lipid screening.[76] Although some studies suggest no difference in lipid screening rates between men and women,[76,81] Rifas-Shiman and colleagues[80] found that women were screened at lower rates than men across all risk levels. Although there is clear evidence for racial and ethnic disparities in CVD prevalence,[6,7,82] outcomes,[6,7] and some treatment modalities,[6,83] evidence for such disparities in lipid screening rates is less consistent. Analysis of data from the Medical Expenditure Panel Survey, which constructs a nationally representative sample with oversampling of Hispanics and non-Hispanic blacks, from both 1996[84] and 2007[85] did not find significant racial or ethnic differences in cholesterol screening rates. In contrast, 2 independent studies using data from the National Health and Nutrition Examination Survey during the 1988–1994[86] and 1999–2006[87] periods conveyed that African Americans and Mexican Americans were less likely than whites to report serum cholesterol screening.

Given the lower absolute benefit from statin treatment in low-risk individuals,[41,49] variation in lipid screening rates based on some clinical factors may reflect appropriate risk stratification by providers. (Rates less than once every 5 years may very well be appropriate for low risk patients.) However, the widespread variation in lipid screening rates based on nonclinical factors suggests a nonsystematic approach to incorporating evidence-based preventive health services in primary care. Although differences between groups or clinics may seem inevitable, as some practices are more efficient in delivering preventive services than others, Solberg and colleagues[78] found significant variation between the delivery of different preventive services within individual clinics. This "marker of haphazard provision of clinical preventive services"[78(p124)] highlights the need for interventions aimed to systematically deliver evidence-based preventive measures, such as lipid screening. Complicating this task is the difficulty of implementing the ATP-III's guidelines in clinical practice as evident by data illustrating that higher-risk patients are more likely to be undertreated for dyslipidemia than those at lower risk. It is suggested that this is related to a lack of provider comfort with the complexity of ATP-III–based risk categorization.[81] Conversely, in a study of 24 primary care offices, higher global patient-centered medical home (PCMH) scores were associated with greater receipt of preventive health services, including lipid screening.[88] In particular, the relational principles of PCMH (such as identifying a personal physician, having continuity of care, and whole person–oriented care) were more strongly associated with lipid screening than the information technology capabilities of PCMH organizational structure.[88]

There are less available data on the current use of ECGs for screening in the primary care setting. In one study of 10 urban academic group internal medicine practices, ECGs were obtained in 4.4% of asymptomatic patients without known CVD.[89] There was significant variability among both group practices and providers, with the rate of ECG performance ranging from 0.8% to 8.6% among the 10 practices and from 0.0% to 24.0% among providers.[89] Clinical predictors of ECG use include older age, male sex, and clinical comorbidities. Additionally, older male providers, those who billed for ECG interpretation, and Medicare as a payment source were associated with obtaining ECGs.[89] Race and ethnicity were not analyzed as predictors of ECG screening.[89] Overall, variation in ECG screening was not well explained by patient characteristics and likely reflects the lack of sufficient evidence for the role of ECG screening in the primary care setting.[89]

IMPACT OF CHANGES WITHIN HEALTH CARE

The true impact of recent transformations within the health care system, such as widespread use of electronic health records (EHR), implementation of the Affordable Care Act (ACA), development of accountable care organization (ACOs), and expansion of PCMH principles, are yet to be seen.

EHR

Advocated for as a facilitator of quality health care delivery, EHRs are becoming increasingly prevalent. Reports of the effects of EHR implementation, however, are mixed.[90–95] Although proponents have pointed to increased use of clinical decision support within the EHR as a benefit, this has not consistently led to improvements in the quality of care[92]; however, EHRs have been used to successfully identify individuals at risk of developing CVD by readily identifying risk-factor clustering.[93]

ACA and ACOs

Although many provisions of the ACA have been implemented, the law will not be fully used until 2018; the effects of many of the recently implemented provisions have not yet been realized. There are several provisions, however, that will likely impact CVD screening and prevention in primary care. A Prevention and Public Health Fund was established by the ACA, which supports prevention and public health programs. Specifically, this fund will be used to increase the primary care workforce and develop programs to prevent tobacco use, obesity, heart disease, stroke and cancer, and to increase immunization rates.[96] Additionally, the ACA requires new health plans and

Medicare to provide coverage for preventive services rated A or B by the USPSTF (including AAA screening for men aged 65–75 years who have ever smoked and cholesterol screening in men older than 35 years or women older than 45 years or younger if at an increased risk for CHD).[96,97] There will also be federal matching payments for preventive services in Medicaid for states that offer A- and B-recommended services with no patient cost sharing.[96]

Through the ACA, the Centers for Medicare and Medicaid Services' Shared Savings Program promotes the growth of ACOs, the aims of which are to improve care for individuals, better the health of populations, and slow the growth of costs. Importantly, prevention is a key component of improving care, bettering health, and slowing growth of costs.[98,99] To accomplish these aims, ACOs must not only effectively manage patients' health care information but also use this information to inform patients about preventive care and increase patients' engagement in prevention through shared decision making.[98]

PCMH

The concept of the PCMH has been present for some time. In 2008, the American Academy of Family Physicians, American Academy of Pediatrics, American College of Physicians, and American Osteopathic Association developed joint principles describing the characteristics of the PCMH.[100] These principles describe a model in which patients have an ongoing relationship with a physician who provides continuous and comprehensive care. This physician leads a team of people who work together to provide care and arrange for care by other professionals when needed. Patients have enhanced access to care and increased options for communication with providers and staff. All of these principles are aligned to improve coordination of care, quality, and safety.[100] Research evaluating principles of the PCMH and the receipt of preventive services found a positive relationship with regard to lipid screening, suggesting that PCMH characteristics of practice organization may facilitate CVD screening best practice.[88]

SUMMARY

Any summary of scientific evidence is somewhat constrained as a particular snapshot in time, and lack of current evidence must not be equated with evidence against effectiveness. Many methods for CVD screening have insufficient evidence to currently recommend use in a general, asymptomatic adult population. This lack of evidence corresponds well with a 2012 Cochrane review evaluating the impact of general health checks (including screening measures) that found general health checks did not improve either overall health or cardiovascular morbidity and mortality.[101] Nonetheless, there is good evidence for some specific CVD screening modalities when used in the proper risk setting. Lipid measurement and abdominal aortic ultrasound, for example, are 2 screening techniques with strong data regarding who benefits from screening and the impact of screening on outcomes. Although current evidence does not support the use of other newer screening modalities for primary prevention of CVD, this may very well change as more high-quality trials are completed in the future.

Risk assessment is a vital first step in determining the appropriate approach to CVD screening. As discussed earlier, even with elevated LDL, younger adults without other risk factors, such as HTN, smoking, or diabetes, will not likely qualify for cholesterol-lowering medications according to the ATP-III's or ACC/AHA's guidelines. In this segment of the population, lipid screening may not be necessary. One study found that prescribed lipid management (ie, lifestyle counseling and medication initiation) was more closely related to pretreatment LDL than to calculated 10-year risk despite a body of research to the contrary, resulting in undertreatment of many intermediate- and high-risk individuals.[81] This finding highlights the importance of moving the assessment of CVD risk factors beyond the traditional focus on LDL and dyslipidemia to a more holistic and individualized approach as outlined by the ACC/AHA's 2013 risk assessment guidelines and championed by the PCMH movement.

Risk assessment tools, such as the Pooled Cohort Equations or Framingham calculator in a US population and SCORE cards or PROCAM calculator in a European population, can facilitate the estimation of risk and open the door for shared decision making regarding interventions to reduce cardiovascular risk. Shared decision-making tools are sometimes built into risk assessment tools (eg, QINTERVENTION tool for use in the United Kingdom: http://qintervention.org/; Mayo Clinic Shared Decision Making National Resource Center Statin/Aspirin Choice tool http://shareddecisions.mayoclinic.org/decision-aids-for-diabetes/cardiovascular-prevention/). These tools are designed to support patient-provider conversations regarding risk factor identification and the potential benefits and harms of screening for and/or treating a health condition. Including patients in the conversation regarding evidence, potential risks, and the various options for CVD screening will provide patients with the knowledge to make informed decisions regarding their health. Further research is needed on the facilitators of and barriers to efforts to implement global risk assessment strategies in a primary care setting.

The absolute benefit of treating risk factors to prevent CVD varies considerably as a function of baseline risk. In light of the current evidence, health organizations should be encouraged to reprioritize quality metrics by shifting the focus away from measuring individual biomarkers to performing global risk assessment to achieve CVD screening best practice.

ACKNOWLEDGMENTS

The authors would like to thank Mary Checovich, Senior Research Specialist with the University of Wisconsin Department of Family Medicine, for her organizational support in the development of this article.

REFERENCES

1. Kochanek KD, Xu J, Murphy SL, et al. Deaths: final data for 2009. Natl Vital Stat Rep 2011;60(3):1–17.
2. Centers for Disease Control and Prevention. Heart disease and stroke prevention addressing the nation's leading killers: at a glance 2011. Prev Chronic Dis 2011. Available at: http://www.cdc.gov/chronicdisease/resources/publications/aag/dhdsp.htm. Accessed May 16, 2013.
3. Cosford PA, Leng GC. Screening for abdominal aortic aneurysm [review]. Cochrane Database Syst Rev 2011;(2):CD002945.
4. Fleming C, Whitlock E, Beil T, et al. Screening for abdominal aortic aneurysm: a best-evidence systematic review for the US Preventive Service Task Force. Ann Intern Med 2005;142:203–11.
5. Khot UN, Khot MB, Bajzer CT, et al. Prevalence of conventional risk factors in patients with coronary heart disease. JAMA 2003;290(7):898–904.
6. Harold JG, Williams KA Sr. President's page: disparities in cardiovascular care: finding ways to narrow the gap. J Am Coll Cardiol 2013;62(6):563–5.

7. Ford ES. Trends in predicted 10-year risk of coronary heart disease and cardio-vascular disease among U.S. adults from 1999 to 2010. J Am Coll Cardiol 2013; 61(22):2249–52.

8. Drewnowski A. Obesity, diets, and social inequalities. Nutr Rev 2009;67(Suppl 1):S36–9.

9. Expert Panel on Detection Evaluation, Treatment of High Blood Cholesterol in Adults. Executive summary of the third report of the National Cholesterol Education Program (NCEP) Expert Panel on Detection, Evaluation, And Treatment of High Blood Cholesterol In Adults (Adult Treatment Panel III). JAMA 2001; 285(19):2486–97.

10. Wood D, De Backer G, Faergeman O, et al. Prevention of coronary heart disease in clinical practice: recommendations of the Second Joint Task Force of European and other Societies on Coronary Prevention. Atherosclerosis 1998; 140(2):199–270.

11. Califf RM, Armstrong PW, Carver JR, et al. 27th Bethesda Conference: matching the intensity of risk factor management with the hazard for coronary disease events. Task Force 5. Stratification of patients into high, medium and low risk subgroups for purposes of risk factor management. J Am Coll Cardiol 1996; 27(5):1007–19.

12. Matheny M, McPheeters M, Glasser A, et al. Systematic review of cardiovascular disease risk assessment tools. Evidence Synthesis No. 85. Rockville (MD): AHRQ Publication; 2011.

13. Barratt A, Wyer PC, Hatala R, et al. Tips for learners of evidence-based medicine: 1. Relative risk reduction, absolute risk reduction and number needed to treat. CMAJ 2004;171(4):353–8.

14. Goff DC Jr, Lloyd-Jones DM, Bennett G, et al. 2013 ACC/AHA guideline on the assessment of cardiovascular risk: a report of the American College of Cardiology/American Heart Association Task Force on Practice Guidelines. Circulation 2013. [Epub ahead of print].

15. James PA, Oparil S, Carter BL, et al. 2014 Evidence-based guideline for the management of high blood pressure in adults: report from the panel members appointed to the Eighth Joint National Committee (JNC 8). JAMA 2014;311(5): 507–20.

16. Sheridan S, Pignone M, Donahue K. Screening for high blood pressure: a review of the evidence for the U.S. Preventive Services Task Force. Am J Prev Med 2003;25(2):151–8.

17. US Preventive Services Task Force. Screening for high blood pressure: US Preventive Services Task Force reaffirmation recommendation statement. Ann Intern Med 2007;147(11):783–6.

18. Emerging Risk Factors Collaboration, Di Angelantonio E, Sarwar N, Perry P, et al. Major lipids, apolipoproteins, and risk of vascular disease. JAMA 2009;302(18): 1993–2000.

19. Akhabue E, Thiboutot J, Cheng JW, et al. New and emerging risk factors for coronary heart disease. Am J Med Sci 2014;347(2):151–8.

20. Humphrey LL, Fu R, Rogers K, et al. Homocysteine level and coronary heart disease incidence: a systematic review and meta-analysis. Mayo Clin Proc 2008; 83(11):1203–12.

21. O'Leary DH, Polak JF, Kronmal RA, et al. Carotid-artery intima and media thickness as a risk factor for myocardial infarction and stroke in older adults. Cardiovascular Health Study Collaborative Research Group. N Engl J Med 1999; 340(1):14–22.

22. Chambless LE, Heiss G, Folsom AR, et al. Association of coronary heart disease incidence with carotid arterial wall thickness and major risk factors: the Atherosclerosis Risk in Communities (ARIC) Study, 1987-1993. Am J Epidemiol 1997; 146(6):483–94.
23. Spence JD. Technology insight: ultrasound measurement of carotid plaque–patient management, genetic research, and therapy evaluation. Nat Clin Pract Neurol 2006;2(11):611–9.
24. Pletcher MJ, Tice JA, Pignone M, et al. Using the coronary artery calcium score to predict coronary heart disease events: a systematic review and meta-analysis. Arch Intern Med 2004;164(12):1285–92.
25. Kramer CK, Zinman B, Gross JL, et al. Coronary artery calcium score prediction of all cause mortality and cardiovascular events in people with type 2 diabetes: systematic review and meta-analysis. BMJ 2013;346:f1654.
26. Moyer VA, US Preventive Serivces Task Force. Screening for coronary heart disease with electrocardiography: US Preventive Services Task Force recommendation statement. Ann Intern Med 2012;157(7):512–8.
27. Ashley EA, Raxwal VK, Froelicher VF. The prevalence and prognostic significance of electrocardiographic abnormalities. Curr Probl Cardiol 2000;25(1): 1–72.
28. Cirino AL, Ho CY. Genetic testing for inherited heart disease. Circulation 2013; 128(1):e4–8.
29. Liao Y, McGee DL, Cooper RS, et al. How generalizable are coronary risk prediction models? Comparison of Framingham and two national cohorts. Am Heart J 1999;137(5):837–45.
30. Orford JL, Sesso HD, Stedman M, et al. A comparison of the Framingham and European Society of Cardiology coronary heart disease risk prediction models in the normative aging study. Am Heart J 2002;144(1):95–100.
31. Okwuosa TM, Greenland P, Ning H, et al. Yield of screening for coronary artery calcium in early middle-age adults based on the 10-year Framingham Risk Score: the CARDIA study. JACC Cardiovasc Imaging 2012;5(9):923–30.
32. Ridker PM, Cook NR. Statins: new American guidelines for prevention of cardiovascular disease. Lancet 2013;382(9907):1762–5.
33. Goff DC Jr, Lloyd-Jones DM, Bennett G, et al. 2013 ACC/AHA Guideline on the Assessment of Cardiovascular Risk: a Report of the American College of Cardiology/American Heart Association Task Force on Practice Guidelines. J Am Coll Cardiol 2013. [Epub ahead of print].
34. The Atherosclerosis Risk in Communities (ARIC) Study: design and objectives. The ARIC investigators. Am J Epidemiol 1989;129(4):687–702.
35. Fried LP, Borhani NO, Enright P, et al. The Cardiovascular Health Study: design and rationale. Ann Epidemiol 1991;1(3):263–76.
36. Friedman GD, Cutter GR, Donahue RP, et al. CARDIA: study design, recruitment, and some characteristics of the examined subjects. J Clin Epidemiol 1988;41(11):1105–16.
37. Govindaraju DR, Cupples LA, Kannel WB, et al. Genetics of the Framingham Heart Study population. Adv Genet 2008;62:33–65.
38. Wilson PW, D'Agostino RB, Levy D, et al. Prediction of coronary heart disease using risk factor categories. Circulation 1998;97(18):1837–47.
39. Assmann G, Cullen P, Schulte H. Simple scoring scheme for calculating the risk of acute coronary events based on the 10-year follow-up of the prospective cardiovascular Munster (PROCAM) study. Circulation 2002;105(3): 310–5.

40. Conroy RM, Pyorala K, Fitzgerald AP, et al. Estimation of ten-year risk of fatal cardiovascular disease in Europe: the SCORE project. Eur Heart J 2003; 24(11):987–1003.

41. Taylor F, Huffman MD, Macedo AF, et al. Statins for the primary prevention of cardiovascular disease. Cochrane Database Syst Rev 2013;(1):CD004816.

42. Pignone MP, Phillips CJ, Atkins D, et al. Screening and treating adults for lipid disorders. Am J Prev Med 2001;20(3 Suppl):77–89.

43. Helfand M, Carson S. Screening for lipid disorders in adults: selective update of 2001 US Preventive Services Task Force Review. Evidence synthesis no. 49. Rockville (MD): AHRQ Publication; 2008.

44. National Cholesterol Education Program Expert Panel on Detection Evaluation, Treatment of High Blood Cholesterol in Adults. Third report of the National Cholesterol Education Program (NCEP) Expert Panel on Detection, Evaluation, and Treatment of High Blood Cholesterol in Adults (Adult Treatment Panel III) final report. Circulation 2002;106(25):3143–421.

45. Stone NJ, Robinson J, Lichtenstein AH, et al. 2013 ACC/AHA guideline on the treatment of blood cholesterol to reduce atherosclerotic cardiovascular risk in adults: a report of the American College of Cardiology/American Heart Association Task Force on Practice Guidelines. Circulation 2013. [Epub ahead of print].

46. Mihaylova B, Emberson J, Blackwell L, et al. The effects of lowering LDL cholesterol with statin therapy in people at low risk of vascular disease: meta-analysis of individual data from 27 randomised trials. Lancet 2012;380(9841):581–90.

47. Taylor F, Ward K, Moore TH, et al. Statins for the primary prevention of cardiovascular disease. Cochrane Database Syst Rev 2011;(1):CD004816.

48. Cooper A, O'Flynn N. Risk assessment and lipid modification for primary and secondary prevention of cardiovascular disease: summary of NICE guidance. BMJ 2008;336(7655):1246–8.

49. Abramson JD, Rosenberg HG, Jewell N, et al. Should people at low risk of cardiovascular disease take a statin? BMJ 2013;347:f6123.

50. Mosca L, Benjamin EJ, Berra K, et al. Effectiveness-based guidelines for the prevention of cardiovascular disease in women–2011 update: a guideline from the American Heart Association. Circulation 2011;123(11):1243–62.

51. Helfand M, Buckley D, Freeman M, et al. Emerging risk factors for coronary heart disease: a summary of systematic reviews conducted for the US Preventive Services Task Force. Ann Intern Med 2009;151:496–507.

52. Helfand M, Buckley D, Fleming C, et al. Screening for intermediate risk factors for coronary heart disease: systematic evidence synthesis. Evidence synthesis No. 73. Rockville (MD): AHRQ Publication; 2009.

53. Buckley DI, Fu R, Freeman M, et al. C-reactive protein as a risk factor for coronary heart disease: a systematic review and meta-analyses for the US Preventive Services Task Force. Ann Intern Med 2009;151(7):483–95.

54. Homocysteine Studies Collaboration. Homocysteine and risk of ischemic heart disease and stroke: a meta-analysis. JAMA 2002;288(16):2015–22.

55. Bonaa KH, Njolstad I, Ueland PM, et al. Homocysteine lowering and cardiovascular events after acute myocardial infarction. N Engl J Med 2006;354(15):1578–88.

56. Lonn E, Yusuf S, Arnold MJ, et al. Homocysteine lowering with folic acid and B vitamins in vascular disease. N Engl J Med 2006;354(15):1567–77.

57. Schnyder G, Roffi M, Flammer Y, et al. Effect of homocysteine-lowering therapy with folic acid, vitamin B12, and vitamin B6 on clinical outcome after percutaneous coronary intervention: the Swiss Heart study: a randomized controlled trial. JAMA 2002;288(8):973–9.

58. Kavousi M, Elias-Smale S, Rutten JH, et al. Evaluation of newer risk markers for coronary heart disease risk classification: a cohort study. Ann Intern Med 2012; 156(6):438–44.
59. van Kempen BJ, Spronk S, Koller MT, et al. Comparative effectiveness and cost-effectiveness of computed tomography screening for coronary artery calcium in asymptomatic individuals. J Am Coll Cardiol 2011;58(16):1690–701.
60. Chou R, Arora B, Dana T, et al. Screening asymptomatic adults with resting or exercise electrocardiography: a review of the evidence for the US Preventive Services Task Force. Ann Intern Med 2011;155:375–85.
61. Austin MA, Hutter CM, Zimmern RL, et al. Genetic causes of monogenic heterozygous familial hypercholesterolemia: a HuGE prevalence review. Am J Epidemiol 2004;160(5):407–20.
62. Wonderling D, Umans-Eckenhausen MA, Marks D, et al. Cost-effectiveness analysis of the genetic screening program for familial hypercholesterolemia in The Netherlands. Semin Vasc Med 2004;4(1):97–104.
63. Nherera L, Marks D, Minhas R, et al. Probabilistic cost-effectiveness analysis of cascade screening for familial hypercholesterolaemia using alternative diagnostic and identification strategies. Heart 2011;97(14):1175–81.
64. United States Preventive Services Task Force. US Preventive Services Task Force. 2013. Available at: http://www.uspreventiveservicestaskforce.org/. Accessed October 21, 2013.
65. US Preventive Services Task Force. US Preventive Services Task Force grade definitions. 2012. Available at: http://www.uspreventiveservicestaskforce.org/uspstf/grades.htm. Accessed May 23, 2013.
66. Greenland P, Alpert JS, Beller GA, et al. 2010 ACCF/AHA guideline for assessment of cardiovascular risk in asymptomatic adults: a report of the American College of Cardiology Foundation/American Heart Association Task Force on Practice Guidelines. J Am Coll Cardiol 2010;56(25):e50–103.
67. Chobanian AV, Bakris GL, Black HR, et al. The seventh report of the Joint National Committee on Prevention, Detection, Evaluation, and Treatment of High Blood Pressure: the JNC 7 report. JAMA 2003;289(19):2560–72.
68. National Cholesterol Education Program-NHLBI, NIH. 2013. Available at: http://www.nhlbi.nih.gov/about/ncep/. Accessed October 21, 2013.
69. Minhas R, Humphries SE, Qureshi N, et al, NICE Guideline Development Group. Controversies in familial hypercholesterolaemia: recommendations of the NICE Guideline Development Group for the identification and management of familial hypercholesterolaemia. Heart 2009;95(7):584–7 [discussion: 587–91].
70. US Preventive Services Task Force. Screening for high blood pressure: US Preventive Services Task Force reaffirmation recommendation statement. 2007. Available at: http://www.uspreventiveservicestaskforce.org/uspstf07/hbp/hbprs.htm. Accessed January 2, 2014.
71. U.S Preventive Services Task Force. Recommendations and rationale: screening for lipid disorders in adults. 2008. Available at: http://www.uspreventiveservicestaskforce.org/uspstf08/lipid/lipidrs.htm. Accessed May 23, 2013.
72. US Preventive Services Task Force. Using nontraditional risk factors in coronary heart disease risk assessment: US Preventive Services Task Force recommendation statement. Ann Intern Med 2009;151:474–82.
73. Lim LS, Haq N, Mahmood S, et al. Atherosclerotic cardiovascular disease screening in adults: American College of Preventive Medicine position statement on preventive practice. Am J Prev Med 2011;40(3):381.e1–10.

74. US Preventive Services Task Force. Screening for abdominal aortic aneurysm: recommendation statement. Ann Intern Med 2005;142:198–202.
75. US Preventive Services Task Force. Screening for coronary heart disease: recommendation statement. 2004. Available at: http://www.uspreventiveservice staskforce.org/3rduspstf/chd/chdrs.htm. Accessed May 23, 2013.
76. McCall-Hosenfeld JS, Weisman CS, Camacho F, et al. Multilevel analysis of the determinants of receipt of clinical preventive services among reproductive-age women. Womens Health Issues 2012;22(3):e243–51.
77. Ma J, Stafford RS. Screening, treatment, and control of hypertension in US private physician offices, 2003-2004. Hypertension 2008;51(5):1275–81.
78. Solberg LI, Kottke TE, Brekke ML. Variation in clinical preventive services. Eff Clin Pract 2001;4(3):121–6.
79. Bertoni AG, Bonds DE, Steffes S, et al. Quality of cholesterol screening and management with respect to the National Cholesterol Education's Third Adult Treatment Panel (ATPIII) guideline in primary care practices in North Carolina. Am Heart J 2006;152(4):785–92.
80. Rifas-Shiman SL, Forman JP, Lane K, et al. Diabetes and lipid screening among patients in primary care: a cohort study. BMC Health Serv Res 2008;8:25.
81. Barham AH, Goff DC Jr, Chen H, et al. Appropriateness of cholesterol management in primary care by sex and level of cardiovascular risk. Prev Cardiol 2009; 12(2):95–101.
82. Allison MA, Ho E, Denenberg JO, et al. Ethnic-specific prevalence of peripheral arterial disease in the United States. Am J Prev Med 2007;32(4):328–33.
83. Rowe VL, Weaver FA, Lane JS, et al. Racial and ethnic differences in patterns of treatment for acute peripheral arterial disease in the United States, 1998-2006. J Vasc Surg 2010;51(4 Suppl):21S–6S.
84. Stewart SH, Silverstein MD. Racial and ethnic disparity in blood pressure and cholesterol measurement. J Gen Intern Med 2002;17(6):405–11.
85. Vaidya V, Partha G, Howe J. Utilization of preventive care services and their effect on cardiovascular outcomes in the United States. Risk Manag Healthc Policy 2011;4:1–7.
86. Nelson K, Norris K, Mangione CM. Disparities in the diagnosis and pharmacologic treatment of high serum cholesterol by race and ethnicity: data from the Third National Health and Nutrition Examination Survey. Arch Intern Med 2002;162(8):929–35.
87. Ford ES, Li C, Pearson WS, et al. Trends in hypercholesterolemia, treatment and control among United States adults. Int J Cardiol 2010;140(2):226–35.
88. Ferrante JM, Balasubramanian BA, Hudson SV, et al. Principles of the patient-centered medical home and preventive services delivery. Ann Fam Med 2010; 8(2):108–16.
89. Stafford RS, Misra B. Variation in routine electrocardiogram use in academic primary care practice. Arch Intern Med 2001;161(19):2351–5.
90. Rabinowitz I, Tamir A. The SaM (Screening and Monitoring) approach to cardiovascular risk-reduction in primary care–cyclic monitoring and individual treatment of patients at cardiovascular risk using the electronic medical record. Eur J Cardiovasc Prev Rehabil 2005;12(1):56–62.
91. Linder JA, Ma J, Bates DW, et al. Electronic health record use and the quality of ambulatory care in the United States. Arch Intern Med 2007;167(13):1400–5.
92. Romano MJ, Stafford RS. Electronic health records and clinical decision support systems: impact on national ambulatory care quality. Arch Intern Med 2011; 171(10):897–903.

93. Hivert MF, Grant RW, Shrader P, et al. Identifying primary care patients at risk for future diabetes and cardiovascular disease using electronic health records. BMC Health Serv Res 2009;9:170.
94. Walsh MN, Yancy CW, Albert NM, et al. Electronic health records and quality of care for heart failure. Am Heart J 2010;159(4):635–42.e1.
95. Zhou L, Soran CS, Jenter CA, et al. The relationship between electronic health record use and quality of care over time. J Am Med Inform Assoc 2009;16(4): 457–64.
96. Kaiser Family Foundation. Health reform implementation timeline. Health Reform 2013. Available at: http://kff.org/interactive/implementation-timeline/. Accessed August 7, 2013.
97. US Preventive Services Task Force. Affordable Care Act: A and B recommendations for preventive services. 2013. Available at: http://www.uspreventiveservices taskforce.org/uspstf/uspsabrecs.htm. Accessed January 2, 2014.
98. Berwick DM. Launching accountable care organizations–the proposed rule for the Medicare Shared Savings Program. N Engl J Med 2011;364(16):e32.
99. Quality Measurement & Health Assessment Group Center for Medicare and Medicaid Services. Quality performance standards narrative measure specifications. Accountable Care Organization 2013 Program Analysis. 2012. Available at: http://www.cms.gov/Medicare/Medicare-Fee-for-Service-Payment/shared savingsprogram/Downloads/ACO-NarrativeMeasures-Specs.pdf.   Accessed August 8, 2013.
100. American Academy of Family Physicians. Joint principles of the Patient-Centered Medical Home. Del Med J 2008;80(1):21–2.
101. Krogsboll L, Jorgensen K, Gronhoj L, et al. General health checks in adults for reducing morbidity and mortality from disease [review]. Cochrane Database Syst Rev 2012;(10):CD009009.

The 2013 American College of Cardiology/American Heart Association Guidelines on Treating Blood Cholesterol and Assessing Cardiovascular Risk

A Busy Practitioner's Guide

Arpeta Gupta, MD[a], Donald A. Smith, MD, MPH[b],*

KEYWORDS

- 2013 ACC/AHA cholesterol guidelines • Pooled cohort equations
- Ten-year ASCVD risk • Statin therapy • Primary prevention of ASCVD
- Blood cholesterol guideline • Cardiovascular risk guideline

KEY POINTS

- The 2013 American College of Cardiology/American Heart Association practice guidelines on the treatment of blood cholesterol and assessment of risk now include stroke in addition to coronary heart disease.
- New risk assessment equations for both 10-year and lifetime risk for atherosclerotic cardiovascular disease (ASCVD) events that include African Americans have been developed.
- Moderate-dose to high-dose statins are recommended for specific groups of persons; those greater than or equal to 21 years of age and low-density lipoprotein cholesterol greater than or equal to 190 mg/dL, and those 40 to 75 years of age with clinical ASCVD, diabetes, or 10-year ASCVD risk greater than or equal to 7.5%.
- New lifetime ASCVD risk equations may be useful in individuals 20 to 59 years of age and with less than 7.5% 10-year risk.
- Intensity of statin therapy can be modified based on probability of adverse statin side effects.

This article originally appeared in Endocrinology and Metabolism Clinics, Volume 43, Issue 4, December 2014.

Disclosure: None (A. Gupta); Site Principal Investigator, Sanofi-Regeneron Odyssey trial (PCSK9 Inhibitor) (D.A. Smith).

[a] Division of Endocrinology, Diabetes, and Bone Diseases, Icahn School of Medicine at Mount Sinai, Box 1055, New York, NY 10029, USA; [b] Mount Sinai Heart, Icahn School of Medicine, Box 1014, 1 Gustave Levy Place, New York, NY 10029-6574, USA

* Corresponding author.

E-mail address: donald.smith@mssm.edu

http://dx.doi.org/10.1016/j.ccol.2015.05.012
2352-7986/15/$ – see front matter © 2015 Elsevier Inc. All rights reserved.

Cardiovascular disease (CVD) remains the leading cause of morbidity and mortality, accounting for every 1 in 3 deaths in the United States.[1] Over the last decade, death rates attributable to CVD declined 31.0% and the number of CVD deaths per year declined by 16.7%. Death rates in 2010 attributable to stroke and coronary heart disease (CHD) were 39.1 and 113.6 down from 60.9 (−33%) and 186.8 (−36%) per 100,000 in 2000, respectively. In diabetic patients from 1990 to 2010 acute myocardial changes decreased 67.8%, stroke 52.7%, and amputations 51.4%.[2] However, in 2010, CVD still accounted for 31.9% of all deaths in the United States. A recent report from a national American clinical laboratory (Quest) reported on low-density lipoprotein (LDL) cholesterol (LDL-C) levels in 150 million Americans from 2000 to 2011. Although there was a steady decline from 2000 to 2008, LDL-C levels remained the same from 2008 to 2011, with no change in the percentage achieving any LDL-C goal levels, including levels less than 100 mg/dL.[3]

On 13 November, 2013, the Joint Task Force of the American College of Cardiology (ACC) and the American Heart Association (AHA) published new atherosclerotic CVD (ASCVD) prevention guidelines as an update to the 2008 guidelines developed by the National Heart, Lung, and Blood Institute.[4] This article restates the guidelines in a simpler format than the original synopsis[5] and discusses further the new risk equations that can help physicians and patients make decisions on lifestyle and medications to significantly reduce patients' lifetime risks of ASCVD.

PARADIGM SHIFT FROM TREAT-TO-TARGET TO INTENSITY OF STATIN THERAPY

For more than a decade, physicians have targeted LDL-C and non–high-density lipoprotein (HDL) cholesterol (non–HDL-C) goals by frequent laboratory testing, adjusting intensity of statin therapy, and using therapeutically unproven combinations of lipid-altering medication added to statin therapy. Unlike Adult Treatment Panel III (ATP-III) guidelines and the recent European and Canadian guidelines, the updated guidelines abandon these targets and recommend treating cholesterol by prescribing the appropriate intensity of statin therapy for those patients who are most likely to benefit. The panel's decision for this recommendation is based on a rigorous systematic review of randomized controlled trials (RCTs), a few of which are listed in **Table 1**; systematic reviews; and meta-analyses (**Table 2**) rather than fewer RCTs and expert opinion, which were used by the ATP-III guidelines. The recommendation is to measure LDL-C at baseline and rule out severe hypertriglyceridemia (≥500 mg/dL), reassess LDL-C 1 to 3 months after statin initiation and every 3 to 12 months thereafter to check for compliance (ie, the stability of the expected percentage decreases in LDL-C). Routine monitoring of alanine aminotransferase (ALT) or creatine phosphokinase (CPK) is no longer recommended in asymptomatic patients. This recommendation translates into less frequent laboratory testing, fewer dose adjustments, and less use of combination lipid therapy.

Previous calculators have defined clinical ASCVD as acute coronary syndromes, myocardial infarction (MI), stable angina, coronary or other arterial revascularization, stroke, transient ischemic attack (TIA), or peripheral arterial disease presumed to be of atherosclerotic origin. The current calculator focuses on so-called hard ASCVD, including first occurrence of nonfatal MI, death from CHD, and nonfatal and fatal stroke.

High-intensity statin therapy is defined as that producing greater than or equal to 50% reduction in LDL-C, with moderate-intensity statin therapy producing 30% to less than 50% reduction. Therefore, high-intensity statin therapy is recommended for groups of patients who are most likely to experience the greatest margin of benefit from the reduction in ASCVD risk given the greater potential for adverse effects.

Moderate-intensity statin therapy is recommended when conditions influencing safety are present (eg, in those >75 years of age), or in primary prevention patients less likely to experience a net benefit from high-intensity statin therapy.

If a less-than-anticipated reduction in LDL-C occurs after initiating a statin, lifestyle and drug adherence should be readdressed. Statin therapy may be uptitrated as tolerated. The addition of nonstatin therapy may also be considered in selected individuals.

Four groups of patients have been identified for whom strong evidence supports the use of statin therapy:

1. Clinical ASCVD
   i. Age less than or equal to 75 years and no safety concerns: high-intensity statin
   ii. Age greater than 75 years or less than or equal to 75 years with safety concerns: moderate-intensity statin
2. Primary prevention: primary LDL-C greater than or equal to 190 mg/dL
   i. Age greater than or equal to 21 years: high-intensity statin
3. Primary prevention: diabetes, age 40–75 years and LDL-C 70–189 mg/dL
   i. Moderate-intensity statin
   ii. Consider high-intensity statin when greater than or equal to 7.5% 10-year ASCVD risk using the pooled cohort equations
4. Primary prevention: no diabetes, age 40–75 years, LDL-C 70–189 mg/dL
   Always engage in a discussion about the risks and benefits of starting statin therapy.
   i. Greater than or equal to 7.5% 10-year ASCVD risk: moderate-intensity or high-intensity statin
   ii. Ten-year ASCVD risk, 5% to less than 7.5%: moderate-intensity statin
   iii. Individuals with less than 5% 10-year ASCVD risk may consider other factors:
      a. LDL-C greater than or equal to 160 mg/dL
      b. Evidence of genetic hyperlipidemias
      c. Family history of premature ASCVD with onset before 55 years of age in a first-degree male relative or before 65 years of age in a first-degree female relative
      d. High-sensitivity C-reactive protein (hs-CRP) greater than or equal to 2 mg/L
      e. Coronary artery calcium (CAC) score greater than or equal to 300 Agatston units or greater than or equal to 75th percentile for age, sex, and ethnicity
      f. Ankle-brachial index (ABI) less than 0.9
      g. High lifetime risk of ASCVD

In summary, all individuals with known CVD qualify to receive statins. For primary prevention, all individuals aged 21 years or older with an LDL-C level of 190 mg/dL or more qualify to receive statin therapy. Otherwise, clinicians should wait until patients are aged 40 years and start statins in those with LDL-C levels as low as 70 mg/dL if they have diabetes or have a calculated 10-year risk score for CVD of 7.5% or higher. For those suspected of having a higher risk than that calculated by the 10-year pooled cohort risk equation, other historical, biochemical, imaging, or risk equation factors listed earlier may be used.

Two groups of patients have not been shown to experience an ASCVD event reduction benefit from the routine initiation of statin therapy: those with New York Heart Association Class II to IV heart failure and those undergoing maintenance hemodialysis.

INCREASE IN ELIGIBILITY FOR STATIN THERAPY

Pencina and colleagues[6] analyzed 3773 National Health and Nutrition Examination Survey (NHANES) participants from 2005 to 2010 for statin eligibility based on the

Table 1
Some important statin trials for LDL-C goal setting

Trial	N	M/F (%)	Mean Age (y)	Medications	Primary vs Secondary Prevention	F/U (y)	Baseline Mean LDL-C mM/L	mg/dL	Achieved LDL-C in Statin Arm mM/L	mg/dL	Events	Relative Risk (CI)
Scandinavian Simvastatin Survival Study[40]	4444	82/18	58	Simvastatin 20/40 vs PBO	Secondary	5.0	4.9	196	3.2	127	All deaths All coronary deaths MI, CHD death Coronary revascularization	0.70 (0.58–0.85) 0.58 (0.46–0.73) 0.73 (0.66–0.80) 0.63 (0.54–0.74)
Heart Protection Study[41]	20,536	72/25	40–80	Simvastatin 40 vs PBO	Primary (DM ± hypertension) and secondary	5.4	3.4	136	2.4	96	Vascular deaths MI, CHD death Any stroke	0.83 (0.75–0.91) 0.73 (0.67–0.79) 0.75 (0.66–0.85)
Treating to New Targets[42]	10,001	81/19	35–75	Atorvastatin 80 vs 10	Secondary	4.9	2.6	101	2.0	77	MI, CHD death Any stroke	0.78 (0.68–0.91) 0.75 (0.59–0.96)
Anglo-Scandinavian Cholesterol Outcomes Trial, Lipid-lowering Arm[43]	10,305	81/19	40–79	Atorvastatin 10 vs PBO	Primary (hypertension + 3 additional RFs)	3.3	3.4	132	2.3	90	MI, CHD death Any stroke	0.64 (0.50–0.83) 0.73 (0.56–0.96)

Study	Population	M/F	Age	Drug/Dose	Prevention						Endpoint	HR (CI)
Collaborative Atorvastatin Diabetes Study[44]	2838 type 2 DM + 1 additional RF + LDL-C ≤160 + LDL-C ≤100	68/32	40–75	Atorvastatin 10 vs PBO	Primary	3.9	3.1	120	2.1	81	Acute CHD, coronary revascularization, stroke	0.63 (0.48–0.83)
											—	0.74 (P<.05)
Justification for the Use of Statins in Prevention: An Intervention Trial Evaluating Rosuvastatin[45]	17,902 LDL-C <130 hs-CRP ≥2.0	62/38	M>50 F>60	Rosuvastatin 20 vs PBO	Primary	1.9	2.8	110	1.4	55	MI, CVA, CV death, hospitalization for angina, revascularization	0.56 (0.46–0.69)
											All-cause mortality	0.80 (0.67–0.97)

Abbreviations: CI, confidence interval; CVA, cerebrovascular accident; DM, diabetes mellitus; F, female; F/U, follow-up; hs-CRP, high-sensitivity C-reactive protein; M, male; MI, myocardial infarction; PAD, peripheral artery disease; PBO, placebo; RF, risk factor.

Data from Refs.[40–45]

Table 2
Meta-analysis: efficacy and safety of intensive lowering of LDL-C from 170,000 participants in 26 randomized trials after ischemic vascular events

Study Design	Trial (n)	Subjects (n)		Baseline Mean LDL-C		LDL-C at 1 y in Statin Arm		F/U (y)	Vascular Events (% per Annum)		Relative Risk Reduction % (CI)	Weighted RRR % per 40 mg/dL (1 mM/L) Lowering LDL-C (CI)
		Primary	Secondary	mM/L	mg/dL	mM/L	mg/dL		PBO	Statin		
Total Vascular Events												
Combined	26	169,138		—	—	—	—	—	—	—		22 (20–24)
More vs less intensive	5	30,593	8659	2.6	101	2.1	81	5.1	5.3	4.5	15 (11–18)	28 (22–34)
Statin vs control	21	129,526	—	3.8	148	2.7	105	4.8	3.6	2.8	22 (19–24)	21 (19–23)
Any Major Coronary Event (Nonfatal MI, CHD Death)												
More vs less intensive	5	—	—	—	—	—	—	—	—	—	13 (7–19)	26 (15–35)
Statin vs control	21	—		—	—	—	—	—	—	—	27 (23–30)	24 (21–27)
Any Stroke												
More vs less intensive	5	—		—	—	—	—	—	—	—	1.4 (4–23)	26 (8–41)
Statin vs control	21	—		—	—	—	—	—	—	—	1.5 (9–20)	15 (10–20)
Revascularization (CABG, PTCA, Unspecified)												
More vs less intensive	5	—		—	—	—	—	—	—	—	19 (15–24)	34 (23–40)
Statin vs control	21	—		—	—	—	—	—	—	—	25 (21–28)	24 (20–27)

Abbreviations: CABG, coronary artery bypass grafting; PTCA, percutaneous transluminal coronary angioplasty.

Data from Cholesterol Treatment Trialists' (CTT) Collaboration, Baigent C, Blackwell L, Emberson J, et al. Efficacy and safety of more intensive lowering of LDL cholesterol: a meta-analysis of data from 170,000 participants in 26 randomised trials. Lancet 2010;376(9753):1670–81. http://dx.doi.org/10.1016/S0140-6736(10)61350-5.

new guidelines and extrapolated their results to 115.4 million US adults between the ages of 40 and 75 years. According to their calculations, 13 million more people would potentially be started on cholesterol-lowering medication under the new guidelines. Reasons for this increase include the reduction of the 10-year risk threshold from 10% to 7.5%, including stroke in the risk equations, and decreasing LDL-C treatment initiation threshold to 70 mg/dL. The investigators also note that most of this increase is in the older population where 87.4% of men and 53.6% of women between the ages of 60 and 75 years are now eligible to receive statin therapy. These numbers are an increase of 33% in men and 21.2% in women in this age group under the ATP-III guidelines. In contrast, the number of adults 40 to 59 years of age eligible for primary prevention therapy is similar between the two guidelines, which suggests that age has a greater impact than other risk factors in the new risk assessment models to such an extent that older men can be encouraged to start statin therapy based on age alone.

RISK ASSESSMENT EQUATIONS

The National Cholesterol Education Program's updated clinical guidelines on the Detection, Evaluation, and Treatment of High Blood Cholesterol in Adults (ATP-III) were published in 2001 and are now widely used by physicians to assess, manage, and follow up patients.[7] These guidelines place strong emphasis on the primary prevention of CVD in adults with multiple risk factors. A calculator to assess the 10-year risk for MI and coronary death (hard CHD) was developed by using data from the Framingham Heart Study. Risk status is determined by a 2-step procedure wherein presence/absence or level of risk factors are first counted giving a total point score from which a 10-year risk assessment is performed with a Framingham scoring sheet. Framingham scoring divides persons with multiple risk factors into those with 10-year risk for CHD of greater than 20%, 10% to 20%, and less than 10%. Intensity of treatment and goals of therapy are then decided based on the category into which that individual is placed (**Table 3**).

An update to the ATP-III guidelines[8] was published in July 2004 based on 5 statin trials: the Heart Protection Study (HPS), the Prospective Study of Pravastatin in the

Table 3
National Cholesterol Education Program Adult Treatment Panel III LDL-C goals for different risk categories

Risk Category	LDL Goal (mg/dL)	LDL Level at Which to Initiate Therapeutic Life Style Changes (mg/dL)	LDL Level at Which to Consider Drug Therapy (mg/dL)
0–1 risk factor	<160	≥160	≥190 (160–189: LDL-lowering drug optional)
2+ risk factors (10-y risk ≤20%)	<130	≥130	10-y risk 10%–20%: 130 10-y risk <10%: 160
CHD or CHD risk equivalents (10-y risk >20%)	<100	≥100	≥130 (100–129: drug optional)

Data from Expert Panel on Detection, Evaluation, and Treatment of High Blood Cholesterol in Adults. Executive summary of the third report of the National Cholesterol Education Program (NCEP) Expert Panel on Detection, Evaluation, and Treatment of High Blood Cholesterol in Adults (Adult Treatment Panel III). JAMA 2001;285(19):2486–97.

Elderly at Risk (PROSPER) study, Antihypertensive and Lipid-lowering Treatment to Prevent Heart Attack Trial Lipid-lowering Trial (ALLHAT-LLT), Anglo-Scandinavian Cardiac Outcomes Trial Lipid-lowering Arm (ASCOT-LLA), and the Pravastatin or Atorvastatin Evaluation and Infection Therapy (PROVE-IT) trial. The recommendation was made to lower LDL-C levels in very-high-risk patients to less than 70 mg/dL. These recommendations did not change the previous ATP-III calculation of risk (**Table 4**).

In 2008, D'Agostino and colleagues[9] proposed an expanded Framingham global CVD score as a more recent sex-specific multivariable calculator for use in the primary care setting for predicting the risk of developing a cardiac event. These more inclusive cardiac events were defined by adding angina, fatal and nonfatal stroke, TIA, claudication, and congestive heart failure to MI and CHD death, which were used in the 2001 and 2004 ATP-III calculators. The investigators evaluated 8491 Framingham study participants (mean age, 49 years; 4522 women) who attended a routine examination between 30 and 74 years of age and were free of CVD. The general CVD algorithm showed good discrimination (C-statistic, 0.763 [men] and 0.793 [women]) and calibration (χ^2, 13.48 in men and 7.79 for the women).

Several statistical criteria were used to assess performance of different risk equations in the new guidelines. A model is well calibrated if it correctly predicts the proportion of patients with given characteristics who develop disease. The modified Hosmer-Lemeshow χ^2 statistic was used for determining calibration. This statistic measures how well predicted and observed disease counts agree. A χ^2 value of greater than 20 or a P value of less than .05 indicates poor calibration, although these quantities depend on the sample size. A model has good discriminatory accuracy if the distribution of predicted risks is much higher in cases than in noncases. A popular measure of discriminatory accuracy is the C index: the probability that a randomly selected case will have a higher predicted risk than a randomly selected noncase. The ideal risk model would have a C index of 1.0; all cases would have predicted risks above a specific cut point value, and all noncases below it. This ideal rarely occurs. A C index between 0.70 and 0.80 is considered moderate to good and 0.80 or greater is considered excellent. The net reclassification index (NRI) measures the ability of a risk factor added to a previous predictive equation to accurately reclassify a person with an event into the stratified group of persons with events, and to accurately reclassify a person without an event into the stratified group of

Table 4
Adult Treatment Panel III and Adult Treatment Panel update guidelines for cholesterol goals

Risk Category	LDL Goal (mg/dL)	Initiate TLC (mg/dL)	Consider Drug Therapy (mg/dL)
Very high risk	<70 (optional)	≥70	≥70
High risk: 10-y risk >20%	<100	≥100	≥100
Moderately high risk: ≥2 risk factors 10-y risk 10%–20%	<130 <100 (optional)	≥130 ≥100 (optional)	≥130
Moderate risk: ≥2 risk factors 10-y risk <10%	<130	≥130	≥160
Low risk: 0–1 risk factor	<160	≥160	≥190

Data from Grundy SM, Cleeman JI, Bairey Merz CN, et al. Implications of recent clinical trials for the National Cholesterol Education Program Adult Treatment Panel III guidelines. J Am Coll Cardiol 2004;44(3):720–32. Available at: http://eresources.library.mssm.edu:2213/10.1016/j.jacc.2004.07.001.

persons without an event minus those who have been accurately classified and now are inaccurately classified.

The new 2013 ACC/AHA Guidelines for the Assessment of Cardiovascular Risk provide race-specific and sex-specific pooled cohort equations to:

1. Predict the 10-year risk for development of ASCVD in non-Hispanic white and African American men and women, 40 to 79 years of age, who are not receiving statin therapy, and who have untreated LDL-C levels of greater than or equal to 70 mg/dL to less than 190 mg/dL; and
2. Assess 30-year or lifetime ASCVD risk in adults 20 to 59 years of age without ASCVD and who are not at high short-term risk

In July 2012, the American Stroke Association[10] called for the inclusion of atherosclerotic stroke along with MI and sudden cardiac death as a high-risk condition and as a cardiovascular event outcome in risk prediction algorithms for vascular disease in order to better identify patients who may benefit from preventive measures. Thus, in contrast with the 2008 Framingham model described earlier, the newly developed risk prediction algorithms expanded the scope of prevention from a more general CVD to hard ASCVD events, including the risk of nonfatal MI, CHD death, and nonfatal and fatal stroke. Revascularization events in the 2008 global CVD score that tend to be influenced by provider preference and those with poor reliability, such as angina and congestive heart failure, were left out of the outcomes.

The new guidelines recommend initiation of statin therapy for primary prevention in patients with predicted 10-year risks of greater than or equal to 7.5%, and consideration of statin therapy in patients with 10-year risks of between 5% and 7.5%. In patients with diabetes, the threshold of greater than or equal to 7.5% can be used to select between high-intensity and moderate-intensity statin regimens.

The new equations apply to non-Hispanic African and non-Hispanic white Americans to predict the 10-year risk of developing a first hard ASCVD event. Because these equations do not include Hispanic white, Asian, and Indian Americans, the Guidelines recommend using the equations for the non-Hispanic white population, with a caution that there might be an overestimation of risk in the Hispanic white population and an underestimation of risk in American Indians.

DEVELOPING THE NEW AMERICAN COLLEGE OF CARDIOLOGY/AMERICAN HEART ASSOCIATION POOLED COHORT 10-YEAR RISK EQUATION

The ACC/AHA Work Group decided to develop new equations for 10-year risk assessment rather than use preexisting algorithms.[11] The decision to do so was based on concerns that the existing risk equations (1) were not able to be generalized to nonwhite community-based cohorts, (2) had narrow end points of hard CHD not accounting for stroke and other atherosclerotic events, (3) did not include diabetes mellitus in the multivariable risk equations, and (4) did not consider novel risk factors beyond the traditional risk factors. Pooled data from 5 community-based, National Heart, Lung and Blood Institute–funded, epidemiologic cohorts of African American and non-Hispanic white men and women with greater than 12 years of follow-up were used to develop the new sex-specific and race-specific equations. These cohorts included the Atherosclerosis Risk in Communities (ARIC) study, the Cardiovascular Health Study (CHS), and the Coronary Artery Risk Development in Young Adults (CARDIA) study, in addition to the original Framingham Heart Study and its Offspring Cohorts Study (**Table 5**).

Table 5
Cohorts used to develop the new sex-specific and race-specific equations

Study	Race	Gender	Total (n)	Age (y)	Location	Total Cholesterol mM/L	mg/dL	HDL-C mM/L	mg/dL	UnRx SBP (mm Hg)	Rx SBP (mm Hg)	Current Smoker (%)	Diabetes (%)	10-y ASCVD Rate (%)
Framingham, Framingham Offspring[46,47]	White	Female	3470	40–74	Framingham, MA	5.79	224	1.50	58	127	148	33	5	3.8
		Male	2995			5.61	217	1.16	45	130	146	34	8	9.5
ARIC[14]	White	Female	5508	44–65	Forsyth County, NC;	5.64	218	1.50	58	114	129	25	6	3.6
		Male	4692		Jackson, MS;	5.43	210	1.11	43	118	129	25	8	9.0
	African	Female	2137	44–66	Minneapolis, MN;	5.59	216	1.50	58	124	133	24	17	7.2
	American	Male	1364		Washington County, MD	5.46	211	1.32	51	128	134	37	15	11.1
CARDIA[13]	White	Female	131	40–42	Birmingham, AL;	4.68	181	1.40	54	105	108	18	2	0.0
		Male	103		Chicago, IL;	4.80	186	1.11	43	113	114	23	3	1.0
	African	Female	110	40–45	Minneapolis, MN;	4.68	181	1.37	53	111	130	27	6	0.9
	American	Male	64		Oakland, CA	4.84	187	1.22	47	117	128	38	3	4.7
CHS[12]	White	Female	2131	65–79	Forsyth County, NC;	5.77	223	1.55	60	130	141	13	10	18.0
		Male	1308		Sacramento County, CA;	5.17	200	1.24	48	132	142	11	15	28.5
	African	Female	394	65–79	Washington County, MD;	5.56	215	1.58	61	137	146	14	22	23.0
	American	Male	219		Pittsburgh, PA	5.17	200	1.34	52	134	144	24	26	24.9
Total			24,626											
	White	Female	11,240											
		Male	9098											
	African	Female	2641											
	American	Male	1647											

Abbreviations: Rx SBP, treated systolic blood pressure; UnRx SBP, untreated systolic blood pressure.
Data from Refs. [12,14,15,46,47]

The CHS[12] was designed to identify risk factors for CHD and stroke in older adults greater than or equal to 65 years of age. In addition to measuring the usual risk factors, particular interest was taken in the measurement of subclinical atherosclerotic disease, which has increased prevalence in the elderly. The CARDIA study[13] was initiated to investigate cardiovascular risk factors in young adults 18 to 30 years of age. The ARIC study[14] was conducted to study the cause of atherosclerosis; its clinical sequelae; and variation in risk factors based on race, sex, place, and time in adults 45 to 64 years of age with a median follow-up of 10 years.

A total of 11,240 white women, 9098 white men, 2641 African American women, and 1647 African American men between the ages of 40 and 79 years and without a history of MI (recognized or unrecognized), stroke, congestive heart failure, percutaneous coronary intervention, coronary bypass surgery, or atrial fibrillation were included.

ASCVD risk estimates included the covariates of age, treated or untreated systolic blood pressure (SBP), total cholesterol, high-density lipoprotein cholesterol (HDL-C), current smoking, and diabetes. Additional risk factors like diastolic BP, family history of ASCVD, moderate or severe chronic kidney disease, and body mass index (BMI) were not included because none of them improved discrimination for 10-year risk prediction when added to the models. Other risk factors like hs-CRP, apolipoprotein B, microalbuminuria, cardiorespiratory fitness, CAC, carotid intimal-medial thickness (CIMT), and ABI were also not included for lack of data because these risk factors and measures of ASCVD were not included in the examined cycles of the studies.

Using the new pooled 10-year risk equations on the 5 populations from which they were derived, internal validation results yielded C-statistics of 0.805 for white women, 0.746 for white men, 0.818 for African American women, and 0.713 for African American men. As seen from the C-statistics, these equations have a good to excellent ability to discriminate in the derivation cohort those who will experience a hard ASCVD event from those who will not.

External validation was performed in 3 populations: the Multi-Ethnic Study of Atherosclerosis (MESA) with a 6-year follow-up; Reasons for Geographic and Racial Differences in Stroke (REGARDS) with a 4-year follow-up; and in the most contemporary data available from ARIC, Framingham original, and Framingham Offspring with a 10-year follow-up. C-statistics ranged from 0.56 (African American men in the REGARDS cohort) to 0.77 (African American women in the MESA cohort). In the 12 cohorts studied (African American and white men and women in the 3 study populations), C-statistics were greater than 0.7 in 6 of 12 cohorts, more than 0.65 in 4 of 12 cohorts, and less than 0.6 in 2 of 12 cohorts. The pooled cohort equations tend to overestimate risk; less so in the lower risk, more so in the higher risk categories (see Table 7 of the Full Work Group Report supplement,[15] http://jaccjacc.cardiosource.com/acc_documents/2013_FPR_S5_Risk_Assessment.pdf)

ASSESSING THE NEW AMERICAN COLLEGE OF CARDIOLOGY/AMERICAN HEART ASSOCIATION POOLED COHORT 10-YEAR RISK EQUATION

Since the release of the new calculator, clinicians have questioned the accuracy of its clinical predictions. Part of the controversy relates to uncertainty in the number of new people who would require statin therapy under these new guidelines. Risk estimators must predict event risk, which closely matches observed risk in populations other than those used for calculating the equations.

Using 3 large-scale primary prevention cohorts (the Women's Health Study, the Physicians' Health Study, and the Women's Health Initiative Observational Study),

Ridker and Cook[16] observed overestimation of risk by 75% to 150% at all levels of 4 gender-specific and race-specific 10-year risk categories.

The investigators of the 2013 ACC/AHA Risk Assessment Guideline, Lloyd-Jones and colleagues defended their position to lower the treatment threshold to 7.5%, which would still provide a buffer with the treatment threshold of 5% shown in trials to provide clinical benefit. Their risk equations overestimate risk mainly in high-risk individuals for whom treatment decision may already have been made rather than low-risk individuals who do not need a statin. The investigators also point out that the 3 primary prevention cohorts used by Ridker and colleagues for their analysis comprised low-risk white populations with remarkably low event rates and hence are not representative of the US population.

REGARDS investigators Muntner and colleagues[17,18] suggest that it is premature to conclude that the new risk equations overestimate risk for the following reasons:

1. The contemporary nature of the MESA and REGARDS cohorts reflects improvements in overall health and lifestyle patterns in the United States over the past 25 years since observations in the original derivation cohort started.
2. In the most recent comparative cohorts, study participants may have been prescribed statins after enrollment based on their baseline test results, leading to altered long-term outcomes.
3. There has been an increased use of revascularization procedures, which can reduce the incidence of hard ASCVD events. Maximum overestimation of risk was therefore observed in the high-risk group.
4. Studies used to develop the risk equations included active surveillance(determining outcomes using periodic telephone calls, searching ASCVD diagnostic codes in the local hospital or regional death records, and documenting out-of-hospital ASCVD events by contact with family or physician) in addition to self-reporting of cardiovascular events. The lack of surveillance components in the contemporary validation studies could lead to under-reporting and be a reason for the overestimation of ASCVD incidence.

In a more recent publication, these same investigators[18] reevaluated the calibration and discrimination of the pooled cohort risk equations in the REGARDS cohort and in participants who could be considered for statin therapy (45–79 years of age, without clinical ASCVD or diabetes, with LDL-C levels between 70 and 189 mg/dL and not taking statins). The equations overestimate risk in the entire REGARDS study population but overestimation of risk was smaller in the subpopulation that would be considered for statin therapy. Further analysis was performed in subjects greater than or equal to 65 years of age who had Medicare claims data available (a form of active surveillance for ASCVD events). In this group the risk equations underestimated ASCVD events (**Table 6**).

RATIONALE FOR CONSTRUCTING MODELS TO ASSESS THE LONG-TERM/LIFETIME RISK FOR A FIRST HARD ATHEROSCLEROTIC CARDIOVASCULAR DISEASE EVENT

The short-term risk equations do not predict the lifetime risk of hard ASCVD events that develop as a result of increasing number or severity of risk factors. The increasing life expectancy of the population would translate into a higher incidence of ASCVD in an older population. Predicting an individual's lifetime risk of developing hard ASCVD events may hence serve in helping individuals decide whether to significantly change lifestyle or to start statins.

Studies of lifetime risk so far have been based on a variety of risk factor stratification strategies defined by categorical definition of risk factors: risk factor absence or

Table 6
Validation of the 10-year risk prediction equations in the REGARDS data

10-y ASCVD Risk (%)	Observed 5-y Incidence Rate/1000 Patient Years	Predicted 5-y Incidence Rate/1000 Patient Years	Calibration Hosmer-Lemeshow χ^2 >20 Poor	Discrimination C-Statistic Moderate–Good (0.70–0.79)
Overall Population (N = 18,498)				
5 to <7.5	4.2	4.8	84.2	0.71
7.5 to <10	5.0	6.8		
≥10	12.6	17.8		
Subgroup for Statin Consideration: No ASCVD, No Diabetes and LDL-C Level 70–189 mg/dL (N = 10,997)				
5 to <7.5	4.8	4.8	19.9	0.72
7.5 to <10	6.1	6.9		
≥10	12	15.1		
Medicare Linked Data (N = 6121)				
<7.5	5.3	4.1	11.4	0.65
7.5 to <10	7.7	6.5		
≥10	18.2	19.3		
Medicare Subgroup for Statin Consideration: No ASCVD, No Diabetes and LDL-C Level 70–189 mg/dL (N = 3333)				
<7.5	5.3	4	5.4	0.71
7.5 to <10	7.9	6.4		
≥10	17.4	16.4		

Data from Muntner P, Colantonio LD, Cushman M, et al. Validation of the atherosclerotic cardiovascular disease pooled cohort risk equations. JAMA 2014;311(14):1406–15. http://dx.doi.org/10.1001/jama.2014.2630.

presence (smoking, diabetes) and 3 to 4 risk factor levels of SBP (including or not including diastolic blood pressure [DBP]) and total cholesterol, HDL-C, and treatment or not of hypertension (treatment means higher lifetime risk, presumably because blood pressure has been higher for longer and thus on-treatment status adds risk to that reported by measured blood pressure level alone). Ten studies were identified with a follow-up of more than 15 years that provided long-term outcomes data in individuals at low or intermediate short-term risk. These studies have shown that young individuals, who have low 10-year predicted risk for CHD despite having a significant risk factor burden, are at a very high risk for developing CHD over their remaining lifespans.[19,20]

The long-term risk assessment for ASCVD is recommended for adults aged 20 to 39 years with LDL-C less than 190 mg/dL and adults 40 to 59 years of age who are free from ASCVD and at low 10-year risk less than 7.5%, not at 10-year risk greater than or equal to 7.5%. The investigators of the new guidelines noted that the Framingham 10-year risk score could not be used to predict lifetime risk because extrapolation from 10-year risk scores underestimate the observed lifetime risk. The lifetime risk score that was developed was able to stratify CHD lifetime risk fairly well in women of all ages but not as well in young men. For example, a 40-year-old woman in the lowest, middle, and highest tertiles of predicted 10-year CHD risk, the remaining lifetime risks for CHD to age 84 years were 12.2%, 25.4%, and 33.2%, respectively. In contrast, the lifetime risks for a 40-year-old man were 38.4%, 41.7%, and 50.7%, respectively.[21]

Pencina and colleagues[22] compared the 10-year and lifetime risks for ASCVD events, and prospectively followed 4506 participants of the Framingham Offspring cohort aged 20 to 59 years and free of CVD at baseline for the development of hard CVD events (coronary death, MI, and fatal and nonfatal stroke). Participants were followed for a maximum of 35 years. The investigators compared the results of 30-year risk estimates obtained by diverse methods: (1) tripling a 10-year risk estimate without accounting for the competing risks (naive approach); (2) estimating 3 event probabilities for each person with the 10-year risk calculators using the baseline age, age plus 10 years, and age plus 20 years, while maintaining the same baseline risk factor levels in all 3 models (combined approach), and calculating the 30-year risk as 1 minus the product of these three 10-year probabilities; (3) a 30-year risk estimate not accounting for competing risks (unadjusted approach); and (4) a 30-year risk estimate accounting for competing risks (adjusted approach). Long-term or lifetime risk estimation models adjusting for competing causes of mortality were shown to be more valid than extrapolation of results from 10-year risk equations.

For the lifetime risk equations in the new guidelines, Lloyd-Jones and colleagues[15] followed 3564 men and 4362 women enrolled in the Framingham Heart and Offspring Study who were free of CVD (MI, coronary insufficiency, angina, stroke, claudication) at 50 years of age. Lifetime risks were estimated to 95 years of age with non-CVD death as a competing event. Compared with participants with greater than or equal to 2 major risk factors, those with optimal levels had substantially lower lifetime risks (5.2% vs 68.9% in men, 8.2% vs 50.2% in women). For a comparative view of the stratified risk factors used in developing the lifetime risk equations and how increasing level of risk factors affects lifetime risk see **Table 7**. Individuals age ≥ 50 years who have a lifetime ASCVD risk double the 10 year coronary-equivalent risk of ≥ 20% would have a high lifetime risk ≥ 40% which is present in 60% of Framingham participants that age. **Table 7** may be helpful in physician/patient understanding of the importance and significance of lifetime risk for middle-aged patients. For other ages, lifetime risk for those in the lowest risk category is given, allowing a discussion

Table 7
Short-term and lifetime ASCVD risk in Framingham subjects aged ≥ 50 years

Risk Category	Subjects (%)	10-y ASCVD Risk (%)	Lifetime ASCVD Risk (M + F) (%)	Lifetime ASCVD Risk: M (%)	Lifetime ASCVD Risk: F (%)
≥2 Major risk factors: TC ≥240 mg/dL, SBP ≥160 mm Hg, DBP ≥100 mm Hg, DM, current smoking	20	10–25	>50	68.9	50.2
1 Major risk factor	40	10	39–50	50.4	38.8
≥1 Increased risk factors: TC 200–239 mg/dL, SBP 140–159 mm Hg, DBP 90–99 mm Hg, no DM, no smoking	23	5	39–46	45.5	39.1
≥1 Nonoptimal risk factors: TC 180–199 mg/dL, SBP 120–139 mm Hg, DBP 80–89 mm Hg, no DM, no smoking	12	<5	27–36	36.4	26.9
Optimal risk factors: TC <180 mg/dL, SBP <120 mm Hg, DBP <80 mm Hg, no DM, no smoking	4	<5	<10	5.2	8.2

Abbreviation: TC, total cholesterol.
Data from Lloyd-Jones DM, Leip EP, Larson MG, et al. Prediction of lifetime risk for cardiovascular disease by risk factor burden at 50 years of age. Circulation 2006;113(6):791–8. http://dx.doi.org/10.1161/CIRCULATIONAHA.105.548206.

with the patient of what lifestyle they may want to change or whether they want to take statins to lower increased lifetime risk.

Because the data for the current lifetime risk estimates are from the Framingham Heart and Offspring Study participants, risks calculated are derived from a non-Hispanic white population. Newer lifetime risk calculators will be forthcoming as reviewed in a meta-analysis of lifetime risks of hard ASCVD events from approximately 250,000 participants (including African Americans) from 18 long-term cohort studies published in 2012.[23]

The investigators of the new guidelines found that lifetime risk equations predicted CHD death with good discrimination (0.76–0.81 women and 0.71–0.75 in men). Pencina and colleagues[22] previously showed that lifetime risk equations have an improved validity when ASCVD risk factors are updated every 4 to 6 years and this is what the new guidelines suggest in terms of periodic reassessment of risk.

The 10-year and lifetime risk calculators can be downloaded at http://my.ame ricanheart.org/cvriskcalculator and http://www.cardiosource.org/en/Science-And-Quality/Practice-Guidelines-and-Quality-Standards/2013-Prevention-Guideline-Tools. aspx (**Fig. 1**).

Also, examples of 10-year and lifetime risk in a 55-year-old white man and woman with total cholesterol of 213 mg/dL, HDL-C 50 mg/dL, untreated SBP of 120 mm Hg, no diabetes, and no smoking are shown in **Fig. 2**.

OTHER MEASUREMENTS

The Work Group tested additional new markers for inclusion in the risk model. These markers included several blood and urine biomarkers (hs-CRP, apolipoprotein B, creatinine [or estimated glomerular filtration rate], and microalbuminuria), several measures of subclinical CVD (CAC, CIMT, ABI), family history, and cardiorespiratory fitness. Thirteen meta-analysis and systematic reviews including studies with at least 10 years of follow-up were reviewed. None of these markers have been evaluated as a screening test in RCTs with clinical events as outcomes. It is the opinion of the Work

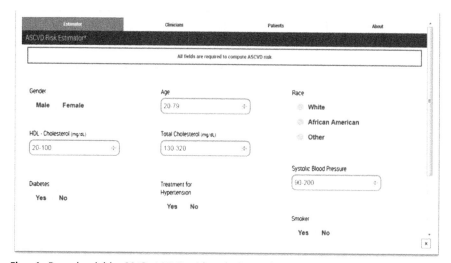

Fig. 1. Downloadable 2013 ASCVD risk calculator. (*From* American Heart Association. Available at: http://my.americanheart.org/professional/StatementsGuidelines/Prevention-Guidelines_UCM_457698_SubHomePage.jsp. Accessed August 13, 2014; with permission.)

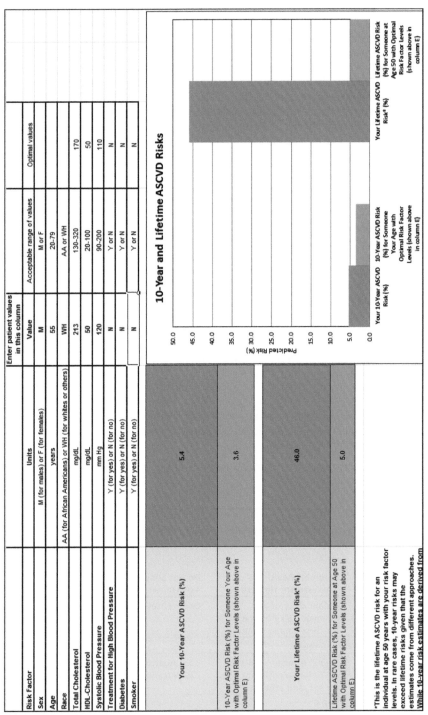

Fig. 2. Sample 10-year and lifetime risks in a 55-year-old white man with total cholesterol level of 213 mg/dL, HDL-C level 50 mg/dL, untreated SBP of 120 mm Hg, no diabetes, and not a smoker.

Group that assessments of family history of premature CVD and measurement of hs-CRP, CAC, and ABI show some promise for clinical utility among the novel risk markers, based on limited data (**Table 8**).

CAC reference values have been developed from the MESA study.[24] Participants were free of clinical CVD and treated diabetes at baseline. They were between 45 and 84 years of age, and identified themselves as white, African American, Hispanic, or Chinese. The calculator can be accessed at http://www.mesa-nhlbi.org/Calcium/input.aspx. The CAC score generated for an individual can be compared with others of the same age, gender, and race/ethnicity who do not have clinical CVD or treated diabetes. A systematic review by Peters and colleagues[25] reported NRI ranging from 14% to 25% for CAC as opposed to −1.4% to 12% for CIMT and 8% to 11% for carotid plaques. Uncertainty remains regarding assessing CAC because:

1. Most studies have assessed CHD outcomes and not hard ASCVD events
2. Widespread CAC screening would increase the risk of radiation exposure and the costs incurred

CAC has been proposed as a class IIb recommendation for individuals at moderate risk for whom a risk-based treatment decision is uncertain. Statin therapy can be initiated in the presence of a significant CAC ($\geq$300 Agatston units or >75th percentile for age/gender group).

ABI can easily be assessed in routine practice and a value of less than 0.9 might support initiation of treatment. In a recently published meta-analysis of CIMT, Den Ruijter and colleagues[26] reported only a small net reclassification improvement of 0.8% (95% confidence interval [CI], 0.1%–1.6%) in 10-year risk prediction of first-time MI or stroke. Problems with CIMT measurement standardization led the Work Group to recommend against use of CIMT in routine medical practice.

STATIN SAFETY

The guidelines recommend moderate-dose statins rather than high-dose statins in individuals for whom high doses would be recommended because of the possibility of adverse effects of high dosage:

1. Individuals with multiple or serious comorbidities, including impaired renal or hepatic function

Table 8
Expert opinion thresholds for use of optional screening tests when risk-based decisions regarding initiation of pharmacologic therapy are uncertain following quantitative risk assessment

Measure	Support Revising Risk Assessment Upward	Do Not Support Revising Risk Assessment
Family history of premature CVD	Male <55 y of age Female <65 y of age (first-degree relative)	Occurrences at older ages only (if any)
hs-CRP	$\geq$2 mg/L	<2 mg/L
CAC score	$\geq$300 Agatston units or $\geq$75th percentile for age, sex, and ethnicity[a]	<300 Agatston units and <75 percentile for age, sex, and ethnicity[a]
ABI	<0.9	$\geq$0.9

[a] For additional information, see http://www.mesa-nhlbi.org/CACReference.aspx.

2. Individuals with a history of previous statin intolerance or muscle disorders
3. Individuals with unexplained ALT increases greater than 3 times the upper limit of normal (ULN)
4. Individuals who use drugs that affect statin metabolism
5. Individuals who are more than 75 years of age

For those of Asian ancestry a lower dose statin at the start of statin therapy may be chosen.

For those with a hemorrhagic stroke, moderate-dose statins may be more appropriate, although on meta-analyses in the trials of more versus less statin there was no significant increase in hemorrhagic stroke (Relative risk [RR], 1.21; 95% CI, 0.85–1.17; P = .3). In the same meta-analysis in trials of statin versus placebo, there was no significant increase in hemorrhagic stroke (RR, 1.15; 95% CI, 0.93–1.41; P = .2) and ischemic stroke incidence was decreased by 20% (RR, 0.80; 95% CI, 0.74–0.87; P = .0001).[27]

A baseline ALT level was measured in the RCTs with statins and is recommended by the guidelines. Patients with increased ALT levels (usually >1.5–2 times the ULN) were excluded from statin trials and manufacturers state that unexplained ALT greater than 3 times the ULN is a contraindication to statin therapy. In RCTs increases in transaminase levels occur at equal rates in subjects on statins and subjects on placebo. No cases of hepatic failure were reported. Thus no follow-up ALT level is necessary unless a person develops symptoms of liver disease, which the guidelines list as fatigue, weakness, loss of appetite, abdominal pain, or significant yellowing of sclera, skin, or urine.

For patients who are concerned about statins as a cause of cancer, the meta-analysis of 170,000 persons in statin randomized trials showed that statins did not increase the incidence of total cancer (RR, 1.00; 95% CI, 0.96–1.04; P = .9), site-specific cancer, or the risk of cancer death.[27]

Statins can produce adverse muscle symptoms in 1% to 5% of subjects in controlled clinical trials and at higher frequencies in observational cohorts such as the one done in France of 8000 outpatients taking high-dose statin, in which muscular symptoms were reported in 10.5% of patients with a median time of onset of 1 month after statin initiation.[28] The management of these patients includes stopping the problematic statin and then rechallenging with a second statin. The Cleveland Clinic showed that 72.5% of intolerant patients were ultimately able to tolerate some regimen of long-term statin therapy.[29] They also used intermittent statin dosing rather than daily dosing in many patients and, although it did not produce as much LDL-C lowering, it nevertheless was better than no statin therapy. Other LDL-C–lowering drugs may be added, such as ezetimibe[30] and bile acid binders, to lower the LDL-C level further but there are no combination studies showing efficacy in reducing ASCVD events. Rhabdomyolysis occurs rarely (<0.06% over a mean treatment period of 4.8 to 5.1 years). A rate of creatine kinase increase greater than 3 times ULN occurs infrequently and at a similar rate in those treated with intensive-dose or moderate-dose statin therapy (0.02% for moderate-dose statin to 0.1% for higher dose statin) over a 1-year to 5-year treatment period.

The guidelines recommend a baseline history of muscle symptoms and, for patients with a family or personal history of muscle symptoms, a baseline CPK is recommended before starting statins. Follow-up CPK levels are not recommended unless a person develops significant muscle symptoms on statins, including pain, tenderness, stiffness, cramping, weakness, or fatigue. Statins would then be stopped until symptoms are relieved. For severe muscle symptoms, testing of CPK, creatinine, and urinalysis for myoglobinuria may be appropriate. Guidelines suggest restarting a patient on the same statin at the same or lower dose for establishment of causality. If symptoms reappear, another statin or use of intermittent day dosing of another statin might be tried. If there is no resolution of muscle symptoms after 2 months in patients stopping statins, a search for another cause should be instituted.

Many persons refuse statins because of a small risk of a diabetes diagnosis with statins compared with placebo. The following provides risk estimates that may be given to patients concerned about this unexplained small increased risk. A recent meta-analysis of 13 trials of statin therapy (including Justification for the Use of Statins in Prevention: An Intervention Trial Evaluating Rosuvastatin [JUPITER]) comparing statin versus placebo or usual care in 91,140 participants without diabetes reported an excess of 174 cases with new-onset diabetes (2226 vs 2052; Hazard Ratio, 1.09; 95% CI, 1.02–1.17).[31] There was no significant heterogeneity among statins, and the numbers needed to treat over 4 years to produce 1 new case of diabetes was 255, or 1 new case per 1000 treated per year compared with placebo. In the 150,000 women in the Women's Health Initiative, mean age 63 years and BMI of 28 kg/m^2, the cumulative incidence of diabetes over 9 years in the 7% of women on statins at years 1 and 3 versus those not on statins was 9.1% versus 6.0%, or an increased risk of diabetes of 3 per 100 over 9 years or 1 per 300 per year.[32] Highest dose statin therapy (atorvastatin 80 or simvastatin 80) versus lower dose statin therapy in 5 trials over 4 years involving 32,752 participants resulted in new-onset diabetes in 8.8% on statins versus 8.0% on moderate-dose statin therapy, or 1 extra case of new diabetes per 500 per year on the highest dose versus lower dose statin therapy. Meanwhile 3.2 CVD events were prevented per year.[33] In the JUPITER trial using Crestor 20 versus placebo for primary prevention in men more than 50 and women more than 60 years of age with LDL-C less than 130 mg/dL, and hs-CRP greater than or equal to 2, subjects without any risk factors for diabetes had no new-onset diabetes on Crestor versus placebo. In those on Crestor with 1 or more risk factors included in the metabolic syndrome, there was an absolute increase of 1 per 100 cases of diabetes but an absolute decrease of 2 per 100 ischemic CVD events.[34] For patients with diabetes, statins may increase hemoglobin A1c (HbA1c) from 0.1% to 0.3%,[35] although one meta-analysis showed no change in HbA1c in 26 statin trials ranging from 4 weeks to 4 years.[36]

The guidelines state and confirm that the potential for ASCVD risk reduction outweighs the risk of diabetes in all but those with the lowest ASCVD risk. Those who develop diabetes on a statin should be counseled on a healthy lifestyle, including achieving and maintaining a healthy body weight, participation in exercise, smoking cessation, and continuation of the statin to reduce the risk of an ASCVD event.

The panel did not find evidence that statins had an adverse effect on cognitive changes or risk of dementia. This finding has been confirmed in 2 recent meta-analyses.[37,38] The first cited a meta-analysis by Richardson and colleagues[38] who searched the US Food and Drug Administration database and found that the reported rates of cognitive-related adverse events were no higher for statins than for 2 drugs not know to cause cognitive impairment: losartan and clopidogrel (1.9 vs 1.6 and 1.9 per million written prescriptions). Thus the guidelines suggest that, for individuals presenting with a confusional state or memory impairment while on statin therapy, it may be reasonable to evaluate the patient for nonstatin causes, such as exposure to other drugs, as well as for systemic and neuropsychiatric causes in addition to the possibility of such an effect associated with statin drug therapy.

The National Lipid Association Task Force on Statin Safety Update 2014 has a supplement in the *Journal of Clinical Lipidology* that provides a more in-depth review of statin safety and management.[39]

SUMMARY

The 2013 ACC/AHA risk assessment and cholesterol treatment guidelines emphasize important core concepts and introduce new concepts for risk assessment. They differ substantially from the previous ATP-III guidelines, particularly with respect to primary prevention of CVD. The ATP-III guidelines place more emphasis on levels of LDL-C to select patients for statin therapy, whereas the new guidelines base the recommendation solely on the 10-year ASCVD predicted risk, as long as the LDL-C level is 70 to 189 mg/dL or higher. High-intensity statin treatment is recommended in all people with known ASCVD irrespective of their LDL-C levels and in those without such disease but at high LDL-C levels greater than or equal to 190 mg/dL or with diabetes with increased ASCVD risk. The guidelines have identified patient groups in which a more intensive treatment is superior to a moderate treatment, and focus on statins as the mainstay of therapy rather than clinically unproven lipid-lowering drug combinations. These steps are important to simplify and improve care for high-risk individuals. It is recommended that clinicians determine an individual's absolute 10-year risk score by standard clinical testing in order to engage in a meaningful clinician-patient discussion regarding the potential for ASCVD risk reduction, treatment adverse effects, drug-drug interactions, and patient preferences. The recommendation to treat individuals with 10-year risks of 7.5% or greater has been boosted by the newest validation study of REGARDS[18]; the validity of lifetime risk prediction algorithms remain controversial but may help in stimulating more serious conversations between doctors and patients at younger ages when 10-year risk is low. According to these new guidelines, more than 30 million people without existing CVD might be candidates for statin therapy. These large numbers should mobilize the medical community to identify potentially modifiable risk factors affected by lifestyle and institute behavioral changes before starting statins in order to further contain the epidemic of CVD. They are intended to guide decision making but not replace clinical judgment.

REFERENCES

1. Go AS, Mozaffarian D, Roger VL, et al. Executive summary: heart disease and stroke statistics–2014 update: a report from the American Heart Association. Circulation 2014;129(3):399–410. http://dx.doi.org/10.1161/01.cir.0000442015. 53336.12.
2. Gregg EW, Li Y, Wang J, et al. Changes in diabetes-related complications in the united states, 1990-2010. N Engl J Med 2014;370(16):1514–23. http://dx.doi.org/ 10.1056/NEJMoa1310799.
3. Kaufman HW, Blatt AJ, Huang X, et al. Blood cholesterol trends 2001-2011 in the United States: analysis of 105 million patient records. PLoS One 2013;8(5): e63416. http://dx.doi.org/10.1371/journal.pone.0063416.
4. Stone NJ, Robinson JG, Lichtenstein AH, et al. 2013 ACC/AHA guideline on the treatment of blood cholesterol to reduce atherosclerotic cardiovascular risk in adults: a report of the American College of Cardiology/American Heart Association Task Force on Practice Guidelines. J Am Coll Cardiol 2014;63(25 Pt B): 2889–934. http://dx.doi.org/10.1016/j.jacc.2013.11.002.
5. Stone NJ, Robinson JG, Lichtenstein AH, et al. Treatment of blood cholesterol to reduce atherosclerotic cardiovascular disease risk in adults: synopsis of the 2013 American College of Cardiology/American Heart Association cholesterol guideline. Ann Intern Med 2014;160(5):339–43. http://dx.doi.org/10.7326/M14-0126.

6. Pencina MJ, Navar-Boggan AM, D'Agostino RB, et al. Application of new choles-terol guidelines to a population-based sample. N Engl J Med 2014;370(15): 1422–31. http://dx.doi.org/10.1056/NEJMoa1315665.
7. Expert Panel on Detection, Evaluation, and Treatment of High Blood Cholesterol in Adults. Executive summary of the third report of the National Cholesterol Education Program (NCEP) Expert Panel on Detection, Evaluation, and Treatment of High Blood Cholesterol in Adults (Adult Treatment Panel III). JAMA 2001; 285(19):2486–97.
8. Grundy SM, Cleeman JI, Bairey Merz CN, et al. Implications of recent clinical trials for the national cholesterol education program adult treatment panel III guidelines. J Am Coll Cardiol 2004;44(3):720–32.http://eresources.library.mssm.edu:2213/10.1016/j.jacc.2004.07.001.
9. D'Agostino RB, Vasan RS, Pencina MJ, et al. General cardiovascular risk profile for use in primary care: the Framingham Heart Study. Circulation 2008;117(6): 743–53. http://dx.doi.org/10.1161/CIRCULATIONAHA.107.699579.
10. Lackland DT, Elkind MS, D'Agostino RS, et al. Inclusion of stroke in cardiovascu-lar risk prediction instruments: a statement for healthcare professionals from the American Heart Association/American Stroke Association. Stroke 2012;43(7): 1998–2027. http://dx.doi.org/10.1161/STR.0b013e31825bcdac.
11. Goff DC Jr, Lloyd-Jones DM, Bennett G, et al. 2013 ACC/AHA guideline on the assessment of cardiovascular risk: a report of the American College of Car-diology/American Heart Association Task Force on Practice Guidelines. J Am Coll Cardiol 2014;63(25 Pt B):2935–59. http://dx.doi.org/10.1016/j.jacc.2013. 11.005.
12. Fried LP, Borhani NO, Enright P, et al. The cardiovascular health study: design and rationale. Ann Epidemiol 1991;1(3):263–76.
13. Friedman GD, Cutter GR, Donahue RP, et al. CARDIA: study design, recruitment, and some characteristics of the examined subjects. J Clin Epidemiol 1988; 41(11):1105–16. pii:0895-4356(88)90080-7.
14. Chambless LE, Folsom AR, Sharrett AR, et al. Coronary heart disease risk predic-tion in the Atherosclerosis Risk in Communities (ARIC) study. J Clin Epidemiol 2003; 56(9):880–90. pii:S0895435603000556.
15. Lloyd-Jones DM, Leip EP, Larson MG, et al. Prediction of lifetime risk for cardio-vascular disease by risk factor burden at 50 years of age. Circulation 2006; 113(6):791–8. http://dx.doi.org/10.1161/CIRCULATIONAHA.105.548206.
16. Ridker PM, Cook NR. Statins: new American guidelines for prevention of cardio-vascular disease. Lancet 2013;382(9907):1762–5. http://dx.doi.org/10.1016/ S0140-6736(13)62388-0.
17. Muntner P, Safford MM, Cushman M, et al. Comment on the reports of over-estimation of ASCVD risk using the 2013 AHA/ACC risk equation. Circulation 2014;129(2):266–7. http://dx.doi.org/10.1161/CIRCULATIONAHA.113.007648.
18. Muntner P, Colantonio LD, Cushman M, et al. Validation of the atherosclerotic cardiovascular disease pooled cohort risk equations. JAMA 2014;311(14): 1406–15. http://dx.doi.org/10.1001/jama.2014.2630.
19. Lloyd-Jones DM, Wilson PW, Larson MG, et al. Lifetime risk of coronary heart disease by cholesterol levels at selected ages. Arch Intern Med 2003;163(16): 1966–72. http://dx.doi.org/10.1001/archinte.163.16.1966.
20. Marma AK, Berry JD, Ning H, et al. Distribution of 10-year and lifetime predicted risks for cardiovascular disease in US adults: findings from the National Health and Nutrition Examination Survey 2003 to 2006. Circ Cardiovasc Qual Outcomes 2010;3(1):8–14. http://dx.doi.org/10.1161/CIRCOUTCOMES.109.869727.

21. Lloyd-Jones DM, Wilson PW, Larson MG, et al. Framingham risk score and prediction of lifetime risk for coronary heart disease. Am J Cardiol 2004;94(1): 20–4. http://dx.doi.org/10.1016/j.amjcard.2004.03.023.

22. Pencina MJ, D'Agostino RB, Larson MG, et al. Predicting the 30-year risk of cardiovascular disease: the Framingham Heart Study. Circulation 2009;119(24): 3078–84. http://dx.doi.org/10.1161/CIRCULATIONAHA.108.816694.

23. Berry JD, Dyer A, Cai X, et al. Lifetime risks of cardiovascular disease. N Engl J Med 2012;366(4):321–9. http://dx.doi.org/10.1056/NEJMoa1012848.

24. McClelland RL, Chung H, Detrano R, et al. Distribution of coronary artery calcium by race, gender, and age: results from the Multi-ethnic Study of Atherosclerosis (MESA). Circulation 2006;113(1):30–7. pii:CIRCULATIONAHA.105.580696.

25. Peters SA, den Ruijter HM, Bots ML, et al. Improvements in risk stratification for the occurrence of cardiovascular disease by imaging subclinical atherosclerosis: a systematic review. Heart 2012;98(3):177–84. http://dx.doi.org/10.1136/heartjnl-2011-300747.

26. Den Ruijter HM, Peters SA, Anderson TJ, et al. Common carotid intima-media thickness measurements in cardiovascular risk prediction: a meta-analysis. JAMA 2012;308(8):796–803. http://dx.doi.org/10.1001/jama.2012.9630.

27. Cholesterol Treatment Trialists' (CTT) Collaboration, Baigent C, Blackwell L, Emberson J, et al. Efficacy and safety of more intensive lowering of LDL cholesterol: a meta-analysis of data from 170,000 participants in 26 randomised trials. Lancet 2010;376(9753):1670–81. http://dx.doi.org/10.1016/S0140-6736(10)61350-5.

28. Bruckert E, Hayem G, Dejager S, et al. Mild to moderate muscular symptoms with high-dosage statin therapy in hyperlipidemic patients–the PRIMO study. Cardiovasc Drugs Ther 2005;19(6):403–14. http://dx.doi.org/10.1007/s10557-005-5686-z.

29. Mampuya WM, Frid D, Rocco M, et al. Treatment strategies in patients with statin intolerance: the Cleveland Clinic experience. Am Heart J 2013;166(3):597–603. http://dx.doi.org/10.1016/j.ahj.2013.06.004.

30. Ballantyne CM, Houri J, Notarbartolo A, et al. Effect of ezetimibe coadministered with atorvastatin in 628 patients with primary hypercholesterolemia: a prospective, randomized, double-blind trial. Circulation 2003;107(19):2409–15. http://dx.doi.org/10.1161/01.CIR.0000068312.21969.C8.

31. Sattar N, Preiss D, Murray HM, et al. Statins and risk of incident diabetes: a collaborative meta-analysis of randomised statin trials. Lancet 2010;375(9716): 735–42. http://dx.doi.org/10.1016/S0140-6736(09)61965-6.

32. Culver AL, Ockene IS, Balasubramanian R, et al. Statin use and risk of diabetes mellitus in postmenopausal women in the Women's Health Initiative. Arch Intern Med 2012;172(2):144–52. http://dx.doi.org/10.1001/archinternmed.2011.625.

33. Preiss D, Seshasai SR, Welsh P, et al. Risk of incident diabetes with intensive-dose compared with moderate-dose statin therapy: a meta-analysis. JAMA 2011; 305(24):2556–64. http://dx.doi.org/10.1001/jama.2011.860.

34. Ridker PM, Pradhan A, MacFadyen JG, et al. Cardiovascular benefits and diabetes risks of statin therapy in primary prevention: an analysis from the JUPITER trial. Lancet 2012;380(9841):565–71. http://dx.doi.org/10.1016/S0140-6736(12) 61190-8.

35. Maki KC, Ridker PM, Brown WV, et al. An assessment by the statin diabetes safety task force: 2014 update. J Clin Lipidol 2014;8(Suppl 3):S17–29. http://dx.doi.org/10.1016/j.jacl.2014.02.012.

36. Zhou Y, Yuan Y, Cai RR, et al. Statin therapy on glycaemic control in type 2 diabetes: a meta-analysis. Expert Opin Pharmacother 2013;14(12):1575–84. http://dx.doi.org/10.1517/14656566.2013.810210.

37. Swiger KJ, Manalac RJ, Blumenthal RS, et al. Statins and cognition: a systematic review and meta-analysis of short- and long-term cognitive effects. Mayo Clin Proc 2013;88(11):1213–21. http://dx.doi.org/10.1016/j.mayocp.2013.07.013.

38. Richardson K, Schoen M, French B, et al. Statins and cognitive function: a systematic review. Ann Intern Med 2013;159(10):688–97. http://dx.doi.org/10.7326/0003-4819-159-10-201311190-00007.

39. Jacobson TA. NLA task force on statin safety–2014 update. J Clin Lipidol 2014; 8(Suppl 3):S1–4. http://dx.doi.org/10.1016/j.jacl.2014.03.003.

40. Randomised trial of cholesterol lowering in 4444 patients with coronary heart disease: The Scandinavian Simvastatin Survival Study (4S). Lancet 1994;344(8934): 1383–9.

41. Heart Protection Study Collaborative Group. MRC/BHF heart protection study of cholesterol lowering with simvastatin in 20,536 high-risk individuals: a randomised placebo-controlled trial. Lancet 2002;360(9326):7–22. pii:S0140-6736(02) 09327-3.

42. LaRosa JC, Grundy SM, Waters DD, et al. Intensive lipid lowering with atorvastatin in patients with stable coronary disease. N Engl J Med 2005;352(14):1425–35. pii:NEJMoa050461.

43. Sever PS, Dahlof B, Poulter NR, et al. Prevention of coronary and stroke events with atorvastatin in hypertensive patients who have average or lower-than-average cholesterol concentrations, in the Anglo-Scandinavian Cardiac Outcomes Trial–Lipid Lowering Arm (ASCOT-LLA): a multicentre randomised controlled trial. Lancet 2003;361(9364):1149–58. pii:S0140-6736(03)12948-0.

44. Colhoun HM, Betteridge DJ, Durrington PN, et al. Primary prevention of cardiovascular disease with atorvastatin in type 2 diabetes in the Collaborative Atorvastatin Diabetes Study (CARDS): multicentre randomised placebo-controlled trial. Lancet 2004;364(9435):685–96. http://dx.doi.org/10.1016/S0140-6736(04) 16895-5.

45. Ridker PM, Danielson E, Fonseca FA, et al. Rosuvastatin to prevent vascular events in men and women with elevated C-reactive protein. N Engl J Med 2008;359(21):2195–207. http://dx.doi.org/10.1056/NEJMoa0807646.

46. Dawber TR, Kannel WB, Lyell LP. An approach to longitudinal studies in a community: the Framingham Study. Ann N Y Acad Sci 1963;107:539–56.

47. Kannel WB, Feinleib M, McNamara PM, et al. An investigation of coronary heart disease in families. The Framingham Offspring Study. Am J Epidemiol 1979; 110(3):281–90.

New Cholesterol Guidelines for the Management of Atherosclerotic Cardiovascular Disease Risk

A Comparison of the 2013 American College of Cardiology/American Heart Association Cholesterol Guidelines with the 2014 National Lipid Association Recommendations for Patient-Centered Management of Dyslipidemia

Bhavin B. Adhyaru, MS, MD[a], Terry A. Jacobson, MD[b],*

KEYWORDS

- Clinical recommendations • Guidelines • Low-density lipoprotein cholesterol (LDL-C)
- Atherosclerotic cardiovascular disease (ASCVD) • Dyslipidemia
- Atherogenic cholesterol

KEY POINTS

- The 2013 American College of Cardiology (ACC)/American Heart Association (AHA) guideline proposes a pooled risk calculator as an improved method to assess quantitative atherosclerotic cardiovascular disease (ASCVD) risk in primary prevention.
- The 2013 ACC/AHA Guideline recommends shifting away from low-density lipoprotein cholesterol (LDL-C) targets and goals and focuses in on the intensity of statin therapy.
- The 2014 National Lipid Association (NLA) recommendations provides a more comprehensive, patient-centered approach to identifying ASCVD risk.

Continued

This article originally appeared in Cardiology Clinics, Volume 33, Issue 2, May 2015.
Conflicts of Interest & Financial Disclosures: Dr T.A. Jacobson is a consultant for Amarin, Amgen, Astra-Zeneca, Merck, and Regeneron/Sanofi.
[a] Division of General Internal Medicine & Geriatrics, Department of Medicine, Emory University School of Medicine, 49 Jesse Hill Jr Drive, Atlanta, GA 30303, USA; [b] Lipid Clinic and Cardiovascular Risk Reduction Program, Department of Medicine, Emory University School of Medicine, 49 Jesse Hill Jr Drive, Atlanta, GA 30303, USA
* Corresponding author.
E-mail address: tjaco02@emory.edu

Clinics Collections 5 (2015) 215–235
http://dx.doi.org/10.1016/j.ccol.2015.05.013
2352-7986/15/$ – see front matter © 2015 Elsevier Inc. All rights reserved.

Continued

- The NLA recommendations emphasizes the use of statins as first-line therapy, and advocate the use of non–high-density lipoprotein cholesterol (HDL-C) and LDL-C as markers of the atherogenic risk.
- The NLA recommendations emphasize the importance of using evidence-based nonstatin therapy to achieve non–HDL-C and LDL-C goals.

THE 2013 AMERICAN COLLEGE OF CARDIOLOGY/AMERICAN HEART ASSOCIATION GUIDELINE ON THE TREATMENT OF BLOOD CHOLESTEROL
Scope and Methodology

Almost one-third of the population in the United States will die as a result of heart attack and stroke associated with atherosclerotic cardiovascular disease (ASCVD), which is currently the leading cause of death in the United States.[1–3]

To provide an update to the 2004 Adult Treatment Panel (ATP) III guidelines,[4,5] the National Heart Lung Blood Institute (NHLBI) formulated a multidisciplinary expert panel consisting of cardiologists, medical subspecialists, and experts in clinical lipidology in 2008.[1] The panel elected to include only randomized controlled trials (RCTs) involving statins, systematic reviews, and metaanalyses for the treatment of blood cholesterol to reduce ASCVD. In the guideline, clinical ASCVD included coronary heart disease (acute coronary syndromes, history of myocardial infarction [MI], stable or unstable angina, coronary or other arterial revascularization), stroke or transient ischemic attack, and peripheral arterial disease presumed to be of atherosclerotic origin. The panel constructed 3 critical questions, and an independent contractor helped search for evidence for each of these critical questions based on inclusion and exclusion criteria. The search included data from 1995 to 2009; however, major RCTs and metaanalyses through July 2013 were included in the discussions of their final recommendations. The RCTs were graded from good to poor quality, with only good or fair quality RCTs included for consideration. The final recommendations were approved by at least a majority of the voting members of the expert panel. In 2013, the NHLBI turned over its recommendations to the American College of Cardiology (ACC) and the American Heart Association (AHA), who were charged with further review and guideline dissemination to the broader provider community. The synthesis of the evidence is based on the NHLBI grading of recommendations (**Table 1**) as well as the ACC/AHA (**Table 2**) classification system.

Groups Benefiting from Statin Therapy ("Statin Benefit Groups")

The ACC/AHA panel found in its review of statin RCTs that there was a consistent reduction in ASCVD events from statin therapy in both secondary and primary prevention. The intensity of statin therapy was defined based on the average expected LDL-C response. As shown in **Table 3**, the 3 types of statin therapy include high intensity (≥50% reduction in LDL-C), moderate intensity (30 to <50% reduction), and low intensity (<30% reduction).

The guideline found 4 major groups where the benefit of a statin on ASCVD risk reduction outweighed the risk of adverse events (**Fig. 1**)[1]:

1. Patients with clinical ASCVD (eg, acute coronary syndromes, history of MI, stable or unstable angina, stroke, transient ischemic attack, or peripheral arterial disease).
2. Patients with primary elevation of LDL-C of 190 mg/dL or higher.

Table 1
NHLBI grading of recommendations

Grade	Strength of Recommendation
A	Strong recommendation There is high certainty based on evidence that the net benefit (benefits minus risk/harm of service/intervention) is substantial.
B	Moderate recommendation There is moderate certainty based on evidence that the net benefit is moderate to substantial, or there is high certainty that the net benefit is moderate.
C	Weak recommendation There is at least moderate certainty based on evidence that there is small net benefit.
D	Recommendation against There is at least moderate certainty based on evidence that it has no net benefit or that risks/harms outweigh benefits.
E	Expert opinion ("There is insufficient evidence or evidence is unclear or conflicting, but this is what the work group recommends.") Net benefit is unclear. Balance of benefits and harms cannot be determined because of no evidence, insufficient evidence, unclear evidence, or conflicting evidence, but the work group thought it was important to provide clinical guidance and make a recommendation. Further research is recommended in this area.
N	No recommendation for or against ("There is insufficient evidence or evidence is unclear or conflicting.") Net benefit is unclear. Balance of benefits and harms cannot be determined because of no evidence, insufficient evidence, unclear evidence, or conflicting evidence, and the work group thought no recommendation should be made. Further research is recommended in this area.

Abbreviation: NHLBI, National Heart Lung Blood Institute.

From Stone NJ, Robinson JG, Lichtenstein AH, et al. 2013 ACC/AHA guideline on the treatment of blood cholesterol to reduce atherosclerotic cardiovascular risk in adults: a report of the American College of Cardiology/American Heart Association Task Force on Practice Guidelines. Circulation 2014;129(25 Suppl 2):S6; with permission.

3. Patients with diabetes (type 1 and 2) aged 40 to 75 years with LDL-C of 70 to 189 mg/dL and without clinical ASCVD.
4. Patients without diabetes or clinical ASCVD and estimated 10-year ASCVD risk of 7.5% or greater.

For primary prevention, in patients age 40 to 75 years with LDL-C of 70 to 189 mg/dL without diabetes or clinical ASCVD, the decision to initiate statin is based on 10-year ASCVD risk using new pooled risk equations (discussed in more detail elsewhere in this article). The data used to identify who would benefit from a statin was based on 3 trials (Air force/Texas coronary atherosclerosis prevention study [AFCAPS-TexCAPS], Primary Prevention of Cardiovascular Disease With Pravastatin in Japan [MEGA], and Justification for the Use of Statins in Primary Prevention: An Intervention Trial Evaluating Rosuvastatin Trial [JUPITER]) that included patients with LDL-C of greater than 70 mg/dL and less than 190 mg/dL in primary prevention. It was determined that patients with a ASCVD risk of 7.5% or higher benefited most from moderate- to high-intensity statin therapy. This value is not an absolute threshold to start statin therapy, but this is when physicians and patients should engage in discussion of the risks and benefits of statin therapy.[6–8]

Table 2
ACC/AHA recommendation classification and level of evidence

		Size of Treatment Effect			
Level		Class I *Benefit > > Risk* Procedure/Treatment Should Be Performed/ Administered	Class IIa *Benefit > > Risk* *Additional Studies With* *Focused Objectives* *Needed* It Is Reasonable to Perform Procedure/ Administer Treatment	Class IIb *Benefit ≥ Risk* *Additional Studies With* *Broad Objectives* *Needed; Additional* *Registry Data Would Be* *Helpful* Procedure/Treatment May Be Considered	Class III No Benefit or CLASS III Harm
					Procedure/Test: Not Helpful / Treatment: No Proven Benefit COR III: No benefit — Procedure/Test Not Helpful, Treatment No Proven Benefit COR III: Harm — Excess Cost W/O Benefit or Harmful, Treatment Harmful to Patients
Estimate of certainty (precision) of treatment effect	Level A Multiple populations evaluated Data derived from multiple randomized clinical trials or metaanalyses	Recommendation that procedure or treatment is useful/effective Sufficient evidence from multiple randomized trials or metaanalyses	Recommendation in favor of treatment or procedure being useful/effective Some conflicting evidence from multiple randomized trials or metaanalyses	Recommendation's usefulness/efficacy less well established Greater conflicting evidence from multiple randomized trials or meta-analyses	Recommendation that procedure or treatment is useful/effective and may be harmful Sufficient evidence from multiple randomized trials or meta-analyses
	Level B Limited populations evaluated Data derived from a single randomized trial or nonrandomized studies	Recommendation that procedure or treatment is useful/effective Evidence from single randomized trial or nonrandomized studies	Recommendation in favor of treatment or procedure being useful/effective Some conflicting evidence from single randomized trial or nonrandomized studies	Recommendation's usefulness/efficacy less well established Greater conflicting evidence from single randomized trial or nonrandomized studies	Recommendation that procedure or treatment is not useful/effective and may be harmful Evidence from single randomized trial or nonrandomized studies
	Level C Very limited populations evaluated Only consensus opinion of experts, case studies, or standard of care	Recommendation that procedure or treatment is useful/evidence Only expert opinion, case studies, or standard of care	Recommendation in favor of treatment or procedure being useful/effective Only diverging expert opinion, case studies, or standard of care	Recommendation's usefulness/efficacy less well established Only diverging expert opinion, case studies, or standard of care	Recommendation that procedure or treatment is not useful/effective and may be harmful Only expert opinion, case studies, or standard of care

Abbreviations: COR, class of recommendation; W/O, without.

From Stone NJ, Robinson JG, Lichtenstein AH, et al. 2013 ACC/AHA guideline on the treatment of blood cholesterol to reduce atherosclerotic cardiovascular risk in adults: a

Table 3
Intensity of statin therapy according to the 2013 American College of Cardiology/American Heart Association Guideline

High-Intensity Statin Therapy	Moderate-Intensity Statin Therapy	Low-Intensity Statin Therapy
Daily dose lowers LDL-C on average, by approximately ≥50%	Daily dose lowers LDL-C on average, by approximately 30% to <50%	Daily dose lowers LDL-C on average, by <30%
Atorvastatin 40–80 mg Rosuvastatin 20–40 mg	Atorvastatin 10–20 mg Rosuvastatin 5–10 mg Simvastatin 20–40 mg Pravastatin 40–80 mg Lovastatin 40 mg Fluvastatin XL 80 mg Fluvastatin 40 mg twice daily Pitavastatin 2–4 mg	Simvastatin 10 mg Pravastatin 10–20 mg Lovastatin 20 mg Fluvastatin 20–40 mg Pitavastatin 1 mg

Abbreviation: LDL-C, low-density lipoprotein cholesterol.
Adapted from Stone NJ, Robinson JG, Lichtenstein AH, et al. 2013 ACC/AHA guideline on the treatment of blood cholesterol to reduce atherosclerotic cardiovascular risk in adults: a report of the American College of Cardiology/American Heart Association task force on practice guidelines. Circulation 2014;129(25 Suppl 2):S25; with permission.

In patients with a 10-year ASCVD risk of 5.0% to 7.4%, a similar amount of evidence supports moderate- to high-intensity statin therapy, although there is evidence that the benefit of a moderate intensity statin outweighs the risk of adverse events in this group. For patients with an ASCVD risk of less than 5% or those not in a statin benefit group (ie, age <40 or age >75), it is important to consider the risks and benefits of statin therapy as well as considering other risk factors that may better inform treatment decisions such as:

- LDL-C of 160 mg/dL or greater
- Family history of premature ASCVD with onset less than 55 years old in first degree male relatives or less than 65 years old in first-degree female relative
- Coronary artery calcium score of 300 Agatston units or more, or greater than 75th percentile
- Highly sensitive C-reactive protein of 2 mg/L or greater
- Ankle-brachial index of less than 0.9
- High lifetime risk at age 20 to 59 years.

Pooled Cohort Risk Equations for Atherosclerotic Cardiovascular Disease Risk Assessment

To determine an individual's risk, the guideline recommends the estimation of a 10-year risk for ASCVD events (CHD and stroke). This differs from the 10-year risk score from the previous National Cholesterol Education Program (NCEP)/ATP III guideline, which only included hard CHD events (nonfatal MI and CHD death).[9] The risk assessment is based on pooled cohort risk assessment and can be calculated by many online calculators and risk prediction apps.[10]

The Framingham 10-year general CVD risk was used as the basis for the development of the pooled cohort risk. However, to make it more generalizable, data from large, racially and geographically diverse cohort studies were included (Atherosclerosis Risk in Communities [ARIC] study, Cardiovascular Health Study, Coronary Artery

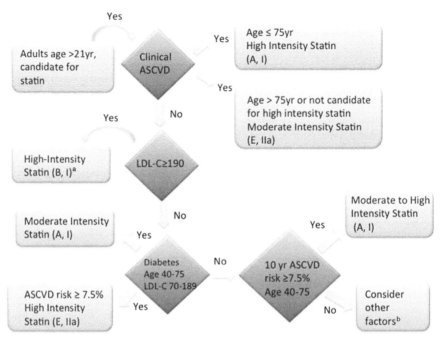

Fig. 1. The major recommendations based on the 2013 American College of Cardiology/ American Heart Association (ACC/AHA) guidelines for atherosclerotic cardiovascular disease (ASCVD) prevention. Recommendations are given with the National Heart Lung Blood Institute (NHLBI) grade and ACC/AHA classification (eg, A, I). [a] Note. For patients >21 years with untreated primary LDL-C >190 mg/dL after maximum intensity of statin, addition of nonstatin drug can be considered (E, IIbC). [b] Consider for additional assessment of ASCVD risk in patients who do not fall within 1 of the 4 statin benefit groups: LDL-C ≥160 mg/dL, family history of premature ASCVD, coronary artery calcium score (CAC) ≥300 Agatston units of 75th percentile, high-sensitivity C-reactive protein ≥2 mg/L, ankle–brachial index <0.9, and high lifetime risk at age 20 to 59. LDL-C, low-density lipoprotein cholesterol. (*Adapted from* Stone NJ, Robinson JG, Lichtenstein AH, et al. 2013 ACC/AHA guideline on the treatment of blood cholesterol to reduce atherosclerotic cardiovascular risk in adults: a report of the American College of Cardiology/American Heart Association Task Force on Practice Guidelines. Circulation 2014;129(25 Suppl 2):S15; with permission.)

Risk Development in Young Adults [CARDIA]) combined with the Framingham original and offspring cohorts.[1] The cohort included 11,240 white women, 9098 white men, 2641 African-American women, and 1647 African-American men. These data were used to develop sex- and race-specific equations to predict the 10-year risk of a first hard ASCVD event. The ATP III panel considered diabetes to be a CHD risk equivalent and for this reason did not include diabetes in their multivariable risk equations. Because a recent metaanalysis did not show that diabetes is a CHD risk equivalent, diabetes was included as an independent predictor variable in the new pooled cohort risk equations.[11]

The pooled cohort had good internal validation, and external validation was performed in the Whites and African-Americans from the Multi-Ethnic Study of Atherosclerosis (MESA)[12] and the Reasons for Geographic And Racial Differences in Stroke Study (REGARDS).[13] The guideline authors did note that even in their external validation there was overprediction of ASCVD risk in all of the groups.[1]

Low-Density Lipoprotein Cholesterol Treatment Targets

The evidence included in the ACC/AHA guideline was based on RCTs that compared a fixed dose or compared high-intensity versus moderate-intensity statins. Based on this, they did not find evidence to support titrating therapy to achieve a specific LDL-C or non–HDL-C goal as recommended by the ATP III. The panel gave no recommendation for or against specific LDL-C or non–HDL-C targets for primary prevention of ASCVD. The panel also argued that, given the lack of evidence to treat to a specific target or that even if lower lipid levels were better (vs the statin dose), the use of multidrug therapy may be harmful and not evidence based.

The guideline provides an approach to monitor statin therapy. They recommend an initial lipid panel followed by a second lipid panel 4 to 12 weeks after initiation of statin therapy to determine adherence and appropriate LDL-C response to therapy (**Fig. 2**). If a patient is already on a statin where the baseline LDL-C is unknown, an LDL-C less than of 100 mg/dL was observed in individuals receiving high-intensity statin therapy in RCTs. If a patient with ASCVD is on a moderate- or low-intensity statin with an LDL-C of less than 100 mg/d, then based on current evidence, that patient would have a greater reduction in ASCVD events if a high-intensity statin was given and tolerated. Therefore, we could conclude based on the ACC/AHA guidelines that, if a patient with ASCVD is on a moderate-intensity statin with LDL-C of less than 100 mg/dL, they still should be switched to a high-intensity statin.

THE 2014 NATIONAL LIPID ASSOCIATION RECOMMENDATIONS FOR PATIENT-CENTERED MANAGEMENT OF DYSLIPIDEMIA
Scope and Methodology

The National Lipid Association (NLA) convened their expert panel to develop a patient-centered approach to the management of dyslipidemia.[2] The guideline was developed with 2 parts, the first discussing the screening and classification of lipoprotein lipid levels, targets for intervention in dyslipidemia, ASCVD risk assessment, atherogenic cholesterol (non-HDL, LDL-C) as targets for therapy, and lifestyle/drug therapies to reduce ASCVD events. The second part addressed lifestyle therapies, special populations including the elderly, children, women, other ethnic groups (Hispanics, Asian Americans, African Americans), patients with HIV, high-risk inflammatory conditions (rheumatoid arthritis), and those with high residual risk on statin therapy.

The guideline was developed to provide an update to the revised ATP III guideline published in 2004 and to consider new evidence from RCT trials involving statin and nonstatin therapy, as well as combination statin therapy. The evidence that was evaluated not only included RCTs, but also metaanalyses, epidemiologic and observational studies, metabolic and genetic studies, and mechanistic investigations. The following core principles were used to develop the guideline:

1. Elevated levels of cholesterol carried by apolipoprotein (Apo) B-containing lipoproteins (non–HDL-C and LDL-C, called atherogenic cholesterol) are a root cause of atherosclerosis, the major underlying process contributing to ASCVD events.
2. Reducing elevated levels of atherogenic cholesterol will lower ASCVD risk in proportion to the extent that atherogenic cholesterol is lowered.
3. The intensity of risk reduction therapy should be adjusted to the patient's absolute risk for an ASCVD event.
4. Both intermediate- and long-term (or lifetime) risk should be considered when assessing potential benefits and hazards of risk reduction therapies.
5. Statin treatment is the primary and most evidence-based modality for reducing ASCVD risk.

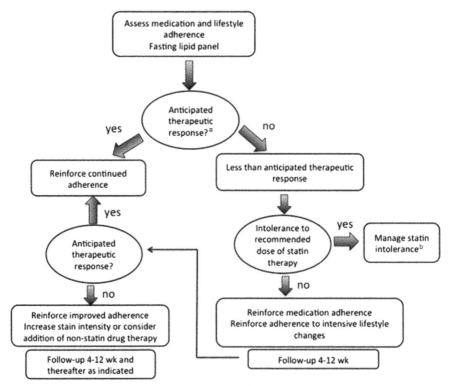

Fig. 2. Monitoring therapeutic response and adherence to statin therapy by the 2013 American College of Cardiology/American Heart Association (ACC/AHA) guidelines. [a] Indicators of anticipated therapeutic response and adherence to selected statin intensity: high-intensity statin therapy reduces LDL-C by approximately ≥50% from the untreated baseline and moderate-intensity statin therapy reduces LDL-C by approximately 30% to <50% from the untreated baseline. [b] Management of statin intolerance: (1) To avoid unnecessary discontinuation of statins, obtain history of prior or current muscle symptoms to establish a baseline before statin therapy; (2) If unexplained severe muscle symptoms, discontinue statin and address possibility of rhabdomyolysis by evaluating a creatine kinase (CK), creatinine, and urinalysis; (3) If mild to moderate muscle symptoms develop during statin therapy, discontinue statin until symptoms can be evaluated, consider other conditions that might increase risk for muscle symptoms (ie, hypothyroidism, reduced renal/hepatic function, vitamin D deficiency), if symptoms resolve give the patient original or lower dose of the same statin to establish a causal relationship, increase dose as tolerated; if persistent muscle symptoms are unrelated to statin therapy, resume statin therapy at the original dose. (*Adapted from* Stone NJ, Robinson JG, Lichtenstein AH, et al. 2013 ACC/AHA guideline on the treatment of blood cholesterol to reduce atherosclerotic cardiovascular risk in adults: a report of the American College of Cardiology/American Heart Association task force on practice guidelines. Circulation 2014;129(25 Suppl 2):S43; with permission.)

6. Lipid targets and goals are important clinical and motivational tools for patients and providers, and LDL-C monitoring is important in assessing adherence to therapy, adequacy of response to therapy, and determining lipid-related residual risk.

Atherogenic Cholesterol (Non–High-Density Lipoprotein Cholesterol and Low-Density Lipoprotein Cholesterol)

Although LDL-C has typically been the primary target of therapy, the NLA consensus was that non–HDL-C is a better primary target than LDL-C. The non–HDL-C comprises cholesterol carried by all potentially atherogenic particles that include LDL, intermediate density lipoproteins, very low-density lipoproteins, and very low-density lipoproteins remnants, chylomicron remnants, and lipoprotein (a). In several metaanalyses of statin[14,15] and nonstatin trials,[16] it was found that non–HDL-C correlated more closely with ASCVD risk than LDL-C both at baseline and during therapy. This may be owing to several factors, including that (1) some triglyceride-rich lipoprotein remnants enter the arterial wall similar to LDL-C, contributing to the initiation and progression of atherosclerosis, (2) non–HDL-C correlates more closely with all Apo-B–containing lipoproteins and with the total burden of all atherogenic particles, and (3) elevated levels of triglycerides and very low-density lipoprotein-C reflect hepatic production of particles with greater atherogenic potential resulting in longer residence time in circulation. Apo-B is an optional secondary target for treatment because it is also a very robust predictor of ASCVD risk during statin therapy.[17,18] Based on population studies, desirable levels for secondary prevention are non–HDL-C of less than 100 mg/dL, LDL-C of less than 70 mg/dL, and Apo B of less than 80 mg/dL.

Assessment of Atherosclerotic Cardiovascular Disease Risk

According to the NLA, risk assessment is based on the identification of high-risk and very high-risk groups, the counting of individual ASCVD risk factors, and the classification of individual risk status as very high risk, high risk, moderate risk, and low risk. These classifications help to determine when to consider drug therapy, what treatment goals to select, and how to match the intensity of therapy to the patient's absolute risk of an ASCVD event. **Table 4** shows the major ASCVD risk factors and **Tables 5** and **6** show treatment goals in relation to risk categories. **Fig. 3** shows a sequential method for identifying a patient's risk.

Individuals with clinical ASCVD and patients with diabetes with 2 or more ASCVD risk factors are at "very high risk" and should have the most aggressive goals for atherogenic cholesterol (non–HDL-C <100 mg/dL, LDL-C <70 mg/dL). Interestingly,

---

Table 4
Major risk factors for atherosclerotic cardiovascular disease according to the National Lipid Association recommendations

Risk Factor	Parameter
Age	Male $\geq$45 y Female $\geq$55 y
Family history of early coronary heart disease	<55 y of age in a male first-degree relative <65 y of age in a female first-degree relative
Current cigarette smoking	
High blood pressure	$\geq$140/$\geq$90 mm Hg or on blood pressure medication
Low high-density lipoprotein cholesterol	Male <40 mg/dL Female <50 mg/dL

From Jacobson TA, Ito MK, Maki KC, et al. National Lipid Association recommendations for patient-centered management of dyslipidemia: part 1 - executive summary. J Clin Lipidol 2014;8(5):479; with permission.

Table 5
Treatment goals for non–HDL-C, LDL-C, and Apo B according to the National Lipid Association Recommendations

Risk Category	Treatment Goals		
	Non–HDL-C (mg/dL)	LDL-C (mg/dL)	Apo B[a] (mg/dL)
Low	<130	<100	<90
Moderate	<130	<100	<90
High	<130	<100	<90
Very high	<100	<70	<80

Abbreviations: Apo B, apolipoprotein B; HDL-C, high-density lipoprotein cholesterol; LDL-C, low-density lipoprotein cholesterol.
[a] Apo B is a secondary, optional target of treatment.
From Jacobson TA, Ito MK, Maki KC, et al. National Lipid Association recommendations for patient-centered management of dyslipidemia: part 1 - executive summary. J Clin Lipidol 2014;8(5):476; with permission.

chronic kidney disease stage 5 represents a group at very high risk of ASCVD; however, data from RCTs have not shown consistent benefits and clinical judgment should be used when deciding treatment for this group.

For patients with 2 major ASCVD risk factors, other major ASCVD risk indicators can be considered (**Box 1**) in clinical decision making, or quantitative risk assessment can be performed to identify those at high risk. The thresholds recommended for commonly used risk scores are shown below. These risk cutpoints differ than the cutpoints in both the 2013 AHA/ACC guidelines and the ATP III guidelines using the Framingham risk calculator. Of note, these cutpoints are not the same as the "statin benefit groups" as outlined in the 2013 AHA/ACC cholesterol guideline. These cutpoints are intended to inform clinical judgment by placing patients into their different risk categories.

1. ATP III Framingham risk calculator: 10% or greater 10-year risk for a hard CHD event.
2. Pooled cohort equations: 15% or greater 10-year risk for a hard ASCVD event.
3. Framingham long-term (30-year to age 80) risk calculator: 45% or greater risk for CVD (MI, CHD death, or stroke).

Treatment Algorithm

First-line pharmacologic treatment for elevated atherogenic cholesterol levels is a moderate- or high-intensity statin (discussed in the ACC/AHA guideline section). For patients with contraindication or intolerance to statin therapy, nonstatin drug therapy may be considered. The nonstatin drug classes for LDL-C reduction include the cholesterol absorption inhibitors, bile acid sequesterants, and nicotinic acid, and the nonstatin drugs for triglyceride reduction include the fibrates, nicotinic acid, and the long-chain omega-3 fatty acids.

If the goal levels of atherogenic cholesterol have not been achieved, the statin dosage may be increased or switched to a more efficacious agent. If, after a trial of the highest tolerable dose of a high-intensity statin, goal levels have not been achieved, the clinician can consider addition of a second cholesterol-lowering agent or referral to a lipid specialist. Once goals have been achieved, response to therapy should be monitored periodically.

Table 6
Criteria for ASCVD risk assessment, treatment goals, and levels at which to consider drug therapy according to the National Lipid Association recommendations

Risk Category	Criteria	Treatment Goal		Consider Drug Therapy	
		Non–HDL-C (mg/dL)	LDL-C (mg/dL)	Non–HDL-C (mg/dL)	LDL-C (mg/dL)
Low	0–1 major ASCVD risk factors	<130	<100	≥190	≥160
	Consider other risk indicators, if known				
Moderate	2 major ASCVD risk factors	<130	<100	≥160	≥130
	Consider quantitative risk scoring				
	Consider other risk indictors[a]				
High	≥3 major ASCVD risk factors	<130	<100	≥130	≥100
	Diabetes				
	0–1 other major ASCVD risk factor				
	No evidence of end organ damage				
	CKD stage 3B or 4				
	LDL-C >190 mg/dL				
	Quantitative risk score reaching the high risk threshold				
Very high	ASCVD	<100	<70	≥100	≥70
	Diabetes				
	≥2 major risk factors or				
	Evidence of end-organ damage[a]				

For patients with ASCVD or diabetes mellitus, consideration should be given to use of moderate- or high-intensity statin therapy, irrespective of baseline atherogenic cholesterol levels.

Note: End-organ damage is indicated by increased albumin/creatinine ratio (≥30 mg/g), CKD, or retinopathy.

Abbreviations: ASCVD, atherosclerotic cardiovascular disease; CKD, chronic kidney disease; HDL-C, high-density lipoprotein cholesterol; LDL-C, low-density lipoprotein cholesterol.

[a] For those at moderate risk, additional testing may be considered for some patients to assist with decisions about risk stratification. These include metabolic syndrome and risk indicators such as (1) severe disturbance in a major ASCVD risk factor such as multipack per day smoking or strong family history of premature coronary heart disease, (2) coronary calcium score of ≥300 Agatston units, (3) LDL-C ≥ 160 mg/dL or non–HDL-C ≥190 mg/dL, (4) high-sensitivity C-reactive protein of ≥2.0 mg/L, (5) lipoprotein (a) ≥50 mg/dL, (6) urine albumin/creatinine ratio ≥30 mg/g.

From Jacobson TA, Ito MK, Maki KC, et al. National Lipid Association recommendations for patient-centered management of dyslipidemia: part 1 - executive summary. J Clin Lipidol 2014;8(5):477; with permission.

There are several adverse events related to statin therapy that have been reported. The most common adverse effects are muscle-related complaints (ie, myalgias, muscle aches, or muscle discomfort) that are related mostly to the dose of the statin than the degree of LDL reduction. Musculoskeletal complaints are common in older patients and in those who are more physically active; therefore, it is important to assess for these causes before attributing symptoms to statin therapy. It is also important to consider other medications and conditions (hypothyroidism), which may interact with statins thus increasing the risk of muscle symptoms.[19,20] There has been a modest increase in the risk of type 2 diabetes observed with statin therapy, and higher intensity statin therapy increases this risk to a greater extent than less intensive regimens. It is recommended to check a hemoglobin A1c level before initiation of a statin and within a

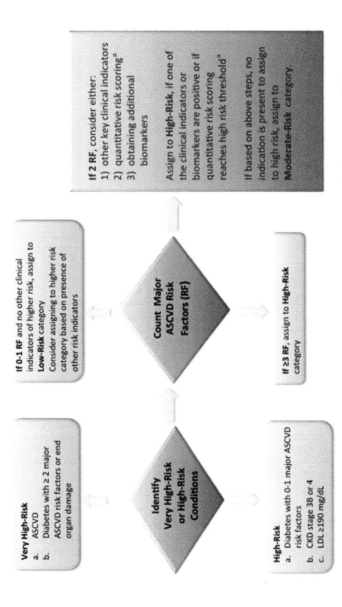

Fig. 3. National Lipid Association sequential steps in atherosclerotic cardiovascular disease (ASCVD) risk assessment. [a] The 10-year Framingham risk is ≥10%; American College of Cardiology/American Heart Association pooled cohort equations 10-year risk is ≥15%; Framingham long-term (30-year to age 80) risk is ≥45%.

Box 1
National Lipid Association risk indicators considered for risk refinement

1. A severe disturbance in a major ASCVD risk factor, such as multipack per day smoking, or strong family history of premature CHD.

2. Indicators of subclinical disease, including coronary artery calcium.

   a. ≥300 Agatston units is considered high risk.

3. LDL-C ≥160 and/or non–HDL-C ≥190 mg/dL.

4. High-sensitivity C-reactive protein ≥2.0 mg/L.

5. Lipoprotein (a) ≥50 mg/dL (protein) using an isoform insensitive assay.

6. Urine albumin/creatinine ratio ≥30 mg/g.

Abbreviations: ASCVD, atherosclerotic cardiovascular disease; CHD, coronary heart disease; HDL-C, high-density lipoprotein cholesterol; LDL-C, low-density lipoprotein cholesterol.

From Jacobson TA, Ito MK, Maki KC, et al. National Lipid Association recommendations for patient-centered management of dyslipidemia: part 1 - executive summary. J Clin Lipidol 2014;8(5):481; with permission.

---

year afterward in those with risk factors for the metabolic syndrome or diabetes.[21–24] Short-term memory impairment has been reported; however, observational studies have failed to find significant evidence for memory loss with those on long-term statin therapy.[23,25] See the articles elsewhere in this issue for a more in-depth discussion about statins and their effects on diabetes risk and cognition.

There are observational data as well as some RCTs comparing lower and higher dosages of statin therapy that suggest that ASCVD event risk reduction is associated with lower levels of atherogenic cholesterol and that greater reductions in atherogenic cholesterol levels are associated with greater ASCVD benefits. The associations between on-treatment levels of LDL-C (and non–HDL-C) follow a log–linear relationship, supporting the view that the primary mechanism of action of statins is through reductions in levels of atherogenic lipoproteins. Until there are further data from RCTs for add-on therapies, the NLA recommends that consideration be given to combination therapy with the highest tolerated statin dose to further lower atherogenic cholesterol (non–HDL-C and LDL-C) to goal levels.

COMPARISON AND CONTRASTS OF THE NEW GUIDELINES

Since its inception, several aspects of the new 2013 ACC/AHA guidelines have been controversial, including the absence of treatment goals, the role of combination therapy on top of statin therapy, and the utility of the pooled cohort equations to assess ASCVD risk.

A recent article reviewing various clinical practice guidelines for lipid management shows major differences in the assessment of risk and treatment targets.[26] Most national and international practice guidelines use LDL-C or non–HDL-C as targets of therapy whereas the 2013 ACC/AHA cholesterol guidelines use LDL-C more as a means of assessing adherence to therapy. The risk assessments vary from using the pooled cohort ASCVD risk equations to the Framingham risk score. This does pose significant challenges to the practicing clinician on how to manage and evaluate a patient's ASCVD risk. Prior studies have shown that few clinicians were actually using the risk prediction engines in primary prevention under the ATP III guidelines and that giving risk prediction scores to clinicians did not improve patient outcomes necessarily.[27–29] Therefore, the NLA guidelines chose not to put a heavy emphasis on quantitative risk scoring, but chose to emphasize the identification of high-risk conditions, the simple counting of cardiovascular risk factors, and the selective use of other risk factor indicators when there is doubt about the necessity for treatment. The NLA guidelines were created to provide a more comprehensive and patient-centered approach to determining an individual's risk and management. Specifically, the NLA recommendations were designed to offer expert advice in where RCT evidence was lacking.

There are some similarities between the guidelines in that both recommend lipid screening for primary prevention at 5-year intervals and lifestyle therapy is advocated as a first step in all treatment algorithms. The goal of therapy for both guidelines is ASCVD risk reduction and moderate- to high-intensity statin is the central focus of pharmacotherapy. Both recommend patient–provider discussion of risk and benefit regarding drug treatment and regular lipid follow-up is warranted to assess adherence to therapy.

There are several other important differences between the guidelines (**Table 7**). One includes the evidence base that was used in forming recommendations. Whereas the ACC/AHA includes only statin RCTs and metaanalyses, the NLA incorporates statin and nonstatin RCTs and metaanalysis, along with observational studies, genetic studies, and mechanistic studies in formulating its recommendations. Although RCTs represent a high quality of evidence, there may be important insights from observational studies, such as assessing ASCVD risk across populations or determining safety signals in large observational cohorts. Finally, for many of the important questions in clinical medicine, there is an absence of RCTs to inform clinical judgment. Therefore, it is important that guidelines give recommendations, even in cases where RCTs are lacking.

Low-Density Lipoprotein Cholesterol Treatment Goals

Other areas of controversy are the importance of treatment targets, whether non–HDL-C is a better target of therapy than LDL-C, and what are the additional benefits of adding nonstatin therapy. The 2013 ACC/AHA guidelines emphasize that RCTs used fixed doses of statins and it therefore should not be assumed that dosage titration is correct. They stress that the evidence suggests that it is the dose of the statin that is more important than either the degree of LDL-C reduction or the obtainment of lipid goals. However, the Treating to New Targets (TNT) trial did show that atorvastatin 80 mg compared with atorvastatin 10 mg did achieve LDL levels (77 vs 100 mg/dL) quite similar to the ATP III goals of therapy (<70 and 100 mg/dL, respectively). This difference in LDL-C was associated with a relative risk reduction in major cardiovascular events of 22% (hazard ratio, 0.78; 95% CI, 0.69–0.89; $P<0.001$; absolute risk reduction, 3.2%).[30]

Combination Statin Therapy

The AHA/ACC guideline refer to several trials wherein the addition of an additional lipid-lowering agent on top of statin therapy did not further lower ASCVD risk. The AIM-HIGH and HPS-2-THRIVE trials studied niacin in combination with statin therapy, but failed to show additional ASCVD risk reduction despite additional LDL-C and non–HDL-C reduction.[31,32] Not discussed in the AHA/ACC guidelines was the fact that both of these high-risk populations studied were already at or near their LDL goals (70 and 63 mg/dL, respectively), despite the additional fact that this limitation of both of these trials has been discussed elsewhere in considerable detail.[33] Similarly, the Action to

Table 7
A comparison of the 2013 ACC/AHA and the 2014 NLA guidelines

	2013 ACC/AHA Guideline	2014 NLA Recommendations
Evidence base	RCTs of statin therapy Metaanalyses and systematic review of RCTs	RCT of statin therapy and nonstatin therapies Meta analyses and systematic review of RCTs Observational and epidemiologic studies Genetic studies Metabolic and mechanistic studies
ASCVD risk assessment	4 major statin benefit groups CV risk calculator based on pooled cohort risk equations (10-year risk and lifetime risk)	Identification of patients with "very high-risk" or "high-risk" conditions Counting of ASCVD risk factors to determine risk factor category If 2 major ASCVD risk factors, consider either: other key clinical criteria, quantitative risk scoring, or obtaining additional biomarkers
Treatment goals and lipid monitoring	No specific LDL-C target or goal of therapy Monitor LDL-C to assess adherence to therapy	Target non–HDL-C and LDL-C based on risk category Use non–HDL-C and LDL-C goals to assess adherence to therapy, adequacy of treatment response, and residual risk related to lipids
Nonstatin therapy	No recommendation for nonstatin therapy except for patients with LDL-C >190 mg/ dL on maximum dose statin therapy, or patients with statin intolerance	If non–HDL-C and LDL-C goals are not met with statin therapy, addition of evidence based nonstatin therapy should be considered

Abbreviations: ACC, American College of Cardiology; AHA, American Heart Association; ASCVD, atherosclerotic cardiovascular disease; CHD, coronary heart disease; CV, cardiovascular; HDL-C, high-density lipoprotein cholesterol; LDL-C, low-density lipoprotein cholesterol; NLA, National Lipid Association; RCT, randomized, controlled trial.

Control Cardiovascular Risk in Diabetes (ACCORD-Lipid) trial did not find additional risk reduction in patients with diabetes mellitus when fenofibrate was added to statin therapy.[34] Again also of note, the patients were already close to their LDL goal (mean of 100.6 mg/dL) before fenofibrate was added and their final LDL values (mean LDL of 81 mg/dL) were no different between placebo and fenofibrate by study end. Despite these results, there is some evidence that fibrates can be considered in select patients with high triglycerides and low HDL-C based on individual trial subgroup analysis and from a metaanalysis that has shown ASCVD risk reduction. However, these findings of benefit in subgroups with high triglycerides and low HDL need to be confirmed prospectively. Finally, it cannot be refuted that, in the prestatin era, clinical trials involving monotherapy with either cholestyramine in the Lipid Research Clinics Coronary Primary Prevention trial, niacin in the Coronary Drug Project, and ileal bypass surgery in the POSCH study all reduced ASCVD risk significantly.[35–38]

Implications of the IMProved Reduction of Outcomes: Vytorin Efficacy International Trial

Excitingly, the recent IMProved Reduction of Outcomes: Vytorin Efficacy International Trial (IMPROVE-IT) study suggests that the addition of ezetimibe to simvastatin is safe and more efficacious than statin therapy alone. This trial was an RCT of 18,144 post-acute coronary syndrome patients with baseline LDL-C of 50 to 125 mg/dL randomized to either simvastatin 40 mg or simvastatin 40 mg plus ezetimibe 10 mg. The primary endpoint was cardiovascular death, MI, hospital admission for unstable angina, stroke, or coronary revascularization 30 days or more after randomization. The absolute risk reduction for the primary endpoint at the end of 5.7 years was 2.0% with a number needed to treat of 50. In addition, the benefit was demonstrated with the achievement of lower LDL-C levels of 50 versus 65 mg/dL, respectively.[39] This is consistent with the Cholesterol Treatment Trialists' metaanalysis of 27 statin trials,[40,41] which showed a greater reduction in risk with larger LDL reductions and no evidence of a threshold level of LDL-C wherein there was no longer a benefit. These new data suggest clearly that there may be additional benefit by further targeting LDL-C and non–HDL-C to lower levels, and that nonstatin therapy can reduce effectively ASCVD risk in combination with-high dose statins. Whether lower doses of statins can be used with ezetimibe in patients who are intolerant to statins needs to be determined.

Atherosclerotic Cardiovascular Disease Risk Assessment

The ASCVD pooled cohort equations remains an important area of controversy. Although a strength of the ACC/AHA guideline is their incorporation of more recent epidemiologic cohorts with greater ethnic diversity, there remain several issues with its validation. A general concern is whether any type of global risk prediction score is needed, given that no trial has ever randomized patients by their absolute risk or tried to tailor or match the intensity of therapy to their absolute risk. For example, the Controlled Rosuvastatin Multinational Trial in Heart Failure (CORONA; heart failure)[42] and A Study to Evaluate the Use of Rosuvastatin in Subjects on Regular Hemodialysis: An Assessment of Survival and Cardiovascular Events (AURORA; hemodialysis)[43] trials included high-risk vascular patients and found no event reduction despite significant reductions in LDL-C. Although the AHA/ACC guidelines appropriately point out that patients with congestive heart failure or on dialysis have not been shown to benefit from statin therapy, it raises some questions about the utility of the equations in certain comorbid patient populations and in populations in where there are few outcomes data, such as Americans of Hispanic or Asian origin. A study by Ridker and Cook[44] showed that the event rate predicted by the ASCVD prediction score systematically overestimated observed risks in external cohorts. Additionally, family history was not included as a part of the ASCVD pooled cohort equations, although it has been shown to be an important risk factor behind smoking and diabetes.[45] The guideline authors also state that even in their external validation in REGARDS and MESA, the pooled cohort equations overestimated 10-year ASCVD risk. The authors of the REGARDS study argue that the overestimation of risk in the REGARDS study may be owing to short follow-up periods, increased use of statin therapy and revascularization, and methodologic issues in identifying ASCVD events.[46,47] Although the REGARDS study is reported by the guideline authors to be confirmatory of the new risk prediction tool, the reliance on patient and family self-report of events, the generalizability of extrapolating 5-year data to 10-year event rates, and the reliance on the

Medicare claims database to be a surrogate for active surveillance limits the use and generalizability of this database.

In addition, a recent study evaluated several ASVD risk assessment models from the ACC/AHA and ATP III on a European cohort (Rotterdam study).[48] They found that all 3 models had poor calibration and all 3 models overestimated ASCVD risk in the Rotterdam cohort. Overall, the study demonstrates that the pooled cohort risk equations may not be generalizable to other populations.

Importance of Shared Decision Making and a Patient-Centered Approach

Ultimately, both guidelines point out that the decision to start statin therapy should be a shared decision between the patient and physician. As noted by Montori and colleagues,[49] the 10-year risk threshold of 7.5% is a value judgment and that the use of shared decision-making tools may help to translate the guidelines into practice.

It is important to recognize that clinical practice guidelines are a tool to help guide a physician in making decisions for his or her patients. They should not be followed uncritically or blindly. A patient-centered approach should be used when applying guidelines. Of note, the 2013 ACC/AHA guideline provided an important paradigm shift by looking at ASCVD risk and focusing in on "statin benefit" groups. They have simplified greatly clinical practice by just focusing clinicians on statin dose and statin intensity. Their focus on starting higher dose statins may seem appropriate based on the lack of statin titration by health care providers. However, the assumption that side effects would be similar with high-intensity versus moderate-intensity statins is not borne out by observational or clinical studies.[22,50,51] Patients enrolled in statin trials tend to be healthier generally than the general population and those with previous side effects to statin therapy, such as those with myalgia, are generally not included in RCTs. The clinical reality for practicing providers is that many patients cannot tolerate a high-intensity statin as initial therapy or need to be titrated slowly based on age or frailty. As in many disease states, titration of therapy to maximally tolerated doses should be an important alternative.

Lipid Targets and Low-Density Lipoprotein Cholesterol Monitoring

The abandonment of target lipid goals takes away an important clinical and motivational tool that providers can use with their patients. Goal setting is an important behavioral tool that providers have used successfully in many disease states, including lifestyle counseling, blood pressure control, and diabetes management. Finally, by indirectly deemphasizing frequent LDL-C monitoring, a major concern is that this might have a significant adverse effect on adherence to lipid-lowering therapy. The recent move by 2015 National Committee for Quality Assurance (NCQA) Healthcare Effectiveness Data and Information Set (HEDIS) to remove baseline LDL-C levels and LDL-C monitoring in patients with CHD or diabetes mellitus, along with similar moves by the ACC/AHA Taskforce on Lipid Performance Measurement, may have unanticipated effects. Such adverse effects include a possible drop in statin adherence and the loss of an important quality indicator, in monitoring the change in a population's LDL-C levels.[52,53]

The NLA provides some alternative perspectives based on evidence that (1) there is utility in treating to LDL-C and non–HDL-C targets; (2) non–HDL-C is a better overall predictor of ASCVD risk than LDL-C both before and on statin therapy; (3) titration of statin therapy may be desirable in certain patient groups, such as those with statin intolerance or those who are frail, elderly, or have significant comorbidities; (4) clinicians and patients may benefit by setting specific lipid goals of therapy based on principles of shared decision making and evidence from behavioral medicine; and (5) frequent lipid monitoring is encouraged to identify patient barriers to statin adherence, encourage patient–provider communication, reward patients for positive changes in compliance to lifestyle and drug therapy, ensure adequate patient response to therapy, and treat lipid-related residual risk. In light of the recent IMPROVE-IT trial, combination nonstatin therapy should be considered in patients not reaching their LDL-C and non–HDL-C goals and the emphasis should be placed back on lipids and not just statin benefit groups.

The Way Forward

Overall, both sets of guidelines complement each other and try to move the needle forward in ASCVD prevention. Given the stakes involved and the growing burden of ASCVD in the United States, it is even more important that all stakeholders including large medical subspecialty organizations (ACC, AHA, NLA, American Diabetes Association, American Association of Clinical Endocrinologists) government and regulatory agencies (Centers for Medicare and Medicaid Services, Medicare, Medicaid, Veteran's Administration, Centers for Disease Control and Prevention), private insurers, primary care (American Academy of Family Physicians, American College of Physicians) and medical subspecialty groups, allied health professionals (nursing, nurse practitioners, pharmacists, dieticians, physician assistants, health educators, public health workers, exercise physiologists, etc), and the general public (consumers, patients, patient advocacy groups) come together to better understand guideline commonalities and remain united in working together to implement the necessary clinical and public health measures needed to reduce ASCVD. Although one can debate the evidence base, disagree on the importance of clinical or expert judgment, or make different decisions based on different biases, preferences, or values, a guideline at its best must be acceptable to major stakeholders and implementable to be effective. An inclusive and transparent process among various stakeholders will ensure broad guideline endorsement, uptake, and adoption. Now is the time for all stakeholders to work together to devise an improved and actionable plan that will center the focus back to the prevention of the leading cause of death and disability in the United States from the ravages of ASCVD.

REFERENCES

1. Stone NJ, Robinson JG, Lichtenstein AH, et al. 2013 ACC/AHA guideline on the treatment of blood cholesterol to reduce atherosclerotic cardiovascular risk in adults: a report of the American College of Cardiology/American Heart Association task force on practice guidelines. Circulation 2014;129(25 Suppl 2):S1–45.
2. Jacobson TA, Ito MK, Maki KC, et al. National Lipid Association recommendations for patient-centered management of dyslipidemia: part 1-executive summary. J Clin Lipidol 2014;8(5):473–88.
3. Go AS, Mozaffarian D, Roger VL, et al. Heart disease and stroke statistics–2014 update: a report from the American Heart Association. Circulation 2014;129(3):e28–292.
4. Grundy SM, Cleeman JI, Merz CN, et al. Implications of recent clinical trials for the national cholesterol education program Adult Treatment Panel III guidelines. Circulation 2004;110(2):227–39.
5. National Cholesterol Education Program Expert Panel on Detection E. Treatment of high blood cholesterol in A. Third report of the National Cholesterol Education Program (NCEP) Expert Panel on Detection, Evaluation, and Treatment of High

Blood Cholesterol in Adults (Adult Treatment Panel III) final report. Circulation 2002;106(25):3143–421.

6. Ridker PM, Danielson E, Fonseca FA, et al. Rosuvastatin to prevent vascular events in men and women with elevated C-reactive protein. N Engl J Med 2008;359(21):2195–207.

7. Downs JR, Clearfield M, Weis S, et al. Primary prevention of acute coronary events with lovastatin in men and women with average cholesterol levels: results of AFCAPS/TexCAPS. Air force/Texas Coronary Atherosclerosis Prevention Study. JAMA 1998;279(20):1615–22.

8. Nakamura H, Arakawa K, Itakura H, et al. Primary prevention of cardiovascular disease with pravastatin in Japan (MEGA Study): a prospective randomised controlled trial. Lancet 2006;368(9542):1155–63.

9. Expert Panel on Detection E. Treatment of high blood cholesterol in a. Executive summary of the third report of the national cholesterol education program (NCEP) expert panel on detection, evaluation, and treatment of high blood cholesterol in adults (Adult Treatment Panel III). JAMA 2001;285(19):2486–97.

10. Association AH. 2013 Prevention guidelines tools. CV risk calculator. 2013. Available at: http://my.americanheart.org/cvriskcalculator. Accessed January 19, 2015.

11. Bulugahapitiya U, Siyambalapitiya S, Sithole J, et al. Is diabetes a coronary risk equivalent? systematic review and meta-analysis. Diabet Med 2009;26(2):142–8.

12. Bild DE, Bluemke DA, Burke GL, et al. Multi-Ethnic Study of Atherosclerosis: objectives and design. Am J Epidemiol 2002;156(9):871–81.

13. Howard VJ, Cushman M, Pulley L, et al. The Reasons for Geographic And Racial Differences in Stroke Study: objectives and design. Neuroepidemiology 2005; 25(3):135–43.

14. Robinson JG, Wang S, Smith BJ, et al. Meta-analysis of the relationship between non-high-density lipoprotein cholesterol reduction and coronary heart disease risk. J Am Coll Cardiol 2009;53(4):316–22.

15. Boekholdt SM, Arsenault BJ, Mora S, et al. Association of LDL cholesterol, non-HDL cholesterol, and apolipoprotein B levels with risk of cardiovascular events among patients treated with statins: a meta-analysis. JAMA 2012;307(12):1302–9.

16. Robinson JG. Are you targeting non-high-density lipoprotein cholesterol? J Am Coll Cardiol 2009;55(1):42–4.

17. Harper CR, Jacobson TA. Using apolipoprotein B to manage dyslipidemic patients: time for a change? Mayo Clin Proc 2010;85(5):440–5.

18. Robinson JG, Wang S, Jacobson TA. Meta-analysis of comparison of effectiveness of lowering apolipoprotein B versus low-density lipoprotein cholesterol and nonhigh-density lipoprotein cholesterol for cardiovascular risk reduction in randomized trials. Am J Cardiol 2012;110(10):1468–76.

19. Abd TT, Jacobson TA. Statin-induced myopathy: a review and update. Expert Opin Drug Saf 2011;10(3):373–87.

20. Toth PP, Thanassoulis G, Williams K, et al. The risk-benefit paradigm vs the causal exposure paradigm: LDL as a primary cause of vascular disease. J Clin Lipidol 2014;8(6):594–605.

21. Harper CR, Jacobson TA. Avoiding statin myopathy: understanding key drug interactions. Clin Lipidol 2011;6(6):665–74.

22. Rosenson RS, Baker SK, Jacobson TA, et al. An assessment by the statin muscle safety task force: 2014 update. J Clin Lipidol 2014;8(Suppl 3):S58–71.

23. Guyton JR, Bays HE, Grundy SM, et al. An assessment by the statin intolerance panel: 2014 update. J Clin Lipidol 2014;8(Suppl 3):S72–81.

24. Cohen JD, Brinton EA, Ito MK, et al. Understanding statin use in America and gaps in patient education (USAGE): an internet-based survey of 10,138 current and former statin users. J Clin Lipidol 2012;6(3):208–15.
25. Rojas-Fernandez CH, Goldstein LB, Levey AI, et al. An assessment by the statin cognitive safety task force: 2014 update. J Clin Lipidol 2014;8(Suppl 3):S5–16.
26. Morris PB, Ballantyne CM, Birtcher KK, et al. Review of clinical practice guidelines for the management of LDL-related risk. J Am Coll Cardiol 2014;64(2):196–206.
27. Jacobson TA, Gutkin SW, Harper CR. Effects of a global risk educational tool on primary coronary prevention: the atherosclerosis assessment via total risk (AVIA-TOR) study. Curr Med Res Opin 2006;22(6):1065–73.
28. Sheridan SL, Viera AJ, Krantz MJ, et al. The effect of giving global coronary risk information to adults: a systematic review. Arch Intern Med 2010;170(3):230–9.
29. Shillinglaw B, Viera AJ, Edwards T, et al. Use of global coronary heart disease risk assessment in practice: a cross-sectional survey of a sample of U.S. physicians. BMC Health Serv Res 2012;12:20.
30. LaRosa JC, Grundy SM, Waters DD, et al. Intensive lipid lowering with atorvastatin in patients with stable coronary disease. N Engl J Med 2005;352(14):1425–35.
31. AIM-HIGH Investigators, Boden WE, Probstfield JL, et al. Niacin in patients with low HDL cholesterol levels receiving intensive statin therapy. N Engl J Med 2011;365(24):2255–67.
32. The HPS2-THRIVE Collaborative Group, Landray MJ, Haynes R, et al. Effects of extended-release niacin with laropiprant in high-risk patients. N Engl J Med 2014; 371(3):203–12.
33. Ginsberg HN, Reyes-Soffer G. Niacin: a long history, but a questionable future. Curr Opin Lipidol 2013;24(6):475–9.
34. The ACCORD Study Group, Ginsberg HN, Elam MB, et al. Effects of combination lipid therapy in type 2 diabetes mellitus. N Engl J Med 2010;362(17):1563–74.
35. Canner PL, Berge KG, Wenger NK, et al. Fifteen year mortality in coronary drug project patients: long-term benefit with niacin. J Am Coll Cardiol 1986;8(6): 1245–55.
36. Buchwald H. Risk reduction and the program on the surgical control of the hyperlipidemias. Circulation 2001;104(9):E47.
37. The lipid research clinics coronary primary prevention trial results. II. The relationship of reduction in incidence of coronary heart disease to cholesterol lowering. JAMA 1984;251(3):365–74.
38. The lipid research clinics coronary primary prevention trial results. I. Reduction in incidence of coronary heart disease. JAMA 1984;251(3):351–64.
39. Kohno T. Report of the American Heart Association (AHA) scientific sessions 2014, Chicago. Circ J 2015;79:34–40.
40. Cholesterol Treatment Trialists' (CTT) Collaboration, Baigent C, Blackwell L, et al. Efficacy and safety of more intensive lowering of LDL cholesterol: a meta-analysis of data from 170,000 participants in 26 randomised trials. Lancet 2010; 376(9753):1670–81.
41. Mihaylova B, Emberson J, Blackwell L, et al. The effects of lowering LDL cholesterol with statin therapy in people at low risk of vascular disease: meta-analysis of individual data from 27 randomised trials. Lancet 2012;380(9841):581–90.
42. Rogers JK, Jhund PS, Perez AC, et al. Effect of rosuvastatin on repeat heart failure hospitalizations: the CORONA trial (Controlled Rosuvastatin Multinational Trial in Heart Failure). JACC Heart Fail 2014;2(3):289–97.
43. Fellstrom BC, Jardine AG, Schmieder RE, et al. Rosuvastatin and cardiovascular events in patients undergoing hemodialysis. N Engl J Med 2009;360(14):1395–407.

44. Ridker PM, Cook NR. Statins: new American guidelines for prevention of cardio-vascular disease. Lancet 2013;382(9907):1762–5.
45. Qureshi N, Armstrong S, Dhiman P, et al. Effect of adding systematic family history enquiry to cardiovascular disease risk assessment in primary care: a matched-pair, cluster randomized trial. Ann Intern Med 2012;156(4):253–62.
46. Muntner P, Safford MM, Cushman M, et al. Comment on the reports of over-estimation of ASCVD risk using the 2013 AHA/ACC risk equation. Circulation 2014;129(2):266–7.
47. Cook NR, Ridker PM. Response to comment on the reports of over-estimation of ASCVD risk using the 2013 AHA/ACC risk equation. Circulation 2014;129(2):268–9.
48. Kavousi M, Leening MJ, Nanchen D, et al. Comparison of application of the ACC/AHA guidelines, Adult Treatment Panel III guidelines, and European Society of Cardiology guidelines for cardiovascular disease prevention in a European cohort. JAMA 2014;311(14):1416–23.
49. Montori VM, Brito JP, Ting HH. Patient-centered and practical application of new high cholesterol guidelines to prevent cardiovascular disease. JAMA 2014;311(5):465–6.
50. Bruckert E, Hayem G, Dejager S, et al. Mild to moderate muscular symptoms with high-dosage statin therapy in hyperlipidemic patients–the PRIMO study. Cardiovasc Drugs Ther 2005;19(6):403–14.
51. Jacobson TA. Statin safety: lessons from new drug applications for marketed statins. Am J Cardiol 2006;97(8A):44C–51C.
52. NCQA updates HEDIS Quality Measure. Available at: http://www.ncqa.org/Newsroom/NewsArchive/2014NewsArchive/NewsReleaseJuly12014.aspx. Accessed January 19, 2015.
53. Drozda JJ, Ferguson TB Jr, Jneid H, et al. 2014 ACC/AHA update of secondary prevention lipid measures: a report of the American College of Cardiology/American Heart Association Task Force on Performance Measures. J Am Coll Cardiol, in press.

Management of Hypertriglyceridemia for Prevention of Atherosclerotic Cardiovascular Disease

Eliot A. Brinton, MD, FAHA, FNLA

KEYWORDS

• Hypertriglyceridemia • Atherosclerosis • Cardiovascular disease • Triglycerides

KEY POINTS

- Mendelian randomization data strongly suggest that hypertriglyceridemia (HTG) causes atherosclerotic cardiovascular disease (ASCVD), and so triglyceride (TG) level–lowering treatment in HTG is now more strongly recommended to address the residual ASCVD risk than has been the case in (generally earlier) published guidelines.
- Fibrates are the best-established agents for TG level lowering and are generally used as first-line treatment of TG levels greater than 500 mg/dL.
- In addition to better ASCVD evidence, potential advantages of omega-3 compared with fenofibrate include that it is a natural product, it lacks any associated myopathy, and it might provide antiinflammatory, mood, cognitive, or other benefits.
- Statins are the best-established agents for ASCVD prevention, and so are usually used as first-line treatment of TG levels less than 500 mg/dL.

EPIDEMIOLOGY AND PATHOPHYSIOLOGY OF HYPERTRIGLYCERIDEMIA

About 40 million US adults have hypertriglyceridemia (HTG), defined as a fasting triglyceride (TG) level more than 200 mg/dL. Of these, about 36 million have a TG level of 200 to 500 mg/dL and about 4 million have a TG level greater than 500 mg/dL.[1] Thus, moderate HTG is common, and very high TG level (>500 mg/dL) is more common than numerically similar cholesterol level increases. Further, the prevalence of HTG has increased several-fold over the past few decades.[2,3] This increase is coincident with, and most likely largely driven by, increasing obesity.[4] Although there is

This article originally appeared in Cardiology Clinics, Volume 33, Issue 2, May 2015.
Atherometabolic Research, Utah Foundation for Biomedical Research, 419 Wakara Way, Suite 211, Salt Lake City, UT 84108, USA
E-mail address: eliot.brinton@utah.edu

Clinics Collections 5 (2015) 237–256
http://dx.doi.org/10.1016/j.ccol.2015.05.014
2352-7986/15/$ – see front matter © 2015 Elsevier Inc. All rights reserved.

some controversy regarding categorization of HTG, most categories have a reasonable consensus, as noted in **Table 1**.

Increase of plasma TG level is related to an excess of one or more of the 3 main types of TG-rich lipoproteins: (1) chylomicrons, (2) very-low-density lipoprotein (VLDL), or (3) intermediate-density lipoprotein (IDL). In the case of chylomicronemia, TG levels usually exceed about 800 mg/dL and may be 10,000 mg/dL or higher.[5] The underlying cause is decreased lipolysis of TG in plasma caused by decreased (or absent) activity of lipoprotein lipase (LPL) in the vascular endothelium. Decreased TG lipolysis also tends to increase the TG content of VLDL and all other TG-rich lipoproteins, but decreased lipolysis has the greatest effect on chylomicrons because they have the greatest TG content. Because the TG/cholesterol ratio in chylomicrons is generally about 10:1, the plasma TG level is usually close to 10-fold higher than the plasma cholesterol level. Nevertheless, the total cholesterol level can far exceed 200 mg/dL in severe chylomicronemia, and so clinicians must always remember to look for severe HTG as a possible hidden cause of hypercholesterolemia.[6] Familial chylomicronemia classically is caused by homozygous deficiency of LPL but is more commonly caused by a combination of other genetic factors, such as absence or severe functional defects in the function of LPL-related factors, such as apolipoproteins C-II, C-III, and V; lipase maturation factor-1; and angiopoietinlike proteins 3, 4, and 8.[5,7] Environmental factors such as central obesity, insulin resistance, and diabetes mellitus can also play important contributory roles in decreasing LPL activity sufficient to cause chylomicronemia, with or without identifiable genetic abnormalities.[5]

In increased VLDL levels, by far the most common type of moderate HTG, the primary cause seems to be hepatic overproduction of VLDL. Two terms for increased VLDL levels are found in the scientific literature but do not seem to be clinically useful. Familial combined hyperlipoproteinemia (FCHL) is a term that has been used for moderate HTG presenting with or without increased cholesterol levels (or even as high cholesterol with normal TG), depending on environmental factors.[8] Familial HTG (FHTG) has been said always to present without hypercholesterolemia and to carry no increased risk of atherosclerotic cardiovascular disease (ASCVD),[9] whereas FCHL was said to increase ASCVD considerably.[8] However, subsequent research has not clearly sustained the original proposed distinctions between FCHL and

Table 1
Categorization of HTG

TG Range (mg/dL)	NCEP ATP-III 2004[1]	AHA Statement 2011[2]	Disease Risk	FDA Approval
<100	Desirable	Optimal	None	No apparent interest
<150		Normal	Dyslipidemia	
150–199	Borderline high	Borderline	More dyslipidemia	
200–499	High	High	↑CVD	Approve if ↓CVD likely
≥500	Very high	Very high	↑CVD and ↑pancreatitis (especially ↑if >2000 mg/dL)	Approve if reasonable safety

Abbreviations: AHA, American Heart Association; CVD, cardiovascular disease; FDA, US Food and Drug Administration; NCEP ATP-III, Third Adult Treatment Panel of the National Cholesterol Education Program.

FHTG, so there is little clinical impetus at present for distinguishing between them. A family history of ASCVD and the presence of hypercholesterolemia added to hypertriglyceridemia increase ASCVD risk, but pure HTG also carries excess risk, even in the absence of a clearly positive family history. Thus, efforts to make the distinction between FCHL and FHTG are probably not clinically beneficial, and treatment should instead be directed according to lipid levels and other standard risk factors.

Increased IDL levels seem to be caused primarily by reduced hepatic clearance of IDL particles caused by impaired binding to the apolipoprotein (apo) B/E receptor. Although IDL levels should be increased with any loss of apo B/E receptor activity, such as familial hypercholesterolemia (which primarily involves decreased low-density lipoprotein [LDL] clearance), in some cases IDL clearance is selectively impaired. This condition is familial dysbetalipoproteinemia (sometimes referred to as type III disease), which is well documented to carry a high risk of ASCVD, beyond that expected from the moderately increased plasma TG levels.[10] It has been thought that dysbetalipoproteinemia is rare, occurring in only 1 in 10,000 in the general population and it has also been thought to require apo E2 homozygosity plus another, as yet unspecified metabolic defect.[10] However, recent studies have shown that apo E2 homozygosity is present only in a small minority of cases and that familial dysbetalipoproteinemia may affect as many as 1 in 200 of the general population.[11,12] However, it is difficult to diagnose dysbetalipoproteinemia. Suspicion of the existence of this disorder should be increased in the presence of roughly equally increased TG and TG levels, both within the range of 150 to 500 mg/dL, in an adult man or postmenopausal woman (uncommon in other demographics), especially if an ASCVD event has already occurred. Presence of palmar xanthomas (orange-yellow color in the palmar creases) is pathognomonic but often absent. The diagnoses can be made by one of several special tests: (1) confirming VLDL cholesterol (VLDL-C) enrichment (documented as a VLDL-C/plasma TG ratio >0.3 by beta-quantification), (2) a broad beta band on lipoprotein electrophoresis, (3) increased IDL levels by density gradient ultracentrifugation or nuclear magnetic resonance, or (4) an increased remnant lipoprotein cholesterol level by direct assay.[11,12]

HYPERTRIGLYCERIDEMIA VERSUS ATHEROSCLEROTIC CARDIOVASCULAR DISEASE: ASSOCIATION AND POTENTIAL CAUSATION

Atherosclerosis is characterized by an accumulation of cholesterol in the artery wall, whereas TG does not accumulate. Further, the relationship between HTG and ASCVD is greatly diminished, and in some settings eliminated, by adjustment for other dyslipidemias (especially low high-density lipoprotein cholesterol [HDL-C] level and increased non–HDL-C level).[13] These two facts are often taken to imply that there is no meaningful causal association between HTG and ASCVD and that patients with HTG need no special consideration in management of ASCVD risk. However, results from many recent studies contain many types of data pointing to a strong and likely causal association. In general populations, TG levels are strong predictors of ASCVD risk. For example, one study found a 32% and 76% increased risk of cardiovascular disease (CVD) in men and women, respectively, for each 88-mg/dL increase in TG independent of HDL-C levels.[14] A large meta-analysis of 29 studies with 262,525 subjects found that HTG related to a 72% increase in CVD risk, even after correction for HDL-C.[15] Further, a more recent and even larger meta-analysis (330,566 subjects in 61 studies) reported a 22% increase in ASCVD for every 88-mg/dL increase in TG.[16] Other data show a curvilinear increase in risk across a range of TG level increases, above a TG level of 200 mg/dL and becoming especially pronounced above 500 mg/dL (**Fig. 1**).[10] Of greater clinical relevance, HTG predicts residual ASCVD

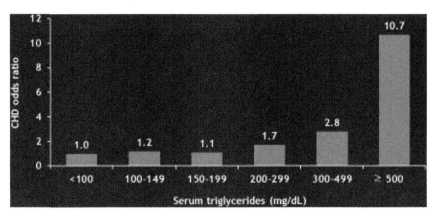

Fig. 1. Coronary heart disease (CHD) risk is greatly increased with TG levels greater than or equal to 500 mg/dL. TG is associated with premature familiar CHD independent of HDL-C. TG odds ratio adjusted for HDL-C; n = 653. N = 1029 controls. (*Adapted from* Hopkins PN, Wu LL, Hunt SC, et al. Plasma triglycerides and type III hyperlipidemia are independently associated with premature familial coronary artery disease. J Am Coll Cardiol 2005;45(7):1003–12; with permission.)

risk in the setting of aggressive statin-based low-density lipoprotein cholesterol (LDL-C) level lowering,[17–19] even with just mild HTG (>150 mg/dL) and even after aggressive statin therapy achieving an LDL-C level of less than 70 mg/dL (**Fig. 2**).[18]

Mechanisms of Accelerated Atherogenesis in Hypertriglyceridemia

First, and most directly, LPL expression by arterial endothelium and artery wall macrophages lipolyze TG from TG-rich lipoproteins, producing free-fatty-acids (FFAs) both on the surface and inside the artery wall. These are proinflammatory,

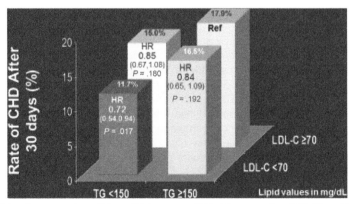

Fig. 2. TG level greater than 150 mg/DL increases CHD risk even when LDL-C level is less than 70 mg/DL on a statin (Pravastatin or Atorvastatin Evaluation and Infection Therapy—Thrombolysis in Myocardial Infarction 22 [PROVE IT-TIMI 22] PROVE IT-TIMI 22 subanalysis). CHD = death, myocardial infarction, and recurrent acute coronary syndrome. HR, hazard ratio. (*Adapted from* Miller M, Cannon CP, Murphy SA, et al. Impact of triglyceride levels beyond low-density lipoprotein cholesterol after acute coronary syndrome in the PROVE IT-TIMI 22 trial. J Am Coll Cardiol 2008;51(7):724–30; with permission.)

proatherogenic, and procoagulant.[20] (see also Ref.[21]) Second, several types of TG-rich lipoproteins are directly atherogenic[22,23] and their presence in excess is most readily signaled by high plasma TG levels. These atherogenic TG-rich lipoproteins are generally called remnants because they have had their TG content reduced by lipolysis by LPL in the plasma compartment. In addition, they lose some TG and become cholesterol enriched by action of cholesteryl-ester transfer protein (CETP), as noted later. One proatherogenic effect of these remnants is that they cause senescence of endothelial precursor cells, which lose their ability to maintain vascular endothelial integrity.[24] Also, remnants stimulate a key early step in atherogenesis by promoting their uptake by artery wall macrophages, which then become foam cells.[25] The increased atherogenicity seen with remnants is thought to operate especially during the postprandial period (during which chylomicrons and also VLDL undergo rapid TG lipolysis), which is associated with increases in endothelial microparticles (which are atherogenic),[26] in inflammatory cytokines (also atherogenic),[27] and in apoptosis of artery wall cells (reflecting and possibly contributing to atherogenesis[28]; see also Ref.[21] for review). Importantly, the association of plasma apolipoprotein B48 levels (reflecting postprandial lipoproteins) with the presence of carotid plaque in diabetes mellitus type 2 (DM2),[29] and the strong and graded association between nonfasting TG levels and increasing ASCVD risk,[30] constitute epidemiologic data strongly supportive of the basic-science evidence for postprandial atherogenesis noted earlier.

In addition, apo C-III, which is associated with HTG by inhibiting LPL activity, also seems to be directly atherogenic by means of proinflammatory effects of activation of vascular endothelial binding to inflammatory cells,[31] and other mechanisms. (see Ref.[32] for review) Apo C-III production seems to be increased by hyperglycemia,[33] possibly explaining in part the increase in ASCVD risk in poorly controlled DM2.

The atherogenicity of lipoprotein remnants (which are rich in both TG and cholesterol) is most clearly seen in the classic disorder of remnant excess, best termed dysbetalipoproteinemia, in which both plasma TG and cholesterol levels are increased comparably, and the risk of ASCVD is very increased (see Ref.[12] for a recent review). Cholesterol enrichment of TG-rich lipoprotein remnants (and thus enhancement of their atherogenicity) also is promoted in most other HTG states, as noted later, although apparently to a lesser degree.

The Atherogenic Dyslipidemia

Another important mechanism linking HTG and ASCVD risk is the effect of HTG on lipoproteins beyond those rich in TG. Core-lipid exchange among major lipoproteins is facilitated by CETP, which moves TG from TG-rich lipoproteins (VLDL, chylomicrons, and chylomicron remnants) to TG-poor lipoproteins (principally LDL and high-density lipoprotein [HDL]). CETP also mediates movement of cholesteryl-ester (CE) in the opposite direction. Movement of CE promotes cholesterol enrichment of remnants, which, as discussed earlier, seems to account for much of their atherogenicity (**Fig. 3**).

The core-lipid exchange process leads to TG enrichment of LDL and HDL. Because of rapid subsequent lipolysis of TG from these lipoproteins, primarily by hepatic lipase, the net effect of this TG transfer is decreased size and increased density of LDL and HDL (see **Fig. 3**).[6,34] The presence of smaller, denser (SD) LDL particles is often accompanied by increased plasma levels of non–HDL-C and of apo B levels, but with average to low LDL-C levels. Counterintuitively, SD LDL particles seem to be more atherogenic per particle than normal-sized LDL, and an excess of SD LDL is associated with increased ASCVD risk.[35–38] The increased atherogenicity seems to result from several mechanisms: (1) increased transport into the subendothelial space (because of smaller size),[39,40] (2) increased binding to arterial proteoglycans (perhaps

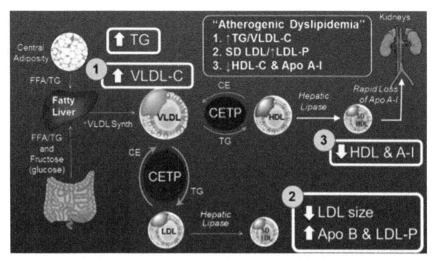

Fig. 3. Causes and atherogenic consequences of hypertriglyceridemia. Apo A-I, apolipoprotein A-I; Apo B, apolipoprotein B; CETP, cholesteryl-ster transfer protein; LDL-P, LDL particle concentration; SD, small, dense. (*Adapted from* Ginsberg HN. Insulin resistance and cardiovascular disease. J Clin Invest 2000;106(4):453–8.)

caused by decreased sialic acid content),[41] (3) increased susceptibility to oxidative modification (perhaps caused by decreased vitamin E content),[42] (4) prolonged plasma residence time caused by decreased affinity to the LDL receptor,[43] (5) increased glycation even in the absence of diabetes mellitus,[44] and (6) an increased tendency to carry atherogenic apoproteins (such as apo C-III).[45] Meanwhile, the presence of SD HDL particles is associated with accelerated renal clearance of apo A-I (lost from HDL as it shrinks) and lower apo A-I levels,[46,47] likely diminishing the overall antiatherogenic function of HDL (see **Fig. 3**).

These 3 HTG-related lipoprotein changes (cholesterol enrichment of TG lipoproteins, SD LDL/increased non–HDL-C and apo B level, and low HDL-C level), constitute the atherogenic dyslipidemia characteristic of most patients with HTG, and can occur even at mildly increased TG levels. Also, it tends to be more pronounced in DM2 and other insulin-resistant states. This dyslipidemia responds poorly to statins and predicts much of the residual ASCVD risk seen with statin monotherapy in patients with HTG, whether the HTG is related to metabolic syndrome[48] or DM2.[19]

Genetic Evidence for a Causal Role of Hypertriglyceridemia in Atherosclerotic Cardiovascular Disease

Concordant with the mechanisms discussed earlier linking HTG with increased atherosclerosis and ASCVD, mendelian randomization studies have recently provided strong evidence that the relationship between TG levels and ASCVD risk is causal. That is, several gene defects associated with moderate HTG are strongly associated with ASCVD.[49,50]

EFFECTS OF TRIGLYCERIDE LEVEL–LOWERING MEDICATIONS ON ATHEROSCLEROTIC CARDIOVASCULAR DISEASE EVENTS: RANDOMIZED CLINICAL TRIALS

Although nearly all medication classes indicated and used for dyslipidemia reduce plasma TG levels (with the notable exception of the bile-acid sequestrants), only fibrates, niacin, and omega-3 are considered to be TG level–lowering drugs. The degree and mechanisms of lipid effects of these agents are of clinical importance, but have been reviewed elsewhere for fibrates,[51] niacin,[52] and omega-3[53] and so are not discussed in this article. Instead, this article reviews a clinically more important issue: their overall risk/benefit ratio (primarily regarding evidence for their ability to reduce the risk of ASCVD events) and the application of those data with regard to priority for clinical use.

Although niacin and omega-3 are available as dietary supplements as well as by prescription, this article focuses on the prescription formulations. This focus is because only prescription products are specifically formulated, reviewed, and regulated for the treatment of disease, and also because randomized clinical trial (RCT) data regarding ASCVD events for these agents are available primarily for the prescription versions.

Randomized Clinical Trials of Fenofibrate

The most recent and most impactful fenofibrate trial is the Action to Control Cardiovascular Risk in Diabetes (ACCORD) trial of cardiovascular disease (ASCVD) effects of intensive glucose level–lowering treatment in patients with DM2, which included a major substudy called ACCORD-Lipid, which was recruited primarily for patients lacking extreme lipid levels.[54] All patients in ACCORD-Lipid were treated with open-label simvastatin then randomized to receive fenofibrate or matching placebo, on which they were followed for several years for ASCVD incidence. There was a modest trend toward an 8% decrease in ASCVD events with fenofibrate but this was far from being statistically significant.[54] However, there was an ASCVD benefit (statistically significant with an interaction P value of .0567) in a prespecified subanalysis of subjects with both HTG (TG level >204 mg/dL) and low HDL-C level (<34 mg/dL) at baseline.[54,55] These same patients had substantially higher ASCVD risk than the others, compared within the placebo arm.[54,55] Thus, although ACCORD-Lipid had only a modest trend to benefit overall, it showed significant ASCVD risk reduction with fenofibrate in patients with the usual lipid indications for that agent. Further, the tolerability and safety of fenofibrate with a statin was excellent and there was no increase in myopathy or reported muscle symptoms,[54] despite a current US Food and Drug Administration (FDA) label warning against increased myopathy risk when fenofibrate is used with statins.

In addition to this finding in ACCORD-Lipid, other major RCTs of fibrates have shown a similar pattern of greater ASCVD benefit in patients with HTG and low HDL-C levels. The primary example is the Fenofibrate Intervention and Event Lowering in Diabetes (FIELD) trial, the only other major trial of fenofibrate effects on ASCVD.[56] As in ACCORD-Lipid, all patients had DM2 and there was little selection for dyslipidemia at baseline. All patients were randomized to receive fenofibrate or matching placebo, but in this study (conducted much sooner after initial availability of statins than was ACCORD) statins were not offered as a part of the study protocol. Nevertheless, statin drop-in therapy occurred, imbalanced in that 17% of placebo-treated subjects but only 8% of fenofibrate-treated subjects (P<.0001) received this incidental statin use, presumably because the primary care physicians were not blinded to lipid levels during the average 5-year study duration. Similar to ACCORD, there was a nonsignificant 11% trend toward decreased ASCVD among all fenofibrate-treated versus placebo-treated subjects.[56] In addition, similar to ACCORD-Lipid, in patients with HTG and low HDL-C levels there was both a much higher ASCVD risk, untreated, and also a statistically significant decrease in ASCVD with fenofibrate (which erased the excess risk).[57]

Note that this greater ASCVD benefit with fenofibrate in patients with HTG/low HDL-C levels has also been seen in the other major ASCVD trials with fibrates (bezafibrate and gemfibrozil).[58] Thus, fibrates in general and fenofibrate in particular seem to decrease risk of ASCVD events in patients with HTG, especially if they have the usual concomitant low HDL-C levels.

Randomized Clinical Trials of Omega-3

Several recent RCTs of prescription ethyl ester omega-3 oil have focused on ASCVD effects, but they used different doses of different agents and found divergent results. The more recent trials used either a prescription formulation of an 85% pure mixture of eicosapentaenoic acid (EPA) with docosahexaenoic acid (DHA), or a comparable nonprescription formulation. One of these was the Risk and Prevention Trial, in which 12,505 subjects were selected for high risk for ASCVD (visible coronary artery disease and/or multiple risk factors) but not selected for HTG or low HDL-C level.[59] The intervention was low-dose (1 g/d) prescription EPA plus DHA (vs 1 g/d olive oil placebo) and there was no ASCVD benefit. Data from dyslipidemic subgroups were not reported.

A similar recent omega-3 trial was Outcome Reduction with Initial Glargine Intervention (ORIGIN), in which 12,536 patients considered to have prediabetes or recent-onset diabetes were randomized to receive the same low dose (1 g/d) of the same prescription EPA plus DHA fish oil as in the Risk and Prevention Trial versus placebo (along with insulin vs control in a 2 × 2 factorial design).[60] No decrease in ASCVD was noted with omega-3 (and no effect of insulin, or interaction between them) but again subjects were not selected for HTG or other dyslipidemia, and dyslipidemic subgroups were not reported.[60] Surprisingly, both the Risk and Prevention Trial and ORIGIN tended to show decreases in TG levels, despite only using very low doses of EPA plus DHA in patients without HTG. The primary focus of these studies and their most robust finding was the lack of ASCVD benefit from low-dose prescription EPA plus DHA.

Another, smaller RCT of omega-3 treatment (N = 4203) focused primarily on prevention of retinal disease but also tracked ASCVD events. It used a nonprescription formulation of EPA plus DHA similar to that used in the ORIGIN and Risk and Prevention Trial and at a comparable dose (in a 2 × 2 factorial design with xanthophylls), and also found no ASCVD benefit.[61]

The earliest of the contemporary ASCVD end point trials of omega-3 was the Japan EPA Lipid Intervention Study (JELIS).[62] In contrast with the others, JELIS studied a higher total dose (1.8 g/d) of omega-3 and used a pure EPA product (icosapent ethyl), such that the EPA dose was 3-fold to 4-fold higher than that of the other recent omega-3 RCTs. More than 18,000 Japanese study subjects were selected for either having had a prior ASCVD event (about one-fifth of subjects) or for having multiple risk factors but no prior event. They were further selected for a total cholesterol level more than 250 mg/dL. During a run-in period, all subjects were given a statin (doses per usual Japanese protocol) to bring their LDL-C levels within Japanese guidelines, with dose uptitration as needed.[62] The baseline LDL-C level of 182 mg/dL was reduced about 25% and subjects were then randomized to the study drug or control arm in an open-label fashion, again as per usual Japanese protocol. All end point adjudication and evaluations were blinded,[62] so the validity of the results of this prospective, open-label, blinded end point evaluation trial is considered roughly comparable with that of a standard double-blind trial. The baseline TG level of about 150 mg/dL was reduced by just 9% with EPA versus about a 3% decrease in the control, and there were no further changes in LDL-C or HDL-C levels. Despite these modest lipid effects, there was a statistically significant 19% reduction in ASCVD events, comparable in both primary and secondary prevention patients.[62] Importantly, safety and tolerability were excellent such that the risk/benefit ratio was favorable. Thus, icosapent ethyl in JELIS was the first agent to show clear RCT evidence of ASCVD benefit as a nonstatin added to a statin, despite current dogma that ezetimibe in the Improved Reduction of Outcomes: Vytorin Efficacy International Trial (IMPROVE-IT) was the first to do so.[63] Further, note that a prespecified subanalysis of 957 subjects in JELIS with HTG levels (>150 mg/dL) and low HDL-C levels (<40 mg/dL) at baseline showed a 53% decrease in ASCVD events versus control.[64] Thus, it seems that intermediate doses of a pure EPA omega-3 can reduce ASCVD when added to statin therapy, especially if the usual lipid indications (mainly HTG) are present.

Randomized Clinical Trials of Niacin

Many RCTs have shown decreased ASCVD with niacin but niacin was generally studied in monotherapy and not separately as a statin adjunct.[65] Two recent RCTs have now suggested that niacin may not reduce ASCVD when added to a statin; however, important design problems and some positive subgroup results make this conclusion tenuous. The first recent RCT with niacin was Atherothrombosis Intervention in Metabolic Syndrome with Low HDL/High Triglycerides: Impact on Global Health Outcomes (AIM-HIGH).[66] Despite appearances to the contrary, AIM-HIGH was not a valid test of the effects of niacin on ASCVD. First, the greater LDL-C level lowering with niacin was largely counterbalanced by greater uptitration of statin dose and increased frequency of ezetimibe use in the control arm. Further, in order to maintain the study blind despite the expected frequent flushing in the treatment arm, the control arm was given low-dose niacin in every placebo tablet, further reducing lipid differences between study arms.[66] Thus, AIM-HIGH was an active comparator study of higher-dose (1500–2000 mg/d) extended-release nicotinic acid (ERNA) plus standard-dose statin and infrequent ezetimibe versus low-dose (100–150 mg/d) immediate-release nicotinic acid plus higher-dose statin and more frequent ezetimibe use.[66] The negative overall results presumably were caused at least in part by this diluted treatment comparison and there was little evidence for harm with high-dose ERNA.[66] Importantly, a post-hoc subanalysis of subjects in AIM-HIGH having both HTG and low HDL-C levels showed a statistically significant 26% reduction in the primary ASCVD end point.[67]

This subgroup finding in AIM-HIGH was not only comparable with that of the subanalyses of the several recent RCTs using fibrates and EPA outlined earlier, but it was also reminiscent of a subanalysis of the largest prior RCT of ASCVD effects of niacin, the Coronary Drug Project (CDP), originally published in 1975.[68] Subjects in CDP were assessed for the presence or absence of the metabolic syndrome, defined by slightly modified criteria because body mass index greater than 28 kg/m² had to substitute for a waist circumference greater than 100 cm (40 inches; all subjects were men and waist had not been measured), and HDL-C levels were available only in 492 of the 3906 subjects.[69] These patients with metabolic syndrome, most of whom had TG levels greater than 150 mg/dL, saw a 78% decrease in nonfatal myocardial infarction with niacin versus only a 24% decrease in patients without the metabolic syndrome.[69] Although the subgroup data in AIM-HIGH and the CDP individually are weak, they are strengthened by their consistency with each other, and also by consistency with subgroup findings in 5 fibrate RCTs and 1 omega-3 RCT (JELIS). Thus, HTG subgroups from a total of 8 RCTs of TG level lowering showed ASCVD benefit.

The most recent niacin RCT, Heart Protection Study 2–Treatment of HDL to Reduce the Incidence of Vascular Events (HPS2-THRIVE), involved 25,673 subjects with prior ASCVD, more than one-third having the metabolic syndrome and an overlapping one-third having DM2.[70] All patients received excellent lipid control with statin monotherapy before randomization, with mean levels of LDL-C, 63 mg/dL; TG, 125 mg/dL; and

HDL-C, 44 mg/dL. However, this meant that the RCT was conducted in patients generally lacking any lipid-related indication for niacin treatment. Another unfortunate design element was that niacin was always given with laropiprant, a prostaglandin blocker with unknown safety or ASCVD effects. The primary composite ASCVD end point was not reduced significantly in the overall study population and so niacin was considered to have been proved incapable of decreasing ASCVD (at least when added to a statin).[70] More than 3400 ASCVD events were included and median follow-up was 3.9 years, suggesting a definitive result. Further, an excess of incident DM2, bleeding, and infection was also seen with ERNA plus laropiprant.

However, several aspects of HPS2-THRIVE weaken the conclusion that niacin does not have a favorable risk/benefit ratio as a TG level–lowering medication in ASCVD prevention. First, among the 57% of subjects who were from Europe (virtually all of whom were white) there was a borderline statistically significant 9% decrease in ASCVD, whereas the 43% of subjects from China (all of eastern Asian descent) had a nonsignificant 2% increase (this result being of borderline significance even by the stringent interaction test).[70] Also of likely clinical importance, there was a strong and statistically significant effect of baseline lipids such that those with LDL-C level greater than 57 mg/dL (most of them) had significantly fewer ASCVD events. Although subjects with HTG and low HDL-C levels were reported not to have ASCVD benefit, the HTG cutoff used was only 150 mg/dL,[70] not the 200 mg/dL cutoff required to see benefit with ERNA plus statin in AIM-HIGH or with fenofibrate plus statin in ACCORD-Lipid. Of potential importance, the ASCVD effects were significantly different between whites and Asian people, being nearly significantly beneficial in the former. Also, the event curves appeared to spread toward greater niacin benefit as the study ended. In addition, with regard to safety, some of the adverse events, such as infection and bleeding, had not been seen in several decades of prior niacin RCTs,[65] or at least not to the degree noted in HPS2-THRIVE,[70] suggesting that they may have resulted from laropiprant. However, neither the adverse events nor the intriguing effects of baseline lipid on ASCVD benefit were reported by racial groups so that the risk/benefit ratio of ERNA plus laropiprant in the divergent white and Asian populations remains unexplored. Thus, although HPS2-THRIVE lessens the priority for niacin use in management of HTG, it leaves many critical questions unanswered, especially in light of the more positive niacin RCT results without laropiprant in patients with HTG.

Summary of Completed Randomized Clinical Trials of Triglyceride Level Lowering Versus Atherosclerotic Cardiovascular Disease

Thus, ASCVD reduction has been shown in several contemporary RCTs (and 1 older trial) of 3 classes of TG level–lowering drugs in patients who entered the studies with HTG and low HDL-C levels. Reliance on study subgroups is a major weakness, but this reliance is required mainly because of the consistent failure of clinical trialists to focus RCTs of TG level–lowering medications on patients who need TG lowering. The 2013 American College of Cardiology (ACC)/American Heart Association (AHA) cholesterol guidelines state that "nonstatin therapies, as compared with statin therapy, do not provide acceptable ASCVD risk reduction benefits compared to their potential for adverse effects in the routine prevention of ASCVD"[71] and "[there are] no data supporting the routine use of nonstatin drugs combined with statin therapy to further reduce ASCVD events."[71] Nevertheless, a large RCT showed that icosapent ethyl can safely decrease ASCVD risk beyond that of statin monotherapy, even without selecting for HTG,[62] and 1 RCT each with fenofibrate (ACCORD-Lipid; Ginsberg, HN. *NEJM*, e-published March 14, 2010[54]) and ERNA[67] showed reduced ASCVD in patient subgroups with baseline HTG and low HDL-C levels. Thus, it is reasonable to strongly consider use of icosapent ethyl (and perhaps other prescription omega-3) and also to consider fenofibrate and/or ERNA as statin adjuncts (or possibly as statin alternates in statin intolerance) for ASCVD prevention in patients with HTG.

Ongoing Randomized Clinical Trials of Triglyceride Level Lowering Versus Atherosclerotic Cardiovascular Disease

Two RCTs of ASCVD effects of omega-3 treatment are now underway. The first is Reduction of Cardiovascular Events With EPA – Intervention Trial (REDUCE-IT, NCT01492361).[72] REDUCE-IT is studying icosapent ethyl, 2 g twice a day with meals, versus a matching mineral oil placebo with a composite of ASCVD events as the primary end point. It will involve about 8000 subjects selected for a prior cardiovascular event or otherwise at high ASCVD risk, and a plasma TG level of more than 150 mg/dL, and this is the first clinical end point RCT, with any agent, to use increased TG levels as a primary entry criterion. Recruitment is nearly complete, treatment will continue for about 4 to 6 years, and the trial is expected to be completed in about December 2017.[72]

The second omega-3 RCT is A Long-term Outcomes Study to Assess Statin Residual Risk Reduction with Epanova in High Cardiovascular Risk Patients with Hypertriglyceridemia (STRENGTH).[73] Epanova, the newly approved carboxylic acid formulation of EPA and DHA, will be given once daily without reference to meals (at an as-yet unstated dose) versus a matching corn oil placebo and with an ASCVD event composite as the primary end point. It plans to involve 13,000 subjects and, like REDUCE-IT, subjects will be selected for high ASCVD risk and HTG. Recruitment is just beginning, treatment is expected to continue for 3 to 5 years, and the trial is expected to be completed in about June 2019.[73]

TREATMENT RECOMMENDATIONS FOR HYPERTRIGLYCERIDEMIA
Current Guidelines for Management of Hypertriglyceridemia

In 2004, an update of the Third Adult Treatment Panel (ATP-III) of the National Cholesterol Education Program (NCEP) carefully reviewed the issue of HTG and reiterated prior advice that fibrates and niacin could be considered for use with or without statin therapy in patients with high TG and/or low HDL-C levels.[74] The National Heart, Lung and Blood Institute (NHLBI) subsequently sponsored a major effort to review new scientific data and to replace ATP-III. However, the range of evidence ordinarily considered in guideline writing was sharply curtailed to allow only a few RCTs of the highest quality, and the scope was limited to hypercholesterolemia. At the end of the 5-year review process, the NHLBI stated that the work would be published simply as an evidentiary review, to serve as the basis for a multiparty effort to create new lipid guidelines.[75] Instead of following this course, as recommended by the sponsor of the writing, the ACC and the AHA chose to publish the review rapidly, just a couple of months later, as a finished guideline,[76] without seeking any further substantive scientific input. Because the 2013 ACC/AHA guidelines focused only on cholesterol and did not review HTG or address its management, they referred physicians to the 2011 AHA statement on HTG management.[6] The 2011 AHA statement is useful as a comprehensive review of causes and dietary and lifestyle treatments of HTG. In sharp contrast with the 2004 ATP-III update, it does not focus on pharmacotherapy or even mention the possible use of TG level–lowering medications for ASCVD prevention with fasting TG levels less than 500 mg/dL. However, the European Atherosclerosis Society also published guidance on management of HTG,[77] just 3 weeks before the 2011 AHA statement. The European guidelines recommend continued consideration of TG level–lowering agents for TG levels remaining in the range of 200 to 500 mg/dL despite statin therapy, just as had the ATP-III update.[74] As noted earlier, the approach recommended by the Europeans seems justified in light of current RCT and mechanistic data.

Dosing of fenofibrate is complicated in that there are 6 different brand names and 8 different formulations currently available in the United States alone, each with its own unique dose (**Table 2**). This situation is further complicated because each of these is available in a one-third dose for renal insufficiency. However, aside from considerations of pill/capsule size, insurance formulary, and price and availability, they all seem to be clinically equivalent. One of these formulations is fenofibric acid, the active metabolite of fenofibrate, which has yet another (seventh) brand name. It is chemically distinct but clinically indistinguishable because impaired conversion from fenofibrate to fenofibric acid has never been described. The sole advantage of fenofibric acid offers is that its FDA label does not warn against concurrent statin use.

Dosing of prescription omega-3 is generally 4 g/d, best given as 2 g twice daily with meals, except the new FFA formulation, which has better bioavailability and so can be given without food and at 2 g/d (albeit with less efficacy). Compared with EPA, DHA can depress LDL-receptor activity[78] and increase LDL-C levels,[79] so icosapent ethyl, being DHA-free, probably has more favorable effects on LDL-C levels than other omega-3 preparations that contain DHA (the other prescription ethyl ester and FFA formulations, as well as all dietary supplements).

Dosing of ERNA is between 500 and 2000 mg per day, generally best tolerated at bedtime and with 325 mg of aspirin to reduce flushing. In patients with little or no flushing, immediate-release niacin can be tried, twice or 3 times daily up to 3 or 4 g/d. ERNA or sustained-release niacin should not be given more than once daily. Niacinamide, nicotinamide, and inositol hexaniacinate should be avoided because they have no lipid benefit.

Diet and Lifestyle Treatment of Hypertriglyceridemia

All of the guidelines and statements discussed earlier mention diet and lifestyle treatment, and HTG is the dyslipidemia most responsive to nonpharmacologic treatments. The 2011 AHA statement on TG provides an excellent review of this subject,[6] the main principles of which are summarized here and in **Table 3**:

1. Sugar intake should be restricted. Most sugars, especially fructose, stimulate hepatic synthesis of FFAs and thus FFA and TG accumulation in the liver. This

Table 2
Available fenofibrate doses

Regular Dose (mg/d)	Reduced Dose[a] (mg/d)	Brand Name
200	67[b]	Lofibra
160	54/50	Lofibra/Triglide
150	50	Lipofen
145	48	Tricor
135	45	Trilipix[c]
130	43	Antara
120	40	Fenoglide
90	30	Antara

See FDA-approved prescribing information for further details.
[a] Primarily for renal or geriatric patients.
[b] Also available at 134 mg.
[c] Fenofibric acid (see text).
Data from Fenofibrate Interchange. Available at: http://www.drugs.com/fenofibrate.html. Accessed January 5, 2015.

Table 3
Diet and lifestyle treatments for hypertriglyceridemia

Intervention	Useful in TG Range	Strength of Effect
↓Sugar intake (especially fructose)	Mainly <800 mg/dL	Moderate
↑Fiber intake	Mainly <800 mg/dL	Weak
↓Fat intake	Only >800 mg/dL	Strong
↑Physical activity	Any TG level	Moderate
Weight loss	Any TG level	Moderate
↓Ethanol intake	Any TG level	Weak to moderate

Adapted from Miller M, Stone NJ, Ballantyne C, et al. Triglycerides and cardiovascular disease: a scientific statement from the American Heart Association. Circulation 2011;123:2292–333.

accumulation drives VLDL production and increases plasma TG level in the mild to moderate range (~100–500 mg/dL). Fructose is prevalent in the Western diet, being about half the content of sucrose (white or brown sugar), of high-fructose corn syrup, and also of honey, and being more than half the content of the sugar in fruit juice and certain other sweeteners, like agave. Thus, restriction of sugar-sweetened beverages, other added sugars, and fruit juice (but not fruit) is usually helpful to reduce TG levels. Nonsugar carbohydrate (starch) has a weak TG level–raising effect, mainly if low in fiber, so restricting total carbohydrates may slightly reduce TG levels.

2. Increase dietary fiber intake. Fiber has a modest effect to blunt TG level increase with sugar and other carbohydrates.
3. Fat intake may need to be restricted. Dietary fat drives chylomicron production and restricting dietary fat is the most effective way to reduce TG levels of more than about 800 mg/dL. Saturated fats are slightly more likely to lead to HTG than unsaturated fats, but fatty fish has a paradoxic effect of lowering TG levels because of the several favorable effects of omega-3 oil on TG metabolism.
4. Physical activity should be increased. Increased exercise tends to reduce TG levels, likely because of increased muscle TG oxidation as a fuel source, improved glucose and insulin metabolism (including increased LPL activity/TG lipolysis), and decreased hepatic TG and FFA content.
5. Weight loss should be encouraged. Whether by decreasing total calories or increasing activity, negative caloric balance reduces TG levels, likely related to improvement in insulin resistance and decreased hepatic TG and FFA content.
6. Restriction of alcohol intake may be beneficial. Ethanol increases TG levels in many patients at any level of intake, and so a trial of decreased consumption is warranted for plasma TG levels of more than about 200 mg/dL in patients who consume more than about 2 servings per week. Tobacco and marijuana have minor TG level–raising effects that are generally not of clinical importance.

Treatment of Secondary Factors in Hypertriglyceridemia

The treatment of secondary factors that promote HTG is always worth consideration in the clinical management of HTG. They are well outlined in the 2011 AHA statement[6] and are summarized here and in **Table 4**:

1. Diabetes mellitus should be prevented or controlled. DM2 and diabetes mellitus type 1 (DM1) contribute to HTG via hyperglycemia and insulin resistance (in the

Table 4
Secondary causes of hypertriglyceridemia to treat to reduce TG levels

Cause	Comment
Hyperglycemia	Control glucose/prevent DM if possible, reduce insulin resistance
Insulin resistance	↓Calories and adiposity, ↑exercise, consider insulin sensitizer medications
Hypothyroidism	Screen and treat if present
Proteinuria and renal insufficiency	Screen and treat if possible
Endogenous hypercortisolism	Consider screening, treat if present
Medications	Reduce dose or discontinue if clinically appropriate
Oral contraceptives	Variable effect
Oral estrogen replacement	Variable effect
Retinoic acid derivatives	Large effect
Systemic glucocorticoids	Large effect
Certain antiretroviral medications	Large effect
Certain antipsychotic medications	Modest effect
Most β-blockers	Weak effect
Thiazide diuretics	Weak effect

Abbreviation: DM, diabetes mellitus.
Adapted from Miller M, Stone NJ, Ballantyne C, et al. Triglycerides and cardiovascular disease: a scientific statement from the American Heart Association. Circulation 2011;123:2292–333.

case of DM2). Treatment of hyperglycemia and prevention of DM2 reduce TG levels.

2. Reduce insulin resistance. Decreasing calories, increasing physical activity, and decreasing weight all seem to work by this mechanism. Treating or preventing DM2 with medications that reduce insulin resistance (such as thiazolidinediones or biguanides) may confer extra TG level–lowering benefit.

3. Screen for hypothyroidism and treat it if present. All patients with HTG should have their serum thyroid stimulating hormone (TSH) levels checked. If the TSH level is increased, levothyroxine replacement lowers TG levels (and is beneficial for many other reasons).

4. Proteinuria and renal insufficiency should be screened for and treated if possible. Both increase TG levels if left uncontrolled.

5. Endogenous hypercortisolism should be considered and treated if present. Although rare, it substantially increases plasma TG level and should always be considered in patients with HTG.

6. Medications that increase TG levels should be decreased or discontinued if possible, including:
   a. Oral contraceptives (primarily the estrogen component)
   b. Oral postmenopausal estrogen replacement
   c. Retinoic acid derivatives
   d. Systemic glucocorticoids
   e. Some antiretroviral medications
   f. Some antipsychotic medications
   g. Most β-blockers (generally only a weak effect)
   h. Thiazide diuretics (generally only a weak effect)

Pharmacotherapy Treatment Recommendations Adjunctive to Current Guidelines

Mendelian randomization data strongly suggest that HTG causes ASCVD, and so TG level–lowering treatment in HTG is now more strongly recommended to address the residual ASCVD risk than has been the case in (generally earlier) published guidelines.[5]

Fibrates are the best-established agents for TG level lowering and are generally used first line for TG levels greater than 500 mg/dL. Fenofibrate is almost always preferred to gemfibrozil because it is far less likely to cause myopathy with concurrent statin use. Two exceptions are patients with severe renal insufficiency not taking a statin or likely to do so in the future, and patients taking fluvastatin, which has no adverse interaction with gemfibrozil.

There are 3 FDA-approved prescription omega-3 products: (1) an ethyl ester mix of EPA and DHA, (2) an ethyl ester pure EPA (icosapent ethyl), and (3) a carboxylic acid mix of EPA and DHA. They are much more expensive to manufacture than fenofibrate and so even the generic ethyl ester EPA/DHA mix may incur higher out-of-pocket cost, even when covered by insurance. Omega-3 (at least icosapent ethyl in JELIS[62]) has been better proved to reduce ASCVD risk as a statin adjunct, and for this reason the class can be strongly considered for first-line use. Also, prescription omega-3 is generally as effective as fenofibrate for TG level lowering and is usually as well tolerated. In addition to better ASCVD evidence, other potential advantages of omega-3 compared with fenofibrate include that it is a natural product, it lacks any associated myopathy, and it might provide antiinflammatory, mood, cognitive, or other benefits, although none of these benefits is in the product label or has been established in an RCT. In light of the positive ASCVD results in JELIS[62] it is unfortunate that no current official lipid guidelines mention this class. Whether the preparation does or does not contain DHA, omega-3 is useful for treatment of HTG, and can be used as first or second line, ahead of or behind fibrates (generally in combination with them).

Niacin is usually reserved for third-line use because it is less well tolerated, may cause or worsen diabetes, and is generally harder to use. Statins are a crucial consideration for management of HTG in addition to the traditional TG level–lowering medications noted earlier. Statins are the best-established agents for ASCVD prevention, and so are usually used as first line for TG levels less than 500 mg/dL. Because they have lesser TG level–lowering efficacy than fibrates and omega-3, statins are generally not used as first line in patients with a fasting TG levels more than 500 mg/dL.

REFERENCES

1. Maki KC, Bays HE, Dicklin MR. Treatment options for the management of hypertriglyceridemia: strategies based on the best-available evidence. J Clin Lipidol 2012;6:413–26.
2. Ford ES, Li C, Zhao G, et al. Hypertriglyceridemia and its pharmacologic treatment among US adults. Arch Intern Med 2009;169:572–8.
3. Christian JB, Bourgeois N, Snipes R, et al. Prevalence of severe (500 to 2,000 mg/dl) hypertriglyceridemia in United States adults. Am J Cardiol 2011;107:891–7.
4. Roger VL, Go AS, Lloyd-Jones DM, et al. Heart disease and stroke statistics–2011 update: a report from the American Heart Association. Circulation 2011;123:e18–209.
5. Hegele RA, Ginsberg HN, Chapman MJ, et al. The polygenic nature of hypertriglyceridaemia: implications for definition, diagnosis, and management. Lancet Diabetes Endocrinol 2014;2:655–66.

6. Miller M, Stone NJ, Ballantyne C, et al. Triglycerides and cardiovascular disease: a scientific statement from the American Heart Association. Circulation 2011;123: 2292–333.

7. Kersten S. Physiological regulation of lipoprotein lipase. Biochim Biophys Acta 2014;1841:919–33.

8. Glueck CJ, Fallat R, Buncher CR, et al. Familial combined hyperlipoproteinemia: studies in 91 adults and 95 children from 33 kindreds. Metabolism 1973;23: 1403–28.

9. Glueck CJ, Tsang R, Fallat R, et al. Familial hypertriglyceridemia: studies in 130 children and 45 siblings of 36 index cases. Metabolism 1973;22:1287–309.

10. Hopkins PN, Wu LL, Hunt SC, et al. Plasma triglycerides and type III hyperlipidemia are independently associated with premature familial coronary artery disease. J Am Coll Cardiol 2005;45:1003–12.

11. Hopkins PN, Nanjee MN, Wu LL, et al. Altered composition of triglyceride-rich lipoproteins and coronary artery disease in a large case-control study. Atherosclerosis 2009;207:559–66.

12. Hopkins PN, Brinton EA, Nanjee MN. Hyperlipoproteinemia type 3: the forgotten phenotype. Curr Atheroscler Rep 2014;16:440.

13. Sarwar N, Sandhu MS, Ricketts SL, et al. Triglyceride-mediated pathways and coronary disease: collaborative analysis of 101 studies. Lancet 2010;375:1634–9.

14. Austin MA, Hokanson JE, Edwards KL. Hypertriglyceridemia as a cardiovascular risk factor. Am J Cardiol 1998;81:7B–12B.

15. Sarwar N, Danesh J, Eiriksdottir G, et al. Triglycerides and the risk of coronary heart disease: 10,158 incident cases among 262,525 participants in 29 western prospective studies. Circulation 2007;115:450–8.

16. Liu J, Zeng FF, Liu ZM, et al. Effects of blood triglycerides on cardiovascular and all-cause mortality: a systematic review and meta-analysis of 61 prospective studies. Lipids Health Dis 2013;12:159.

17. Sacks FM, Alaupovic P, Moye LA, et al. VLDL, apolipoproteins B, CIII, and E, and risk of recurrent coronary events in the Cholesterol and Recurrent Events (CARE) trial. Circulation 2000;102:1886–92.

18. Miller M, Cannon CP, Murphy SA, et al. Impact of triglyceride levels beyond low-density lipoprotein cholesterol after acute coronary syndrome in the PROVE IT-TIMI 22 trial. J Am Coll Cardiol 2008;51:724–30.

19. Drexel H, Aczel S, Marte T, et al. Factors predicting cardiovascular events in statin-treated diabetic and non-diabetic patients with coronary atherosclerosis. Atherosclerosis 2010;208:484–9.

20. Wang L, Gill R, Pedersen TL, et al. Triglyceride-rich lipoprotein lipolysis releases neutral and oxidized FFAs that induce endothelial cell inflammation. J Lipid Res 2009;50:204–13.

21. Goldberg IJ, Eckel RH, McPherson R. Triglycerides and heart disease: still a hypothesis? Arterioscler Thromb Vasc Biol 2011;31:1716–25.

22. Ginsberg HN. New perspectives on atherogenesis: role of abnormal triglyceride-rich lipoprotein metabolism. Circulation 2002;106:2137–42.

23. Schlaich MP, Grassi G, Lambert GW, et al. European Society of Hypertension Working Group on Obesity Obesity-induced hypertension and target organ damage: current knowledge and future directions. J Hypertens 2009;27: 207–11.

24. Liu L, Wen T, Zheng XY, et al. Remnant-like particles accelerate endothelial progenitor cells senescence and induce cellular dysfunction via an oxidative mechanism. Atherosclerosis 2009;202:405–14.

25. Mahley RW, Innerarity TL, Rall SC Jr, et al. Lipoproteins of special significance in atherosclerosis. Insights provided by studies of type III hyperlipoproteinemia. Ann N Y Acad Sci 1985;454:209–21.

26. Ferreira AC, Peter AA, Mendez AJ, et al. Postprandial hypertriglyceridemia increases circulating levels of endothelial cell microparticles. Circulation 2004; 110:3599–603.

27. Norata GD, Grigore L, Raselli S, et al. Post-prandial endothelial dysfunction in hypertriglyceridemic subjects: molecular mechanisms and gene expression studies. Atherosclerosis 2007;193:321–7.

28. Shin HK, Kim YK, Kim KY, et al. Remnant lipoprotein particles induce apoptosis in endothelial cells by NAD(P)H oxidase-mediated production of superoxide and cytokines via lectin-like oxidized low-density lipoprotein receptor-1 activation: prevention by cilostazol. Circulation 2004;109:1022–8.

29. Tanimura K, Nakajima Y, Nagao M, et al. Association of serum apolipoprotein B48 level with the presence of carotid plaque in type 2 diabetes mellitus. Diabetes Res Clin Pract 2008;81:338–44.

30. Langsted A, Freiberg JJ, Tybjaerg-Hansen A, et al. Nonfasting cholesterol and triglycerides and association with risk of myocardial infarction and total mortality: the Copenhagen City Heart Study with 31 years of follow-up. J Intern Med 2011;270:65–75.

31. Zheng C, Azcutia V, Aikawa E, et al. Statins suppress apolipoprotein CIII-induced vascular endothelial cell activation and monocyte adhesion. Eur Heart J 2013;34: 615–24.

32. Ginsberg HN, Brown WV. Apolipoprotein CIII: 42 years old and even more interesting. Arterioscler Thromb Vasc Biol 2011;31:471–3.

33. Caron S, Verrijken A, Mertens I, et al. Transcriptional activation of apolipoprotein CIII expression by glucose may contribute to diabetic dyslipidemia. Arterioscler Thromb Vasc Biol 2011;31:513–9.

34. Ginsberg HN. Insulin resistance and cardiovascular disease. J Clin Invest 2000; 106:453–8.

35. Lamarche B, Tchernof A, Moorjani S, et al. Small, dense low-density lipoprotein particles as a predictor of the risk of ischemic heart disease in men. Prospective results from the Québec Cardiovascular Study. Circulation 1997;95: 69–75.

36. St-Pierre AC, Ruel IL, Cantin B, et al. Comparison of various electrophoretic characteristics of LDL particles and their relationship to the risk of ischemic heart disease. Circulation 2001;104:2295–9.

37. Hirano T, Ito Y, Koba S, et al. Clinical significance of small dense low-density lipoprotein cholesterol levels determined by the simple precipitation method. Arterioscler Thromb Vasc Biol 2004;24:558–63.

38. Rizzo M, Kotur-Stevuljevic J, Berneis K, et al. Atherogenic dyslipidemia and oxidative stress: a new look. Transl Res 2009;153:217–23.

39. Packard C, Caslake M, Shepherd J. The role of small, dense low density lipoprotein (LDL): a new look. Int J Cardiol 2000;74(Suppl 1):S17–22.

40. Berneis KK, Krauss RM. Metabolic origins and clinical significance of LDL heterogeneity. J Lipid Res 2002;43:1363–79.

41. Anber V, Griffin BA, McConnell M, et al. Influence of plasma lipid and LDL-subfraction profile on the interaction between low density lipoprotein with human arterial wall proteoglycans. Atherosclerosis 1996;124:261–71.

42. Goulinet S, Chapman MJ. Plasma LDL and HDL subspecies are heterogenous in particle content of tocopherols and oxygenated and hydrocarbon carotenoids.

Relevance to oxidative resistance and atherogenesis. Arterioscler Thromb Vasc Biol 1997;17:786–96.

43. Nigon F, Lesnik P, Rouis M, et al. Discrete subspecies of human low density lipo-proteins are heterogeneous in their interaction with the cellular LDL receptor. J Lipid Res 1991;32:1741–53.

44. Younis N, Charlton-Menys V, Sharma R, et al. Glycation of LDL in non-diabetic people: Small dense LDL is preferentially glycated both in vivo and in vitro. Atherosclerosis 2009;202:162–8.

45. Zheng C, Khoo C, Furtado J, et al. Apolipoprotein C-III and the metabolic basis for hypertriglyceridemia and the dense low-density lipoprotein phenotype. Circu-lation 2010;121:1722–34.

46. Brinton EA, Eisenberg S, Breslow JL. Increased apo A-I and apo A-II fractional catabolic rate in patients with low high density lipoprotein-cholesterol levels with or without hypertriglyceridemia. J Clin Invest 1991;87:536–44.

47. Brinton EA, Eisenberg S, Breslow JL. Human HDL cholesterol levels are deter-mined by apoA-I fractional catabolic rate, which correlates inversely with esti-mates of HDL particle size. Effects of gender, hepatic and lipoprotein lipases, triglyceride and insulin levels, and body fat distribution. Arterioscler Thromb 1994;14:707–20.

48. Rizzo M, Spinas GA, Cesur M, et al. Atherogenic lipoprotein phenotype and LDL size and subclasses in drug-naive patients with early rheumatoid arthritis. Athero-sclerosis 2009;207:502–6.

49. Do R, Willer CJ, Schmidt EM, et al. Common variants associated with plasma tri-glycerides and risk for coronary artery disease. Nat Genet 2013;45:1345–52.

50. Jørgensen AB, Frikke-Schmidt R, Nordestgaard BG, et al. Loss-of-function mutations in APOC3 and risk of ischemic vascular disease. N Engl J Med 2014;371:32–41.

51. Chapman M. Fibrates: therapeutic review. Br J Diabetes Vasc Dis 2006;6:11–20.

52. Kamanna VS, Kashyap ML. Nicotinic acid (niacin) receptor agonists: will they be useful therapeutic agents? Am J Cardiol 2007;100:S53–61.

53. McKenney JM, Sica D. Role of prescription omega-3 fatty acids in the treatment of hypertriglyceridemia. Pharmacotherapy 2007;27:715–28.

54. Ginsberg HN, Elam MB, Lovato LC, et al. Effects of combination lipid therapy in type 2 diabetes mellitus. N Engl J Med 2010;362:1563–74.

55. Ginsberg HN. The ACCORD (Action to Control Cardiovascular Risk in Diabetes) Lipid trial: what we learn from subgroup analyses. Diabetes Care 2011;34(Suppl 2):S107–8.

56. Keech A, Simes RJ, Barter P, et al. Effects of long-term fenofibrate therapy on car-diovascular events in 9795 people with type 2 diabetes mellitus (the FIELD study): randomised controlled trial. Lancet 2005;366:1849–61.

57. Scott R, O'Brien R, Fulcher G, et al. Effects of fenofibrate treatment on cardiovas-cular disease risk in 9,795 individuals with type 2 diabetes and various compo-nents of the metabolic syndrome: the Fenofibrate Intervention and Event Lowering in Diabetes (FIELD) study. Diabetes Care 2009;32:493–8.

58. Sacks FM, Carey VJ, Fruchart JC. Combination lipid therapy in type 2 diabetes. N Engl J Med 2010;363:692–4 [author reply: 694–5].

59. Risk, Prevention Study Collaborative Group, Roncaglioni MC, Tombesi M, et al. n-3 fatty acids in patients with multiple cardiovascular risk factors. N Engl J Med 2013;368:1800–8.

60. ORIGIN Trial Investigators, Bosch J, Gerstein HC, et al. n-3 fatty acids and car-diovascular outcomes in patients with dysglycemia. N Engl J Med 2012;367:309–18.

61. Writing Group for the AREDS2 Research Group, Bonds DE, Harrington M, et al. Effect of long-chain omega-3 fatty acids and lutein + zeaxanthin supplements on cardiovascular outcomes: results of the Age-related Eye Disease Study 2 (AREDS2) randomized clinical trial. JAMA Intern Med 2014;174: 763–71.

62. Yokoyama M, Origasa H, Matsuzaki M, et al. Effects of eicosapentaenoic acid on major coronary events in hypercholesterolaemic patients (JELIS): a randomised open-label, blinded endpoint analysis. Lancet 2007;369:1090–8.

63. Cannon C. Improved Reduction of Outcomes: Vytorin Efficacy International Trial (IMPROVE-IT). Chicago: AHA Scientific Sessions; 2014.

64. Saito Y, Yokoyama M, Origasa H, et al. Effects of EPA on coronary artery disease in hypercholesterolemic patients with multiple risk factors: sub-analysis of primary prevention cases from the Japan EPA Lipid Intervention Study (JELIS). Atherosclerosis 2008;200:135–40.

65. Bruckert E, Labreuche J, Amarenco P. Meta-analysis of the effect of nicotinic acid alone or in combination on cardiovascular events and atherosclerosis. Atherosclerosis 2010;210:353–61.

66. Boden WE, Probstfield JL, Anderson T, et al. Niacin in patients with low HDL cholesterol levels receiving intensive statin therapy. N Engl J Med 2011;365: 2255–67.

67. Guyton JR, Slee AE, Anderson T, et al. Relationship of lipoproteins to cardiovascular events: The AIM-HIGH trial (atherothrombosis intervention in metabolic syndrome with low HDL/high triglycerides and impact on global health outcomes). J Am Coll Cardiol 2013;62:1580–4.

68. Group TCDPWR. Clofibrate and niacin in coronary heart disease. JAMA 1975; 231:360–81.

69. Canner PL, Furberg CD, McGovern ME. Benefits of niacin in patients with versus without the metabolic syndrome and healed myocardial infarction (from the coronary drug project). Am J Cardiol 2006;97:477–9.

70. HPS2-THRIVE Collaborative Group, Landray MJ, Haynes R, Hopewell JC, et al. Effects of extended-release niacin with laropiprant in high-risk patients. N Engl J Med 2014;371:203–12.

71. Stone NJ, Robinson JG, Lichtenstein AH, et al. 2013 ACC/AHA guideline on the treatment of blood cholesterol to reduce atherosclerotic cardiovascular risk in adults: a report of the American College of Cardiology/American Heart Association Task Force on Practice Guidelines. Circulation 2014;129:S1–45.

72. Reduction of Cardiovascular Events with EPA - Intervention Trial (REDUCE-IT). Available at: https://clinicaltrials.gov/ct2/show/NCT01492361?term=reduce-it&rank=1. Accessed January 6, 2015.

73. Outcomes Study to Assess STatin Residual Risk Reduction with EpaNova in HiGh Cardiovascular Risk PatienTs with Hypertriglyceridemia (STRENGTH). Available at: https://clinicaltrials.gov/ct2/show/NCT02104817?term=epanova&rank=4. Accessed January 6, 2015.

74. Grundy SM, Cleeman JI, Merz CN, et al. Implications of recent clinical trials for the national cholesterol education program adult treatment panel III guidelines. Circulation 2004;110:227–39.

75. Gibbons GH, Shurin SB, Mensah GA, et al. Refocusing the agenda on cardiovascular guidelines: an announcement from the National Heart, Lung, and Blood Institute. J Am Coll Cardiol 2013;62:1396–8.

76. Stone N, Robinson J, Lichtenstein, et al. 2013 ACC/AHA guideline on the treatment of blood cholesterol to reduce atherosclerotic cardiovascular risk in

adults: a report of the American College of Cardiology/American Heart Association Task Force on Practice Guidelines. Circulation 2013;1–84.

77. Chapman MJ, Ginsberg HN, Amarenco P, et al. Triglyceride-rich lipoproteins and high-density lipoprotein cholesterol in patients at high risk of cardiovascular disease: evidence and guidance for management. Eur Heart J 2011;32:1345–61.

78. Ishida T, Ohta M, Nakakuki M, et al. Distinct regulation of plasma LDL cholesterol by eicosapentaenoic acid and docosahexaenoic acid in high fat diet-fed hamsters: participation of cholesterol ester transfer protein and LDL receptor. Prostaglandins Leukot Essent Fatty Acids 2013;88:281–8.

79. Wei MY, Jacobson TA. Effects of eicosapentaenoic acid versus docosahexaenoic acid on serum lipids: a systematic review and meta-analysis. Curr Atheroscler Rep 2011;13:474–83.

Lipid-Modifying Treatments for Heart Failure

Is Their Use Justified?

John G.F. Cleland, MD, PhD, FRCP, FESC[a,*], Kate Hutchinson, MBChB[b],
Pierpaolo Pellicori, MD[b], Andrew Clark, MD, MA, FRCP[b]

KEYWORDS

- Fibrates • Polyunsaturated fatty acids • Statins • Heart failure

KEY POINTS

- Most patients with heart failure have atherosclerotic disease either as a cause of ventricular dysfunction or as a concomitant problem.
- Sudden death may be the most common presentation of myocardial infarction amongst patients with heart failure.
- Meta-analyses of trials of fibrates in cardiovascular disease identified no reduction in all-cause or cardiovascular mortality or heart failure events; there are no large trials of fibrates in patients with heart failure, but what evidence exists suggests no benefit.
- Meta-analyses of trials of polyunsaturated fatty acids in cardiovascular disease failed to show an effect on all-cause mortality but did suggest a small reduction in cardiac deaths (9% reduction in relative risk). There is equivocal evidence of benefit in patients with heart failure.
- Meta-analysis shows that statins reduce all-cause and cardiovascular mortality and heart failure events in patients with or at high risk of cardiovascular disease.

INTRODUCTION

There are theoretical arguments for and against lipid-modifying therapy for patients with heart failure but little conclusive clinical evidence that it provides substantial benefit or causes significant harm. However, one of the curses of modern therapeutics

This article originally appeared in Heart Failure Clinics, Volume 10, Issue 4, October 2014.
Disclosure: Professor J.G.F. Cleland received honoraria for participation in the CORONA trial. No other relevant disclosures.
Professor J.G.F. Cleland is supported, in part, by the NIHR cardiovascular Biomedical Research Unit at the Royal Brompton and Harefield NHS Foundation Trust and Imperial College, London.
[a] National Heart & Lung Institute, Royal Brompton & Harefield Hospitals, Imperial College, London UB9 6JH, UK; [b] Department of Cardiology, Hull York Medical School, Castle Hill Hospital, Kingston-upon-Hull HU6 5JQ, UK
* Corresponding author. Department of Cardiology, Harefield Hospital, Imperial College, Hill End Road, Harfield, Middlesex UB9 6JH, UK.
E-mail address: j.cleland@imperial.ac.uk

Clinics Collections 5 (2015) 257–274
http://dx.doi.org/10.1016/j.ccol.2015.05.015

is polypharmacy. In a bygone era, the pharmacopoeia consisted of agents that were safe and ineffective (placebo) and those that might be effective but with varying degrees of toxicity. Placebo does not prevent spontaneous recovery and may have psychological benefits and therefore often appears effective. The low benefit/risk ratio of interventions in this era gave rise to the old adage, "primum non nocere." Now that we have many more medicines, many of which are safe and effective, primum non nocere is no longer a tenable position, at least for serious diseases such as heart failure that rarely remit, because medicine practiced in this way is, paradoxically, quite likely to cause harm. A patient given too many medicines is likely not to take them all and may experience drug interactions. When faced with a plethora of choices, the motto of modern medicine for serious disease is "primum efficatum." Once an agent is shown to be effective, the penalty in terms of side effects, risk, and harm can be weighed. Of course, the power of placebo and concept of primum non nocere might still apply when the disease is likely to resolve spontaneously or causes little disability or when no effective treatments exist. Some medical disciplines are contaminated by agents upon which the medical community wastes huge amounts of money, for example, aspirin for long-term prophylaxis of cardiovascular disease,[1,2] most hypoglycemic agents for type-2 diabetes,[3] and vitamin and mineral supplements for osteoporosis.[4] The purpose of this report is to explore these issues with respect to lipid-modifying agents in patients with heart failure.

Most patients with heart failure have atherosclerosis, which is often the primary cause of their heart failure. Progression of atherosclerosis, which may impair blood flow to heart, brain, kidney, and skeletal muscle, and plaque rupture, leading to acute coronary and cerebrovascular syndromes, could be important pathways for the progression of heart failure, morbidity, and death.[5] Stabilizing plaque either by reducing its cholesterol content or by reducing inflammatory activity could reduce acute vascular events. Causing plaque to regress could reduce ischemia. Hyperlipidemia can also impair microvascular function that can be improved by lipid-lowering therapies.[6] Some authorities believe that all patients with heart failure due to left ventricular systolic dysfunction, regardless of its etiology, have myocardial ischemia, caused by epicardial coronary artery disease, microvascular dysfunction, elevated ventricular filling pressures, or potentially all three.[7]

Fatty acids are an important energy substrate for the myocardium but may be less efficient than glucose and lactate and may increase proton production, lowering cellular pH and impairing cell function. Diverting the myocardial energy substrate from lipids to carbohydrates might be beneficial.[8] Theoretically, lipid lowering might have beneficial effects on myocardial function. Lipid-modifying therapies may also have ancillary effects on inflammatory systems that might also improve myocardial function, encourage repair, reduce fibrosis, and increase electrical stability. However, higher plasma concentrations of arachidonic acid and some long-chain fatty acids, such as docosahexaenoic acid are associated with a lower incidence of heart failure.[9,10]

On the other hand, cholesterol decreases as heart failure progresses and a low cholesterol level is a bad prognostic sign in heart failure. This decrease may just reflect the metabolic stress of a patient who is in the process of dying from heart failure, but there is some concern that circulating lipid fractions may bind endotoxins absorbed from the gut.[11] Lowering cholesterol might impair this natural defense mechanism, cause cytokine activation, increase inflammation, and accelerate the progression of heart failure.[12] Moreover, statins can interfere with the synthesis of coenzyme Q10, an essential component of the mitochondrial respiratory chain.[13] Recent evidence suggests that coenzyme Q10 supplements may have a beneficial effect on prognosis in patients with heart failure.[14]

Lowering cholesterol might be both beneficial and harmful; in some patients the benefit will outweigh the harm; in others, harm and benefit will be similar, and the patient will derive no benefit. In some, harm may outweigh benefit. This article focuses on treatments designed to modify lipids; fibrates, statins and omega-3 fatty acids.

FIBRATES

There are no substantial randomized, controlled trials of fibrates in patients with heart failure. Node and colleagues[15] investigated the effects of bezafibrate on amino-terminal probrain natriuretic peptide (NT-proBNP) in 108 patients with New York Heart Association (NYHA) class III heart failure enrolled in the Bezafibrate Infarction Prevention study, a study of secondary prevention after a myocardial infarction. After 2 years of follow-up, plasma concentrations of NT-proBNP were similar in patients assigned to bezafibrate or placebo. In the overall population (with or without heart failure), the study was neutral.

Both the Veterans Affairs study of gemfibrozil[16] and the Action to Control Cardiovascular Risk in Diabetes (ACCORD) of fenofibrate[17] suggested fewer heart failure events in the actively managed group but no effect on all-cause or cardiovascular mortality. A meta-analysis of more than 45,000 patients in randomized, controlled trials of fibrates for the primary or secondary prevention of cardiovascular disease suggested no effect on all-cause or cardiovascular mortality or heart failure outcomes but a substantial effect on microvascular complications such as retinopathy among diabetic patients.[18]

There is little evidence to support the use of fibrates in patients with heart failure and insufficient trial evidence to confirm that they are either ineffective or safe.

OMEGA-3 FATTY ACIDS OR POLYUNSATURATED FATTY ACIDS

Overall, omega-3 fatty acids seem safe in patients with or at risk of cardiovascular disease, but the evidence of benefit is inconclusive. However, benefit may be modified depending on the country where the research was conducted. Most of the positive trials of omega-3 fatty acids come from Italy, a country where a lot of olive oil is used. Olive oil has commonly been used as the placebo intervention in trials of omega-3 fatty acids. However, in countries with low consumption of omega-3, olive oil may not be a placebo, although whether the dose of placebo olive oil is high enough to have a clinical effect is disputed.[19] In countries where olive oil consumption is high, a little extra olive oil might truly be a placebo, and the effect of omega-3 might become apparent.

The Gruppo Italiano per lo Studio della Sopravvivenza nell' Infarto miocardico (GISSI)-prevenzione trial[20] was a large (n = 11,324) randomized, double-blind trial comparing olive oil capsules with polyunsaturated fatty acids (PUFA) in patients with a recent myocardial infarction. The study found a reduction in mortality but not in nonfatal cardiovascular events. The major impact on mortality seemed to be caused by a reduction in sudden death, which many attributed to a reduction in ventricular arrhythmias but could also have been in part caused by a reduction in coronary events. A genuine reduction in coronary events combined with a reduction in prehospital arrhythmic mortality (patients who die before they reach the hospital cannot get a diagnosis) could account for the lack of effect on nonfatal events. The effect was greatest in patients with a reduced left ventricular ejection fraction, but perhaps only because this is a group with a higher rate of events. These observations triggered a second large study, GISSI-Heart Failure (HF) trial, which investigated the effects of rosuvastatin and PUFA on mortality.

GISSI-HF[21] included 6975 patients with NYHA class II to IV heart failure with or without a reduced left ventricular ejection fraction and randomized them, double-blind, to n-3

PUFA (1 g/d) or placebo. Patients not indicated for or already receiving a statin were then rerandomized to rosuvastatin or placebo (see later discussion). The coprimary outcome measures were all-cause mortality and the composite of death or admission to hospital for cardiovascular reasons. The median follow-up was 3.9 years (interquartile range, 3.0–4.5).

More than 40% of patients were older than 70 years, about half had known ischemic heart disease, and use of guideline-indicated treatment, apart perhaps from β-blockers, was good (**Table 1**). Taking PUFA had no effect on heart rate or blood pressure and did not change total, high- or low-density lipoprotein cholesterol, although it did reduce triglycerides (P<.0001). A substudy suggested that PUFA could improve left ventricular ejection fraction, although the absolute difference from placebo was less than 1% at 3 years.[22]

Overall, 955 (27%) patients assigned to PUFA died, and 1014 (29%) of those assigned to placebo (olive oil) (adjusted hazard ratio [HR], 0.91; 95.5% confidence interval [CI], 0.833–0.998; P = .041), a result of borderline statistical significance (**Fig. 1**). Most deaths were cardiovascular (**Table 2**), but the reduction in cardiovascular death was not significant because of the slightly smaller number of events. Among causes of death, the reduction in sudden death was probably greatest (7.8% vs 8.7%). There were no subgroup interactions, but patients with left ventricular ejection fraction greater than 40% may have obtained less benefit. A cardiovascular admission or death occurred in 1981 (57%) patients assigned to PUFA and 2053 (59%) in those

Table 1
Patient characteristics in the GISSI-HF trial

	Placebo	n-3 PUFA
N	3481	3494
Age (y)	67	67
Age >70 y	43%	42%
Women	21%	22%
Ischemic heart disease	50%	49%
Dilated cardiomyopathy	28%	30%
NYHA II	63%	64%
Body mass index (kg/m²)	27	27
Systolic blood pressure (mm Hg)	126	126
Atrial fibrillation	16%	16%
Left ventricular ejection fraction >40%	9%	10%
Defibrillator	7%	7%
Diuretics	90%	90%
Angiotensin-converting enzyme inhibitor or angiotensin II receptor blockers	93%	94%
β-blockers	65%	65%
Spironolactone	40%	39%
Digoxin	37%	37%
Anti-coagulants	28%	29%
Statins	23%	22%

From Tavazzi L, Maggioni AP, Marchioli R, et al. Effect of n-3 polyunsaturated fatty acids in patients with chronic heart failure (the GISSI-HF trial): a randomised, double-blind, placebo-controlled trial. Lancet 2008;372(9645):1225; with permission.

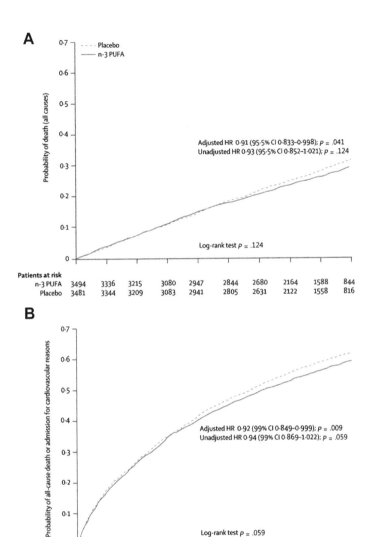

Fig. 1. Kaplan-Meier curves for time to all-cause death (*A*) and for time to all-cause death or admission to hospital for cardiovascular reasons (*B*). (*From* Tavazzi L, Maggioni AP, Marchioli R, et al. Effect of n-3 polyunsaturated fatty acids in patients with chronic heart failure (the GISSI-HF trial): a randomised, double-blind, placebo-controlled trial. Lancet 2008;372(9645):1226; with permission.)

assigned to placebo (adjusted HR, 0.92; 99% CI, 0.849–0.999; *P* = .009). However, there was no reduction in hospitalization for heart failure (HR, 0.94).

In absolute terms, 56 patients needed to be treated for a median duration of 3.9 years to avoid one death or 44 to avoid the composite event. Similar numbers of patients withdrew from PUFA and placebo, mostly by choice rather than because

Table 2 Causes of death		
	n-3 PUFA (N = 3494) (%)	Placebo (N = 3481) (%)
Total mortality	955 (27.3)	1014 (29.1)
Acute myocardial infarction	20 (0.6)	25 (0.7)
Worsening heart failure	319 (9.1)	332 (9.5)
Presumed arrhythmic	274 (7.8)	304 (8.7)
Stroke	50 (1.4)	44 (1.3)
Other cardiovascular reasons	49 (1.4)	60 (1.7)
Neoplasia	107 (3.1)	112 (3.2)
Other noncardiovascular reasons	97 (2.8)	102 (2.9)
Not known	39(1.1)	35 (1.0)

From Tavazzi L, Maggioni AP, Marchioli R, et al. Effect of n-3 polyunsaturated fatty acids in patients with chronic heart failure (the GISSI-HF trial): a randomised, double-blind, placebo-controlled trial. Lancet 2008;372(9645):1227; with permission.

of adverse reactions. However, a small trial of patients with heart failure due to non-ischemic cardiomyopathy randomized 43 patients to placebo, 1 g/d or 4 g/d of PUFA. PUFA improved vascular function, markers of inflammation and left ventricular ejection fraction in a dose-dependent manner. Perhaps the dose of PUFA used in the studies conducted so far has been too low.[23]

These results should be interpreted in the wider context of trials of PUFA in populations at risk of heart failure such as those with or at high risk of cardiovascular disease. A meta-analysis including almost 70,000 patients identified no effect on all-cause mortality but suggested a small reduction (HR, 0.91; 95% CI, 0.85–0.98) in cardiac deaths. However, in a subgroup of trials conducted in patients with implanted defibrillators, a substantial effect on all-cause mortality (HR, 0.69; 95% CI, 0.39–1.23) could not be excluded.[24]

Current guidelines from the European Society of Cardiology give a class IIb, level of evidence B recommendation for PUFA,[25] a fairly weak recommendation that seems warranted by the totality of the evidence. Guidelines from the American Heart Association/American College of Cardiology give a stronger recommendation: class IIa, level of evidence B.[26]

STATINS (3-HYDROXY-3-METHYLGLUTARYL-COENZYME-A REDUCTASE INHIBITORS)

Many have been intrigued by the rather low incidence of myocardial infarction in clinical trials of heart failure despite the high prevalence of ischemic heart disease.[5,27,28] This low incidence could be because coronary events are uncommon and contribute little to the progression of disease or mortality. Alternatively, we know that many patients have coronary events but do not have typical symptoms. Cardiac denervation as a consequence of diabetes or previous cardiac damage may modify symptoms and might account for why many patients with worsening heart failure have elevated biomarkers of cardiac damage in the absence of classical symptoms of myocardial ischemia or infarction. Another important reason why the incidence of myocardial infarction may be so low is that patients with preexisting cardiac dysfunction may be much more likely to die suddenly of arrhythmias or shock before they can get medical attention and a diagnosis of infarction.[29] Thus, statins could reduce further silent cardiac damage as well as overt vascular events and sudden death. Statins might also have other effects, such as improving microvascular function or reducing myocardial inflammation.[12,30]

Observational studies suggest that patients treated with statins have a better outcome than those who are not, after adjusting for measured confounders such as age and ischemic heart disease.[31–34] However, many unmeasured confounders make such adjusted observational analyses unreliable. The effect seemed to be mainly on sudden death, although it is unclear whether this is vascular or arrhythmic sudden death. Patients without known coronary artery disease also seemed to benefit.[33]

Smaller randomized, controlled trials suggested that statins could reduce cholesterol and some markers of inflammation such as soluble tumor necrosis factor receptor-1 and C-reactive protein but not others such as interleukin-6.[35,36] Atorvastatin also reduced endothelin-1 but not brain natriuretic peptide.[35] Effects on ventricular function have been variable,[22,36–38] with some randomized studies reporting improvement even in patients without coronary disease[36] and reductions in natriuretic peptides.[37] Some small trials even suggested a reduction in sudden death and overall mortality.[39]

The next level of evidence comes from subgroup analyses of large clinical trials in populations that contained some patients with heart failure. The Treating to New Targets (TNT) Study compared two doses of atorvastatin, 80 mg/d and 10 mg/d, in patients with coronary disease.[40] Patients had to have stable coronary disease and a left ventricular ejection fraction greater than 30%. Hospitalizations for heart failure in the overall population (10,001) were reduced from 3.3% to 2.4% (HR, 0.74; 95% CI, 0.59–0.94; $P<.0116$) with higher-dose statin over a median follow-up of 4.9 years. The rate of hospitalization for heart failure seems low in both arms, suggesting that many cases were missed. The higher the baseline cholesterol, the greater was the risk of a heart failure event and the greater the difference in effect between doses. Of 10,001 patients enrolled, only 7.8% had some degree of heart failure at baseline, but it must have been very mild, as only about 50% of them were prescribed a diuretic. The effect of the higher dose of atorvastatin on hospitalization for heart failure was more marked in patients with a history of heart failure at baseline: 17.3% versus 10.6% in the 10-mg and 80-mg arms, respectively (HR, 0.59; 95% CI, 0.4–0.88; $P<.009$).

Finally, three substantial studies, two with rosuvastatin, a hydrophilic agent, and one with pitavastatin, a lipophilic agent, have been conducted; all were neutral for their primary endpoint.

GISSI-HF

The GISSI-HF trial investigated the safety and efficacy of rosuvastatin 10 mg/d in 4574 patients with symptomatic heart failure, irrespective of age or left ventricular ejection fraction and included patients both with and without ischemic heart disease. Patients with a recent vascular event or with a serum creatinine level greater than 221 μmol/L were excluded. The coprimary outcome measures were all-cause mortality and the composite of death or admission to hospital for cardiovascular reasons. The median follow-up was 3.9 years (interquartile range, 3.0–4.4).

More than 40% of patients were older than 70 years, about half had known ischemic heart disease, and use of guideline-indicated treatment, apart perhaps from β-blockers (63%), was good. Taking rosuvastatin reduced C-reactive protein and low-density lipoprotein cholesterol levels (from 3.16 mmol/L to 2.15 mmol/L; $P<.0001$)[41] but had no effect on high-density lipoprotein cholesterol or left ventricular ejection fraction.[22]

There were 657 (29%) deaths in patients assigned to rosuvastatin (29%) compared with 644 (28%) in those assigned to placebo (*P* = .76) (**Fig. 2**). The composite outcome of death or admission to the hospital for cardiovascular reasons occurred in 1305 (57%) patients assigned to rosuvastatin and 1283 (56%) assigned to placebo. All other

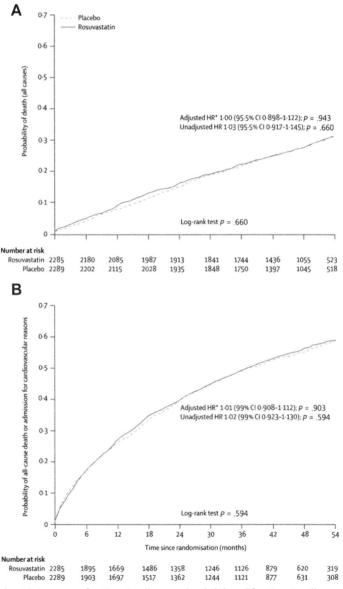

Fig. 2. Kaplan-Meier curves for time to all-cause death (*A*) and for time to all-cause death or admission for cardiovascular reasons (*B*). (*From* Gissi-HF Investigators, Tavazzi L, Maggioni AP, et al. Effect of rosuvastatin in patients with chronic heart failure (the GISSI-HF trial): a randomised, double-blind, placebo-controlled trial. Lancet 2008;372(9645):1234; with permission.)

secondary endpoints were neutral as were all subgroup analyses. Similar numbers of patients stopped rosuvastatin and placebo.

CORONA

The CORONA (Controlled rosuvastatin multinational study in heart failure) trial[42] investigated the safety and efficacy of rosuvastatin 10 mg/d in 5011 patients older than 60 years with symptomatic heart failure and at least some evidence of ischemic heart disease. Left ventricular ejection fraction had to be less than 40% unless the patient was in NYHA class II, in which case it had to be less than 35%. Patients with a recent vascular event or with a serum creatinine level greater than 221 μmol/L were excluded. The primary outcome was nonfatal myocardial infarction or stroke or cardiovascular death. The median follow-up was 33 months (**Table 3**).

More than 40% of patients were aged older than 75 years, and most were on full contemporary guideline-indicated therapy. Taking rosuvastatin reduced C-reactive protein, triglyceride, and low-density lipoprotein cholesterol levels (from 3.54 mmol/L to 1.96 mmol/L; $P<.0001$) and increased levels of high-density lipoprotein cholesterol.

The primary composite endpoint occurred in 732 (29%) patients assigned to placebo and 692 (28%) assigned to rosuvastatin (HR, 0.92; 95% CI, 0.83–1.02; $P = .12$), and all-cause mortality was 759 (30%) and 728 (29%), respectively (HR, 0.95; 95% CI, 0.86–1.05; $P = 0.31$) (**Fig. 3**). A non-prespecified outcome of nonfatal or fatal myocardial infarction or stroke was slightly lower in patients assigned to rosuvastatin (HR, 0.84; 95% CI, 0.70–1.00; $P = .05$). There were fewer hospitalizations for

Table 3
Patient characteristics in the CORONA trial

	Placebo	Rosuvastatin
N	2497	2514
Age (y)	73	73
Age >75 y	41%	41%
Women	24%	24%
NYHA II	37%	37%
Body mass index (kg/m²)	27	27
Systolic blood pressure (mm Hg)	129	129
Atrial fibrillation	23%	24%
Defibrillator	3%	3%
Diuretics	88% (75% loop)	89% (76% loop)
Angiotensin-converting enzyme inhibitor or angiotensin II receptor blockers	92%	91%
β-blockers	75%	75%
Aldosterone antagonist	39%	39%
Digoxin	32%	34%
Anticoagulants	34%	36%
NT-proBNP (ng/L)	1404 (600–2960)	1522 (626–3247)
Total cholesterol	5.4	5.4
Low-density lipoprotein cholesterol	3.6	3.5

Data from Kjekshus J, Apetrei E, Barrios V, et al. Rosuvastatin in older patients with systolic heart failure. N Engl J Med 2007;357(22):2250–1; with permission.

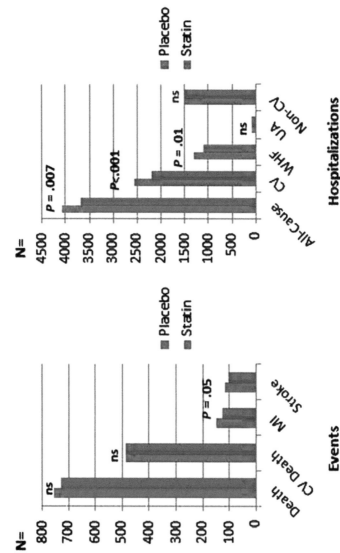

Fig. 3. Events in the CORONA study. Left hand panel shows all-cause and cardiovascular (CV) mortality, myocardial infarction, and stroke (*P* = .05 for the difference between placebo and rosuvastatin on myocardial infarction and stroke combined). Right hand panel shows the number of hospitalization events; all-cause, cardiovascular, worsening heart failure (WHF), unstable angina (UA), and noncardiovascular. (*From* Kjekshus J, Apetrei E, Barrios V, et al. Rosuvastatin in older patients with systolic heart failure. N Engl J Med 2007;357(22):2248–61; with permission.)

cardiovascular causes, including worsening heart failure, in the rosuvastatin group (2193) than the placebo group (2564; *P*<.001; see **Fig. 3**). Withdrawals and adverse effects were similar in each group.

A prespecified subgroup analysis identified little heterogeneity in the results. However, when results were analyzed by tercile of NT-proBNP, patients in the lowest third had the lowest rate of events but the greatest reduction in risk with rosuvastatin. A subsequent analysis, in which the data were combined with those from the Heart Protection study (N = 20,536), comparing simvastatin with placebo in a broad range of older patients at high risk of vascular disease, suggested that the greatest relative benefit of statins was among those with the lowest NT-proBNP.[43] As NT-proBNP increased, the population risk increased, but the relative benefit of simvastatin decreased. Combining the data from CORONA completed the picture, predicting no effect of statins on major vascular events or mortality when values exceeded approximately 800 ng/L (the upper limit of the lower tertile of values in CORONA; **Fig. 4**). However, a reduction in hospitalizations was still observed even with higher NT-proBNP values. An analysis of serum coenzyme Q10 concentrations found that lower levels were associated with a poorer prognosis, but this was explained by greater age and frailty of the patients. Rosuvastatin reduced serum coenzyme Q10, but its effects were similar regardless of baseline or change in serum levels of Q10.[13]

PEARL

The PEARL (Pitavastatin Heart Failure) study enrolled 574 patients with chronic heart failure and randomized them to placebo or pitavsatatin, a lipophilic statin. Pitavastatin failed to reduce the primary composite outcome (cardiac death or hospitalization for worsening heart failure - hazard ratio 0.92, 95% CI 0.63–1.35, *P* = 0.672). However, a strong interaction between assigned treatment and left ventricular ejection fraction

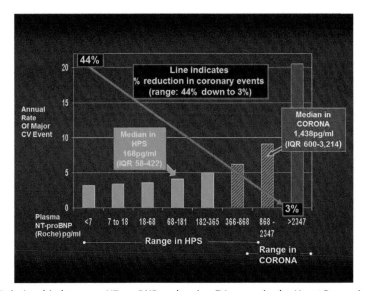

Fig. 4. Relationship between NT-proBNP and major CV events in the Heart Protection Study and CORONA. (*From* Cleland JG, Squire I, Ng L. Interpretation of amino-terminal pro-brain natriuretic peptide levels in the HPS and the CORONA study. J Am Coll Cardiol 2008;52(13):1104; with permission.)

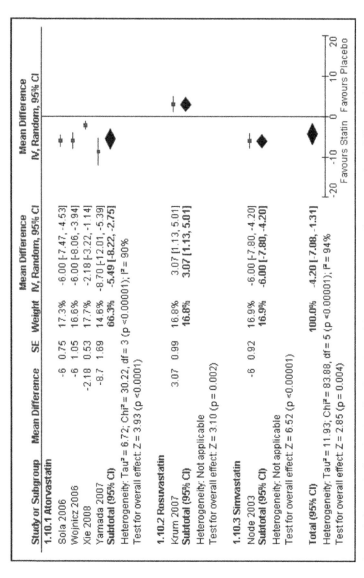

Fig. 5. Effect of statins on left ventricular ejection fraction. Since this report, GISSI-HF also reported no difference between rosuvastatin and placebo. (*From* Lipinski MJ, Cauthen CA, Biondi-Zoccai GG, et al. Meta-analysis of randomized controlled trials of statins versus placebo in patients with heart failure. Am J Cardiol 2009;104(12):1713; with permission.)

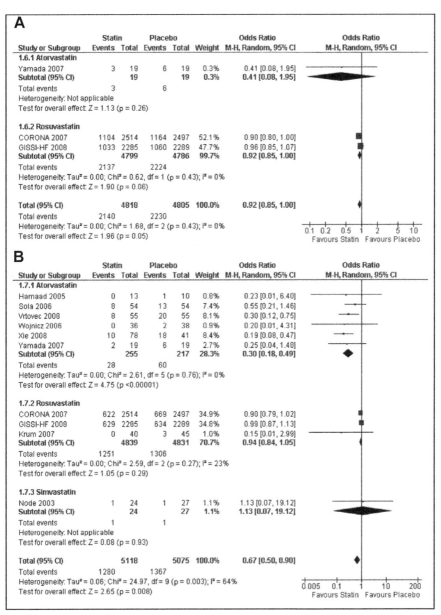

Fig. 6. Comparison of hospitalization outcomes of patients with HF randomized to statin therapy or placebo found no overall benefit for statins compared with placebo for (*A*) hospitalization for cardiovascular causes but found a significant improvement in (*B*) hospitalization for worsening HF for statins compared with placebo. (*From* Lipinski MJ, Cauthen CA, Biondi-Zoccai GG, et al. Meta-analysis of randomized controlled trials of statins versus placebo in patients with heart failure. Am J Cardiol 2009;104(12):1712; with permission.)

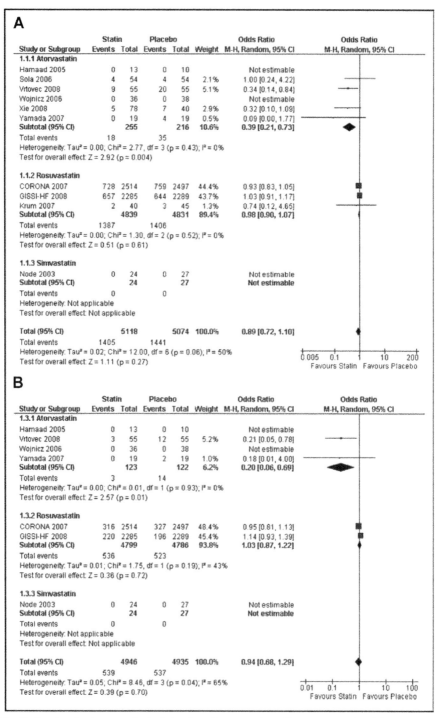

Fig. 7. Randomized, controlled trials of statins reporting all-cause mortality (*A*) or sudden death (*B*) in patients with heart failure. (*From* Lipinski MJ, Cauthen CA, Biondi-Zoccai GG, et al. Meta-analysis of randomized controlled trials of statins versus placebo in patients with heart failure. Am J Cardiol 2009;104(12):1711; with permission.)

was observed ($P = 0.004$); those with an ejection fraction $\geq$30% gained substantial benefit (hazard ratio 0.53, 95% CI 0.31–0.90, $P = 0.018$) with possible harm in those with lower ejection fractions. If ejection fraction is used as a surrogate measure for natriuretic peptides (patients with a markedly depressed ejection fraction are more likely to have increased plasma concentrations of natriuretic peptides), then these results are rather consistent with those from CORONA.[44]

A meta-analysis, not including the PEARL study, identified 10 randomized, controlled trials of statins that enrolled 10,192 patients with heart failure, although more than 95% of patients enrolled were in trials of rosuvastatin.[45] This suggested that simvastatin and atorvastatin but not rosuvastatin might improve left ventricular ejection fraction (**Fig. 5**) and that atorvastatin might be associated with a greater reduction in hospitalization (**Fig. 6**) and a reduction in all-cause mortality (**Fig. 7**) driven by a reduction in sudden death. There are at least 5 possible explanations for these possible differences. First, they may reflect the play of chance, especially given the small numbers of patients and events in trials of atorvastatin. There may be publication bias; small neutral trials often fail to get submitted for or accepted for publication. It is possible that larger doses of statins are more effective, but doses that had similar effects on cholesterol were used in trials of rosuvastatin and atorvastatin. It is possible that patients in trials of atorvastatin were less sick and had lower NT-proBNP. Had patients been matched, then each agent might have been similarly affected. Finally, there might really be an important difference between agents. Atorvastatin and simvastatin are lipophilic but rosuvastatin is not. Greater lipophilicity should lead to higher myocardial concentrations that may account for observed differences. The PEARL study suggests this is not the case.

SUMMARY

So far, lipid-modifying interventions have shown little evidence of benefit in patients with heart failure. The evidence to support the use of fibrates and PUFA in the general population is weak or absent, and patients with heart failure may fare no better. However, for statins, there is clear evidence of benefit in patients that have cardiac damage subsequent to a myocardial infarction but not once the patient has heart failure. There must be a transition point, as many patients occupy a gray area between cardiac dysfunction and heart failure; a sedentary life can conceal heart failure for an extended period. NT-proBNP seems a useful way to stratify patients who are likely to get a mortality benefit from the use of statins; values less than 800 ng/L are associated with benefit. However, statins seem safe and may reduce the risk of hospitalization even in patients with higher levels of NT-proBNP. There might also be differences between statins.

REFERENCES

1. Cleland JG. Is aspirin useful in primary prevention? Eur Heart J 2013;34:3412–8.
2. Cleland JG. Chronic aspirin therapy for the prevention of cardiovascular events: a waste of time or worse? Nat Clin Pract Cardiovasc Med 2006;3(5):234–5.
3. Cleland JG, Atkin SL. Thiazolidinediones, deadly sins, surrogates and elephants. Lancet 2007;370(9593):1103–4.
4. Cleland JG, Witte KK, Steel S. Calcium supplements in people with osteoporosis. BMJ 2010;341:c3856.
5. Cleland JG, Massie BM, Packer M. Sudden death in heart failure: vascular or electrical? Eur J Heart Fail 1999;1:41–5.

6. Tousoulis D, Antoniades C, Bosinakou E, et al. Effects of atorvastatin on reactive hyperaemia and the thrombosis–fibrinolysis system in patients with heart failure. Heart 2005;91:27–31.

7. Unverferth DV, Magorien RD, Lewis RP, et al. The role of subendocardial ischemia in perpetuating myocardial failure in patients with non-ischemic congestive cardiomyopathy. Am Heart J 1983;105:176–9.

8. Tuunanen H, Engblom E, Naum A, et al. Trimetazidine, a metabolic modulator, has cardiac and extracardiac benefits in idiopathic dilated cardiomyopathy. Circulation 2008;118(12):1250–8.

9. Yamagishi K, Nettleton JA, Folsom AR. Plasma fatty acid composition and incident heart failure in middle-aged adults: the Atherosclerosis Risk in Communities (ARIC) Study. Am Heart J 2008;156(5):965–74.

10. Lavie CJ, Milani RV, Mehra MR, et al. Omega-3 polyunsaturated fatty acids and cardiovascular diseases. J Am Coll Cardiol 2009;54(7):585–94.

11. Rauchhaus M, Clark AL, Doehner W, et al. The relationship between cholesterol and survival in patients with chronic heart failure. J Am Coll Cardiol 2003;42:1933–40.

12. Cleland JG, Loh H, Windram J, et al. Threats, opportunities and statins in the modern management of heart failure. Eur Heart J 2006;27(6):641–3.

13. McMurray JJ, Dunselman P, Wedel H, et al, on behalf of the CORONA Study Group. Coenzyme Q10, rosuvastatin, and clinical outcomes in heart failure. J Am Coll Cardiol 2010;56:1196–204.

14. First drug to improve heart failure mortality in over a decade: coenzyme Q10 decreases all-cause mortality by half in randomized double blind trial. Eur Heart J 2013;34(32):2496–7.

15. Node K, Inoue T, Boyko V, et al. Long-term effects of peroxisome proliferator-activated receptor ligand bezafibrate on N-terminal pro-B type natriuretic peptide in patients with advanced functional capacity impairment. Cardiovasc Diabetol 2009;8:5.

16. Rubins HB, Robins SJ, Collins D, et al. Gemfibrozil for the secondary prevention of coronary heart disease in men with low levels of high-density lipoprotein cholesterol. Veterans Affairs High-Density Lipoprotein Cholesterol Intervention Trial Study Group. N Engl J Med 1999;341(6):410–8.

17. Ginsberg HN, Elam MB, Lovato LC, et al. Effects of combination lipid therapy in type 2 diabetes mellitus. N Engl J Med 2010;362(17):1563–74.

18. Jun M, Foote C, Lv J, et al. Effects of fibrates on cardiovascular outcomes: a systematic review and meta-analysis. Lancet 2010;375(9729):1875–84.

19. Cleland JG, Joseph A, Pellicori P. Fish oil vs olive oil for postoperative atrial fibrillation. JAMA 2013;309(9):871.

20. Dietary supplementation with n-3 polyunsaturated fatty acids and vitamin E after myocardial infarction: results of the GISSI-Prevenzione trial. Gruppo Italiano per lo Studio della Sopravvivenza nell'Infarto miocardico. Lancet 1999;354(9177):447–55.

21. Tavazzi L, Maggioni AP, Marchioli R, et al. Effect of n-3 polyunsaturated fatty acids in patients with chronic heart failure (the GISSI-HF trial): a randomised, double-blind, placebo-controlled trial. Lancet 2008;372(9645):1223–30.

22. Ghio S, Scelsi L, Latini R, et al. Effects of n-3 polyunsaturated fatty acids and of rosuvastatin on left ventricular function in chronic heart failure: a substudy of GISSI-HF trial. Eur J Heart Fail 2010;12(12):1345–53.

23. Moertl D, Hammer A, Steiner S, et al. Dose-dependent effects of omega-3-polyunsaturated fatty acids on systolic left ventricular function, endothelial

function, and markers of inflammation in chronic heart failure of nonischemic origin: A double-blind, placebo-controlled, 3-arm study. Am Heart J 2011; 161(5):915.e1–9.

24. Rizos EC, Ntzani EE, Bika E, et al. Association between omega-3 fatty acid supplementation and risk of major cardiovascular disease events: a systematic review and meta-analysis. JAMA 2012;308(10):1024–33.

25. McMurray JJ, Adamopoulos S, Anker SD, et al. ESC guidelines for the diagnosis and treatment of acute and chronic heart failure 2012: the task force for the diagnosis and treatment of acute and chronic heart failure 2012 of the European Society of Cardiology. Developed in collaboration with the Heart Failure Association (HFA) of the ESC. Eur J Heart Fail 2012;14:803–69.

26. Yancy CW, Jessup M, Bozkurt B, et al. 2013 ACCF/AHA guideline for the management of heart failure: a report of the American College of Cardiology Foundation/American Heart Association task force on practice guidelines. J Am Coll Cardiol 2013;62(16):e147–239.

27. Cleland JG, Thygesen K, Uretsky BF, et al. Cardiovascular critical event pathways for the progression of heart failure. A report from the ATLAS study. Eur Heart J 2001;22:1601–12.

28. Khand AU, Gemmell I, Rankin AC, et al. Clinical events leading to the progression of heart failure: insights from a national database of hospital discharges. Eur Heart J 2001;22:153–64.

29. Uretsky B, Thygesen K, Armstrong PW, et al. Acute coronary findings at autopsy in heart failure patients with sudden death: Results from the assessment of treatment with lisinopril and survival study (ATLAS) trial. Circulation 2000;102:611–6.

30. Windram J, Loh PH, Rigby AS, et al. Relationship of high-sensitivity C-reactive protein to prognosis and other prognostic markers in outpatients with heart failure. Am Heart J 2007;153(6):1048–55.

31. Krum H, Latini R, Maggioni AP, et al. Statins and symptomatic chronic systolic heart failure: a post-hoc analysis of 5010 patients enrolled in Val-HeFT. Int J Cardiol 2007;119(1):48–53.

32. Mozaffarian D, Nye R, Levy WC. Statin therapy is associated with lower mortality among patients with severe heart failure. Am J Cardiol 2004;93:1124–9.

33. Go AS, Lee WY, Yang J, et al. Statin therapy and risks for death and hospitalization in chronic heart failure. JAMA 2006;296(17):2105–11.

34. Huan LP, Windram JD, Tin L, et al. The effects of initiation or continuation of statin therapy on cholesterol level and all-cause mortality after the diagnosis of left ventricular systolic dysfunction. Am Heart J 2007;153(4):537–44.

35. Mozaffarian D, Minami E, Letterer RA, et al. The effects of atorvastatin (10 mg) on systemic inflammation in heart failure. Am J Cardiol 2005;96(12):1699–704.

36. Sola S, Mir MQ, Lerakis S, et al. Atorvastatin improves left ventricular systolic function and serum markers of inflammation in nonischemic heart failure. J Am Coll Cardiol 2006;47(2):332–7.

37. Yamada T, Node K, Mine T, et al. Long-term effect of atorvastatin on neurohumoral activation and cardiac function in patients with chronic heart failure: a prospective randomized controlled study. Am Heart J 2007;153(6):1055–8.

38. Wojnicz R, Wilczek K, Nowalany-Kozielska E, et al. Usefulness of atorvastatin in patients with heart failure due to inflammatory dilated cardiomyopathy and elevated cholesterol levels. Am J Cardiol 2006;97(6):899–904.

39. Vrtovec B, Okrajsek R, Golicnik A, et al. Atorvastatin therapy may reduce the incidence of sudden cardiac death in patients with advanced chronic heart failure. J Card Fail 2008;14(2):140–4.

40. Khush KK, Waters DD, Bittner V, et al. Effect of high-dose atorvastatin on hospitalizations for heart failure: subgroup analysis of the Treating to New Targets (TNT) study. Circulation 2007;115(5):576–83.

41. Gissi-HF Investigators, Tavazzi L, Maggioni AP, et al. Effect of rosuvastatin in patients with chronic heart failure (the GISSI-HF trial): a randomised, double-blind, placebo-controlled trial. Lancet 2008;372(9645):1231–9.

42. Kjekshus J, Apetrei E, Barrios V, et al, CORONA Group. Rosuvastatin in older patients with systolic heart failure. N Engl J Med 2007;357(22):2248–61.

43. Cleland JG, Squire I, Ng L. Interpretation of amino-terminal pro-brain natriuretic peptide levels in the HPS and the CORONA study. J Am Coll Cardiol 2008; 52(13):1104–5.

44. Takano H, Mizuma H, Kuwabara Y, et al. Effects of Pitavastatin in Japanese Patients With Chronic Heart Failure: the Pitavastatin Heart Failure Study (PEARL Study). Circ J 2013;77(4):917–25.

45. Lipinski MJ, Cauthen CA, Biondi-Zoccai GG, et al. Meta-analysis of randomized controlled trials of statins versus placebo in patients with heart failure. Am J Cardiol 2009;104(12):1708–16.

Managing Residual Risk After Myocardial Infarction Among Individuals with Low Cholesterol Levels

Lisandro D. Colantonio, MD, MSc[a],*, Vera Bittner, MD, MSPH, FNLA[b]

KEYWORDS

- Myocardial infarction ● Disease management ● Secondary prevention
- Lipid-lowering medications ● Statins ● Ezetimibe

KEY POINTS

- About half of individuals with an acute myocardial infarction (MI) have a low-density lipoprotein cholesterol (LDL-C) level of less than 100 mg/dL.
- Management of individuals with MI and low LDL-C should include cardiac rehabilitation, lifestyle changes, evidence-based post-MI pharmacologic treatment, and adequate control of concomitant coronary risk factors.
- All individuals with a prior MI are recommended to take high-intensity statins (moderate intensity for those ≥75 years of age).
- Ezetimibe can be used as adjunctive lipid-lowering therapy among individuals with an MI and low LDL-C, particularly if they have inadequate response or intolerance to recommended intensity of statins.
- Little evidence exists to support the use of lipid-lowering medications other than ezetimibe in combination with statins among individuals with a prior MI.

INTRODUCTION

Despite substantial improvements in the last 50 years, coronary heart disease (CHD) remains an important cause of morbidity and mortality in the United States and globally.[1] Lipid-lowering medications, particularly statins, have been a core element

This article originally appeared in Cardiology Clinics, Volume 33, Issue 2, May 2015.
Disclosures: V. Bittner has received research support from NIH grant R01 HL080477, Amgen, AstraZeneca, Bayer Healthcare, Janssen Pharmaceuticals, Pfizer, Sanofi Aventis. She has participated in advisory panels for Amgen and Eli Lilly.
[a] Department of Epidemiology, University of Alabama at Birmingham, 1530 3rd Avenue South, RPHB 217C, Birmingham, AL 35294, USA; [b] Division of Cardiovascular Disease, Department of Medicine, University of Alabama at Birmingham, 701 19th Street South, LHRB 310, Birmingham, AL 35294, USA
* Corresponding author.
E-mail address: lcolantonio@uab.edu

of primary and secondary prevention of CHD over the past decades. In 2001, the Third Report of the National Cholesterol Education Program, Expert Panel on Detection, Evaluation, and Treatment of High Blood Cholesterol in Adults (ATP-III) recommended a low-density lipoprotein cholesterol (LDL-C) of less than 100 mg/dL as a therapeutic target in high-risk individuals.[2] An optional therapeutic target of an LDL-C of less than 70 mg/dL was suggested later for very high-risk patients, including those with acute coronary syndrome (ACS) and an LDL-C of less than 100 mg/dL at the time of the event.[3] An increasing number of patients present with LDL-C levels below these targets, but remain at risk for a recurrent event. In this article, we review the current evidence and guidelines on the post-acute event management of individuals with myocardial infarction (MI) and LDL-C of less than 100 mg/dL.

EPIDEMIOLOGY AND SIGNIFICANCE

Cholesterol levels have declined in the United States as awareness of cholesterol as a CHD risk factor and use of statins have increased.[4] As a consequence, the population presenting with MI in the current era is enriched by individuals with low LDL-C. Using data from the Get With The Guidelines program, Sachdeva and colleagues[5] reported that about one-half of individuals hospitalized for MI in 2000 through 2006 had an LDL-C level of less than 100 mg/dL, and 17.6% had an LDL-C of less than 70 mg/dL.

Individuals with an acute MI have an increased risk for recurrent coronary events and death. About 11% of all men and 22% of all women 45 to 64 years of age with a first MI will have a recurrent event or fatal CHD within 5 years (**Fig. 1**).[1] Overall, 14.8% of individuals with a history of atherosclerotic disease will have an MI, stroke, revascularization, or cardiovascular death within 1 year.[6] These figures highlight the importance of considering residual risk among individuals with CHD, including those with low LDL-C levels.

Several factors are associated with risk for a recurrent MI or death in addition to blood cholesterol levels (**Box 1**). A formal appraisal of this residual risk could be performed using the Framingham risk prediction equations for subsequent coronary events, the CRUSADE long-term risk score, or the GRACE prediction tool.[7–9] However, these prediction models have not been incorporated into current guidelines and their applicability to individuals on "optimal medical therapy" is unclear.

Lifestyle changes and evidence-based pharmacologic therapy can effectively reduce risk among individuals with CHD. However, several investigators have shown that prescription of evidence-based post-MI pharmacologic therapy (both in hospital and at discharge) remains inadequate and that adherence to such therapy in the outpatient setting is suboptimal.[10,11] For example, only about 27% of Medicare beneficiaries fill a prescription for high-intensity statins after discharge for an MI.[12]

CURRENT GUIDELINES FOR POST-MYOCARDIAL INFARCTION MANAGEMENT AND SUPPORTING EVIDENCE

Current secondary prevention guidelines in the United States, UK, and Canada emphasize the importance of cardiac rehabilitation, lifestyle changes, and evidence-based post-MI pharmacologic therapy, as well as treatment for complications and other comorbidities in the management of individuals with established CHD.[13–16] Guidelines also emphasize the importance of a shared patient–provider decision-making process, in accordance with the principle of autonomy.

Cardiac Rehabilitation and Lifestyle Changes

Current guidelines recommend referral to and participation in cardiac rehabilitation for all MI survivors.[13,14,16] This recommendation is based on prior clinical trials showing

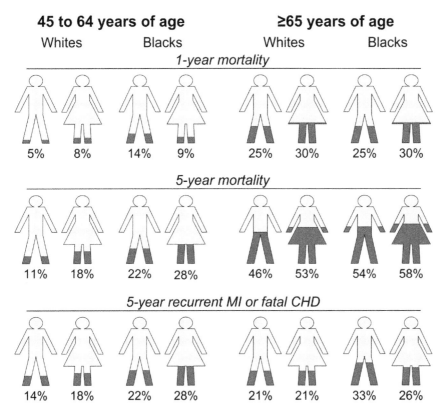

Fig. 1. Risk for all-cause mortality and recurrent myocardial infarction (MI) or coronary heart disease (CHD) death among individuals with a first MI. (*Data from* Go AS, Mozaffarian D, Roger VL, et al. Heart disease and stroke statistics 2014 update: a report from the American Heart Association. Circulation 2014;129:e231.)

Box 1
Factors associated with residual risk for death or recurrent event in secondary prevention for MI

Older age[7,55]

Male sex[55]

Social deprivation[56]

Increased body mass index[55]

Diabetes mellitus[7,55]

Hypertension[7,55]

Heart failure or high Killip class at the presentation of prior MI[9]

Smoking[7,55]

Elevated apolipoprotein B[55]

Reduced apolipoprotein A-I and HDL-C[42,55]

Chronic kidney disease, elevated urea nitrogen, and elevated creatinine[9,55,57]

Anhedonia, depressive mood, anxiety, stress, and type D personality[58–61]

Abbreviations: HDL-C, high-density lipoprotein cholesterol; MI, myocardial infarction.

that exercise-based post-MI cardiac rehabilitation is associated with a lower risk for reinfarction (odds ratio [OR], 0.53; 95% CI, 0.38–0.76), cardiac mortality (OR, 0.64; 95% CI, 0.46–0.88), and all-cause mortality (OR, 0.74; 95% CI, 0.58–0.95) compared with no exercise.[17] An observational study of 1692 individuals with MI showed that those engaged in cardiac rehabilitation were less likely to discontinue prescribed medication, including statins (hazard ratio [HR], 0.66; 95% CI, 0.45–0.92) and β-blockers (HR, 0.70; 95% CI, 0.49–0.98).[18]

Recommendations for lifestyle changes include increasing physical activity, adopting a healthier diet, weight management, and limited alcohol consumption (**Table 1**). Among smokers, smoking status should be assessed at every encounter and smoking cessation counseling should be provided. For those who express their desire to quit, proper support should be offered, including pharmacologic therapy. Current US guidelines also recommend avoiding exposure to air pollution and second-hand smoke.[13]

Evidence-Based Post-Myocardial Infarction Pharmacologic Treatment

Antiplatelet therapy

Several studies have shown that antiplatelet therapy is effective in reducing the risk for vascular events after an MI.[19] Low-dose aspirin (75–150 mg/d) has been shown to be as effective as higher doses and similar to other antiplatelet drugs, and is considered the first choice in current guidelines.[13–15]

Dual antiplatelet therapy (DAPT) is more effective than aspirin alone among individuals with ACS, although the excess risk for bleeding needs to be counterbalanced. In a

Table 1 Recommendations for lifestyle changes according to current guidelines	
Guidelines	**Recommendations**
Increasing physical activity	
2012 US guidelines[a,13]	Perform 30–60 min of moderate-intensity aerobic activity 5–7 days per week.
2013 NICE guidelines (UK)[14]	Exercise 20–30 min a day to the point of slight breathlessness.
2014 CCS guidelines (Canada)[15]	A total of 150 min of moderate to vigorous physical activity cumulated per week.
Adopting a healthier diet	
2012 US guidelines[a,13]	Diet high in fresh fruits, whole grains, and vegetables, with low saturated fat (<7% total calories), cholesterol (<200 mg/dL per day) and trans fat (<1% total calories), and reduced sodium intake.
2013 NICE guidelines (UK)[14]	Mediterranean-style diet.
Limited alcohol consumption	
2012 US guidelines[a,13]	1 drink per day for nonpregnant women and 1–2 drinks per day for men.
2013 NICE guidelines (UK)[14]	No more than 21 and 14 units of alcohol per week for men and nonpregnant women, respectively.

Abbreviations: CCS, Canadian Cardiovascular Society; NICE, National Institute of Health and Care Excellence.
  [a] Guidelines from the American College of Cardiology Foundation, American Heart Association, American College of Physicians, American Association for Thoracic Surgery, Preventive Cardiovascular Nurses Association, Society for Cardiovascular Angiography, Society of Thoracic Surgeons.

metaanalysis of 5 clinical trials comparing aspirin plus clopidogrel versus aspirin monotherapy for secondary prevention, DAPT was associated with a reduced risk for MI (OR, 0.82; 95% CI, 0.75–0.89), stroke (OR, 0.82; 95% CI, 0.73–0.93), and all-cause mortality (OR, 0.94; 95% CI, 0.89–0.99), but increased risk of major bleeding (OR, 1.26; 95% CI, 1.11–1.41).[20]

In the PLATO study, 18,624 individuals with ACS who received aspirin if tolerated were assigned randomly to ticagrelor or clopidogrel.[21] After 12 months follow-up, the risk for MI, stroke or cardiovascular death was lower among those who received ticagrelor (9.8%; HR, 0.84; 95% CI, 0.77–0.92) compared with those assigned to clopidogrel (11.7%), with a similar risk for major bleeding.

Indefinite antiplatelet therapy with aspirin is recommended for all MI survivors.[13,14] The 2013 NICE guidelines recommend DAPT with aspirin/ticagrelor for all individuals with ACS for up to 12 months.[14] The 2014 American College of Cardiology (ACC)/ American Heart Association (AHA) guidelines recommend DAPT with aspirin plus either clopidogrel or ticagrelor for up to 12 months for the management of patients with non–ST-elevation ACS.[16] For those who received drug-eluting stents, DAPT could be extended for up to 30 months according to a recently published clinical trial.[22]

Renin–angiotensin system inhibition

Angiotensin-converting enzyme (ACE) inhibitors reduce cardiovascular risk after MI regardless of the presence of left ventricular dysfunction (LVD).[23,24] In the HOPE study, 9297 individuals without heart failure (HF) but with history of MI, atherosclerotic disease or 2 or more risk factors, including diabetes, were randomly assigned to ramipril 10 mg/d or placebo.[23] After 5 years of follow-up, 14.4% of participants assigned to ramipril had an MI, stroke, or cardiovascular death compared with 17.8% in the control group (P<.001).

The ONTARGET study showed noninferiority of angiotensin-receptor blockade with telmisartan versus ACE inhibition with ramipril to prevent cardiovascular events among 25,620 individuals with atherosclerotic disease without HF.[25] After a median follow-up of 56 months, the risk for death from cardiovascular causes, MI, stroke, or hospitalization for HF among individuals assigned to ramipril or telmisartan was 16.5% and 16.7% (relative risk [RR], 1.01; 95% CI, 0.94–1.09), respectively. The RR associated with telmisartan monotherapy was statistically lower than the noninferiority boundary of 1.13 (P = .003) defined a priori. In this study, combined therapy with telmisartan/ramipril was not superior to ramipril monotherapy (RR, 0.99; 95% CI, 0.92–1.07) and was associated with hypotensive symptoms, renal impairment, and hyperkalemia.

Current US guidelines recommend indefinite therapy with ACE inhibitors for individuals with CHD who have hypertension, diabetes, LVD (<40%), or stable chronic kidney disease and consider it reasonable for individuals with CHD and other vascular disease.[13,16] In contrast, UK and Canadian guidelines recommend ACE inhibition for all individuals with CHD.[14,15] Guidelines agree that angiotensin-receptor blockade should be offered to those with intolerance to ACE inhibitors.[13–15]

β-Blocker therapy

β-Blockers have been a cornerstone in the management of individuals with CHD for decades. In the BHAT study, 3828 individuals with a recent MI (5–21 days after the event) were assigned randomly to propranolol or placebo.[26] After 25.1 months of follow-up, participants assigned to propranolol had a lower risk for all-cause mortality (7.2% vs 9.8%; P<.01), CHD mortality (6.2% vs 8.5%; P<.01), and sudden death

(3.3% vs 4.6%; P<.05) compared with those who received placebo. Similar results were found in the Norwegian timolol study, in which β-blockade reduced the risk for sudden death (7.7% vs 13.9%, P<.001) and reinfarction (14.4% vs 20.1%; P<.001) versus placebo after 33 months of follow-up among 1884 individuals with a recent MI.[27]

Recent studies have questioned the role of β-blockers for secondary prevention in the era of revascularization and statin therapy. Bangalore and colleagues[28] conducted a metaanalysis of 60 randomized, controlled trials with more than 100 participants comparing β-blockers versus placebo, no treatment, or other active treatment among individuals with an MI. β-Blockers were associated with a lower risk for all-cause mortality (RR, 0.86; 95% CI, 0.79–0.94) in studies conducted in the pre-revascularization era (ie, studies with <50% of participants receiving revascularization or a combination of aspirin plus statins), but not in studies conducted in the revascularization era (RR, 0.98; 95% CI, 0.92–1.05). Although β-blockers were associated with a lower risk for recurrent MI in studies conducted in the revascularization era (RR, 0.72; 95% CI, 0.62–0.83), they were also associated with an increased risk for HF (RR 1.10; 95% CI, 1.05–1.16) and cardiogenic shock (RR, 1.29; 95% CI, 1.18–1.40).

In the CHARISMA study initiated in 2002, β-blocker users versus nonusers had lower risk for nonfatal MI, stroke, or cardiovascular death after propensity score adjustment when comparing individuals with a prior MI (7.1% vs 10.2%, respectively; HR, 0.69; 95% CI, 0.50–0.94) but not among those with atherosclerotic disease without MI (6.7% vs 6.2%; HR, 1.06; 95% CI, 0.82–1.38).[29] β-Blockade did not reduce all-cause mortality in either group.

Current guidelines recommend initiation of β-blockade within 24 hours in patients with ACS who do not have signs of acute HF or increased risk for cardiogenic shock or high-degree heart block.[16] β-Blockade is recommended to be continued for up to 3 years for individuals without LVD.[13] Among those with clinically stable LVD, β-blockade with carvedilol, metoprolol succinate, or bisoprolol is recommended to be continued indefinitely given its association with reduced mortality.[13,15]

Statin therapy

Statin therapy after MI reduces major coronary events by 22% (95% CI, 16%–26%) per 1 mm/L (39 mg/dL) reduction in LDL-C.[30] Furthermore, data suggest that individuals with baseline low LDL-C benefit as well. In the Heart Protection Study, participants with a baseline LDL-C of less than 100 mg/dL who were randomly assigned to simvastatin 40 mg/d had a significantly lower risk for nonfatal MI, CHD death, stroke, or revascularization compared with those who received placebo (16.4% vs 21.0%; P<.001).[31]

Several post–ATP-III clinical trials have shown that universal high-intensity statin therapy in secondary prevention is more effective than less intensive therapy, regardless of LDL-C levels.[32–34] In a meta-analysis using individual data from 5 clinical trials, participants assigned to high-intensity statin therapy had lower risk for nonfatal MI, stroke, coronary revascularization, or CHD death compared with those receiving less intensive therapy (4.5% vs 5.3% annually; RR, 0.85; 95% CI, 0.82–0.89).[35] The same association was observed among individuals with an LDL-C level of less than 77 mg/dL at baseline (4.6% vs 5.2% annual risk; RR, 0.71; 95% CI, 0.52–0.98).

Based on this evidence, the 2013 ACC/AHA treatment guidelines recommend high-intensity statin therapy (see definition in **Table 2**) after an MI for those under age 75 without contraindications, regardless of prior therapy or cholesterol levels at the time of the event.[36] For older individuals or those with comorbidities preventing high-intensity statin therapy, moderate-intensity treatment is appropriate. According

Table 2
High-, moderate- and low-intensity statins according to the 2013 ACC/AHA guideline on the treatment of blood cholesterol

Intensity	Generic Drug	Daily Dose (mg)
High-intensity (reduction in LDL-C ≥50% on average)	Atorvastatin	40 or 80
	Rosuvastatin	20 or 40
Moderate-intensity (reduction in LDL-C by ≥30% to <50% on average)	Atorvastatin	10 or 20
	Rosuvastatin	5 or 10
	Simvastatin	20 or 40
	Pravastatin	40 or 80
	Lovastatin	40
	Fluvastatin XL	80
	Fluvastatin	40 twice a day
	Pitavastatin	2 or 4
Low-intensity (reduction in LDL-C by <30% on average)	Simvastatin	10
	Pravastatin	10 or 20
	Lovastatin	20
	Fluvastatin	20 or 40
	Pitavastatin	1

Abbreviations: ACC, American College of Cardiology; AHA, American Heart Association; LDL-C, low-density lipoprotein cholesterol.

Data from Stone NJ, Robinson JG, Lichtenstein AH, et al. 2013 ACC/AHA guideline on the treatment of blood cholesterol to reduce atherosclerotic cardiovascular risk in adults: a report of the American College of Cardiology/American Heart Association Task Force on Practice Guidelines. Circulation 2014;129:S13.

to the guidelines, it is reasonable to add a nonstatin lipid-lowering medication when recommended doses of statins cannot be achieved because of intolerance or if the reduction in LDL-C is less than expected (<50% or <30% vs untreated levels for high- and moderate-intensity therapy, respectively).

Complications and Comorbidities

In addition to lifestyle changes and post-MI pharmacologic treatment, current guidelines emphasize investigation and treatment of complications and comorbidities that may increase cardiovascular risk, including coronary disease with indication for revascularization, diabetes, hypertension, LVD, HF, and chronic kidney disease.[13–16] In addition, US guidelines also recommend annual influenza and pneumococcal vaccination, and management of stress and depression.[13]

MANAGING SERUM LIPIDS IN THE CONTEMPORARY ERA

Meta-analyses and subgroup analyses of individual statin trials suggest that individuals who achieve LDL-C levels well below 100 mg/dL have better outcomes than those who have higher on treatment LDL-C levels, giving rise to the notion that "lower is better."[35] Based on these results, addition of nonstatin lipid-lowering medications may be considered for individuals with a prior MI who are receiving appropriate statin therapy.

The IMPROVE-IT study presented in November 2014 at the AHA Scientific Sessions provides evidence to support the use of combined lipid-lowering therapy for secondary prevention.[37] In this study, 18,144 individuals with ACS and low LDL-C (≤125 mg/dL or ≤100 mg/dL if prior statin therapy; mean LDL-C, 95 mg/dL) were randomized to simvastatin/ezetimibe 40/10 mg/d or simvastatin 40 mg/d (with simvastatin uptitrated to

80 mg if required). After 7 years of follow-up, the simvastatin/ezetimibe group had a 2% absolute risk reduction (32.7% vs 34.7%, $P = .02$) in the primary endpoint of MI, unstable angina, coronary revascularization beyond 30 days, and stroke or cardiovascular death, corresponding with a number needed to treat of 50 participants to prevent 1 event. There were significant reductions in components of this endpoint, including MI, stroke, and combined MI, stroke, or cardiovascular death. However, there were no differences in all-cause or cardiovascular mortality.

Niacin and bile acid sequestrants are other lipid-lowering medications that can reduce LDL-C modestly. Both niacin and bile acid sequestrants, separately or in combination, could be used among individuals with intolerance to statins.[13,36] However, there is limited evidence that adding these medications to recommended doses of statins reduces cardiovascular events.

Proprotein convertase subtilisin kexin type 9 (PCSK9) is a protein that downregulates LDL-C receptors in the liver and is responsible for maintaining serum LDL-C levels. Prior studies have shown that treatment with statin and ezetimibe increases the expression of PCSK9, which may reduce their effectiveness.[38] Recently developed PCSK9 inhibitors reduce LDL-C by about 40% to 70%.[39] These drugs could be used in the future among individuals with familial hypercholesterolemia or statin intolerance, or simply as an adjunct to statins. Several phase III trials are ongoing to assess the efficacy of PCSK9 inhibitors to reduce CHD risk (NCT01764633, NCT01975376, NCT01975389, NCT01663402).

Other Lipid Targets

In addition to LDL-C, other lipid markers are associated with increased risk for recurrent events, including low high-density lipoprotein cholesterol (HDL-C) and high triglycerides.[40,41] Abnormal values for these lipid markers are common among individuals on statin therapy. For example, although 17.6% of patients with MI studied by Sachdeva and colleagues[5] had LDL-C of less than 70 mg/dL at the time of their hospitalization, only 1.4% had both LDL-C of less than 70 mg/dL and HDL-C of 60 mg/dL or higher. Importantly, on statin treatment levels of HDL-C and triglycerides were predictive of cardiovascular events in post hoc analyses of the TNT and PROVE IT-TIMI 22 studies, respectively.[42,43]

Older studies have suggested that fibrates can reduce coronary risk among those with low HDL-C or high triglycerides.[44] However, there are no trials to document incremental benefit from fibrates on statin background therapy. In particular, gemfibrozil use is not recommended in combination with statins because of increased risk for hepatotoxicity and rhabdomyolysis.[45] Two large trials (FIELD and ACCORD) failed to show a benefit of fenofibrate as monotherapy or when added to statins, respectively, among individuals with diabetes.[46,47]

Niacin also increases HDL-C and reduces triglycerides. However, 2 large clinical trials (AIM-HIGH and HPS2-THRIVE) failed to show a benefit when niacin was added to statin background therapy, including among individuals with low HDL-C.[48,49] Importantly, niacin therapy was associated with an increased risk for serious adverse events, including infections.[49,50]

Although trials have shown no effect of adding fibrate or niacin to statin background therapy overall, some subgroup analyses suggest that those with both low HDL-C and high triglycerides may have benefitted.[46,51] Prospective clinical trials are needed to confirm these findings.

Cholesteryl ester transfer protein (CETP) inhibitors substantially increase HDL-C while reducing LDL-C levels to varying degrees. Two outcomes studies with torcetrapib and dalcetrapib were stopped early because of increased risk for cardiovascular

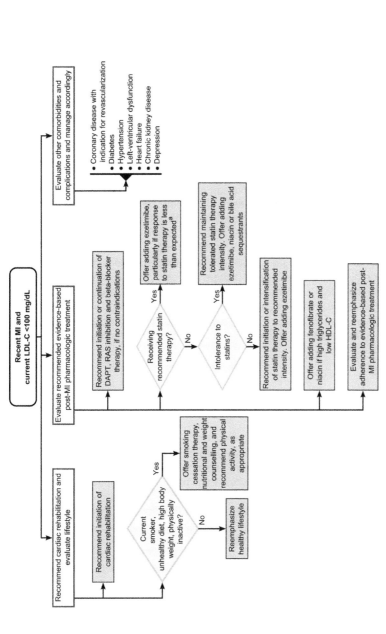

Fig. 2. Summary of evidence-based recommendations and guidelines for management of individuals with MI and LDL-C of less than 100 mg/dL. DAPT, dual antiplatelet therapy; HDL-C, high-density lipoprotein cholesterol; LDL-C, low-density lipoprotein cholesterol; MI, myocardial infarction; RAS, renin–angiotensin system. [a] Less than 50% or less than 30% versus untreated levels for high- and moderate-intensity statins, respectively.

events and all-cause mortality or futility to show benefits for the primary outcome, respectively.[52,53] Trials with other CETP inhibitors are ongoing (NCT01252953, NCT01687998).

SUMMARY

The 2013 ACC/AHA guideline on the treatment of blood cholesterol to reduce atherosclerotic cardiovascular risk in adults has introduced a new paradigm in the management of serum lipids among individuals with MI. All individuals less than 75 years of age with a prior MI are recommended to receive high-intensity statin therapy, regardless of LDL-C levels. A subsequent study suggests that ezetimibe could be considered as adjunctive therapy among individuals on statins. Efforts to further reduce CHD risk among those receiving high-intensity statin therapy with or without ezetimibe should focus on maintaining good adherence to their lipid-lowering regimen, attendance at cardiac rehabilitation, adoption of healthier lifestyles, use of evidence-based post-MI pharmacologic treatment, and achieving adequate control of concomitant cardiovascular risk factors such as hypertension or diabetes (**Fig. 2**).

The high "residual" risk for cardiovascular events among IMPROVE-IT participants on simvastatin/ezetimibe (32.7% after 7 years of follow-up), who had mean LDL-C, HDL-C, and triglycerides of 53, 49, and 126 mg/dL, respectively, suggests that much of this risk in contemporary post-ACS populations is mediated by factors other than dyslipidemia. Given the burden of atherosclerosis generally present at the time of an MI, even the best evidence-based therapy currently available is unlikely to completely eliminate this residual risk. Primordial and primary prevention hold the key to future population health. The recently outlined new paradigm of early atherosclerosis treatment to arrest the disease process should be tested in future trials.[54]

REFERENCES

1. Go AS, Mozaffarian D, Roger VL, et al. Heart disease and stroke statistics–2014 update: a report from the American Heart Association. Circulation 2014;129: e28–292.
2. Expert Panel on Detection, Evaluation, and Treatment of High Blood Cholesterol in Adults. Executive summary of The Third Report of The National Cholesterol Education Program (NCEP) Expert Panel on Detection, Evaluation, and Treatment of High Blood Cholesterol in Adults (Adult Treatment Panel III). JAMA 2001;285: 2486–97.
3. Smith SC Jr, Allen J, Blair SN, et al. AHA/ACC guidelines for secondary prevention for patients with coronary and other atherosclerotic vascular disease: 2006 update: endorsed by the National Heart, Lung, and Blood Institute. Circulation 2006;113:2363–72.
4. Carroll MD, Lacher DA, Sorlie PD, et al. Trends in serum lipids and lipoproteins of adults, 1960-2002. JAMA 2005;294:1773–81.
5. Sachdeva A, Cannon CP, Deedwania PC, et al. Lipid levels in patients hospitalized with coronary artery disease: an analysis of 136,905 hospitalizations in get with the guidelines. Am Heart J 2009;157:111–7.e2.
6. Steg PG, Bhatt DL, Wilson PW, et al. One-year cardiovascular event rates in outpatients with atherothrombosis. JAMA 2007;297:1197–206.
7. D'Agostino RB, Russell MW, Huse DM, et al. Primary and subsequent coronary risk appraisal: new results from the Framingham study. Am Heart J 2000;139: 272–81.

8. Roe MT, Chen AY, Thomas L, et al. Predicting long-term mortality in older patients after non-ST-segment elevation myocardial infarction: the CRUSADE long-term mortality model and risk score. Am Heart J 2011;162:875–83.e1.
9. Fox KA, Dabbous OH, Goldberg RJ, et al. Prediction of risk of death and myocardial infarction in the six months after presentation with acute coronary syndrome: prospective multinational observational study (GRACE). BMJ 2006;333:1091.
10. Arnold SV, Spertus JA, Masoudi FA, et al. Beyond medication prescription as performance measures: optimal secondary prevention medication dosing after acute myocardial infarction. J Am Coll Cardiol 2013;62:1791–801.
11. Olomu AB, Stommel M, Holmes-Rovner MM, et al. Is quality improvement sustainable? Findings of the American College of Cardiology's Guidelines Applied in Practice. Int J Qual Health Care 2014;26:215–22.
12. Rosenson RS, Kent ST, Brown TM, et al. Underutilization of high intensity statin therapy following hospitalization for coronary heart disease. J Am Coll Cardiol 2015;65(3):270–7.
13. Fihn SD, Gardin JM, Abrams J, et al. 2012 ACCF/AHA/ACP/AATS/PCNA/SCAI/STS Guideline for the diagnosis and management of patients with stable ischemic heart disease: a report of the American College of Cardiology Foundation/American Heart Association Task Force on Practice Guidelines, and the American College of Physicians, American Association for Thoracic Surgery, Preventive Cardiovascular Nurses Association, Society for Cardiovascular Angiography and Interventions, and Society of Thoracic Surgeons. J Am Coll Cardiol 2012;60:e44–164.
14. National Institute for Health and Care Excellence. Secondary prevention in primary and secondary care for patients following a myocardial infarction. Clinical guideline 172. London: National Institute for Health and Care Excellence (NICE); 2013. Available at. http://www.gserve.nice.org.uk/ourguidance/reference.jsp?textonly=true.
15. Mancini GB, Gosselin G, Chow B, et al. Canadian Cardiovascular Society guidelines for the diagnosis and management of stable ischemic heart disease. Can J Cardiol 2014;30:837–49.
16. Amsterdam EA, Wenger NK, Brindis RG, et al. 2014 AHA/ACC guideline for the management of patients with non-ST-elevation acute coronary syndromes: A report of the American College of Cardiology/American Heart Association Task Force on Practice Guidelines. J Am Coll Cardiol 2014;64(24):e139–228.
17. Lawler PR, Filion KB, Eisenberg MJ. Efficacy of exercise-based cardiac rehabilitation post-myocardial infarction: a systematic review and meta-analysis of randomized controlled trials. Am Heart J 2011;162:571–84.e2.
18. Shah ND, Dunlay SM, Ting HH, et al. Long-term medication adherence after myocardial infarction: experience of a community. Am J Med 2009;122:961.e7–13.
19. Antithrombotic Trialists' Collaboration. Collaborative meta-analysis of randomised trials of antiplatelet therapy for prevention of death, myocardial infarction, and stroke in high risk patients. BMJ 2002;324:71–86.
20. Helton TJ, Bavry AA, Kumbhani DJ, et al. Incremental effect of clopidogrel on important outcomes in patients with cardiovascular disease: a meta-analysis of randomized trials. Am J Cardiovasc Drugs 2007;7:289–97.
21. Wallentin L, Becker RC, Budaj A, et al. Ticagrelor versus clopidogrel in patients with acute coronary syndromes. N Engl J Med 2009;361:1045–57.
22. Mauri L, Kereiakes DJ, Yeh RW, et al. Twelve or 30 months of dual antiplatelet therapy after drug-eluting stents. N Engl J Med 2014;371(23):2155–66.

23. Yusuf S, Sleight P, Pogue J, et al. Effects of an angiotensin-converting-enzyme inhibitor, ramipril, on cardiovascular events in high-risk patients. The Heart Outcomes Prevention Evaluation Study Investigators. N Engl J Med 2000;342:145–53.
24. Fox KM. Efficacy of perindopril in reduction of cardiovascular events among patients with stable coronary artery disease: randomised, double-blind, placebo-controlled, multicentre trial (the EUROPA study). Lancet 2003;362:782–8.
25. Yusuf S, Teo KK, Pogue J, et al. Telmisartan, ramipril, or both in patients at high risk for vascular events. N Engl J Med 2008;358:1547–59.
26. A randomized trial of propranolol in patients with acute myocardial infarction. I. Mortality results. JAMA 1982;247:1707–14.
27. Timolol-induced reduction in mortality and reinfarction in patients surviving acute myocardial infarction. N Engl J Med 1981;304:801–7.
28. Bangalore S, Makani H, Radford M, et al. Clinical outcomes with beta-blockers for myocardial infarction: a meta-analysis of randomized trials. Am J Med 2014;127:939–53.
29. Bangalore S, Bhatt DL, Steg PG, et al. β-Blockers and cardiovascular events in patients with and without myocardial infarction: post hoc analysis from the CHARISMA trial. Circ Cardiovasc Qual Outcomes 2014;7(6):872–81.
30. Baigent C, Keech A, Kearney PM, et al. Efficacy and safety of cholesterol-lowering treatment: prospective meta-analysis of data from 90,056 participants in 14 randomised trials of statins. Lancet 2005;366:1267–78.
31. Heart Protection Study Collaborative Group. MRC/BHF Heart Protection Study of cholesterol lowering with simvastatin in 20,536 high-risk individuals: a randomised placebo-controlled trial. Lancet 2002;360:7–22.
32. Cannon CP, Braunwald E, McCabe CH, et al. Intensive versus moderate lipid lowering with statins after acute coronary syndromes. N Engl J Med 2004;350:1495–504.
33. Pedersen TR, Faergeman O, Kastelein JJ, et al. High-dose atorvastatin vs usual-dose simvastatin for secondary prevention after myocardial infarction: the IDEAL study: a randomized controlled trial. JAMA 2005;294:2437–45.
34. LaRosa JC, Grundy SM, Waters DD, et al. Intensive lipid lowering with atorvastatin in patients with stable coronary disease. N Engl J Med 2005;352:1425–35.
35. Baigent C, Blackwell L, Emberson J, et al. Efficacy and safety of more intensive lowering of LDL cholesterol: a meta-analysis of data from 170,000 participants in 26 randomised trials. Lancet 2010;376:1670–81.
36. Stone NJ, Robinson JG, Lichtenstein AH, et al. 2013 ACC/AHA guideline on the treatment of blood cholesterol to reduce atherosclerotic cardiovascular risk in adults: a report of the American College of Cardiology/American Heart Association Task Force on Practice Guidelines. Circulation 2014;129:S1–45.
37. IMPROVE-IT: Ezetimibe/simvastatin vs simvastatin monotherapy on CV outcomes after ACS. Cardiosource, American College of Cardiology, 2014. Available at: http://www.cardiosource.org/news-media/publications/cardiology-magazine/2014/11/improve-it-ezetimibe-simvastatin-vs-simvastatin-monotherapy-on-cv-outcomes-after-acs.aspx?WT.mc_id=Twitter. Accessed November 18, 2014.
38. Gouni-Berthold I, Berthold HK, Gylling H, et al. Effects of ezetimibe and/or simvastatin on LDL receptor protein expression and on LDL receptor and HMG-CoA reductase gene expression: a randomized trial in healthy men. Atherosclerosis 2008;198:198–207.
39. Hochholzer W, Giugliano RP. Does it make sense to combine statins with other lipid-altering agents following AIM-HIGH, SHARP and ACCORD? Curr Atheroscler Rep 2013;15:290.

40. Nguyen SV, Nakamura T, Kugiyama K. High remnant lipoprotein predicts recurrent cardiovascular events on statin treatment after acute coronary syndrome. Circ J 2014;78:2492–500.
41. Sirimarco G, Labreuche J, Bruckert E, et al. Atherogenic dyslipidemia and residual cardiovascular risk in statin-treated patients. Stroke 2014;45:1429–36.
42. Barter P, Gotto AM, LaRosa JC, et al. HDL cholesterol, very low levels of LDL cholesterol, and cardiovascular events. N Engl J Med 2007;357:1301–10.
43. Miller M, Cannon CP, Murphy SA, et al. Impact of triglyceride levels beyond low-density lipoprotein cholesterol after acute coronary syndrome in the PROVE IT-TIMI 22 trial. J Am Coll Cardiol 2008;51:724–30.
44. Jun M, Foote C, Lv J, et al. Effects of fibrates on cardiovascular outcomes: a systematic review and meta-analysis. Lancet 2010;375:1875–84.
45. Graham DJ, Staffa JA, Shatin D, et al. Incidence of hospitalized rhabdomyolysis in patients treated with lipid-lowering drugs. JAMA 2004;292:2585–90.
46. Ginsberg HN, Elam MB, Lovato LC, et al. Effects of combination lipid therapy in type 2 diabetes mellitus. N Engl J Med 2010;362:1563–74.
47. Tonkin A, Hunt D, Voysey M, et al. Effects of fenofibrate on cardiovascular events in patients with diabetes, with and without prior cardiovascular disease: the Fenofibrate Intervention and Event Lowering in Diabetes (FIELD) study. Am Heart J 2012;163:508–14.
48. Boden WE, Probstfield JL, Anderson T, et al. Niacin in patients with low HDL cholesterol levels receiving intensive statin therapy. N Engl J Med 2011;365:2255–67.
49. Landray MJ, Haynes R, Hopewell JC, et al. Effects of extended-release niacin with laropiprant in high-risk patients. N Engl J Med 2014;371:203–12.
50. Anderson TJ, Boden WE, Desvigne-Nickens P, et al. Safety profile of extended-release niacin in the AIM-HIGH trial. N Engl J Med 2014;371:288–90.
51. Guyton JR, Slee AE, Anderson T, et al. Relationship of lipoproteins to cardiovascular events: the AIM-HIGH Trial (Atherothrombosis Intervention in Metabolic Syndrome With Low HDL/High Triglycerides and Impact on Global Health Outcomes). J Am Coll Cardiol 2013;62:1580–4.
52. Barter PJ, Caulfield M, Eriksson M, et al. Effects of torcetrapib in patients at high risk for coronary events. N Engl J Med 2007;357:2109–22.
53. Schwartz GG, Olsson AG, Abt M, et al. Effects of dalcetrapib in patients with a recent acute coronary syndrome. N Engl J Med 2012;367:2089–99.
54. Robinson JG, Gidding SS. Curing atherosclerosis should be the next major cardiovascular prevention goal. J Am Coll Cardiol 2014;63:2779–85.
55. Mora S, Wenger NK, Demicco DA, et al. Determinants of residual risk in secondary prevention patients treated with high- versus low-dose statin therapy: the Treating to New Targets (TNT) study. Circulation 2012;125:1979–87.
56. Buckley BS, Simpson CR, McLernon DJ, et al. Five year prognosis in patients with angina identified in primary care: incident cohort study. BMJ 2009;339:b3058.
57. Weiner DE, Tighiouart H, Stark PC, et al. Kidney disease as a risk factor for recurrent cardiovascular disease and mortality. Am J Kidney Dis 2004;44:198–206.
58. Davidson KW, Burg MM, Kronish IM, et al. Association of anhedonia with recurrent major adverse cardiac events and mortality 1 year after acute coronary syndrome. Arch Gen Psychiatry 2010;67:480–8.
59. Denollet J, Pedersen SS, Vrints CJ, et al. Usefulness of type D personality in predicting five-year cardiac events above and beyond concurrent symptoms of stress in patients with coronary heart disease. Am J Cardiol 2006;97:970–3.

60. Rosengren A, Hawken S, Ounpuu S, et al. Association of psychosocial risk factors with risk of acute myocardial infarction in 11119 cases and 13648 controls from 52 countries (the INTERHEART study): case-control study. Lancet 2004; 364:953–62.
61. Ye S, Muntner P, Shimbo D, et al. Behavioral mechanisms, elevated depressive symptoms, and the risk for myocardial infarction or death in individuals with coronary heart disease: the REGARDS (Reason for Geographic and Racial Differences in Stroke) study. J Am Coll Cardiol 2013;61:622–30.

Lifestyle Intervention
Nutrition Therapy and Physical Activity

Alison B. Evert, MS, RD, CDE[a],*, Michael C. Riddell, PhD[b]

KEYWORDS

- Medical nutrition therapy • Weight loss • Carbohydrate • Lifestyle intervention
- Physical activity • Exercise

KEY POINTS

- An individualized nutrition plan should be discussed with patients in a series of encounters with a registered dietitian starting at the time of diabetes diagnosis.
- Diabetes meal planning approaches should include instruction on a variety of topics including carbohydrate counting, healthy food choices, glycemic index, Mediterranean-style diet, low and high sodium foods, low-fat and low-carbohydrate diets.
- Early engagement in physical activity halts or slows the progression of type 2 diabetes development. Activities should include aerobic activities (at least 150 minutes per week) and resistance training 2-3 days per week.
- Accommodation to permit physical activity engagement for all patients with obesity and or diabetes should be performed.
- For patients attempting to lose weight, a mild to moderate daily energy deficit is needed (10-25% relative caloric restriction).

INTRODUCTION

Diabetes and obesity are major health concerns in the United States.[1-5] It is estimated that more than 3 out of every 4 adults with diabetes are overweight.[6] In a nationally representative sample of US adults, the prevalence of diabetes was found to increase with increasing weight classes.[7] The survey revealed that nearly one-fourth of adults with diabetes in this sample had poor glycemic control (defined as hemoglobin A1c [HbA1c] level >8.0%) and nearly half were considered obese.[7] Being obese with diabetes increases insulin resistance and negatively affects glucose tolerance, thereby making glycemic targets more difficult to achieve pharmacologically.

This article originally appeared in Medical Clinics, Volume 99, Issue 1, January 2015.
[a] Diabetes Education Programs, Diabetes Care Center, University of Washington Medical Center, 4245 Roosevelt Way Northeast, 3rd Floor, Seattle, WA 98105, USA; [b] Muscle Health Research Center, School of Kinesiology and Health Science, Bethune College, York University, 4700 Keele Street, 3rd Floor, Toronto, Ontario M3J1P3, Canada
* Corresponding author.
E-mail address: atevert@u.washington.edu

Public health authorities and medical professionals have recommended weight loss as a therapeutic strategy for patients who are obese or who are overweight with co-morbid conditions such as diabetes for several years.[8] The 1998 Clinical Guidelines on the Identification, Evaluation, and Treatment of Overweight and Obesity in Adults state that, "the initial goal of weight loss therapy should be to reduce body weight by approximately 10% from baseline."[9] Recommended weight-loss strategies included a low-calorie diet to create a deficit of 500 to 1000 kcal/d, behavior therapy, and increased physical activity. More recently, lifestyle intervention strategies have been incorporated into clinically effective diabetes prevention trials around the world.[5,10,11] These strategies have also been found to be integral components of the treatment and management of type 2 diabetes, with documented improvements in weight, depression scores, quality of life, and various biochemical markers of health status.[12,13] Lifestyle intervention seems to be particularly beneficial early in the natural history of type 2 diabetes, before loss of beta cell function and mass becomes so extensive that multidrug pharmacotherapy is required to achieve optimal glycemic control.[14,15]

As type 2 diabetes progresses over the years with the continued loss of beta cell function and enduring insulin resistance, medications are often added to the treatment plan to achieve optimal glycemic control. From a lifestyle perspective, a reduced energy intake with an emphasis on nutrient-dense, fiber-rich foods (**Box 1**) along with regular physical activity should be priorities for all individuals living with type 2 diabetes.[2] However, people with diabetes, as well as their health care providers, are reluctant to initiate the use of medication for fear of weight gain. Referral to a registered dietitian (RD) for nutrition therapy has been shown to help mitigate this unwanted side effect of treatment.[16-20] In addition, successful lifestyle intervention typically reduces the reliance on pharmacologic agents to achieve glycemic targets.[12] Therefore, regardless of duration of diabetes in years, nutrition therapy remains a key treatment strategy.

Because of the importance of physical activity in enhancing weight loss and supporting weight maintenance, and the increasingly strong evidence that increased physical activity and fitness level can affect health independently of body mass index,[21] it is important to have interventions available that can lead to sustained changes in physical activity. The role of physical activity in treatment of type 2 diabetes is elaborated later in this article.

Box 1
Nutrient-dense foods

Nutrient density is a measure of the amount of nutrients a food contains compared with the number of calories. A food is more nutrient dense when the level of nutrients is high in relation to the number of calories the food contains.

Nutrient-dense food choices include the following:

• Grains, especially whole grains

• Fruits and vegetables: fresh, frozen, or canned with so-called lite sodium

• Fat-free or low-fat milk or dairylike products

• Lean protein sources or meat alternatives such as beans, lentils, and unsalted nuts

• Substitute unsaturated (liquid fats such as olive, canola, corn, safflower oil) for foods higher in saturated (solid fats) or *trans* fats as much as possible.

NONPHARMACOLOGIC TREATMENT OPTIONS: LIFESTYLE INTERVENTION: NUTRITION THERAPY

In a recent position statement for the management of hyperglycemia in type 2 diabetes the American Diabetes Association (ADA) and European Association for the Study of Diabetes endorse a patient-centered approach.[22] At diagnosis, before initiating pharmacotherapy, highly motivated patients with HbA1c already near target levels (eg, 7.5%) should be given the opportunity to participate in lifestyle change for a period of 3 to 6 months. Individuals with moderate hyperglycemia or in whom lifestyle changes are anticipated to be unsuccessful could be started on an antihyperglycemic agent (usually metformin) at diagnosis, which can later be modified or possibly discontinued if lifestyle changes are successful. Pharmacologic treatment options for type 2 diabetes are discussed in detail elsewhere in this issue.

Diabetes Nutrition Therapy: How Is It Provided?

People with diabetes should ideally be referred to an RD, and preferably one who is knowledgeable and skilled in providing diabetes medical nutrition therapy (MNT) soon after diagnosis.[23] Another option is participation in a comprehensive diabetes self-management education (DSME) program that includes instruction on nutrition.[23] Many insurance plans and Medicare cover MNT and DSME. These services require a referral or prescription from the health care provider and it is important to confirm coverage in advance of receiving service. Some insurance plans require preauthorization before diabetes self-management or nutrition consultation services are covered. Medicare typically covers up to 10 hours of initial DSME and 3 hours of MNT, and up to 2 hours of each type of service in subsequent years. However, national data in the United States indicate that only about a half of all persons with diabetes receive diabetes education and even fewer see an RD.[6] One study of more than 18,000 people with diabetes revealed that only 9.1% had at least 1 nutrition visit within a 9-year period.[24]

Diabetes Medical Nutrition Therapy: The Process

MNT is based on an assessment of lifestyle changes that would assist the person with diabetes in achieving and maintaining clinical goals[3] and has been shown to be effective in diabetes management.[2] The Academy of Nutrition and Dietetics Evidence-Based Nutrition Practice Guidelines recommend the following structure for the implementation of MNT for adults with diabetes[25]:

- A series of 3 to 4 encounters with RDs lasting from 45 to 90 minutes
  - The series of encounters should begin at diagnosis of diabetes or at first referral to an RD for MNT for diabetes and should be completed within 3 to 6 months.
- The RD should determine whether additional MNT encounters are needed.
- At least 1 follow-up encounter is recommended annually to reinforce lifestyle changes and to evaluate and monitor outcomes that indicate the need for changes in MNT or medications.
  - An RD should determine whether additional MNT encounters are needed.

The RD prioritizes nutrition therapy based on a thorough nutrition assessment of the individual. Once an assessment has been completed, the RD determines the nutrition diagnosis, which includes the presence of, risk of, or potential for developing a nutritional deficit that can be addressed by nutrition therapy. Nutrition interventions are specific actions to remedy the nutrition diagnosis and can include clinical and behavioral goals collaboratively agreed on with the person with diabetes, as well as specific nutrition intervention strategies. These strategies might include selecting a meal-planning strategy such as carbohydrate counting or the plate method, or education on topics such as how to read food labels, portion control, or tips for eating out. In addition, monitoring outcomes and providing ongoing support are also key components of MNT.

Individualization of the Eating Plan

The ADA 2013 position statement, *Nutrition Therapy: Recommendations for the Management of Adults with Diabetes* recommends the development of an individualized eating plan as needed to achieve treatment goals with ongoing support and encouragement to assist with health behavior change.[2] The eating plan should be based on the individual's personal and cultural preferences, literacy and numeracy, and readiness to change, because there is no single eating plan that meets the needs of all adults with diabetes. Food choices should not be limited unnecessarily but should be guided by scientific evidence and the need to delay or prevent complications of diabetes.

In the past a nutrition prescription included a specified calorie level and macronutrient percentage. However, despite efforts since 1994 to promote the individualization of the meal plan, the ADA diet continues to be prescribed. A recent systematic review found that there continues to be no ideal macronutrient distribution for the nutritional management of diabetes.[26] Research has also shown that a wide variety of diabetes meal-planning approaches and eating patterns can be clinically effective, with many including a reduced energy component.[2] Examples include carbohydrate counting, healthy food choices, glycemic index, as well as eating patterns such as the Mediterranean-style diet, Dietary Approach to Stop Hypertension, vegan or vegetarian, and low-fat and low-carbohydrate diets.

NONPHARMACOLOGIC TREATMENT OPTIONS: LIFESTYLE INTERVENTION: PHYSICAL ACTIVITY

Regular physical activity can help people with type 2 diabetes achieve a variety of goals,[27,28] including:

- Increased cardiorespiratory fitness and vigor
- Improved glycemic control
- Decreased insulin resistance
- An improved lipid profile
- Reduced blood pressure
- Maintenance of a healthy body mass after weight loss
- Less depression and anxiety
- Less sleep apnea
- Less medication use
- An overall improved quality of life

However, it is doubtful whether increased physical activity provides significant protection against premature mortality from heart disease and stroke in patients already diagnosed with type 2 diabetes.[12] Nonetheless, a healthful eating plan and regular exercise when implemented soon after diagnosis in a real-world health care setting improves markers of inflammation and the cardiovascular risk profile in patients with type 2 diabetes.[29] In adolescents with type 2 diabetes, regular physical activity is associated with lower HbA1c levels, lower body mass index, and higher HDL-cholesterol levels but not lower medication use.[30]

Definitions and Types of Activity

Physical activity is defined as any body movement caused by the contraction of skeletal muscle that substantially increases energy expenditure.[31] Physical activity comes in a variety of forms and may be performed during a person's occupation or as a leisure activity. It can also be performed at a range of intensities and this is typically expressed either in absolute terms (eg, metabolic equivalents, mL/kg/min, kcal/min), or in relative terms (eg, percent heart rate reserve, percent maximal oxygen consumption [Vo_{2max}], ratings of perceived exertion scale).

Exercise is a structured form of physical activity that can be prescribed as a therapeutic dose with a recommended type, intensity, and volume (ie, duration and frequency). Aerobic exercise, such as walking, bicycling, or jogging, is physical activity that involves continuous, rhythmic movements of large muscle groups lasting for at least 10 minutes at a time. Resistance exercise is physical activity involving brief repetitive exercises with weights, weight machines, resistance bands, or the person's own body weight to increase muscle strength (eg, pushups, sit-ups, and pull-ups). Flexibility exercise, such as lower back or hamstring stretching, is a form of activity that enhances the ability of joints to move through their full ranges of motion.

Recommendations on Type, Intensity, and Volume of Exercise

The American College of Sports Medicine and the ADA joint Position Stands recommendations suggest both aerobic and resistance-type exercise for people with prediabetes or type 2 diabetes.[32] A summary of recommendations is shown in **Table 1**. A goal of 150 minutes per week of accumulated moderate-intensity aerobic exercise is recommended for all patients with diabetes as long as this volume of exercise can be tolerated by the individual.[32] In general, aerobic exercise in the form of brisk walking on level ground, cycling, or recumbent cycling for those with joint pain with walking, are preferred activities for overweight/obese elderly patients with diabetes.[33]

Table 1
American College of Sports Medicine and the ADA recommendations for aerobic and resistance-type exercise for people with prediabetes or type 2 diabetes (PMID: 21115771)

Definitions, Examples and Frequency	Intensity	Examples
Aerobic exercise: rhythmic, repeated, and continuous movements of large muscle groups for at least 10 min at a time	Moderate: 50%–70% of person's maximum heart rate, or 40%–60% of heart rate reserve, or about 4–6 metabolic equivalents	Brisk walking (9–12 min per km [15–20 min per mile]), dancing, continuous swimming, biking, raking leaves, water aerobics
Performed daily or every other day	Vigorous: >70% of a person's maximum heart rate, or	Jogging, walking up an incline, aerobics, team
Total amount = 150–175 min/wk (moderate to vigorous intensity)	60%–85% of heart rate reserve, or about 6–8 metabolic equivalents	sports (soccer, hockey, basketball), fast swimming, fast dancing
Resistance exercise: activities that use muscular strength to move against a weight or against a load[a]	Start with 1 set of 10–15 repetitions at moderate weight	Exercise with weight machines
Performed 2–3 times per week	Progress to 2 sets of 10–15 repetitions	Weight lifting
	Progress to 3 sets of 8 repetitions at heavier weight	Sit-ups, pull-ups (assisted), and pushups (modified if necessary)

[a] Initial instruction and periodic supervision by a qualified exercise professional are recommended.

More vigorous activities, such as walking up hills or jogging, can be encouraged for middle-aged and younger patients. In addition, resistance exercise performed 2 or 3 times per week provides additional benefits that complement those of aerobic training (eg, increased lean mass and strength, reduced body fat, increased resting metabolic rate).[34,35]

TREATMENT RESISTANCE AND COMPLICATIONS: NUTRITION THERAPY AND PHYSICAL ACTIVITY

It is essential that people with diabetes are actively involved with health professionals to collaboratively develop appropriate nutrition interventions and an individualized eating pattern that they can implement. Multiple encounters to provide education and counseling initially and on a continued basis are also essential.[36] Because of the progressive nature of type 2 diabetes, nutrition therapy recommendations often need to be adjusted over time based on changes in life circumstance, preferences, and disease course. Progression of diabetes complications may be modified by improving glycemic control, reducing blood pressure, and reducing fat intake.[2]

Because cardiovascular disease (CVD) is a common cause of death among individuals with and without diabetes, nutrition recommendations similar to those for the general population to manage CVD risk factors should be followed. The Dietary Guidelines for Americans 2010 recommendations include reducing saturated fats to less than 10% of calories, aiming for 300 mg of dietary cholesterol per day, and limiting *trans* fat as much as possible.[37] In people with type 2 diabetes, a Mediterranean-style, monounsaturated fatty acid–rich eating pattern may also benefit glycemic control and CVD risk factors and can, therefore, be recommended as an effective alternative to a lower-fat, higher-carbohydrate eating pattern.[2,14,38–40]

Evidence from 2 meta-analyses shows no clear benefits for individuals with diabetic neuropathy on renal parameters from protein-restricted diets.[41,42] Therefore reducing protein intake to less than the usual intake for people with diabetes and diabetic kidney disease (either microalbuminuria or macroalbuminuria) is not recommended because it does not alter glycemic measures, cardiovascular risk measures, or the course of glomerular filtration rate decline.[2]

Although regular physical activity is clearly beneficial for patients with diabetes, compliance with recommendations is often poor. Compared with physical activity advice only, supervised programs involving both aerobic and resistance exercise are associated with better improvements in glycemic control in people with type 2 diabetes.[43] Supervision helps with instruction, safety, motivation, and the capacity to overcome any physical barriers. Unsupervised exercise programs usually fail to improve glycemic control on their own, but can be associated with improved HbA1c levels if they are done with dietary intervention.[43] Exercise dropout remains a major limitation, with ~ 60% of patients failing to maintain both aerobic and resistance-type exercises after a lifestyle intervention.[44] However, motivational interviewing following a lifestyle intervention improves the maintenance of physical activity in people with type 2 diabetes.[45]

Although having diabetes increases the risk of having underlying CVD and other comorbidities, there is little evidence to suggest that moderate-intensity exercise triggers adverse cardiovascular events or worsens disease complications in people with diabetes.[46] Nonetheless, before beginning a program of vigorous physical activity, people with diabetes should be assessed for conditions that might increase risks associated with certain types of exercise or predispose them to injury.[33] Before establishing an exercise prescription, health care providers should pay attention to and talk to patients about the following relative contraindications for vigorous exercise[46]:

- Severe autonomic neuropathy (symptoms during exertion may include dizziness)
- Severe peripheral neuropathy (feet should be inspected regularly and proper footwear is required)
- Proliferative retinopathy (should be treated before starting resistance exercise or vigorous aerobic exercise)
- CVD (symptoms may or may not include dyspnea, or chest discomfort)
- Musculoskeletal issues (back, hip, and/or knee problems)

Initial physical assessment before initiating a new program of vigorous exercise should include a resting electrocardiogram and possibly a stress test for individuals with possible CVD.[27] Patients with severe autonomic neuropathy, severe peripheral neuropathy, preproliferative or proliferative retinopathy, and unstable angina should be stabilized and exercise only at a low intensity for brief periods (eg, 10–15 minutes of walking) under appropriate supervision. This type of activity may be best done in a cardiac rehabilitation setting.[47,48] Patients with severe peripheral neuropathy should be instructed to inspect their feet daily, especially on days in which they are physically active, and to wear appropriate footwear.[33] Patients with movement disorders, pain, or any physical limitations should be supervised by a qualified exercise professional.

The risk of hypoglycemia during exercise is of concern for all patients with diabetes who are taking insulin or insulin secretagogues (sulfonylureas and meglitinides). Reductions in insulin administration or oral secretagogues may be needed once the new exercise pattern is established. Patients should be encouraged to monitor their blood glucose levels regularly and to treat hypoglycemia accordingly. As a general rule, patients should indicate in their log books the level of blood glucose just before initiating an exercise session (eg, walking, physically demanding chores) and following every 30 to 45 minutes of sustained activity. Hypoglycemia can be prevented and/or treated by the consumption of 15 to 30 g of fast-acting carbohydrate before exercise or when hypoglycemia develops. If hypoglycemia develops regularly with increased activity levels, perhaps because of a change in routine, then a reduction in exogenous insulin (or oral hypoglycemic agent) should be considered. Patients taking insulin can reduce mealtime insulin by 25% to 50% at the meal before exercise if the activity follows after a meal.[49] Reductions in basal insulin should also be made if the activity is particularly prolonged or regular (every day).

Education on the treatment of mild hypoglycemia includes the assessment of the individual's ability to recognize foods that contain carbohydrate and how these foods affect blood glucose. Based on the 2013 ADA/Endocrine Society Scientific Statement, as a starting point the treatment of hypoglycemia should include carrying carbohydrate foods such as glucose tablets, as well as education on how to use them[50]:

- Take 15 g of glucose or half a cup of fruit juice
- Wait 15 minutes
- Remeasure blood glucose level
- Repeat if hypoglycemia persists

People with diabetes may be more susceptible to adverse events associated with hot environments, perhaps because of reduced capacity to dissipate heat.[51] Thus, elderly patients in particular and those with autonomic neuropathy, cardiac disease, or pulmonary disease should take care to avoid heat-related illness. Precautions may include exercising indoors in cool environments or outdoors in the early or later hours of the day during hot or sunny days.

EVALUATION OF OUTCOME: NUTRITION THERAPY AND PHYSICAL ACTIVITY

Diabetes nutrition therapy has been found to be an effective component of a comprehensive group education program or an individualized session.[23] Evidence from meta-analyses, randomized controlled trials, and observational studies shows that nutrition therapy improves metabolic outcomes such as HbA1c, lipids, and blood pressure in people with diabetes.[13,14,16,36,52] Individualized education sessions or group education programs including nutrition therapy have shown HbA1c reductions of 0.5% to 2% for type 2 diabetes.[2–4,16,17,53,54]

The evaluation of exercise interventions can be performed by conducting an initial assessment of exercise fitness and body composition. Maximal exercise testing on a motorized treadmill or cycle ergometer can be useful for exercise prescription and postintervention assessment. This is best done before an intervention, because the appropriate exercise intensity can be prescribed and assessed more accurately when the maximum heart rate or Vo_{2max} is determined from exercise testing by a qualified clinical exercise physiologist or equivalent health care expert. Estimating target heart rate or work rate from age-predicted calculations is simpler but is prone to measurement error and medication interactions with the cardiovascular system. Exercise testing can also be useful for risk stratification, given that lower aerobic capacity and the presence of ischemic changes on electrocardiogram are each associated with higher risks of cardiovascular and overall morbidity and mortality in diabetes[55,56] and in prediabetes.[57] Exercise testing may also help detect coronary disease and allow the aerobic exercise prescription to be below the ischemic threshold. Several other assessments should be considered both as a baseline and as outcome follow-up[58]:

- An assessment of fall risk (eg, the Timed Up and Go Test, Functional Reach Test, Berg Balance Scale, Dynamic Gait Index)
- Baseline physical activity level (pedometer/accelerometer)
- Body composition (bioelectrical impedance, waist circumference)
- Muscle strength (manual muscle testing, handgrip dynamometer, or repetition maximal testing of certain muscle groups)

LONG-TERM RECOMMENDATIONS: CLINICAL PRIORITIES: NUTRITION THERAPY AND PHYSICAL ACTIVITY

The ADA 2013 nutrition therapy recommendations provide a summary of priority topics for persons with diabetes[2]:

- Portion control with emphasis on choosing nutrient-dense, high-fiber foods, whenever possible, instead of processed foods with added sodium, fat, and sugars.
- Carbohydrate-containing foods and beverages are the greatest determinant of the postmeal blood glucose excursions in people with diabetes, along with the capacity to secrete endogenous insulin. Therefore it is important for individuals with diabetes to know what foods contain carbohydrates (starchy vegetables, whole grains, fruit, milk and milk products, vegetables, and sugar) and how the various forms of carbohydrate influence their glycemia.

- For individuals trying to lose weight, a mild to moderate daily energy deficit is needed (10%–25% relative caloric restriction). Modest weight loss (of >6 kg or ~7.0%–8.5% loss of initial body weight) may provide clinical benefits such as improved glycemia, blood pressure, and/or lipid levels in some individuals with diabetes, especially those early in the disease process. Intensive lifestyle interventions (counseling about nutrition therapy, physical activity, and behavior change) with ongoing support are recommended to achieve and sustain a modest energy deficit until a goal weight is achieved.
- Limitation of any caloric sweetener, including high-fructose corn syrup and sucrose, reduces risk of worsening the cardiometabolic risk profile and weight gain.[2] The term free fructose refers to the consumption of fructose that is naturally occurring in foods such as fruit, and does not include the fructose that is found in the form of the disaccharide sucrose or the fructose in high-fructose corn syrup.[2] It seems that free fructose is not more harmful than other forms of sugar unless it is consumed in excessive amounts (>12% of the total caloric intake).[59,60]
- The selection of lean protein sources and meat alternatives and the substitution of foods high in unsaturated fat (liquid oils) should be preferred rather than those high in *trans* or saturated fats. Fat quality seems to be more in important than quantity.
- Micronutrients, vitamins, herbal products, and supplements are not recommended for management of diabetes because of a lack of evidence at this time. However, without well-designed clinical trials to prove efficacy, the benefit of pharmacologic doses of micronutrients and supplements is unknown, and findings from small clinical and animal studies is frequently extrapolated to clinical practice.[61]
- Use of nonnutritive sweeteners (NNS), also commonly referred to as artificial sweeteners, continues to be an area of much debate and misinformation. The US Food and Drug Administration has reviewed several types of hypocaloric sweeteners (eg, aspartame, sucralose, saccharin, and sugar alcohols) for safety and has approved them for consumption by the general public, including people with diabetes.[62] **Table 2** shows the acceptable daily intake of popular nonnutritive sweeteners (based on a 70-kg [150-lb] adult). Research supports that nonnutritive sweeteners do not produce a glycemic effect; however, foods containing

Table 2
Acceptable daily intake of popular nonnutritive sweeteners (based on 70-kg [150-lb] adult)

Type of Sweetener	Acceptable Daily Intake[a] (mg/kg Body Weight)	Amount of Diet Soda/Day (355-mL [12-ounce] can)	Amount of Artificial Sweetener (Packets)
Aspartame	50	17	97
Saccharin	5	2	9
Sucralose	5	5	68
Acesulfame K	15	26	20
Stevia	0–4	[b]	30

[a] The US Food and Drug Administration sets an acceptable daily intake (ADI) for each sweetener, which is the maximum amount considered safe to consume each day during a person's lifetime. The ADI is set at about 100 times less than the smallest amount that might cause health concerns, based on studies done in laboratory animals.
[b] Product information not available; sodas containing Stevia are not widely available.

NNSs may affect glycemia based on other ingredients in the product.[63] In a recently published meta-analysis that included 15 randomized controlled trials, the use of NNSs and other low-calorie sweeteners (LCSs) such as sugar alcohols was associated with lower body weight, BMI, and waist circumference when substituted for calorically dense alternatives. The meta-analysis also included 9 cohort studies that reported that the use of NNSs and LCSs were associated with less weight gain but a slightly greater BMI.[64]

- The recommendation for the general population to limit sodium intake to less 2300 mg/d is also appropriate for individuals with diabetes. Lower levels should only be considered on an individual basis for people with diabetes and hypertension.
- Moderate alcohol consumption (1 drink/d or less for adult women and 2 drinks/d or less for adult men) has minimal acute or long-term effects on blood glucose and may have beneficial effects on cardiovascular risk. To reduce the risk of hypoglycemia for individuals using insulin or insulin secretagogues, alcohol should be consumed with food.

Key strategies for individuals requiring medications or insulin include:

- Eating moderate amounts of carbohydrate at meals (and snacks, if desired)
- Not skipping meals
- If on a multiple-daily injection plan or an insulin pump, take mealtime insulin before eating
- If on a premixed or fixed insulin plan, meals need to be eaten at similar times every day and contain similar amounts of carbohydrate that match set doses of insulin

According to the ADA/American College of Sports Medicine position statement[32] and the guide to prescribing physical activity for patients with diabetes by Colberg[65]:

- At least 2.5 h/wk of moderate to vigorous physical activity should be undertaken as part of lifestyle changes to prevent type 2 diabetes onset in high-risk adults.
- Persons with type 2 diabetes should undertake at least 150 min/wk of moderate to vigorous aerobic exercise spread over at least 3 days during the week, with no more than 2 consecutive days between bouts of aerobic activity.
- In addition to aerobic training, persons with type 2 diabetes should undertake moderate to vigorous resistance training at least 2 to 3 d/wk.
- Supervised and combined aerobic and resistance training may confer additional health benefits, although milder forms of physical activity (such as yoga) have shown mixed results.
- Persons with type 2 diabetes are encouraged to increase their total daily unstructured physical activity.
- Flexibility training may be included but should not be undertaken in place of other recommended types of physical activity.
- Although hyperglycemia can be worsened by exercise in type 1 diabetic individuals who are insulin deficient and ketotic (caused by missed or insufficient insulin), few persons with type 2 diabetes develop such a profound degree of insulin deficiency. As such, individuals with type 2 diabetes may engage in physical activity, using caution when exercising with blood glucose levels exceeding 300 mg/dL (16.7 mmol/L) without ketosis, provided they are feeling well and are adequately hydrated.
- Known CVD is not an absolute contraindication to exercise. Individuals with angina classified as moderate or high risk should likely begin exercise in a supervised cardiac rehabilitation program.

- Patients with intermittent claudication are advised to walk at a speed that induces claudication pain within 3 to 5 minutes. Walking should be stopped when claudication pain is rated as moderate and the patient should rest until the claudication pain has resolved. At that point, the patient should resume walking until moderate claudication pain is induced again. The walking exercise program should begin with exercise and rest cycles of at least 30 minutes and should progress to 60 minutes.[66]
- Individuals with peripheral neuropathy and without acute ulceration may participate in moderate weight-bearing exercise. Comprehensive foot care including daily inspection of feet and use of proper footwear (correct sizing and with custom-made foot beds with some cushioning, if feasible) is recommended for prevention and early detection of sores or ulcers. In general, shoes should:
  o Fit well
  o Be made out of breathable material
  o Have a firm heel
  o Have hook and loop type fasteners or shoelaces
  o Have good shock absorption
  o Not be bent or twisted
  o Have no seams in the toe box
  o Stabilize overpronation or oversupination
- Moderate walking likely does not increase risk of foot ulcers or reulceration in patients with peripheral neuropathy.
- Individuals with cardiac autonomic neuropathy should be screened and receive physician approval and possibly an exercise stress test before exercise initiation. Exercise intensity is best prescribed using the heart rate reserve method with direct measurement of maximal heart rate.
- In individuals with proliferative or preproliferative retinopathy or macular degeneration, careful screening and physician approval are recommended before initiating an exercise program. Activities that greatly increase intraocular pressure, such as high-intensity aerobic or resistance training (with large increases in systolic blood pressure) and head-down activities, are not advised with uncontrolled proliferative disease, nor are jumping or jarring activities, all of which increase hemorrhage risk.
- Individuals with nephropathy often have exercise intolerance. However, exercise training improves cardiovascular risk profile, muscle mass, physical function, and quality of life in individuals with kidney disease[67] and may even be undertaken during dialysis sessions. Animal models suggest that regular exercise delays the progression of diabetic nephropathy[68,69] although good evidence for this in humans is currently lacking. The presence of microalbuminuria per se does not necessitate exercise restrictions.
- Patients with knee pain from osteoarthritis and obesity should be encouraged to participate in modified exercise programs to help with weight loss and improvements in pain, physical function, mental health, and quality of life.[70] Walking, if tolerated, should be encouraged, as should resistance exercise as long as the affected joints are not overly stressed. Other exercise modes, such as recumbent cycling and aquatic exercises, may also help limit knee pain.
- Efforts to promote physical activity should focus on developing self-efficacy and fostering social support from family, friends, and health care providers. Encouraging mild or moderate physical activity may be most beneficial to adoption and maintenance of regular physical activity participation. Lifestyle interventions may have some efficacy in promoting physical activity behavior.

Box 2
The 5 As

Assess: establish current physical activity level and readiness for change (consider the frequency, intensity, duration, and type of activity)

• Not active, not thinking about physical activity

• Not active, ready for physical activity

• Active and ready to maintain or progress

Advise: strongly encourage all patients to get more active by reviewing the health risks of inactivity and the benefits of physical activity. Advise on the appropriate amount and type of physical activity.

Agree: collaboratively develop goals and a personalized action plan. Provide individually relevant exercise prescriptions, time frames, and monitoring of strategies to meet the goals.

Assist: identify personal barriers and strategies to overcome barriers. Identify connections and resources for exercise and physical activity in the community.

Arrange: specify plan for follow-up at diabetes-focused visits with telephone calls or email reminders. Review physical activity level at subsequent visits and provide advice to achieve the next level of activity.

Adapted from Glynn TJ, Manley MW. How to help your patients stop smoking: a National Cancer Institute manual for physicians. Bethesda (MD): National Cancer Institute; 1989. NIH publication no. 89-3064.

To help facilitate changes in physical activity and eating habits, diabetes health care professionals can incorporate the use of the so-called 5 As (assess, advise, agree, assist, and arrange). This approach does not require a lot of training and offers a simple framework that can be integrated with other education and counseling resources. The 5 As concept was introduced by the National Cancer Institute as a guide to help physicians counsel their patients about smoking cessation.[71] This framework has since been expanded to address broader issues of health behavior change and to give care providers the flexibility of addressing important lifestyle topics in a manner ranging from simple to in-depth (depending on time, training, and resources). **Box 2** provides an example of how to use the 5 As for development of a physical activity prescription[71,72]:

FUTURE CONSIDERATIONS/SUMMARY

Lifestyle intervention for the treatment of type 2 diabetes should focus on a reduced energy intake with modification of food choices (increased whole grains, fiber, vegetables, and fruit; reduced total and saturated fat, sugar, and refined grains) and increased physical activity (150 min/wk of aerobic exercise plus strength training 2–3 times per week). In order to be successful another critical component of lifestyle intervention is the use of behavior modification, such as motivational interviewing, self-monitoring, and individualized goal setting, to support long-term results.

REFERENCES

1. Centers for Disease Control and Prevention. National diabetes fact sheet, United States. 2014. Available at: http://www.cdc.gov/diabetes/pubs/statsreport14.htm. Accessed May 23, 2014.

2. Evert AB, Boucher JL, Cypress M, et al. Nutrition therapy recommendations for the management of adults with diabetes. Diabetes Care 2013;36:3821–42.
3. Franz MJ, Powers MA, Leontos C, et al. The evidence for medical nutrition therapy for type 1 and type 2 diabetes in adults. J Am Diet Assoc 2010;110:1852–89.
4. Academy of Nutrition and Dietetics. Diabetes type 1 and 2 for adults evidence-based nutrition practice guidelines. 2008. Available at: http://www.adaevidencelibrary.com/topic.cfm?cat=3253. Accessed May 23, 2014.
5. Diabetes Prevention Program Research Group (DPP). Reduction in the incidence of type 2 diabetes with lifestyle intervention or metformin. N Engl J Med 2011;346:393–403.
6. Ali MK, Bullard KM, Saaddine JB, et al. Achievement of goals in US diabetes care. 1999–2010. N Engl J Med 2013;368:1613–24.
7. Nguyen NT, Nguyen XM, Lane J, et al. Relationship between obesity and diabetes in a US adult population: findings from the National Health and Nutrition Examination Survey, 1999-2006. Obes Surg 2011;21:351–5.
8. Clinical guidelines on the identification, evaluation, and treatment of overweight and obesity in adults–the evidence report. National Institutes of Health. Obes Res 1998;6:51S–209S.
9. National Heart, Lung, and Blood Institute; Clinical Guidelines on the Identification, Evaluation, and Treatment of Overweight and Obesity in Adults. The Evidence Report NHLBI Obesity Education Initiative Expert Panel on the Identification, Evaluation, and Treatment of Obesity in Adults (US). Bethesda (MD):1998 Sep. Report No 98-4083.
10. Lindstrom J, Ilanne-Parikka P, Peltonen M, et al, Finnish Diabetes Prevention Study Group. Sustained reduction in the incidence of type 2 diabetes by lifestyle intervention: follow-up of the Finnish Diabetes Prevention Study. Lancet 2006;368:1673–9.
11. Li G, Zhang P, Wang J, et al. The long-term effect of lifestyle interventions to prevent diabetes in the China Da Qing Diabetes Prevention Study: a 20-year follow-up study. Lancet 2008;371:1783–9.
12. Look AHEAD Research Group. Cardio-vascular effects of intensive lifestyle intervention in type 2 diabetes. N Engl J Med 2013;369:145–54.
13. Look AHEAD Research Group. Impact of intensive lifestyle intervention on depression and health-related quality of life in type 2 diabetes: the Look AHEAD Trial. Diabetes Care 2014;37:1544–53.
14. Esposito K, Maiorino MI, Ciotola M, et al. Effects of a Mediterranean-style diet on the need for antihyperglycemic drug therapy in patients with newly diagnosed type 2 diabetes: a randomized trial. Ann Intern Med 2009;151:306–14.
15. Feldstein AC, Nichols GA, Smith DH, et al. Weight change in diabetes and glycemic and blood pressure control. Diabetes Care 2008;31:1960–5.
16. Andrews RC, Cooper AR, Montgomery AA, et al. Diet or diet plus physical activity versus usual care in patients with newly diagnosed type 2 diabetes: the early ACTID randomized controlled trial. Lancet 2011;378:129–39.
17. Coppell KJ, Kataoka M, Williams SM, et al. Nutritional intervention in patients with type 2 diabetes who are hyperglycaemic despite optimized drug treatment—Lifestyle Over and Above Drugs in Diabetes (LOADD) study: randomized controlled trial. BMJ 2010;341:c3337.
18. Battista MC, Labonté M, Ménard J, et al. Dietitian-coached management in combination with annual endocrinologist follow up improves global metabolic and cardiovascular health in diabetic participants after 24 months. Appl Physiol Nutr Metab 2012;37:610–20.

19. Banister NA, Jastrow ST, Hodges V, et al. Diabetes self-management training program in a community clinic improves patient outcomes at modest cost. J Am Diet Assoc 2004;104:807–10.
20. Barratt R, Frost G, Millward DJ, et al. A randomized controlled trial investigating the effect of an intensive lifestyle intervention v. standard care in adults with type 2 diabetes immediately after initiating insulin therapy. Br J Nutr 2008;99: 1025–31.
21. Lee DC, Sui X, Church TS, et al. Changes in fitness and fatness on the development of cardiovascular disease risk factors hypertension, metabolic syndrome, and hypercholesterolemia. J Am Coll Cardiol 2012;59:665–72.
22. Inzucchi SE, Bergenstal RM, Buse JB, et al, American Diabetes Association (ADA), European Association for the Study of Diabetes (EASD). Management of hyperglycemia in type 2 diabetes: a patient-centered approach. Position statement of the American Diabetes Association (ADA) and the European Association for the Study of Diabetes (EASD). Diabetes Care 2012;35:1364–79.
23. American Diabetes Association. Standards of medical care in diabetes–2014. Diabetes Care 2014;37(Suppl 1):S14–90.
24. Robbins JM, Thatcher GE, Webb DA, et al. Nutritionist visits, diabetes classes, and hospitalization rates and charges: the Urban Diabetes Study. Diabetes Care 2008;31:655–60.
25. Lacey K, Pritchett E. Nutrition care process and model: ADA adopts road map to quality care and outcomes management. J Am Diet Assoc 2003;103: 1061–72.
26. Wheeler ML, Dunbar SA, Jaacks LM, et al. Macronutrients, food groups and eating patterns in the management of diabetes: a systematic review of the literature, 2010. Diabetes Care 2012;35:434–45.
27. Canadian Diabetes Association Clinical Practice Guidelines Expert Committee, Sigal RJ, Armstrong MJ, et al. Physical activity and diabetes. Can J Diabetes 2013;7(Suppl 1):S40–4.
28. Steinberg H, Jacovino C, Kitabchi AE. Look inside look ahead: why the glass is more than half-full. Curr Diab Rep 2014;7:500.
29. Thompson D, Walhin JP, Batterham AM, et al. Effect of diet or diet plus physical activity versus usual care on inflammatory markers in patients with newly diagnosed type 2 diabetes: the Early ACTivity In Diabetes (ACTID) randomized, controlled trial. J Am Heart Assoc 2014;3:e000828.
30. Herbst A, Kapellen T, Schober E, et al, for the DPV-Science-Initiative. Impact of regular physical activity on blood glucose control and cardiovascular risk factors in adolescents with type 2 diabetes mellitus - a multicenter study of 578 patients from 225 centres. Pediatr Diabetes 2014. http://dx.doi.org/10.1111/pedi. 12144.
31. Balducci S, Sacchetti M, Haxhi J, et al. Physical exercise as therapy for type 2 diabetes mellitus. Diabetes Metab Res Rev 2014;30(Suppl 1):13–23.
32. Colberg SR, Sigal RJ, Fernhall B, et al, American College of Sports Medicine, American Diabetes Association. Exercise and type 2 diabetes: the American College of Sports Medicine and the American Diabetes Association: joint position statement executive summary. Diabetes Care 2010;33:2692–6.
33. Colberg SR, Sigal RJ. Prescribing exercise for individuals with type 2 diabetes: recommendations and precautions. Phys Sportsmed 2014;39:13–26.
34. Church TS, Blair SN, Cocreham S, et al. Effects of aerobic and resistance training on hemoglobin A1c levels in patients with type 2 diabetes: a randomized controlled trial. JAMA 2010;304(20):2253–62.

35. Sigal RJ, Kenny GP, Boulé NG, et al. Effects of aerobic training, resistance training, or both on glycemic control in type 2 diabetes: a randomized trial. Ann Intern Med 2007;147(6):357–69.
36. Pastors JG, Franz MJ. Effectiveness of medical nutrition therapy in diabetes. In: Franz MJ, Evert AB, editors. American Diabetes Association guide to nutrition therapy for diabetes. Alexandria (VA): American Diabetes Association; 2012. p. 1–18.
37. US Department of Health and Human Services and US Department of Agriculture. Dietary guidelines for Americans, 2010. [Internet]. Available at: www.health.gov/dietaryguidelines/. Accessed 12 July 7, 2014.
38. Schwingshackl L, Strasser B, Hoffmann G. Effects of monounsaturated fatty acids on glycaemic control in patients with abnormal glucose metabolism: a systematic review and meta-analysis. Ann Nutr Metab 2011;58:290–6.
39. Itsiopoulos C, Brazionis L, Kaimakamis M, et al. Can the Mediterranean diet lower HbA1c in type 2 diabetes? Results from a randomized cross-over study. Nutr Metab Cardiovasc Dis 2011;21:740–7.
40. Brehm BJ, Lattin BL, Summer SS, et al. One-year comparison of a high-monounsaturated fat diet with a high-carbohydrate diet in type 2 diabetes. Diabetes Care 2009;32:215–20.
41. Pan Y, Guo LL, Jin HM. Low-protein diet for diabetic nephropathy: a meta-analysis of randomized controlled trials. Am J Clin Nutr 2008;88:660–6.
42. Robertson L, Waugh N, Robertson A. Protein restriction for diabetic renal disease. Cochrane Database Syst Rev 2007;(4):CD002181.
43. Umpierre D, Ribeiro PA, Kramer CK, et al. Physical activity advice only or structured exercise training and association with HbA1c levels in type 2 diabetes: a systematic review and meta-analysis. JAMA 2011;305:1790–9.
44. Tulloch H, Sweet SN, Fortier M, et al. Exercise facilitators and barriers from adoption to maintenance in the diabetes aerobic and resistance exercise trial. Can J Diabetes 2013;37:367–74.
45. Armstrong MJ, Campbell TS, Lewin AM, et al. Motivational interviewing-based exercise counselling promotes maintenance of physical activity in people with type 2 diabetes. Can J Diabetes 2013;37(Suppl 4):S3.
46. Riddell MC, Burr J. Evidence-based risk assessment and recommendations for physical activity clearance: diabetes mellitus and related comorbidities. Appl Physiol Nutr Metab 2011;36(Suppl 1):S154–89.
47. Colberg SR, Vinik AI. Exercising with peripheral or autonomic neuropathy: what health care providers and diabetic patients need to know. Phys Sportsmed 2014;42(1):15–23.
48. Armstrong MJ, Martin BJ, Arena R, et al. Patients with diabetes in cardiac rehabilitation: attendance and exercise capacity. Med Sci Sports Exerc 2014;46(5):845–50.
49. Rabasa-Lhoret R, Bourque J, Ducros F, et al. Guidelines for premeal insulin dose reduction for postprandial exercise of different intensities and durations in type 1 diabetic subjects treated intensively with a basal-bolus insulin regimen (ultralente-lispro). Diabetes Care 2001;24:625–30.
50. Seaquist ER, Anderson J, Childs B, et al. Hypoglycemia and diabetes: a report of a workgroup of the American Diabetes Association and the Endocrine Society. Diabetes Care 2013;36:1384–95.
51. Yardley JE, Stapleton JM, Sigal RJ, et al. Do heat events pose a greater health risk for individuals with type 2 diabetes? Diabetes Technol Ther 2013;15:520–9.

52. Pi-Sunyer X, Blackburn G, Brancati FL, et al. Reduction in weight and cardiovascular disease risk factors in individuals with type 2 diabetes: on-year results of the Look AHEAD trial. Diabetes Care 2007;30:1374–83.

53. Metz JA, Stern JS, Kris-Etherton P, et al. A randomized trial of improved weight loss with a prepared meal plan in overweight and obese patients: impact on cardiovascular risk reduction. Arch Intern Med 2000;160:2150–8.

54. Nield L, Moore HJ, Hooper L, et al. Dietary advice for treatment of type 2 diabetes mellitus in adults. Cochrane Database Syst Rev 2007;(3):CD004097.

55. Church TS, LaMonte MJ, Barlow CE, et al. Cardiorespiratory fitness and body mass index as predictors of cardiovascular disease mortality among men with diabetes. Arch Intern Med 2005;16:2114–20.

56. Lyerly GW, Sui X, Lavie CJ, et al. The association between cardiorespiratory fitness and risk of all-cause mortality among women with impaired fasting glucose or undiagnosed diabetes mellitus. Mayo Clin Proc 2009; 84:780–6.

57. McAuley PA, Artero EG, Sui X, et al. Fitness, fatness, and survival in adults with pre-diabetes. Diabetes Care 2014;37:529–36.

58. Hansen D, Peeters S, Zwaenepoel B, et al. Exercise assessment and prescription in patients with type 2 diabetes in the private and home care setting: clinical recommendations from AXXON (Belgian Physical Therapy Association). Phys Ther 2013;93:597–610.

59. Sievenpiper JL, Carleton AJ, Chatha S, et al. Heterogeneous effects of fructose on blood lipids in individuals with type 2 diabetes: systematic review and meta-analysis of experimental trials in humans. Diabetes Care 2009;32: 1930–7.

60. Livesey G, Taylor R. Fructose consumption and consequences for glycation, plasma triacylglycerol, and body weight: meta-analyses and meta-regression models of intervention studies. Am J Clin Nutr 2008;88:1419–37.

61. Nuemiller JJ. Micronutrients and diabetes. In: Franz MJ, Evert AB, editors. American Diabetes Association guide to nutrition therapy for diabetes. Alexandria (VA): American Diabetes Association; 2012. p. 41–68.

62. US Department of Agriculture. Nutritive and nonnutritive sweetener resources [Internet]. National Agricultural Library, Food and Nutrition Information Center. 2013. Available at: http://fnic.nal.usda.gov/food-composition/nutritive-and-nonnutritive-sweetener-resources. Accessed May 23, 2014.

63. Gardner C, Wylie-Rosett J, Gidding SS, et al, American Heart Association Nutrition Committee of the Council on Nutrition, Physical Activity and Metabolism, Council on Arteriosclerosis, Thrombosis and Vascular Biology, Council on Cardiovascular Disease in the Young, American Diabetes Association. Nonnutritive sweeteners: current use and health perspectives: a scientific statement from the American Heart Association and the American Diabetes Association. Diabetes Care 2012;35:1798–808.

64. Miller PE, Perez V. Low-calorie sweeteners and body weight and composition: a meta-analysis of randomized controlled trials and prospective cohort studies. Am J Clin Nutr 2014;100:765–77.

65. Colberg SR. Exercise and diabetes. A clinician's guide to prescribing physical activity. Alexandria (VA): American Diabetes Association; 2013.

66. Brunelle CL, Mulgrew JA. Exercise for intermittent claudication. Phys Ther 2011; 91:997–1002.

67. Smith AC, Burton JO. Exercise in kidney disease and diabetes: time for action. J Ren Care 2012;38(Suppl 1):52–8.

68. Tufescu A, Kanazawa M, Ishida A, et al. Combination of exercise and losartan enhances renoprotective and peripheral effects in spontaneously type 2 diabetes mellitus rats with nephropathy. J Hypertens 2008;26:312–21.
69. Ghosh S, Khazaei M, Moien-Afshari F, et al. Moderate exercise attenuates caspase-3 activity, oxidative stress, and inhibits progression of diabetic renal disease in db/db mice. Am J Physiol Renal Physiol 2009;296:F700–8.
70. Foy CG, Lewis CE, Hairston KG, et al, Look AHEAD Research Group. Intensive lifestyle intervention improves physical function among obese adults with knee pain: findings from the Look AHEAD trial. Obesity (Silver Spring) 2011;19:83–93.
71. Glynn TJ, Manley MW. How to help your patients stop smoking: a National Cancer Institute manual for physicians. Bethesda (MD): National Cancer Institute; 1989. NIH publication no. 89–3064.
72. Estabrooks PA, Glasgow RE, Dzewaltowski DA. Physical activity promotion through primary care. JAMA 2003;289:2913–6.

Statins and Diabetes

Kevin C. Maki, PhD[a],*, Mary R. Dicklin, PhD[a], Seth J. Baum, MD[b]

KEYWORDS

- Statins • High intensity statins • Diabetes mellitus • Glucose • Glycemia
- Dyslipidemia • Cardiovascular disease • Coronary heart disease

KEY POINTS

- Statin use is associated with a modest increase in risk for new-onset type 2 diabetes mellitus compared with placebo or usual care.
- The risk for diabetes seems to be greater for intensive-dosage statin therapy, and to be most evident in those with major risk factors for diabetes.
- The cardiovascular benefits of statin therapy outweigh the potential risk for diabetes development, with several cardiovascular events generally prevented for each excess case of diabetes.
- No changes to clinical practice have been recommended, other than measuring glycated hemoglobin or fasting glucose in patients at elevated diabetes risk before and within 1 year of initiating therapy.
- The American Diabetes Association guidelines should be followed for screening and diagnosis, and lifestyle modification is emphasized for the prevention or delay of diabetes mellitus.

INTRODUCTION

Statins are first-line drug therapy for the management of dyslipidemia and have been shown to reduce the risks for myocardial infarction, stroke, and cardiovascular death,[1–3] but clinical trial data suggest a modest, yet statistically significant, increase in the incidence of new-onset type 2 diabetes mellitus (T2DM) with statin use.[4–10]

This article originally appeared in Cardiology Clinics, Volume 33, Issue 2, May 2015.
Disclosures: Dr K.C. Maki discloses that in the past 12 months he has received consulting fees and/or research grants from AbbVie, Amarin, AstraZeneca, and Trygg Pharmaceuticals. Dr M.R. Dicklin has nothing to disclose. Dr S.J. Baum discloses that in the past 12 months he has received consulting/speaking fees from Aegerion, Genzyme, Sanofi, AstraZeneca, and Merck Pharmaceuticals.

[a] Metabolic Sciences, Midwest Center for Metabolic & Cardiovascular Research, 489 Taft Avenue, Suite 202, Glen Ellyn, IL 60137, USA; [b] Division of Medicine, Charles E. Schmidt College of Biomedical Science, Florida Atlantic University, 777 Glades Road, Boca Raton, FL 33431, USA
* Corresponding author.
E-mail address: kmaki@mc-mcr.com

Clinics Collections 5 (2015) 307–320
http://dx.doi.org/10.1016/j.ccol.2015.05.018
2352-7986/15/$ – see front matter © 2015 Elsevier Inc. All rights reserved.

Diabetes mellitus is a common condition affecting nearly 10% of the US population[11] and is increasing in prevalence worldwide.[12] In 2012, the US Food and Drug Administration added a statement to the labels of statin medications indicating that increases in glycated hemoglobin (HbA$_{1C}$) and fasting glucose levels have been reported with statin use.[13] In 2014, the National Lipid Association Statin Diabetes Safety Task Force reviewed the published evidence relating statin use to the hazard of diabetes mellitus or worsening glycemia, and provided practical guidance on how to manage this issue in clinical practice.[10] This paper provides a brief overview of the literature regarding statin use and T2DM risk and summarizes the findings and guidance from the National Lipid Association Expert Panel. The terms T2DM and diabetes are used synonymously throughout the article.

CLINICAL TRIAL EVIDENCE REGARDING STATIN USE AND DIABETES
West of Scotland Coronary Prevention Study

The West of Scotland Coronary Prevention Study (WOSCOPS) was one of the first clinical trials to draw attention to a possible association, albeit inverse in that trial, between T2DM risk and statin use.[14] An examination of the incidence of new-onset diabetes mellitus among 5974 subjects receiving pravastatin in WOSCOPS indicated that pravastatin therapy was associated with a lesser risk for development of diabetes mellitus, defined as a blood glucose level of 7.0 mmol/L or greater (126 mg/dL).[14] Subjects assigned to receive pravastatin had a 30% reduction in the risk for developing diabetes, compared with placebo, in multivariate analysis (hazard ratio [HR], 0.70; 95% CI, 0.50–0.99; $P = .042$). Because these analyses were post hoc and not predefined, it was acknowledged that they should be considered hypothesis generating and interpreted with caution.

Justification for the Use of Statins in Prevention: an Intervention Trial Evaluating Rosuvastatin

The WOSCOPS results sparked interest in pursuing a formal, prospective analysis of the relationship between T2DM risk and statin use. The Justification for the Use of Statins in Prevention: an Intervention Trial Evaluating Rosuvastatin (JUPITER) was a study of 17,802 apparently healthy men and women with low-density lipoprotein cholesterol levels of less than 130 mg/dL and high-sensitivity C-reactive protein levels of 2.0 mg/L or more treated with rosuvastatin 20 mg/d or placebo (n = 8901 in each group) and followed for a median of 1.9 years.[4] The study included protocol-specified comparisons of glucose changes and physician-reported T2DM incidence between treatments. The results of JUPITER indicated that there were no differences between treatment groups in incidence of newly diagnosed glycosuria (rosuvastatin, n = 36; placebo, n = 32) or fasting blood glucose concentrations. A difference between groups in median HbA$_{1C}$ concentration, although small, was detected, with a significantly higher value observed in the rosuvastatin group (5.9% vs 5.8% in the placebo group; $P = .001$). Furthermore, in the rosuvastatin group, there were significantly ($P = .01$) more cases of physician-reported diabetes (not adjudicated by the endpoint committee) among subjects receiving rosuvastatin (270 reports) versus subjects receiving placebo (216 reports; **Table 1**).

A follow-up analysis from JUPITER included stratification of participants on the basis of whether they had none or at least 1 of the following 4 major risk factors for developing diabetes: the metabolic syndrome, impaired fasting glucose, body mass index of 30 kg/m^2 or greater, or HbA$_{1C}$ of greater than 6% (see **Table 1**).[5] Of the participants, 6095 had no major diabetes mellitus risk factors and 11,508 had at least 1 diabetes

Table 1
Risk for developing T2DM with rosuvastatin treatment according to the number of diabetes risk factors in JUPITER

Event and Hazard Ratio	Placebo (n = 8901)	Rosuvastatin (n = 8901)	Difference	P-Value
New T2DM (All)	216 (2.4%)	270 (3.0%)	+54	.01
New T2DM (0 DM RF)	12 (0.2%)	12 (0.2%)	0	.99
New T2DM (≥1 DM RF)	204 (1.7%)	258 (2.1%)	+54	.01
HR (95% CI) 0 DM RF	—	0.99 (0.45, 2.21)	−1%	—
HR (95% CI) ≥1 DM RF	—	1.28 (1.07, 1.54)	+28%	—

There were 6095 patients with no major diabetes mellitus risk factors and 11,508 with ≥1 risk factor. Diabetes mellitus risk factors included the metabolic syndrome, impaired fasting glucose, body mass index of ≥30 kg/m², and glycated hemoglobin of >6%.
Abbreviations: CI, confidence interval; HR, hazard ratio; JUPITER, Justification for Use of Statins in Prevention: an Intervention Trial Evaluating Rosuvastatin; RF, risk factors; T2DM, type 2 diabetes mellitus.
Data from Ridker PM, Pradhan A, MacFadyen JG, et al. Cardiovascular benefits and diabetes risks of statin therapy in primary prevention: an analysis from the JUPITER trial. Lancet 2012;380:565–71.

risk factor. During follow-up, there were 54 more new cases of T2DM in rosuvastatin-treated subjects with at least 1 diabetes risk factor compared with placebo-treated subjects with at least 1 diabetes risk factor (258 and 204 cases, respectively; P = .01). Importantly, all of the excess cases of T2DM with rosuvastatin occurred in patients with at least 1 major diabetes risk factor. There was no difference between treatment groups in the number of new T2DM cases among subjects with no diabetes risk factors (12 cases in each). The HRs (95% CIs) for developing diabetes associated with rosuvastatin use compared with placebo among subjects with none versus at least 1 diabetes risk factor were 0.99 (0.45–2.21) and 1.28 (1.07–1.54), respectively. These results suggest that risk for developing diabetes while on statin therapy may be limited to those with major T2DM risk factors.

Although the risk for developing diabetes was increased modestly, the risk for the primary cardiovascular endpoint (myocardial infarction, stroke, arterial revascularization, hospitalization for unstable angina, or death from cardiovascular causes) in JUPITER was reduced substantially with rosuvastatin overall and in subjects with and without major diabetes risk factors (**Table 2**). In those with at least 1 risk factor, rosuvastatin treatment was associated with a 39% reduction in the primary endpoint (HR, 0.61; 95% CI, 0.47–0.79; P = .0001), and among subjects with no diabetes risk factors, rosuvastatin treatment was associated with a 52% reduction in the primary endpoint (HR, 0.48; 95% CI, 0.33–0.68; P = .0001).[4,5]

Metaanalyses of Statin Clinical Trials and the Risk:Benefit Ratio

Because of the apparent conflicting findings for new-onset diabetes between the WOSCOPS and JUPITER trials of statin therapy, metaanalyses of clinical trials have been conducted to further examine the association.[7,8,15] Sattar and colleagues[7] identified 13 statin trials with 91,140 participants, of whom 4278 (statin treated [n = 2226] and control treated [n = 2052]) developed diabetes during a mean of 4 years of follow-up (**Fig. 1**). Statin therapy was associated with 9% increased odds for incident diabetes (odds ratio, 1.09; 95% CI 1.02–1.17) with little heterogeneity between trials (I^2 = 11%). Although the power was limited to detect differences regarding the association with T2DM among 5 statins—rosuvastatin, atorvastatin, pravastatin,

Table 2
Risk for the primary cardiovascular endpoint with rosuvastatin treatment according to the number of diabetes risk factors in JUPITER

Event and HR	Placebo (n = 8901)	Rosuvastatin (n = 8901)	Difference	P-Value
1° CVD endpoint (All)	251 (2.8%)	142 (1.6%)	−109	.0001
1° CVD endpoint (0 DM RF)	91 (1.5%)	44 (0.7%)	−47	.0001
1° CVD endpoint (≥1 DM RF)	157 (1.3%)	96 (0.8%)	−61	.0001
HR (95% CI) 0 DM RF	—	0.48 (0.33, 0.68)	−52%	
HR (95% CI) ≥1 DM RF	—	0.61 (0.47, 0.79)	−39%	

There were 6095 patients with no major diabetes mellitus risk factors and 11,508 with ≥1 risk factor. Diabetes mellitus risk factors included metabolic syndrome, impaired fasting glucose, body mass index of ≥30 kg/m², and glycated hemoglobin of >6%.
Abbreviations: 1°, primary; CI, confidence interval; CVD, cardiovascular disease; DM, diabetes mellitus; HR, hazard ratio; JUPITER, Justification for Use of Statins in Prevention: an Intervention Trial Evaluating Rosuvastatin; RF, risk factor.
Data from Ridker PM, Danielson E, Fonseca FA, et al. JUPITER Study Group. Rosuvastatin to prevent vascular events in men and women with elevated C-reactive protein. N Engl J Med 2008;359:2195–207; and Ridker PM, Pradhan A, MacFadyen JG, et al. Cardiovascular benefits and diabetes risks of statin therapy in primary prevention: an analysis from the JUPITER trial. Lancet 2012;380:565–71.

simvastatin, and lovastatin—it is important to recognize that no differences were identified. The number of patients that would need to be treated for 4 years to produce 1 excess case of T2DM was estimated to be 255 (95% CI, 150–852). The benefit associated with each 1 mmol/L (38.7 mg/dL) decrease in low-density lipoprotein cholesterol over 4 years of statin use, based on an analysis of the Cholesterol Treatment Trialists' group, was reported to be a prevention of 5.4 coronary heart disease events (including myocardial infarction and fatal coronary heart disease).[1] The inclusion of revascularizations and strokes in this analysis roughly doubles the cardiovascular benefit.[2] Thus, when comparing risk and benefit for statin use, as many as 5 to 10 major adverse cardiovascular events might be prevented for each excess case of T2DM associated with use of statin therapy in those with T2DM risk, similar to the average risk among those in the statin trials evaluated.

In another metaanalysis, Preiss and colleagues[8] identified 5 statin trials that compared intensive- with moderate-dosage statin therapy. These included 32,752 participants, of whom 2749 (intensive dosage statin treated [n = 1449] and moderate dosage statin treated [n = 1300]) developed diabetes, and of whom 6684 (intensive dosage statin treated [n = 3134] and moderate dosage statin treated [n = 3550]) experienced a cardiovascular event during a mean follow-up of 4.9 years. The statin therapies defined as intensive dosage in this metaanalysis were atorvastatin 80 mg and simvastatin 80 mg, and the moderate dosage statin therapies were pravastatin 40 mg, simvastatin 10 to 40 mg, and atorvastatin 10 mg. There were 2.0 additional cases of T2DM in the intensive dosage group per 1000 patient-years, and 6.5 fewer cardiovascular events in the intensive dosage group per 1000 patient-years. Odds ratios (95% CIs) for new-onset diabetes and cardiovascular events, respectively, for those receiving intensive dosage compared with moderate dosage statin therapy were 1.12 (1.04–1.22) and 0.84 (0.75–0.94; Fig. 2). The number of patients who would need to be treated for 1 year with intensive dosage statin therapy versus moderate dosage statin therapy to produce 1 excess case of T2DM was estimated to be 498,

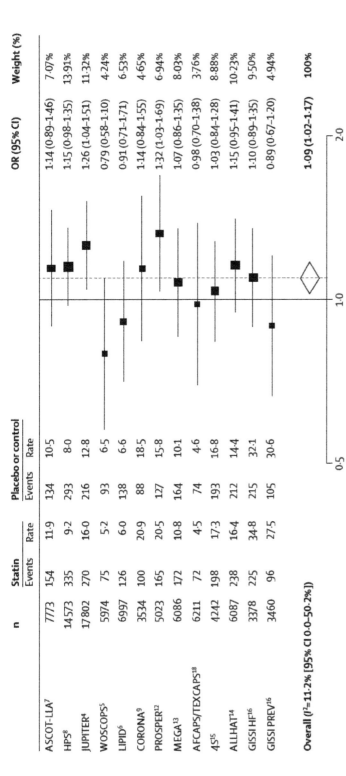

	n	Statin		Placebo or control		OR (95% CI)	Weight (%)
		Events	Rate	Events	Rate		
ASCOT-LLA[7]	7773	154	11·9	134	10·5	1·14 (0·89–1·46)	7·07%
HPS[8]	14573	335	9·2	293	8·0	1·15 (0·98–1·35)	13·91%
JUPITER[4]	17802	270	16·0	216	12·8	1·26 (1·04–1·51)	11·32%
WOSCOPS[5]	5974	75	5·2	93	6·5	0·79 (0·58–1·10)	4·24%
LIPID[6]	6997	126	6·0	138	6·6	0·91 (0·71–1·71)	6·53%
CORONA[9]	3534	100	20·9	88	18·5	1·14 (0·84–1·55)	4·65%
PROSPER[22]	5023	165	20·5	127	15·8	1·32 (1·03–1·69)	6·94%
MEGA[13]	6086	172	10·8	164	10·1	1·07 (0·86–1·35)	8·03%
AFCAPS/TEXCAPS[18]	6211	72	4·5	74	4·6	0·98 (0·70–1·38)	3·76%
4S[5]	4242	198	17·3	193	16·8	1·03 (0·84–1·28)	8·88%
ALLHAT[14]	6087	238	16·4	212	14·4	1·15 (0·95–1·41)	10·23%
GISSI HF[16]	3378	225	34·8	215	32·1	1·10 (0·89–1·35)	9·50%
GISSI PREV[16]	3460	96	27·5	105	30·6	0·89 (0·67–1·20)	4·94%
Overall (I²=11·2% [95% CI 0·0–50·2%])						1·09 (1·02–1·17)	100%

Fig. 1. Statin therapy and incident diabetes in cardiovascular endpoint trials.[7] 4S, Scandinavian Simvastatin Survival Study; AFCAPS/TEXCAPS, Air Force/ Texas Coronary Atherosclerosis Prevention Study; ALLHAT, Antihypertensive and Lipid-Lowering Treatment to Prevent Heart Attack Trial; ASCOT-LLA, Anglo-Scandinavian Cardiac Outcomes Trial – Lipid-Lowering Arm; CI, confidence interval; CORONA, Controlled Rosuvastatin Multinational Trial in Heart Failure; GISSI-HF, Gruppo Italiano per lo Studio della Sopravvivenza nell'Insufficienza Cardiaca; JUPITER, Justification for Use of Statins in Prevention: an Intervention Trial Evaluating Rosuvastatin; LIPID, Long-term Intervention with Pravastatin in Ischemic Disease; MEGA, Management of Elevated Cholesterol in the Primary Prevention Group of Adult Japanese; OR, odds ratio; PROSPER, Prospective Study of Pravastatin in the Elderly at Risk; WO-SCOPS, West of Scotland Coronary Prevention Study. (*From* Sattar N, Preiss D, Murray HM, et al. Statins and risk of incident diabetes: a collaborative meta-analysis of randomized statin trials. Lancet 2010;375:737; with permission.)

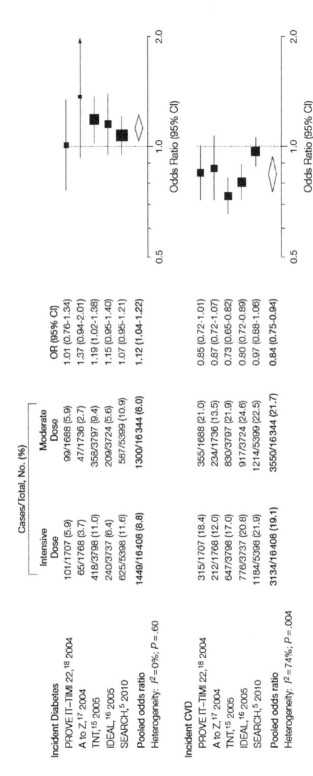

Fig. 2. Metaanalysis of new-onset diabetes and first major cardiovascular events in clinical trials of intensive versus moderate dosage statin therapy. A to Z, Aggrastat to Zocor; CI, confidence interval; CVD, cardiovascular disease; IDEAL, Incremental Decrease in End Points Through Aggressive Lipid Lowering; OR, odds ratio; PROVE IT-TIMI 22, Pravastatin or Atorvastatin Evaluation and Infection Therapy – Thrombolysis in Myocardial Infarction; SEARCH, Study of the Effectiveness of Additional Reductions in Cholesterol and Homocysteine; TNT, Treating to New Targets. (*From* Preiss D, Seshasai SR, Welsh P, et al. Risk of incident diabetes with intensive-dose compared with moderate-dose statin therapy: a meta-analysis. JAMA 2011;305:2560; with permission.)

and the number of patients that would need to be treated for 1 year with intensive versus moderate dosage statin therapy to prevent 1 cardiovascular event was 155. Accordingly, 3.2 cardiovascular events would be prevented for each excess case of diabetes with intensive versus moderate dosage statin therapy.

The results of these metaanalyses indicate that statin use is associated with a modest, but statistically significant, increase in risk for the development of T2DM of approximately 10% to 12% overall. T2DM risk with statin therapy is somewhat greater for more intensive dosage statin regimens and the increase in risk seems likely to be more pronounced (25%–30%) in those with major T2DM risk factors.[5,8,9] However, available data indicate that several fewer major cardiovascular events should be expected to occur for each excess case of new-onset diabetes associated with statin therapy, or intensification of statin therapy.

The definition of intensity with regard to statin therapies is somewhat complicated. The American College of Cardiology/American Heart Association 2013 cholesterol guidelines[16] defined high-intensity statins as regimens that reduce low-density lipoprotein cholesterol by at least 50%, and included rosuvastatin 20 and 40 mg and atorvastatin 40 and 80 mg (although according to the largest study of atorvastatin, a 40 mg dosage reduced low-density lipoprotein cholesterol by just 48%[17]). Simvastatin 80 mg was placed in the moderate category. This is different from the definition of intensive dosage therapy used in the Preiss metaanalysis.[8]

Three studies have compared 2 dosages of the same statin: Treating to New Targets (80 vs 10 mg atorvastatin),[18] Aggrastat to Zocor (80 vs 20 mg simvastatin),[19] and the Study of the Effectiveness of Additional Reductions in Cholesterol and Homocysteine (80 vs 20 mg simvastatin).[20] However, there are no studies that compare statins at similar degrees of efficacy. Thus, although the available data support the view that higher intensity (efficacy) regimens increase risk for diabetes more than lower intensity (efficacy) regimens, additional research is needed to determine whether there are differences between statins with regard to diabetogenicity at similar degrees of low-density lipoprotein cholesterol reduction.

Observational Studies of the Relationship Between Statin Use and Diabetes Risk

Data from randomized, clinical trials are very useful for assessing hazards and benefits of therapies, but may have limitations, including relatively short follow-up periods, minimal enrollment of those at greatest risk for ancillary outcomes, and lack of standardized methods for ascertainment of adverse outcomes such as incident T2DM. Therefore, it is also useful to consider results from observational studies. For the association between initiation of statin therapy and new-onset T2DM, the observational data have been consistently supportive of the findings from clinical trials.[21–24] For example, an analysis of electronic medical records from 500 general practices in the UK, including data from 285,864 men and women from 2000 to 2010, indicated that during 1.2 million person-years of follow-up there were 13,455 cases of T2DM, and that statin initiation was associated with increased risk for T2DM (HR [95% CI] of 1.45 [1.39–1.50] before adjusting for potential confounders and 1.14 [1.10–1.19] after adjustment).[21] A systematic review and metaanalysis of 90 observational studies of statin use from 1988 to 2012, which examined the unintended effects of statins, reported an increased risk of diabetes for patients exposed to statins of 31% (odds ratio, 1.31; 95% CI, 0.99–1.73).[24]

Corrao and colleagues[22] investigated the relationship between adherence to statin therapy and risk for developing diabetes in a cohort of 115,708 persons in Italy who started taking statins during 2003 and 2004 and were followed until 2010. Adherence to the statin was assessed by the proportion of days covered with statins (exposure) based on pharmacy refill records. During follow-up, 11,154 subjects were diagnosed with diabetes. Compared with patients with very low adherence (proportion of days covered, <25%), those with low (26%–50%), intermediate (51%–75%), and high (≥75%) adherence to statin therapy had increased risks for developing diabetes (HRs [95% CIs] of 1.12 [1.06–1.18], 1.22 [1.14–1.27], and 1.32 [1.26–1.39], respectively; **Fig. 3**).

The greater risk for diabetes associated with the use of higher intensity statins that has been shown in clinical trials[8] has also been confirmed in observational studies of statin use and diabetes. In an examination of 8 population-based cohort studies and a metaanalysis from 6 Canadian provinces and 2 international databases from the United States and the UK, Dormuth and colleagues[23] measured the incremental increase in new-onset diabetes associated with taking higher versus lower intensity statins in 136,966 secondary prevention patients between 1997 and 2011. In the first 2 years of regular statin use, there was a significant increase in the risk of new-onset diabetes with higher intensity statins compared with lower intensity agents (fixed

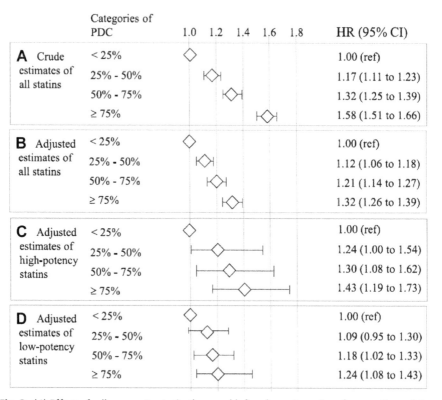

Fig. 3. (*A*) Effect of adherence to statin therapy (defined as categories of proportion of days covered) on HRs for the development of diabetes. (*B–D*) Adjusted estimates were made for age (continuous), sex, first-line statin therapy, concomitant use of other drugs, history of cardiovascular disease, categories of Charlson comorbidity index score, number of cholesterolemia tests, and number of outpatient specialist visits. CI, confidence interval; HR, hazard ratio; PDC, proportion of days covered; ref, reference. (*From* Corrao G, Ibrahim B, Nicotra F, et al. Statins and the risk of diabetes: evidence from a large population-based cohort study. Diabetes Care 2014;37:2229; with permission.)

effect rate ratio, 1.15; 95% CI, 1.05–1.26). It was estimated that 342 secondary prevention patients needed to be treated with a higher intensity statin instead of a lower intensity statin for 2 years to produce 1 additional case of diabetes.

Mechanisms for Causality Between Use of Statins and Increased Diabetes Risk

Major causal factors for T2DM include insulin resistance (peripheral and hepatic) and a defect in the ability of pancreatic β cells to provide sufficient insulin to maintain normal blood glucose levels.[25,26] In combination, these defects result in an imbalance between the rate at which glucose enters the circulation from the liver, intestine, and kidney, and the rate at which glucose is removed from the circulation by the tissues, producing hyperglycemia. To date, there have been relatively few clinical investigations of the effects of statin therapy on determinants of glucose homeostasis.[27–30] Results from studies in animal models and cell cultures suggest a number of cellular mechanisms may be involved, but none of these has been sufficiently demonstrated in humans.[31–33]

In a systematic review and metaanalysis, Baker and colleagues[28] examined the effects of statin treatment on insulin sensitivity in nondiabetic patients, and found no significant class effect of statins in 16 studies. However, subset analyses suggested a modest increase in insulin sensitivity with pravastatin, a modest decrease with simvastatin, and no difference from the comparison conditions for atorvastatin or rosuvastatin. Most of the studies considered in the Baker metaanalysis did not use reference methods for the measurement of insulin sensitivity, and many were also small and likely to be underpowered. A study by Lamendola and colleagues[27] that did use a reference method (modified insulin suppression test) reported no difference in the steady-state plasma glucose concentration for rosuvastatin versus baseline or versus the change with gemfibrozil treatment in 39 insulin-resistant, nondiabetic patients with combined dyslipidemia.

Swerdlow and colleagues[15] recently investigated whether the increase in new-onset T2DM with statin use may be explained by inhibition of 3-hydroxy-3-methylglutaryl coenzyme A reductase (HMGCR). Associations between single nucleotide polymorphisms of the HMGCR gene (rs17238484 and rs12916) that produce lower HMGCR activity and T2DM risk were assessed using data from 223,463 individuals in 43 genetic studies. These HMGCR variants were associated with higher mean (95% CI) plasma glucose concentration (0.23% [95% CI, 0.02–0.44]), and with higher risk of T2DM (odds ratio [95% CI] per rs17238484-G allele of 1.02 [1.00–1.05] and per rs12916-T allele of 1.06 [1.03–1.09]). These findings suggest that the effect of statins on T2DM risk is caused, at least in part, by HMGCR inhibition, and support the hypothesis that the intensity of HMGCR inhibition is important for diabetes risk, but it is unknown whether this effect is independent of the reduction in low-density lipoprotein cholesterol.

At present, the evidence regarding a potential mechanistic link between statin therapy and increased risk for insulin sensitivity or the development of diabetes mellitus are mixed. Additional studies are needed urgently to assess possible influences of statins on hepatic and peripheral insulin sensitivity and pancreatic β cell function, particularly in patients with major T2DM risk factors.

Impact of Statin Therapy on Glycemic Control in Patients with Diabetes Mellitus

Although there have been many clinical outcomes trials that enrolled subjects with diabetes, relatively few of these have reported the effects of statins on glycemic control.[34–38] In the Heart Protection Study, 40 mg/d simvastatin (n = 10,269) or placebo (n = 10,267) was administered to high-risk patients,[34,35] 5963 of whom had been diagnosed with diabetes. Plasma HbA$_{1C}$ measured at study entry in a random sample of the diabetic subjects (n = 1087) indicated mean (standard error of the mean) values of 6.99% (0.11) for simvastatin and 7.06% (0.10) for placebo; follow-up values 4 to 6 years later were 7.14% (0.06) and 7.17% (0.06), respectively. There was no difference between groups for the increase in HbA$_{1C}$ (simvastatin 0.15% [0.09] vs placebo 0.12% [0.09]).

In the Collaborative Atorvastatin Diabetes Study, which administered 10 mg/d atorvastatin (n = 1410) or placebo (n = 1428) to patients with T2DM, but without evidence of clinical cardiovascular disease, mean HbA$_{1C}$ increased from 7.9% (1.4) to 8.3% (1.5) and from 7.8% (1.4) to 8.1% (1.5) after 4 years of treatment with atorvastatin and placebo, respectively.[36] This outcome was suggestive of a modestly greater increase in HbA$_{1C}$ with atorvastatin, but the results may have been biased or confounded by dropout or changes in the use of medication(s) for glycemic control. In the Atorvastatin in Factorial with Omega-3 EE90 Risk Reduction in Diabetes trial, which administered atorvastatin 20 mg/d and omega-3-acid ethyl esters 2 g/d, using a 2-by-2 factorial design, to patients with T2DM, but without known cardiovascular disease, mean HbA$_{1C}$ at baseline was 7.0% in both groups, and 4 months later had increased by 0.3% among subjects taking atorvastatin relative to placebo (P<.0001).[37]

In a metaanalysis of 26 randomized, controlled trials of statin therapy in 3232 subjects with T2DM, Zhou and colleagues[38] assessed the influence of statin therapy on glycemic control and reported unremarkable increases in HbA$_{1C}$ (weighted mean difference, 0.04%; 95% CI, -0.08 to 0.16; I^2 = 45.7%) and fasting plasma glucose (2.25 mg/dL; 95% CI, -3.50 to 7.99; I^2 = 46%). When examined by specific statin, atorvastatin therapy was associated with a modest increase in HbA$_{1C}$ (weighted mean difference, 0.20%; 95% CI, 0.08–0.31), and simvastatin therapy was associated with a modest reduction in HbA$_{1C}$ (weighted mean difference, -0.26%; 95% CI, -0.48 to -0.04). There were no effects observed for cerivastatin, lovastatin, or rosuvastatin (no results for fluvastatin, pravastatin, and pitavastatin were reported).

The JUPITER trial, although it did not include subjects with diabetes, suggested a slightly greater increase from baseline in HbA$_{1C}$ among subjects assigned to rosuvastatin treatment (mean [standard deviation] 0.30% [0.35]) compared with placebo (0.22% [0.40]; P<.001).[4,39] There was no change in fasting serum glucose between the treatment groups (mean [standard deviation] 3 [18.3] mg/dL for rosuvastatin vs 2 [17.3] mg/dL for placebo).

In summary, few data exist regarding the effects of statin therapy on glycemic control in patients with diabetes mellitus. However, the available results suggest that if there is an adverse effect, it is sufficiently small that it is likely to be easily managed by changing the medication regimen for glycemia management. Research is also needed to determine the effects of statin discontinuation on management of glycemic control, that is, if a patient stops taking a statin after statin-associated deterioration in glycemia, would plasma glucose and HbA$_{1C}$ return to their prestatin levels?

Clinical Guidance

The guidelines for screening and the criteria for the diagnosis of T2DM in the asymptomatic patient as outlined in the *Standards of Medical Care in Diabetes* from the American Diabetes Association,[40,41] and recommended by the National Lipid Association Statin Diabetes Task Force,[10] are listed below.

Criteria for Screening

- Testing to detect T2DM and prediabetes (fasting glucose, HbA$_{1C}$ or a 75 g oral glucose tolerance test) in asymptomatic, nonpregnant people should be

considered in adults of any age who are overweight or obese (body mass index $\geq$25 kg/m^2 or $\geq$23 kg/m^2 in Asian Americans) and who have 1 or more of the additional risk factors for diabetes listed:
- o Physical inactivity,
- o First-degree relative with T2DM,
- o High-risk race/ethnicity,
- o Hypertension or history of cardiovascular disease,
- o Polycystic ovary syndrome, delivery of a baby weighing greater than 9 pounds, or diagnosed with gestational diabetes,
- o High triglycerides and/or low high-density lipoprotein cholesterol,
- o Impaired fasting glucose, impaired glucose tolerance, or HbA$_{1C}$ of 5.7 or more, and
- o Another condition associated with insulin resistance.
- In those without risk factors, testing should begin at age 45 years.
- If tests are normal, repeat testing at 3-year intervals or less is reasonable. However, testing should be repeated within 1 year of starting a statin.

Screening should occur before initiation of statin therapy in those with at least 1 major diabetes risk factor, although clinicians should not generally delay the initiation of statin therapy to await results from screening tests in a patient for whom statin therapy is indicated. Managing diabetes risk factors to prevent diabetes is of utmost importance whether or not a patient is taking a statin. Medical nutrition therapy directed at weight loss (often 5%–10% of body weight) in those who are overweight or obese and regular physical activity (at least 150 minutes per week of walking or equivalent activities and limiting the amount of time spent being sedentary by breaking up extended amounts of time spent sitting) are central to efforts to prevent diabetes.[40,41] Regularly monitoring weight and preventing weight gain in patients taking a statin are particularly important.

Potential Use of Nonstatin Add-On Therapy as an Alternative to Statin Intensification in Primary Prevention

The results from the IMProved Reduction of Outcomes: Vytorin Efficacy International Trial (IMPROVE-IT) study supported the cardiovascular benefit of lipid lowering with a Nieman-Pick C1-Like 1 protein inhibitor (ezetimibe) as add-on therapy to a statin in 18,444 patients after acute coronary syndromes.[42,43] The results for ezetimibe as a statin add-on were consistent with effects predicted from studies of statin therapy,[1,44] producing an approximate 10% reduction in major adverse cardiovascular outcomes with a reduction of approximately 0.43 mmol/L (16.7 mg/dL) in low-density lipoprotein cholesterol. Notably, no excess risk for diabetes was observed with ezetimibe plus simvastatin compared with placebo plus simvastatin.[43] These results suggest that the combination of a statin with ezetimibe may be a reasonable alternative to intensification of statin therapy in primary prevention patients with major T2DM risk factors, although it should be emphasized that this strategy has not been tested directly in clinical trials.

SUMMARY

- Statin use is associated with a modest increase in risk ($\sim$10%–12%) for new-onset T2DM, compared with placebo or usual care.
- Intensive dosage statin therapy seems to increase diabetes risk beyond that of moderate dosage statin therapy.

- Excess risk for diabetes with statin use is most clearly evident in those with major risk factors for diabetes.
- The cardiovascular benefits of statin therapy outweigh the potential risk for diabetes development, with several cardiovascular events prevented for each excess case of diabetes.
- Statin therapy should continue to be recommended when appropriate for the reduction of cardiovascular disease event risk.
- Lifestyle modification should be emphasized to all patients for whom statin therapy is recommended to:
  ○ Reduce cardiovascular risk, and
  ○ Attenuate the increase in diabetes risk.
- Patients with risk factors for diabetes should be screened, generally with fasting glucose or HbA_{1C}, ideally before starting statin therapy, within 1 year of initiation, and at intervals no longer than 3 years thereafter.

REFERENCES

1. Cholesterol Treatment Trialists' (CTT) Collaboration, Baigent C, Blackwell L, Emberson J, et al. Efficacy and safety of more intensive lowering of LDL cholesterol: a meta-analysis of data from 170,000 participants in 26 randomised trials. Lancet 2010;376:1670–81.
2. Cholesterol Treatment Trialists' (CTT) Collaborators, Mihaylova B, Emberson J, Blackwell L, et al. The effects of lowering LDL cholesterol with statin therapy in people at low risk of vascular disease: meta-analysis of individual data from 27 randomised trials. Lancet 2012;380:581–90.
3. Taylor R. Banting Memorial Lecture 2012: reversing the twin cycles of type 2 diabetes. Diabet Med 2013;30:267–75.
4. Ridker PM, Danielson E, Fonseca FA, et al, JUPITER Study Group. Rosuvastatin to prevent vascular events in men and women with elevated C-reactive protein. N Engl J Med 2008;359:2195–207.
5. Ridker PM, Pradhan A, MacFadyen JG, et al. Cardiovascular benefits and diabetes risks of statin therapy in primary prevention: an analysis from the JUPITER trial. Lancet 2012;380:565–71.
6. Rajpathak SN, Kumbhani DJ, Crandall J, et al. Statin therapy and risk of developing type 2 diabetes: a meta-analysis. Diabetes Care 2009;32:1924–9.
7. Sattar N, Preiss D, Murray HM, et al. Statins and risk of incident diabetes: a collaborative meta-analysis of randomized statin trials. Lancet 2010;375: 735–42.
8. Preiss D, Seshasai SR, Welsh P, et al. Risk of incident diabetes with intensive-dose compared with moderate-dose statin therapy: a meta-analysis. JAMA 2011;305:2556–64.
9. Waters DD, Ho JE, DeMicco DA, et al. Predictors of new-onset diabetes in patients treated with atorvastatin: results from 3 large randomized clinical trials. J Am Coll Cardiol 2011;57:1535–45.
10. Maki KC, Ridker PM, Brown WV, et al. An assessment by the statin diabetes safety task force: 2014 update. J Clin Lipidol 2014;8:S17–29.
11. National Center for Chronic Disease Prevention and Health Promotion. Division of Diabetes Translation. National Diabetes Statistics Report. 2014. Available at: http://www.cdc.gov/diabetes/pubs/statsreport14/national-diabetes-report-web.pdf. Accessed February 24, 2015.

12. International Diabetes Federation. IDF Diabetes Atlas. 6th edition. 2014. Available at: http://www.idf.org/sites/default/files/Atlas-poster-2014_EN.pdf. Accessed February 24, 2015.

13. Food and Drug Administration. FDA drug safety communication: important safety label changes to cholesterol lowering statin drugs. Available at: http://www.fda.gov/Drugs/DrugSafety/ucm293101.htm. Accessed November 6, 2013.

14. Freeman DJ, Norrie J, Sattar N, et al. Pravastatin and the development of diabetes mellitus: evidence for a protective treatment effect in the West of Scotland Coronary Prevention Study. Circulation 2001;103:357–62.

15. Swerdlow DJ, Preiss D, Kuchenbaecker KB, et al. HMG-coenzyme A reductase inhibition, type 2 diabetes, and bodyweight: evidence from genetic analysis and randomised trials. Lancet 2015;385:351–61.

16. Stone NJ, Robinson JG, Lichtenstein AH, et al. 2013 ACC/AHA guideline on the treatment of blood cholesterol to reduce atherosclerotic cardiovascular risk in adults: a report of the American College of Cardiology/American Heart Association Task Force on Practice Guidelines. J Am Coll Cardiol 2014;63(25 Pt B): 2889–934.

17. Jones PH, Davidson MH, Stein EA, et al. Comparison of the efficacy and safety of rosuvastatin versus atorvastatin, simvastatin, and pravastatin across doses (STELLAR Trial). Am J Cardiol 2003;92:152–60.

18. LaRosa JC, Grundy SM, Waters DD, et al. Intensive lipid lowering with atorvastatin in patients with stable coronary disease. N Engl J Med 2005;352:1425–35.

19. de Lemos JA, Blazing MA, Wiviott SD, et al. Early intensive vs a delayed conservative simvastatin strategy in patients with acute coronary syndromes: phase Z of the A to Z trial. JAMA 2004;292:1307–16.

20. Study of the Effectiveness of Additional Reductions in Cholesterol and Homocysteine (SEARCH) Collaborative Group, Armitage J, Bowman L, et al. Intensive lowering of LDL cholesterol with 80 mg versus 20 mg simvastatin daily in 12,064 survivors of myocardial infarction: a double-blind randomised trial. Lancet 2010;376:1658–69.

21. Danaei G, Garcia Rodriquez LA, Fernandez Cantero O, et al. Statins and risk of diabetes: an analysis of electronic medical records to evaluate possible bias due to differential survival. Diabetes Care 2013;36:1236–40.

22. Corrao G, Ibrahim B, Nicotra F, et al. Statins and the risk of diabetes: evidence from a large population-based cohort study. Diabetes Care 2014;37:2225–32.

23. Dormuth CR, Filion KB, Paterson JM, et al. Canadian network for observational drug effect studies investigators. Higher potency statins and the risk of new diabetes: multicenter, observational study of administrative databases. BMJ 2014; 348:g3244.

24. Macedo AF, Taylor FC, Casas JP, et al. Unintended effects of statins from observational studies in the general population: systematic review and meta-analysis. BMC Med 2014;12:51.

25. Gerich JE. Measurements of renal glucose release. Diabetes 2001;50:905.

26. DeFronzo RA. Banting Lecture. From the triumvirate to the ominous octet: a new paradigm for the treatment of type 2 diabetes mellitus. Diabetes 2009;58:773–95.

27. Lamendola C, Abbasi F, Chu JW, et al. Comparative effects of rosuvastatin and gemfibrozil on glucose, insulin, and lipid metabolism in insulin-resistant, nondiabetic patients with combined dyslipidemia. Am J Cardiol 2005;95:189–93.

28. Baker WL, Talati R, White CM, et al. Differing effect of statins on insulin sensitivity in non-diabetics: a systematic review and meta-analysis. Diabetes Res Clin Pract 2010;87:98–107.

29. Abbas A, Milles J, Ramachandran S. Rosuvastatin and atorvastatin: comparative effects on glucose metabolism in non-diabetic patients with dyslipidemia. Clin Med Insights Endocrinol Diabetes 2012;5:13–30.
30. Sato H, Carvalho G, Sato T, et al. Statin intake is associated with decreased insulin sensitivity during cardiac surgery. Diabetes Care 2012;35:2095–9.
31. Sampson UK, Linto MF, Fazio S. Are statins diabetogenic? Curr Opin Cardiol 2011;26:342–7.
32. Banach M, Malodobra-Mazur M, Gluba A, et al. Statin therapy and new-onset diabetes: molecular mechanisms and clinical relevance. Curr Pharm Des 2013;19: 4904–12.
33. Goldstein MR, Mascitelli L. Do statins cause diabetes? Curr Diab Rep 2013;13: 381–90.
34. Heart Protection Study Collaborative Group. MRC/BHF Heart Protection Study of cholesterol lowering with simvastatin in 20,536 high-risk individuals: a randomised placebo-controlled trial. Lancet 2002;360:7–22.
35. Collins R, Armitage J, Parish S, et al, Heart Protection Study Collaborative Group. MRC/BHF Heart Protection Study of cholesterol lowering with simvastatin in 5963 people with diabetes: a randomized placebo-controlled trial. Lancet 2003;361: 2005–16.
36. Colhoun HM, Betteridge DJ, Durrington PN, et al, CARDS Investigators. Primary prevention of cardiovascular disease with atorvastatin in type 2 diabetes in the Collaborative Atorvastatin Diabetes Study (CARDS): multicenter randomized placebo-controlled trial. Lancet 2004;364:685–96.
37. Holman RR, Paul S, Farmer A, et al, Atorvastatin in Factorial with Omega 3 EE90 Risk Reduction in Diabetes Study Group. Atorvastatin in Factorial with Omega-3 EE90 Risk Reduction in Diabetes (AFORRD): a randomised controlled trial. Diabetologia 2009;52:50–9.
38. Zhou Y, Yuan Y, Cai RR, et al. Statin therapy on glycaemic control in type 2 diabetes: a meta-analysis. Expert Opin Pharmacother 2013;14:1575–84.
39. Astra Zeneca. Clinical briefing document – Endocrine and Metabolic Drugs Advisory Committee meeting for rosuvastatin (Crestor). Available at: http://www.fda.gov/downloads/AdvisoryCommittees/CommitteesMeetingMaterials/Drugs/EndocrinologicandMetabolicDrugsAdvisoryCommittee/UCM193833.pdf. Accessed November 5, 2013.
40. American Diabetes Association. Standards of medical care in diabetes – 2014. Diabetes Care 2014;37(Suppl 1):S14–80.
41. American Diabetes Association. Standards of medical care in diabetes – 2015. Diabetes Care 2015;38(Suppl 1):S1–90.
42. Katsiki N, Theocharidou E, Karagiannis A, et al. Ezetimibe therapy for dyslipidemia: an update. Curr Pharm Des 2013;19:3107–14.
43. Cannon CP on behalf of the IMPROVE IT Investigators. IMPROVE-IT Trial: A comparison of ezetimibe/simvastatin versus simvastatin monotherapy on cardiovascular outcomes after acute coronary syndromes. Late-breaking clinical trial abstracts and clinical science special reports abstracts from the American Heart Association's Scientific Sessions 2014. Circulation. 2014;130:2105–2126.
44. Cholesterol Treatment Trialists' (CTT) Collaborators, Baigent C, Keech A, Kearney PM, et al. Efficacy and safety of cholesterol-lowering treatment: prospective meta-analysis of data from 90,056 participants in 14 randomised trials of statins. Lancet 2005;366:1267–78.

Lipid-Associated Rheumatologic Syndromes

Eyal Kedar, MD, Gregory C. Gardner, MD*

KEYWORDS

- Hyperlipidemia • Tendon xanthoma • Lipid liquid crystals • Arthritis

KEY POINTS

- Tendon xanthomas are associated with Type II and III hyperlipidemia and their presence is a marker for an increase the risk of cardiovascular disease.
- Arthritis associated with hyperlipidemia may affect one or multiple joints and is likely a periarthritis in most cases.
- Lipid liquid crystal arthritis is self-limited inflammatory arthritis characterized by the presence of positively birefringent spherules in the synovial fluid.
- There is an association between hyperlipidemia and gout that is likely both environmental and genetic.
- Statins have been implicated in the development of autoimmune disease including a recently described necrotizing myopathy.

INTRODUCTION

Lipid-associated musculoskeletal syndromes are uncommon problems seen in the rheumatologist's office. The rheumatologist, however, may be the first clinician to recognize the manifestations of a lipid-associated syndrome and initiate proper investigation and therapy. Khachadurian[1] was one of the first to report that patients with hyperlipidemia experienced musculoskeletal symptoms. The single-author article from the American University in Beirut reported that 10 of 18 patients homozygous for familial type II hyperlipidemia had attacks of acute migratory polyarthritis lasting up to a month that resembled acute rheumatic fever, as well as tendon xanthomata. No other explanation for the arthritis was uncovered, and the implication was that the hyperlipidemia was the cause of the attacks.[1] Since then a variety of reports covering this topic and expanding on the musculoskeletal manifestations of hyperlipidemia has been published. This article reviews the current literature regarding

This article originally appeared in Rheumatic Disease Clinics, Volume 39, Issue 2, May 2013.
Disclosures: Dr Kedar is supported by an NIH training grant. Dr Gardner has no disclosures related to this article.
Division of Rheumatology, University of Washington, Box 356428, Seattle, WA 98195, USA
* Corresponding author.
E-mail address: rheumdoc@uw.edu

http://dx.doi.org/10.1016/j.ccol.2015.05.019
2352-7986/15/$ – see front matter © 2015 Elsevier Inc. All rights reserved.

lipid-associated syndromes involving joints and tendons, and also reviews the data regarding the relationship of hyperlipidemia with hyperuricemia and gout. Finally, drug-induced rheumatologic illness related to lipid-lowering therapy is briefly discussed.

LIPOPROTEINS AND THE CURRENT CLASSIFICATION OF DYSLIPIDEMIA

The 5 major types of hyperlipidemia are classified by their relevant forms of lipoprotein dysmetabolism under the Fredrickson classification system (**Table 1**).[2] A proper understanding of this system requires a brief review of the 5 major lipoproteins and their basic functions.[3]

Lipoproteins are assemblies of lipids (triglycerides and/or cholesterol, in the case of the lipoproteins discussed in this article) and protein (referred to as apolipoproteins or apoproteins), which serve to transport lipids in the body. Lipid metabolism can be broadly characterized as being under the control of both endogenous and exogenous pathways. The lipoprotein associated with exogenous (dietary) lipid metabolism is the chylomicron, which is mainly a carrier of triglycerides but which also carries, to a significantly lesser extent, cholesterol esters. Chylomicrons are formed in enterocytes and are transported through the lymphatic system to the circulation, where they are broken down by lipoprotein lipase into free fatty acids (from triglycerides) and apoproteins. Ultimately, the remaining chylomicron remnants are taken up by hepatocytes and their contents reprocessed (eg, remaining triglycerides can be packaged for reexport into the circulation as part of very low-density lipoproteins [VLDLs]).

Endogenous pathways of lipid metabolism refer to the processing of hepatically derived lipids, and begin with export of VLDLs from the liver. As with chylomicrons, VLDLs carry triglycerides and, to a lesser extent, cholesterol, and are broken down in the periphery by lipoprotein lipase to yield, among other elements, a combination of free fatty acids and apoproteins. The result is the formation of smaller, denser VLDL "remnants" (also referred to as intermediate-density lipoproteins [IDLs]), which in turn can be broken down further by hepatic lipase to yield IDL remnants known as low-density lipoproteins (LDLs). As the VLDL is broken down, it becomes denser and more enriched in cholesterol, as evidenced by LDL's main role as a carrier of cholesterol rather than triglycerides.

High-density lipoprotein (HDL), like LDL, is chiefly a carrier of cholesterol. Its main role is to absorb excess cholesterol from intracellular pools and to transport this

Table 1
Fredrickson/World Health Organization classification of dyslipidemias

Type	Elevated Lipoprotein(s)	Lipids Elevated
I	Chylomicrons	Triglycerides
IIa	LDL	Cholesterol
IIb	LDL, VLDL	Cholesterol > triglycerides
III	IDL (VLDL remnants), chylomicrons	Cholesterol and triglycerides
IV	VLDL	Triglycerides
V	VLDL, chylomicrons	Triglycerides > cholesterol

Abbreviations: IDL, intermediate-density lipoprotein; LDL, low-density lipoprotein; VLDL, very low-density lipoprotein.
Data from Fredrickson DS. An international classification of hyperlipidemias and hyperlipoproteinemias. Ann Intern Med 1971;75(3):471–2; and Durrington P. Dyslipidaemia. Lancet 2003;362(9385):717–31.

cholesterol, via a combination of direct and indirect pathways, back to the liver or to steroidogenic tissues such as the adrenals, ovaries, and testes. This transport can be done directly via interaction with scavenger cholesterol receptors on target tissues, or indirectly via initial transfer of cholesterol esters to LDL, which in turn delivers these esters to the tissues.

The roles of the 5 major lipoproteins (in order of decreasing size and increasing density) can be summarized as follows:

- Chylomicrons: large lipoproteins that carry dietary, or exogenous, lipids (triglycerides > cholesterol)
- VLDLs: carriers of hepatically derived, or endogenous, lipids (triglycerides > cholesterol)
- IDLs (also referred to as VLDL remnants): carriers of endogenous cholesterol and triglycerides
- LDLs: carriers of endogenous cholesterol
- HDLs: absorb excess cholesterol from intracellular pools and return this cholesterol to the liver and steroidogenic tissues (adrenals, ovaries, and testes)

HYPERLIPIDEMIA AND TENDINOPATHY

Of the major classes of hyperlipidemia, types II and III have been shown to be associated with xanthomatous disease, and type II has been associated with tendinopathy.[4] Type II hyperlipidemia is characterized by elevation of LDL levels (see **Table 1**) and has 2 known subtypes (types IIa and IIb). It can be inherited as a familial disease or present as a polygenic or sporadic disorder. Patients homozygous for familial type II hyperlipidemia have mutations in both LDL receptor (LDLR) alleles, and develop tendon xanthomata that can be either symptomatic or asymptomatic.[4,5] These xanthomata are collections of lipid-laden macrophages that typically develop over the Achilles tendons (although other tendon areas, including the triceps tendons, may also be involved) and that, in homozygotes, typically develop in childhood.[6] In addition, type II homozygotes may develop fever and a migratory polyarthritis that mimics rheumatic fever, which was first reported by Khachadurian[1] and is discussed in more depth in the next section. Of note, there was no clear relationship between the observed joint pains and the locations of xanthomata.[1,5]

Tendon xanthomata are also found in patients who have type II heterozygous hyperlipidemia (**Fig. 1**). Xanthomata present later in life than in homozygotes (who typically die of cardiovascular disease before the age of 30 years), are present at

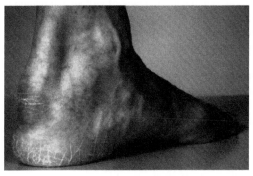

Fig. 1. Achilles tendon xanthoma in a patient with type II heterozygous hyperlipidemia. (*From* Durrington P. Dyslipidaemia. Lancet 2003;362(9385):719; with permission.)

a comparatively lower frequency, and are not present in all patients.[7] As with their homozygous counterparts, these xanthomata can be asymptomatic. The Achilles tendon is the most common location of xanthomata in patients with type II hyperlipidemia, and Mathon and colleagues[7] reported that 18% of 73 patients with familial heterozygous type II hyperlipidemia had Achilles pain and 11% had evidence of Achilles tendinitis.[8] In a controlled cross-sectional study, Beeharry and colleagues[9] reported that 46.6% of 133 patients with familial heterozygous type II hyperlipidemia had had 1 or more episodes of Achilles pain, compared with 6.9% of 87 unaffected controls. The patients were also significantly much more likely to report the pain as severe or very severe, with pain lasting an average of 4 days, and more likely than the controls to seek medical attention for the Achilles symptoms. One of the early studies of symptomatic Achilles tendon involvement reported that tendinitis could be unilateral or bilateral, that patients could have up to 12 attacks per year, and that one patient had 4 to 5 attacks per year for 40 years.[10] The presence of tendon xanthomata is an independent risk factor for cardiovascular disease and indicates the need for more aggressive lipid-lowering therapy.[11] In a meta-analysis of xanthoma formation, heterozygous type II hyperlipidemia, and cardiovascular risk, Oosterveer and colleagues[12] found that the presence of xanthomata conferred a 3.2-fold higher risk for cardiovascular disease. Increasing age, male gender, and levels of LDL cholesterol and triglycerides increased the risk of developing xanthomata. The xanthoma has a composition similar to that of atheroma, and treatment-associated regression of xanthomata with either statins or fibrates may be a marker of atheroma regression.[8] Achilles tendon xanthomata are easily detected by ultrasonography or magnetic resonance imaging (MRI) before they may be detectable clinically. Ultrasonography, in turn, is the easiest and most cost-effective way of detecting xanthomata, and can also be used to quantitatively measure treatment-associated xanthoma regression.[8]

Type III hyperlipidemia (familial dysbetalipoproteinemia) is an autosomal recessive disorder involving 2 apoprotein E2 alleles that results in elevated levels of IDL (VLDL remnants) and chylomicrons and, in turn, elevated cholesterol and triglyceride levels. Tuberoeruptive xanthomata (which typically involve the extensor surfaces) and plantar crease xanthomata (xanthomata palmare striatum) are typical of this disorder.[3,4] These xanthomata are asymptomatic and do not involve joint or tendon areas.[3,13] Of note, reports have shown that close to half of these patients have asymptomatic hyperuricemia, with actual gout attacks being rare.[4,14]

Beyond familial forms of hyperlipidemia, secondary forms (such as hyperlipidemia secondary to diabetes or thyroid disease) can also present with xanthomata.[15] Rheumatic symptoms (such as joint pains) associated with several of the secondary hyperlipidemias are common, but in light of a lack of studies examining the causes of these symptoms as well as the clinical heterogeneity and genetic complexity of the underlying diseases, clear associations have not been found.[5]

Two final entities that deserve note are cerebrotendinous xanthomatosis and sitosterolemia, both of which are rare autosomal recessive disorders of lipid metabolism associated with tendon xanthomata but not actual tendinitis or arthritis.[6] Cerebrotendinous xanthomatosis involves a mutation in the sterol 27-hydroxylase gene, which leads to accumulation of dihydrocholesterol (cholestanol). It is associated with asymptomatic xanthomata of the Achilles tendons that appear in the second to fourth decades of life, as well as a variety of other symptoms including cataracts, diarrhea, vascular disease, cerebellar ataxia, and dementia.[6,16]

Sitosterolemia involves excessive intestinal absorption, and subsequent increased plasma levels, of plant sterols. Patients develop asymptomatic tendon xanthomata as well as accelerated atherosclerosis.[6]

HYPERLIPIDEMIA-ASSOCIATED ARTHRITIS

The 1968 report of Khachadurian has been the basis for the association of hyper-lipidemia with arthritis.[1] Of 18 young homozygous patients with familial type II hyper-lipidemia, 10 were reported to develop self-limited attacks of migratory polyarthritis that could be severe enough to cause the sufferer to be bedridden. In the 10 affected patients, Khachadurian ruled out acute rheumatic fever and hyperuricemia in all cases as a cause of the arthritis. Sedimentation rates and C-reactive protein could be elevated and the patient could be febrile as well. The sedimentation rate often remained elevated between attacks of arthritis. The joints were described as being swollen, but the one attempted arthrocentesis from a swollen knee was unsuccessful in that no fluid was obtained. A photo of a patient's hands included in the report shows marked fullness around the metacarpophalangeal joints, and proximal interphalangeal (PIP) joints in particular are described as being xanthomatous. All of the patients included in this report had xanthomata. The lack of obtainable synovial fluid and the appearance of the hands raise the question of a periarthritis rather than a true arthritis.

A much more detailed report of the arthritis of hyperlipidemia was published in 1978 by Rooney and colleagues.[17] These investigators followed 41 patients with familial hyperbetalipoproteinemia for up to 4 years, noting the symptoms and joints involved, and reporting on fluid obtained during arthrocentesis and even doing xenon clearance from joints assumed to be inflamed. Again a transient migratory polyarthritis was noted, which affected both large and small joints in up to 10 of these patients, lasting 3 to 12 days. The pain was moderate to severe and in no case was the arthritis attribut-able to acute rheumatic fever of gout. Synovial fluid was obtained from 6 swollen joints; in all cases the fluid had 200 or fewer white blood cells (WBCs) per cm^3 and was reported to have normal viscosity. Bacteriologic and crystal analyses were nega-tive in all patients. Xenon clearance for affected joints was also normal, suggesting to the investigators that the arthritis was in all cases actually a periarthritis. In a case report of a male patient with swelling of PIP joints and familial hypercholesterolemia, MRI revealed periarticular fat deposition, which by appearance may have been capsular in location but certainly not intra-articular.[18] Fine-needle aspiration of the periarticular lipid accumulation at the PIP joints in a young girl with familial hypercho-lesterolemia demonstrated the presence of abundant foam cells (ie, macrophages laden with lipids and found in atherosclerotic plaques as well as xanthomata of skin and tendons).[6,19] Foam cells are metabolically active and may produce cytokines and other proinflammatory molecules, or possibly metabolize the internalized lipid to cause it to become phlogistic.[20] These activities may contribute to periarticular inflammation seen in affected patients. A patient with a similar periarticular deposition of lipid is shown in **Fig. 2**.

Although the weight of evidence favors a periarthritis, at least one report has docu-mented an inflammatory synovial fluid in a patient with type II hyperlipidemia arthritis.[10] The patient was a 23-year-old with episodes of oligoarthritis affecting the knees and ankles beginning at age 20 years. Synovial fluid analysis from a swollen knee demonstrated 5400 WBCs with the majority being neutrophils, and with no other apparent cause of the arthritis.

Patients who develop arthritis/periarthritis typically have familial type II hyperlipid-emia. As previously mentioned, these patients are also those who have a tendency to develop tendon xanthomata. Many of the early reports were in patients with the rare homozygous form of disease. Mathon and colleagues,[7] in a cross-sectional study of patients with heterozygous familial hypercholesterolemia, found that 7% of 73 affected patients reported at least 1 episode of a monoarthritis or an oligoarthritis,

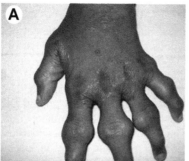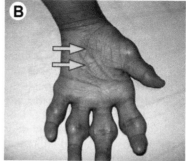

Fig. 2. (*A*) Dorsal view of the hand showing marked periarticular fullness around he PIP joints in a patient with Type II hyperlipidemia. (*B*) Palmar view of the same hand showing palmar xanthomata (*arrows*) in addition to the periarticular fullness. (*From* Sharma A, Dogra S, Mahajan R, et al. An unusual cause of joint swelling. Lancet 2010;375:1109; with permission.)

whereas 4% reported a more classic migratory polyarticular syndrome. The onset is not generally before age 20 years in these patients, in comparison with childhood onset in patients with homozygous disease. In addition, at the time the patients were examined there was no evidence of joint abnormality, despite numerous attacks in some patients, confirming the nondestructive nature of the arthritis/periarthritis.

Although the majority of the case report/case series literature has focused on type II patients, type IV patients have also been reported to develop episodic arthritis. Twenty-four patients with type IV hyperlipidemia described by Goldman and colleagues[21] and Buckingham and colleagues[22] were reported to have an acute to subacute pauciarthritis of large and small joints that could not be explained by another cause (in particular, gout). In some cases of the Goldman series pain could be severe, but in others it was mild and persistent. Goldman and colleagues also reported that the evidence of inflammation was often less than the reported level of pain. The synovial fluid was noninflammatory in 2 knee effusions aspirated by Goldman and colleagues, whereas synovial fluid obtained from 2 patients in the Buckingham series was described as mildly inflammatory.

The results of epidemiologic studies give a mixed picture of arthritis and hyperlipidemia. In 1978 Welin and colleagues[23] reported on a relatively large cohort of men from Sweden born in either 1913 or 1923, and included data on their lipid profiles and clinical information. In a comparison with men with normal lipid levels they could not find a relationship between any of the subtypes of hyperlipidemia and increased musculoskeletal manifestations, although the overall numbers in each subtype of hyperlipidemia were small. Wysenbeek and colleagues[24] reported an increase in foot and ankle pain in 69 patients with type IIa hyperlipidemia compared with 33 controls, but no increase in inflammatory-type manifestations. Klemp and colleagues[25] conducted a comparison between 88 patients with adult and juvenile familial forms of hyperlipidemia (type II) or a mixed form (elevated cholesterol and triglycerides) and 88 controls. Adults with familial forms of hyperlipidemia were found to have an excess of xanthomata and Achilles tendinitis, whereas the mixed form of hyperlipidemia demonstrated an excess of xanthomata, Achilles tendinitis, and oligoarthritis compared with controls. The juvenile form of hyperlipidemia was not found to have excess musculoskeletal manifestations in comparison with controls, and migratory polyarthritis, though reported by 5 patients in the adult group and none of the controls, was reported to be not significant. It is possible that the small number in each group

(48 adult type II, 16 juvenile type II, and 24 mixed) was too inadequate to reveal this rare complication. Large well-controlled studies aimed at answering prevalence questions regarding hyperlipidemia and arthritis are currently lacking.

Anecdotal experience regarding treatment further implicates hyperlipidemia as a cause of joint symptoms. In general, arthritis and musculoskeletal symptoms have been reported to respond to lipid-lowering therapy in both type II and type IV patients.[5,6,19]

LIPID LIQUID CRYSTAL ARTHRITIS

Lipid liquid crystal arthritis is an uncommonly reported cause of acute arthritis. The attacks have a gout-like quality in that they usually affect single, typically large joints, and resolve within days without therapy or in response to nonsteroidal anti-inflammatories (NSAIDs), colchicine, or corticosteroid injections. Acute-phase reactants are often elevated during the attack as well.[26,27] Lipid liquid crystals are identified in synovial fluid under compensated polarized light as strongly positively birefringent spherules resembling beach balls (**Fig. 3**).[28] Such crystals are found both extracellularly and intracellularly in association with, in most cases, a neutrophil-predominant synovial fluid leukocytosis. The crystals stain with Sudan black, dissolve with alcohol/ether 1:1 mixture or xylol, are resistant to urate and ethylenediaminetetraacetic acid, and are alizarin red–negative, implicating lipids as the source of the spherules (rather than the usual causes of gout-like joint swelling).[26,28,29] The positively birefringent spherules do have some resemblance to talc crystals, but at least one report compared talc crystals under polarizing compensated microscopy and pointed out that talc can be easily distinguished from the lipid liquid spherules. The etiology and incidence of this unusual syndrome are still uncertain.

There have been at least 14 cases reported in the English literature, and 7 additional cases from Swiss and Mexican publications (**Table 2**). The first case was described by Weinstein in 1980 in a 48-year-old woman who was hospitalized with an acutely swollen knee, which on arthrocentesis demonstrated 27,800 WBCs, 90% neutrophils, and 8200 red blood cells (RBCs).[30] With polarized light microscopy, up to 10% of the synovial fluid neutrophils contained Maltese-cross inclusions that were Sudanophilic. No other crystals or abnormalities were noted in the synovial fluid or culture, nor were

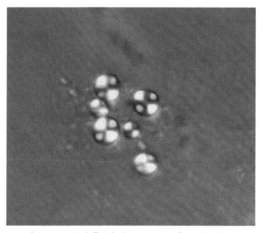

Fig. 3. Lipid liquid crystal in synovial fluid. (*Courtesy of* G. Gardner, MD, Seattle, WA.)

Table 2
Details of 21 cases of lipid liquid arthritis

Case No., Authors,[Ref.] Year	Demographics	Joint or Joints	Course
1. Weinstein,[30] 1980	48-y-old Female	Knee	Resolved in 5 d without therapy
2. Schlesinger et al,[36] 1982	14-y-old Male	Polyarthritis of small and large joints	Acute symptoms improved with NSAIDs; spherules present at 2 mo
3. Reginato et al,[31] 1985	41-y-old Female	Wrist	Resolved in 5 d with colchicine
4. Reginato et al,[31] 1985	21-y-old Female	Knee	Resolved by day 14 with NSAID
5. Reginato et al,[31] 1985	54-y-old Female	Knee	Resolved by day 10 with NSAID
6. Trostle et al,[33] 1986	33-y-old Female	Knee	Resolved in 5 d with colchicine
7. Ugai et al,[34] 1988	36-y-old Male	Knee (PVNS)	Surgery to remove PVNS
8. Ugai et al,[34] 1988	30-y-old Female	Knee (PVNS)	Surgery to remove PVNS
9. Gardner and Terkeltaub,[28] 1989	58-y-old Female	Knee	Resolved in 5 d with NSAID
10. Astorga and Carvajal,[26] 1990	34-y-old Female	Knee	Resolved in 10 d with NSAID
11. Rivest et al,[29] 1992	52-y-old Female	Polyarthritis of MCPs, wrists, elbows (history of RA)	Resolved by day 14 with NSAID; spherules still present at 1 mo
12. Park et al,[37] 1997	Male	Left third MTP then left transverse tarsal joint	Resolved in 14 d with NSAID
13. Hackeng et al,[27] 2000	31-y-old Male	Knee	Resolved in 14 d with NSAID
14. Dylewski,[38] 2005	44-y-old Female	Knee	NSAID followed by steroid injection with resolution in 8 d
15–21	Uncertain	Monoarthritis	Uncertain

Abbreviations: MCP, metacarpophalangeal joint; MTP, metatarsophalangeal joint; NSAID, nonsteroidal anti-inflammatory drug; PVNS, pigmented villonodular synovitis; RA, rheumatoid arthritis.

Cases 15–20 *from* Van Linthoudt D. L'arthrite a cristaux de lipids liquids. Rev Med Suisse 2010;6:2034–7; and Koya P, Marin E, Ricardo R, et al. Monoarthritic asosiada a critales liquidos lipidicos: reporte de seis casos y estudio in vitro de fagocitosis inducida por lipomas artificiales [abstract]. Rev Mex Reumatol 1990;5(Suppl 1):52.

there any serologic data to explain the acute arthritis. Repeat arthrocentesis on day 2 of hospitalization found that the cell count had risen to 38,000, but by day 4 the synovial fluid cell count had dropped to 10,600. Pain and swelling lasted a total of 5 days and resolved without any specific therapy other than the repeated arthrocenteses. The patient reported intermittent swelling in the knee that lasted 2 days per episode (over 2 years of follow-up). Most of the subsequent cases are similar, and the data regarding these are summarized in **Table 2**.

In addition to using laboratory methods to demonstrate the lipid nature of the Maltese crosses, some literature included additional investigation. Reginato and colleagues[31] described 3 cases of acute arthritis associated with intracellular and extracellular Maltese-cross lipid spherules. On electron microscopy of synovial fluid cells, they reported gray lipid droplets and multilayered lamellated inclusions in phagocytic vacuoles that were similar to lipid liquid crystals reported by others. These investigators were the first to refer to the Maltese crosses as lipid liquid crystals. Liquid crystals have properties between those of a liquid and those of solid crystal.[32] A liquid crystal may flow like a liquid, but its molecules may be oriented in a crystalline fashion. Using a polarized light microscope, different liquid crystal phases will appear to have distinct textures, indicating that the molecules of the liquid crystal may be oriented in different, phase-specific directions.

Trostle and colleagues[33] extended the observations of Reginato and colleagues when they performed a synovial biopsy on a patient with acute lipid liquid crystal arthritis. The biopsy showed nonspecific lining cell hyperplasia, with rare lymphocytes and some prominence of the endothelium and perivascular cells. Maltese-cross bodies and irregularly shaped birefringent rod-like material was seen in the neutrophils adherent to the synovium. Some of the irregular birefringent rod-like material was also seen in the synovial lining cells. On electron microscopy, the neutrophils contained lipid droplets as well as multilaminated concentric arrays within phagocytic vacuoles, and some lipid droplets were coated with finely granular protein-like material. Both groups noted that there were lipid droplets as well as lipids in the form of lipid liquid crystals in phagocytic cells.

Two cases reported by Ugai and colleagues[34] may provide further insight into the etiology of lipid liquid crystals. Both patients had pigmented villonodular synovitis with associated abundant RBCs, and the presence of positively birefringent Maltese-cross spherules both in the synovial fluid and inside macrophages. Neither patient had an acute arthritis, but both had chronic joint swelling. The synovial fluids did have a leukocytosis but the cell differentials were different to those seen in patients with the more acute form of the arthritis. The predominant cells were lymphocytes and macrophages, with small numbers of neutrophils noted as well. The investigators speculated that the source of the lipid liquid crystals were the lipid membranes from the degenerating RBCs. Indeed, Choi and colleagues[35] were able to induce an acute synovitis in rabbits by injecting autologous RBCs in knee joints, with subsequent demonstration of lipid liquid crystal formation within the synovial fluid.

Although the majority of patients reported had an acute monoarthritis, 2 patients presented with a polyarthritis. One patient had poorly controlled rheumatoid arthritis and presented a pseudoseptic characterization involving multiple joints, with WBCs as numerous as 120,000/cm^3.[29] The polyarthritis responded symptomatically to naproxen, but 1 month later synovial fluid continued to show intracellular and extracellular lipid liquid crystals. The other patient with polyarthritis had an undefined chronic illness.[36] The inflammatory cells in the synovial fluid were 100% macrophages, and lipid liquid crystals persisted at 2 months after initial presentation (by which point the severe initial symptoms had subsided). These 2 patients illustrate the point that the lipid liquid crystals, like both pyrophosphate crystals and urate crystals, may be present in synovial fluid without being overtly phlogistic.

The authors suspect that lipid liquid crystal–associated arthritis is more common than the 21 cases suggest. Its self-limited nature in most patients and its response to NSAIDs mean that many cases probably go unrecognized, given the requirement that synovial fluid in affected patients must be examined under polarized light to make the diagnosis. The mechanism of formation of lipid liquid crystals is not entirely clear, but they have been seen in the synovial fluid of patients with rheumatoid arthritis along with cholesterol crystals, suggesting that local lipid saturation may be an important requirement for formation.[39] The source of the lipids my well be the breakdown of cell membranes, as suggested by their presence in the patients with pigmented villonodular synovitis and the data advocating that experimental hemarthrosis leads to the development of lipid liquid crystals.[35] Injecting liposomes into knee joints of rabbits results in acute synovitis and the formation of lipid liquid crystals, suggesting a direct phlogistic potential of the lipids.[40] In addition, Simkin and colleagues[41] have reported on 2 patients with pancreatitis-associated arthritis characterized by elevated intra-articular free fatty acids. Like Choi and colleagues,[40] they were able to induce an acute arthritis in rabbit knees by injecting them with free fatty acids, suggesting that it is this component of the lipid that (at least in part) causes the acute arthritis. Like other crystalline causes of acute arthritis, lipid liquid crystals can be seen in asymptomatic joints as well, therefore factors other than the presence of the spherules/lipids likely contribute to the inflammatory process.

HYPERLIPIDEMIA AND GOUT

There is a known association between hyperlipidemia (and the metabolic syndrome in general) and gout.[42] A recent prospective cohort study of 1606 Chinese patients with gout showed a significant association of hyperlipidemia (as well as both hypertension and obesity) with gout, with hazard ratios of 1.12 and 1.7, respectively, for men and women with hyperlipidemia.[43] In another recent multicenter study of 312 patients with gout in Turkey, 30.1% of the patients had some form of hyperlipidemia.[44]

The association of gout with the metabolic syndrome, and hyperlipidemia in particular, is likely the result of a combination of genetic and environmental factors.[44] Recently, the particular association with coronary artery disease, as well the increased risk of myocardial infarction in young patients with gout, has come to increased attention,[45] as has the long-known association of diet and gout.[46]

Beyond the association of gout with secondary hyperlipidemia, there is also a known relationship with some of the primary hyperlipidemias. As noted earlier, reports have shown that half of patients with type III hyperlipidemia (familial dysbetalipoproteinemia) have asymptomatic hyperuricemia.[4,14] Even better described, however, is the association with type IV hyperlipidemia whereby there are elevated levels of VLDL and, in turn, hypertriglyceridemia. When this disorder occurs in a family it is termed familial hypertriglyceridemia.[3,4] These patients can experience recurrent gout attacks,[4,47] although it is unclear whether the hyperlipidemia is a cause of or merely an association with gout, and vice versa.[5]

RHEUMATOLOGIC DISEASE INDUCED BY LIPID-LOWERING THERAPY

Beyond the well-known association of statins with myalgias and myopathy, these medications have also been implicated as a cause of drug-induced autoimmune disease. In a 1993 review of musculoskeletal manifestations of hyperlipidemia, Careless and Cohen[5] noted that there had been several cases of drug-induced lupus associated with statins and 1 case ascribed to clofibrate. These cases were associated with antihistone antibodies, and resolved with immunosuppressive therapy and withdrawal of the medication. Autoantibodies resolved over time as well, suggesting a drug-associated syndrome.

In a 2005 review of the literature for reports of autoimmune disease associated with statins, 28 cases of statin-induced autoimmune diseases were identified.[48] This cohort included 10 cases of systemic lupus erythematosus, 3 cases of subacute cutaneous lupus erythematosus, 14 cases of dermatomyositis and polymyositis, and 1 case of lichen planus pemphigoides. Autoimmune hepatitis was also noted in

2 patients with coexisting systemic lupus erythematosus. Patients were treated for a mean of 12.8 months before symptoms appeared within a range of 1 month to 6 years. Most required immunosuppressive therapy, and 2 patients died of pulmonary complications as a result of their drug-induced syndrome (1 lupus, 1 myositis). More recently, de Jong and colleagues[49] preformed a case/noncase study based on individual case safety reports listed in the World Health Organization global individual case safety reports database (VigiBase). This study identified 3362 cases of lupus-like syndrome in the database, and found that statins were associated with 3.2% of these. As statin use increases, such rare manifestations may be seen in larger numbers and will become important for rheumatologists to recognize.

Finally, a recently described immune-mediated necrotizing myopathy associated with antibodies directed against 3-hydroxy-3-methyl-glutaryl coenzyme-A (HMG CoA) reductase has been described and associated with statin use.[50,51] The myopathy is characterized as a subacute, severe, symmetric, proximal myopathy with elevated creatine kinase levels, which shows little inflammation on biopsy and requires immunosuppressive therapy for control. This form of myopathy is reported to respond to steroids and methotrexate, but in some cases has required rituximab or intravenous immunoglobulin. Manifestations persist after withdrawal of the drugs. Up to 6% of patients treated with statins may demonstrate antibodies, although most do not have evidence of myopathy. Statins upregulate the expression of HMG CoA reductase in muscle cells, and regenerating muscle cells express high levels of these molecules, perpetuating the syndrome even when the statin is no longer present. Patients with other rheumatologic diseases can also express these antibodies, and an HMG CoA reductase antibody-associated myopathy may also spontaneously occur without exposure to statins. More information on this form of myopathy is certain to be forthcoming.

SUMMARY

Although patients with lipid-associated rheumatologic disorders present relatively infrequently, it is likely that most clinical rheumatologists will encounter these conditions during their career. The proper diagnosis and treatment of these patients will relieve their suffering, and in some cases, prevent future complications of hyperlipidemia. However, a complete understanding of the pathophysiologic mechanisms by which these conditions develop remains to be elucidated.

REFERENCES

1. Khachadurian AK. Migratory polyarthritis in familial hypercholesterolemia (type II hyperlipoproteinemia). Arthritis Rheum 1968;11(3):385–93.
2. Fredrickson DS. An international classification of hyperlipidemias and hyperlipoproteinemias. Ann Intern Med 1971;75(3):471–2.
3. Durrington P. Dyslipidaemia. Lancet 2003;362(9385):717–31.
4. Fishel B, Rosenbach TO, Yaron M, et al. Hyperlipidemias and rheumatic manifestations. Clin Rheumatol 1986;5(1):75–9.
5. Careless DJ, Cohen MG. Rheumatic manifestations of hyperlipidemia and antihyperlipidemia drug therapy. Semin Arthritis Rheum 1993;23(2):90–8.
6. Handel ML, Simons L. Rheumatic manifestations of hyperlipidaemia. Best Pract Res Clin Rheumatol 2000;14(3):595–8.
7. Mathon G, Gagné C, Brun D, et al. Articular manifestations of familial hypercholesterolaemia. Ann Rheum Dis 1985;44(9):599–602.
8. Tsouli SG, Kiortsis DN, Argyropoulou MI, et al. Pathogenesis, detection and treatment of Achilles tendon xanthomas. Eur J Clin Invest 2005;35(4):236–44.

9. Beeharry D. Familial hypercholesterolaemia commonly presents with Achilles tenosynovitis. Ann Rheum Dis 2006;65(3):312–5.

10. Glueck CJ, Levy RI, Frederickson DS. Acute tendinitis and arthritis. A presenting symptom of familial type II hyperlipoproteinemia. JAMA 1968;206(13):2895–7.

11. Civeira F. Tendon xanthomas in familial hypercholesterolemia are associated with cardiovascular risk independently of the low-density lipoprotein receptor gene mutation. Arterioscler Thromb Vasc Biol 2005;25(9):1960–5.

12. Oosterveer DM, Versmissen J, Yazdanpanah M, et al. Differences in characteristics and risk of cardiovascular disease in familial hypercholesterolemia patients with and without tendon xanthomas: a systematic review and meta-analysis. Atherosclerosis 2009;207(2):311–7.

13. Sharma D, Thirkannad S. Palmar xanthoma—an indicator of a more sinister problem. Hand (N Y) 2009;5(2):210–2.

14. Morganroth J, Levy RI, Fredrickson DS. The biochemical, clinical, and genetic features of type III hyperlipoproteinemia. Ann Intern Med 1975;82(2):158–74.

15. Parker F. Xanthomas and hyperlipidemias. J Am Acad Dermatol 1985;13(1):1–30.

16. Moghadasian MH, Salen G, Frohlich JJ, et al. Cerebrotendinous xanthomatosis: a rare disease with diverse manifestations. Arch Neurol 2002;59(4):527–9.

17. Rooney PJ, Third J, Madkour MM, et al. Transient polyarthritis associated with familial hyperbetalipoproteinaemia. Q J Med 1978;47(187):249–59.

18. Alfadhli E. Cholesterol deposition around small joints of the hands in familial hypercholesterolemia mimicking "Bouchard's and Heberden's nodes" of osteoarthritis. Intern Med 2010;49(15):1675–6.

19. Chakraborty PP, Mukhopadhyay S, Achar A, et al. Migratory polyarthritis in familial hypercholesterolemia (type IIa hyperlipoproteinemia). Indian J Pediatr 2010;77(3):329–31.

20. McLaren JE, Michael DR, Ashlin TG, et al. Cytokines, macrophage lipid metabolism and foam cells: implications for cardiovascular disease therapy. Prog Lipid Res 2011;50(4):331–47.

21. Goldman JA, Glueck CJ, Abrams NR, et al. Musculoskeletal disorders associated with type-IV hyperlipoproteinaemia. Lancet 1972;2(7775):449–52.

22. Buckingham RB, Bole GG, Bassett DR. Polyarthritis associated with type IV hyperlipoproteinemia. Arch Intern Med 1975;135(2):286–90.

23. Welin L, Larsson B, Svärdsudd K, et al. Serum lipids, lipoproteins and musculoskeletal disorders among 50- and 60-year-old men. An epidemiologic study. Scand J Rheumatol 1978;7(1):7–12.

24. Wysenbeek AJ, Shani E, Beigel Y. Musculoskeletal manifestations in patients with hypercholesterolemia. J Rheumatol 1989;16(5):643–5.

25. Klemp P, Halland AM, Majoos FL, et al. Musculoskeletal manifestations in hyperlipidaemia: a controlled study. Ann Rheum Dis 1993;52(1):44–8.

26. Astorga GP, Carvajal PR. Lipid spherule associated arthritis. J Rheumatol 1990; 17(12):1720.

27. Hackeng CM, de Bruijn LA, Douw CM, et al. Presence of birefringent, maltese-cross-appearing spherules in synovial fluid in a case of acute monoarthritis. Clin Chem 2000;46(11):1861–3.

28. Gardner GC, Terkeltaub RA. Acute monoarthritis associated with intracellular positively birefringent Maltese cross appearing spherules. J Rheumatol 1989; 16(3):394–6.

29. Rivest C, Hazeltine M, Gariepy G, et al. Acute polyarthritis associated with birefringent lipid microspherules occurring in a patient with longstanding rheumatoid arthritis. J Rheumatol 1992;19(4):617–20.

30. Weinstein J. Synovial fluid leukocytosis associated with intracellular lipid inclusions. Arch Intern Med 1980;140(4):560–1.
31. Reginato AJ, Schumacher HR, Allan DA, et al. Acute monoarthritis associated with lipid liquid crystals. Ann Rheum Dis 1985;44(8):537–43.
32. Chandrasekhar S. Cholesteric lipid crystals. Liquid crystals. England: Cambridge University Press; 1992.
33. Trostle DC, Schumacher HR, Medsger TA, et al. Lipid microspherule-associated acute monoarticular arthritis. Arthritis Rheum 1986;29(9):1166–9.
34. Ugai K, Kurosaka M, Hirohata K. Lipid microspherules in synovial fluid of patients with pigmented villonodular synovitis. Arthritis Rheum 1988;31(11):1442–6.
35. Choi SJ, Schumacher HR, Clayburne G. Experimental haemarthrosis produces mild inflammation associated with intracellular Maltese crosses. Ann Rheum Dis 1986;45(12):1025–8.
36. Schlesinger PA, Stillman MT, Peterson L. Polyarthritis with birefringent lipid within synovial fluid macrophages: case report and ultrastructural study. Arthritis Rheum 1982;25(11):1365–8.
37. Park YB, Lee SK, Song CH, et al. Acute monoarthritis associated with positively birefringent maltese cross appearing lipid spherules in a hyperlipidemic diabetic patient. Yonsei Med J 1997;38:236–9.
38. Dylewski J. Acute monoarticular arthritis caused by Maltese cross-like crystals. Canadian Medical Association Journal 2005;172:741–2.
39. Ettlinger RE, Hunder GG. Synovial effusions containing cholesterol crystals report of 12 patients and review. Mayo Clin Proc 1979;54(6):366–74.
40. Choi SJ, Schumacher HR, Clayburne G, et al. Liposome-induced synovitis in rabbits. Light and electron microscopic studies. Arthritis Rheum 1986;29(7):889–96.
41. Simkin PA, Brunzell JD, Wisner D, et al. Free fatty acids in the pancreatic arthritis syndrome. Arthritis Rheum 1983;26(2):127–32.
42. Stamp LK, Chapman PT. Gout and its comorbidities: implications for therapy. Rheumatology 2012;52(1):34–44.
43. Chen JH, Yeh WT, Chuang SY, et al. Gender-specific risk factors for incident gout: a prospective cohort study. Clin Rheumatol 2011;31(2):239–45.
44. Oztürk MA, Kaya A, Senel S, et al. Demographic and clinical features of gout patients in Turkey: a multicenter study. Rheumatol Int 2012. [Epub ahead of print].
45. Kuo CF, Yu KH, See LC, et al. Risk of myocardial infarction among patients with gout: a nationwide population-based study. Rheumatology 2012;52(1):111–7.
46. Kedar E, Simkin PA. A perspective on diet and gout. Adv Chronic Kidney Dis 2012;19(6):392–7.
47. Struthers GR, Scott DL, Bacon PA, et al. Musculoskeletal disorders in patients with hyperlipidaemia. Ann Rheum Dis 1983;42(5):519–23.
48. Noël B. Lupus erythematosus and other autoimmune diseases related to statin therapy: a systematic review. J Eur Acad Dermatol Venereol 2007;21(1):17–24.
49. de Jong HJ, Cohen Tervaert JW, Saldi SR, et al. Association between statin use and lupus-like syndrome using spontaneous reports. Semin Arthritis Rheum 2011;41(3):373–81.
50. Liang C, Needham M. Necrotizing autoimmune myopathy. Curr Opin Rheumatol 2011;23(6):612–9.
51. Mammen AL, Chung T, Christopher-Stine L, et al. Autoantibodies against 3-hydroxy-3-methylglutaryl-coenzyme A reductase in patients with statin-associated autoimmune myopathy. Arthritis Rheum 2011;63(3):713–21.

Fatty Acid Requirements in Preterm Infants and Their Role in Health and Disease

Camilia R. Martin, MD, MS[a,b,]*

KEYWORDS

- Long-chain polyunsaturated fatty acids • Docosahexaenoic acid • Arachidonic acid
- Eicosapentaenoic acid • Linoleic acid • Lipid emulsions

KEY POINTS

- There is selective uptake and transfer of free long-chain polyunsaturated fatty acids (LCPUFAs) from the maternal circulation to the developing fetus.
- LCPUFAs are critical for many biological processes, principally organogenesis (especially of the brain and retina) and regulating inflammation.
- Current nutritional practices are unable to meet the intrauterine fetal accretion rates of LCPUFAs in the early postnatal period for preterm infants.
- Inadequate postnatal delivery of LCPUFAs results in early, rapid deficits in critical fatty acids, notably docosahexaenoic acid and arachidonic acid.
- Altered postnatal LCPUFA levels and n-6/n-3 fatty acid ratios in the preterm infant are associated with chronic lung disease and late-onset sepsis.
- Current scientific literature, including both animal and human data, support the role of LCPUFA supplementation in preventing disease and optimizing health in the preterm infant.
- The optimal strategy to delivery LCPUFAs to preterm infants to emulate recommended fetal accretion rates, maintain birth levels of fatty acids and their relative ratios, prevent early deficits in fatty acid levels, and achieve clinical benefit without potential harm remains to be defined.

INTRODUCTION

Enhancing somatic growth through our knowledge of macronutrient requirements (carbohydrates, proteins, and fats) is only one aspect of fully extracting the potential of nutrition to optimize health in preterm infants. The composition and balance of

This article originally appeared in Clinics in Perinatology, Volume 41, Issue 2, June 2014.
[a] NICU, Department of Neonatology, Beth Israel Deaconess Medical Center, Harvard Medical School, 330 Brookline Avenue, Rose-318, Boston, MA 02215, USA; [b] Division of Translational Research, Beth Israel Deaconess Medical Center, Harvard Medical School, 330 Brookline Avenue, Boston, MA 02215, USA
* NICU, Department of Neonatology, Beth Israel Deaconess Medical Center, Harvard Medical School, 330 Brookline Avenue, Rose-318, Boston, MA 02215.
E-mail address: cmartin1@bidmc.harvard.edu

Clinics Collections 5 (2015) 335–354
http://dx.doi.org/10.1016/j.ccol.2015.05.020
2352-7986/15/$ – see front matter © 2015 Elsevier Inc. All rights reserved.

the individual building blocks within the macronutrients (sugars, amino acids, and fatty acids) are equally essential to understand. These building blocks often serve as bioactive molecules regulating many biological processes, such as organ development, metabolic homeostasis, and immune responsiveness.

Provision of fats is part of a balanced nutritional diet that delivers high-energy content, enhances gluconeogenesis, and prevents essential fatty acid deficiency. A large percentage of dietary fats are in the forms of triglycerides: 3 fatty acids on a glycerol backbone. Enzymatic hydrolysis releases the fatty acids from the glycerol backbone, allowing for trafficking and incorporation of the fatty acids into cell membranes, their primary site of action.

There is an extensive and evolving scientific literature showing the pleiotropic effects of fatty acids in health and disease. However, this literature is considerably more expansive for the adult than for the neonate. Despite this situation, strong evidence exists to support the beneficial role of fatty acids in neonatal health, especially in the preterm infant, and the need for ongoing efforts to further understand their mechanisms of action and to identify best nutritional or therapeutic strategies for delivery.

PLACENTAL TRANSFER AND FETAL ACQUISITION OF LONG-CHAIN POLYUNSATURATED FATTY ACIDS

Placental Transfer of Long-Chain Polyunsaturated Fatty Acids

Long-chain polyunsaturated fatty acids (LCPUFAs) are critical for the development of the fetal brain and retina. The importance of fetal acquisition of these critical fatty acids is highlighted by the presence of specific mechanisms allowing for maternal and placental transfer of fatty acids to the developing fetus. Although placental mechanisms for transfer are necessary, the synthesis of LCPUFAs in the placenta is limited, as it is in the developing fetus; thus, the maternal circulation is still considered the major source of LCPUFAs.[1–3]

Two major pathways have been proposed to facilitate the transfer of fatty acids from the maternal circulation, across the placenta, to the developing fetus: passive diffusion and protein-mediated transport (**Fig. 1**).[1,4,5] Maternal lipoproteins, triglycerides and phospholipids, are converted by placental lipoprotein lipase and endothelial lipase to form nonesterified or free fatty acids. Maternally derived free fatty acids are then transported into the placenta by passive diffusion or via protein-mediated transport. Transport proteins essential for the latter pathway include fatty acid transport proteins (FATP) 1– 6, of which FATP-4 seems to be of particular significance, because expression of this protein is directly correlated with docosahexaenoic acid (DHA) content in cord blood phospholipids,[6] placental plasma membrane fatty acid binding protein, and fatty acid translocase/CD36 (FAT/CD36). Once in the placenta, additional fatty acid binding proteins carry the fatty acid to the fetal interface, where FATP and FAT/CD36 deliver the free fatty acid to the fetal circulation.

Unique to this environment is the selective update and accumulation of LCPUFAs in the placenta and the fetal circulation, a phenomenon termed biomagnification. Labeled carbon studies tracking the transfer of fatty acids from the maternal to fetal circulation have shown higher DHA (22:6 n-3) content in cord blood versus maternal plasma, again emphasizing the unique role of the placenta in selectively transferring sufficient quantities of LCPUFAs to support the needs of the developing fetus (**Fig. 2**).[2,7]

Fetal Acquisition of LCPUFAs

The delivery of LCPUFAs substantially increases during the third trimester, coinciding with continued organ development and rapid fetal growth. Fetal accretion is targeted

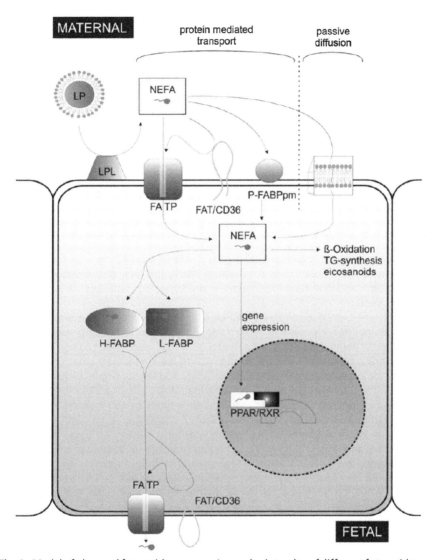

Fig. 1. Model of placental fatty acid transport. A complex interplay of different fatty acid transport proteins orchestrates fatty acid uptake by placental cells. Within the cell, NEFA are bound by different fatty acid binding proteins and have multiple functions like energy generation, TG, and eicosanoid synthesis, and activation of nuclear transcription factors like PPAR/RXR. FAT, fatty acid translocase; FATP, fatty acid transport protein; H-FABP, heart-fatty acid binding protein; L-FABP, liver-fatty acid binding protein; LP, lipoprotein; LPL, lipoprotein lipase; NEFA, nonesterified fatty acid; P-FABPpm, placental plasma membrane fatty acid binding protein; PPAR, peroxisome proliferator activated receptor; RXR, retinoid X receptor. (*Reprinted from* Hanebutt FL, Demmelmair H, Schiessl B, et al. Long-chain polyunsaturated fatty acid (LC-PUFA) transfer across the placenta. Clin Nutr 2008;27:688; with permission.)

to the brain, retina, and other lean tissues and organs. However, another important depot of fatty acids in the developing fetus is adipose tissue (**Fig. 3**). This reservoir is important to sustaining fatty acid requirements in organ development after delivery and throughout early infancy.[4] It is estimated that the delivery of long-chain fatty acids

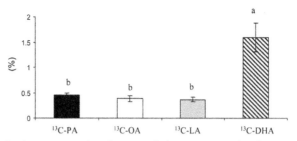

Fig. 2. Mean ratios between cord and maternal plasma area under the curve concentration of ^{13}C-fatty acids, expressed as percentages (n = 11). ^{13}C-PA, [^{13}C]palmitic acid; ^{13}C-OA, [^{13}C] oleic acid; ^{13}C-LA, [^{13}C]linoleic acid. (*Reprinted from* Gil-Sanchez A, Larque E, Demmelmair H, et al. Maternal-fetal in vivo transfer of [^{13}C]docosahexaenoic and other fatty acids across the human placenta 12 h after maternal oral intake. Am J Clin Nutr 2010;92:120; with permission.)

to support optimal fetal accretion is 43 mg/kg/d of DHA and 212 mg/k/d of arachidonic acid (20:4 n-6; AA) (**Table 1**).[8] In the preterm infant, this lack of accretion may have both short-term and long-term implications in predisposing to disease, as is discussed in the next section.

The most well-understood roles of LCPUFAs in the developing fetus are to support brain and retinal development. Approximately 55% of the brain comprises lipid, with the gray matter being 35% lipid, white matter 50% lipid, and myelin nearly 80% lipid.[9] LCPUFAs are a critical component of many of these lipid-based structural components, providing cell membrane structural integrity and fluidity within the phospholipid bilayer along with mediation of cell signaling pathways important in modulating the production of proteins that regulate neuronal differentiation and maturation, cell survival, and protection against oxidative stress.[2,10] Within the retina, DHA is concentrated in the outer segment of rod photoreceptors, playing an important role in differentiation and survival as well as the incorporation and function of the visual pigment rhodopsin.[10]

Much is discussed regarding the accretion of DHA in the fetal brain and retina; however, AA is the predominant fatty acid in the developing brain and retina until

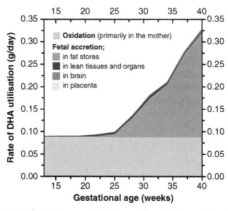

Fig. 3. Change in the rate of DHA use with stage of gestation. (*Reprinted from* Haggarty P. Fatty acid supply to the human fetus. Annu Rev Nutr 2010;30:239; with permission.)

Table 1
Estimates of the fatty acid accretion rate during the last trimester of pregnancy

	Per Day (mg/d)[a]	Per kg Body Weight Per Day (mg/kg/d)[b]
LA (18:2n-6)[c]	184	106
AA (20:4n-6)	368	212
LNA (18:3n-3)	7	4
DHA (22:6n-3)	75	43

[a] Adapted from Giorgieff and Innis [35]; the intrauterine estimate assumes tissue AA to be two-fold higher than LA [20,21]; the intrauterine estimate assumes that (1) DHA represents 90% of total n-3 fatty acids in all tissue except "other 0 tissue" [20,21], (2) the fatty acid composition of "other tissue" (20) is equal to that of skeletal muscle and that skeletal muscle contains 4.5% n-3 fatty acids [37], and (3) DHA represents 69% of total n-3 fatty acids in skeletal muscle [37].[8]
[b] Assumes weight between 25 and 41 weeks of gestation similar to Ref. [38].[8]
[c] Linoleic acid (LA), linolenic acid (LNA), arachidonic acid (AA), and docosahexaenoic acid (DHA).
Reprinted from Lapillonne A, Jensen CL. Reevaluation of the DHA requirement for the premature infant. Prostaglandins Leukot Essent Fatty Acids 2009;81:145; with permission.

approximately 37 and 32 weeks of gestation, respectively (**Fig. 4**).[11] Thus, AA is likely critical to the biological development and function of these organs. Similar to DHA, AA plays important roles in cell division, differentiation, and cell signaling.[12] In addition, adequate AA is important in infant growth.[13,14]

Effect of Prematurity on Systemic Levels of LCPUFAs

Preterm delivery leads to an abrupt cessation in the maternal transfer of critical fatty acids. The early termination of fatty acid delivery coupled with the lack of adipose tissue stores make the preterm infant especially vulnerable to alterations in systemic fatty acids and fully dependent on postnatal nutritional replacement strategies while in the intensive care unit. The current parenteral and enteral nutritional management strategies fail to meet the LCPUFA fetal accretion requirements and thus do not allow preservation of levels that would have been otherwise seen if the infant had remained in utero for the final trimester of pregnancy.

Whether evaluating whole blood or plasma fatty acid levels, preterm infants show a decline in DHA and AA and a concomitant increase in linoleic acid (18:2 n-6; LA) levels (expressed as mol%) within the first postnatal week (**Fig. 5**).[15,16] In addition, the ratios

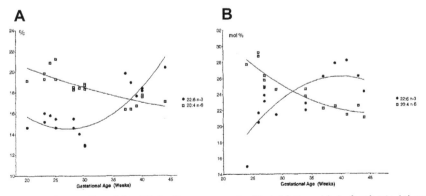

Fig. 4. DHA (22:6n-3) and AA (20:4n-6) as a percent of total fatty acids in forebrain (*A*) and retina (*B*). (*Adapted from* Martinez M. Tissue levels of polyunsaturated fatty acids during early human development. J Pediatr 1992;120:S131; with permission.)

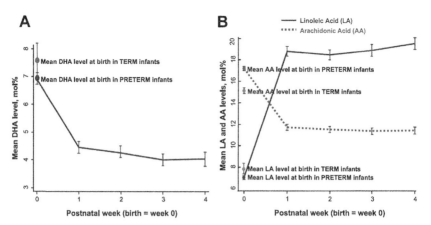

Fig. 5. (A) DHA levels in preterm infants decrease soon after birth and plateau by the first postnatal week. (B) LA levels in preterm infants increase soon after birth, and AA levels decrease soon after birth; both LA and AA plateau by the first postnatal week. (From Martin CR, Dasilva DA, Cluette-Brown JE, et al. Decreased postnatal docosahexaenoic and arachidonic acid blood levels in premature infants are associated with neonatal morbidities. J Pediatr 2011;159:746; with permission.)

of these fatty acids relative to each other are driven in the opposite direction of what is observed during the in utero period and at birth.

The rapid changes in fatty acid levels observed within the first postnatal week in preterm infants are principally driven by the current nutritional practices in the intensive care unit. Specifically, reliance on a parenteral lipid emulsion that is not tailored for the specific needs of the preterm infant and the delayed provision of enteral feedings that do not have sufficient fatty acid content (or delivery strategy) necessary to maintain LCPUFA birth levels lead to the observed profound alterations in systemic fatty acid levels.

Contribution of Parenteral Nutritional Practices to Altered Postnatal LCPUFA Levels

In the United States and much of North America, the principal lipid emulsion used for early delivery of fats to preterm infants is IntraLipid (20%, Fresenius Kabi/Baxter, Bad Homburg, Germany). Compared with the other available lipid emulsions (**Table 2**),[17] IntraLipid is 100% soybean oil, thus providing large amounts of LA but little to no DHA and AA. This lipid emulsion, approved by the US Food and Drug Administration (FDA) in 1972, was originally developed for use in the adult population. However, this product was subsequently applied to the neonatal and pediatric population, especially because no alternative has been approved for use in these specialized populations. Although provision of IntraLipid and thus the essential fatty acids LA and α linolenic acid (18:3 n-3) may be sufficient for adults dependent on parenteral nutrition, the provision alone of essential fatty acids is not adequate for the preterm population. The rationale for providing essential fatty acids alone relies on the presumption that the metabolic conversion of these fatty acids to downstream LCPUFAs is intact (**Fig. 6**).[18] Although not fully elucidated, it remains controversial whether desaturase and elongase activities are sufficient in the preterm infant to efficiently metabolize the precursor essential fatty acids to downstream LCPUFAs at a rate that meets their overall LCPUFA requirements.[19–21] In addition, it is not known how the unique metabolic state of the critically ill preterm infant affects overall fatty acid requirements. Regardless, it is self-evident that the provision of IntraLipid in the preterm infant is insufficient to maintain levels of LCPUFAs that emulate the patterns observed during the third trimester of pregnancy and at birth.

Contribution of Enteral Nutritional Practices to Altered Postnatal LCPUFA Levels

Not uncommonly, the preterm infant is provided with enteral feedings in a slow step-wise manner, such that the time to full enteral feedings to meet total energy require-ments does not occur until, on average, the second postnatal week.[16] Thus, the enteral approach to administering fatty acids is unlikely to prevent the changes in sys-temic fatty acid levels that occur within the first postnatal week.[22] LCPUFAs are pre-sent in breast milk, but there is tremendous interindividual and intraindividual variation in mother's own milk and reduced levels in donor milk; thus, the levels that are present in human milk are unlikely to meet the total requirements of the preterm infant.[23,24] In the United States, preterm formulas have been supplemented with DHA and AA since 2002, but the current levels are not sufficient to prevent the early postnatal decline in these fatty acid levels. Furthermore, the bioavailability of these supplemental fatty acids is compromised by developmentally impaired lipolysis and absorption observed in preterm infants.[8]

HEALTH CONSEQUENCES OF ALTERED LCPUFA LEVELS IN PRETERM INFANTS

The changes in systemic fatty acid levels and n-6/n-3 ratios are directly linked to acute neonatal morbidities.[16] In a cohort of preterm infants less than 30 weeks of gestation, for every 1 mol% decline in whole blood DHA levels, there was a 2.5-fold increase in the odds of developing chronic lung disease (CLD). For every 1 mol% decline in AA, there was a 40% increase in the hazard ratio of developing late-onset sepsis. In addi-tion, a positive change in the LA/DHA ratio was associated with an increase in the risk of both CLD and late-onset sepsis. These results are consistent with the biological role of LCPUFAs, especially DHA and AA, in regulating inflammation and immunity.

Although much has been described regarding the importance of DHA and AA in brain and retinal development, a direct causal link of low levels of these fatty acids to poor neurodevelopment has not been firmly established, especially given the many other competing risks for impaired neurodevelopment in the ill preterm infant. However, animal and human data on LCPUFA deprivation provide support for a critical role of LCPUFAs in neurodevelopment.

In weaning rats, 15 weeks of an n-3 deprivation diet resulted in a decrease in brain-derived neurotropin factor (BDNF) in the frontal cortex.[25] BDNF is an important signaling protein, which promotes Akt activation and, in turn, upregulates the CREB and mTOR pathways. Both CREB and mTOR are responsible for regulating gene expression and synthesis of proteins that are involved in neuroprotection, syn-aptic plasticity, actin organization, cell growth, and survival.[26,27] Nutritional modula-tion of BDNF is of clinical significance in the preterm infant. At birth, plasma BDNF levels in the preterm infant are lower than levels measured in term infants,[28] and the disparity in these levels may be exacerbated by the inadequate provision of n-3 fatty acids as a result of the current nutritional management strategies in the postnatal period of a preterm infant. Thus, the combination of low birth levels of BDNF and deprivation of critical LCPUFAs may place the preterm infant at risk for abnormal brain development.

In nonhuman primate models, plasma levels of fatty acids parallel the levels of these fatty acids in the brain.[29] As a result, the changes in whole blood and plasma levels of DHA and AA in the preterm infant previously described[15,16] are likely to result in changes in fatty acid composition in the developing preterm brain. Supportive of

Table 2
Commercially available intravenous fat emulsion products in the United States and outside the United States

Product Name	Manufacturer/Distributor	Lipid Source	Concentrations of Selected FA, % by Weight				n-6/n-3 Ratio	α-Tocopherol (mg/L)	Phytosterols (mg/L)
			Linoleic	α-Linolenic	EPA	DHA			
IVFE available in United States									
Intralipid	Fresenius Kabi/Baxter	100% soybean oil	44–62	4–11	0	0	7:1	38	348 ± 33
Liposyn III	Hospira	100% soybean oil	54.5	8.3	0	0	7:1	NA	NA
IVFE available only outside the United States									
Intralipid	Fresenius Kabi	100% soybean oil	44–62	4–11	0	0	7:1	38	348 ± 33
Ivelip	Baxter Teva	100% soybean oil	52	8.5	0	0	7:1	NA	NA
Lipovenoes	Fresenius Kabi	100% soybean oil	54	8	0	0	7:1	NA	NA
Lipovenoes 10% PLR	Fresenius Kabi	100% soybean oil	54	8	0	0	7:1	NA	NA
Intralipos 10%	Mitsubishi Pharma Guangzhou/Tempo Green Cross Otsuka Pharmaceutical Group	100% soybean oil	53	5	0	0	7:1	NA	NA
Lipofundin-N	B. Braun	100% soybean oil	50	7	0	0	7:1	180 ± 40	NA

Soyacal	Grifols Alpha Therapeutics	100% soybean oil	46.4	8.8	0	0	7:1	NA	NA
Intrafat	Nihon	100% soybean oil	NA	NA	0	0	7:1	NA	NA
Structolipid 20%[b]	Fresenius Kabi	64% soybean oil 36% MCT	35	5	0	0	7:1	6.9	NA
Lipofundin MCT/LCT	B. Braun	50% soybean oil 50% MCT oil	27	4	0	0	7:1	85 ± 20	NA
Lipovenoes MCT	Fresenius Kabi	50% soybean oil 50% MCT oil	25.9	3.9	0	0	7:1	NA	NA
ClinOleic 20%	Baxter	20% soybean oil 80% olive oil	18.5	2	0	0	9:1	32	327 ± 8
Lipoplus	B. Braun	40% soybean oil, 50% MCT, 10% fish oil	25.7	3.4	3.7	2.5	2.7:1	190 ± 30	NA
SMOFlipid	Fresenius Kabi	30% soybean oil, 30% MCT, 25% olive oil, 15% fish oil	21.4	2.5	3.0	2.0	2.5:1	200	47.6
Omegaven	Fresenius Kabi	100% fish oil	4.4	1.8	19.2	12.1	1:8	150–296	0

Abbreviations: EPA, eicosapentaenoic acid; FA, fatty acid; IVFE, intravenous fat emulsion; MCT, medium-chain triglyceride; n-6/n-3 ratio, ratio of ω-6 fatty acids to ω-3 fatty acids; NA, not available.

[a] References 1, 10, 26, 37.[17]

[b] Fat source uses structured lipids.

Reprinted from Vanek VW, Seidner DL, Allen P, et al. ASPEN position paper: clinical role for alternative intravenous fat emulsions. Nutr Clin Pract 2012;27:156; with permission.

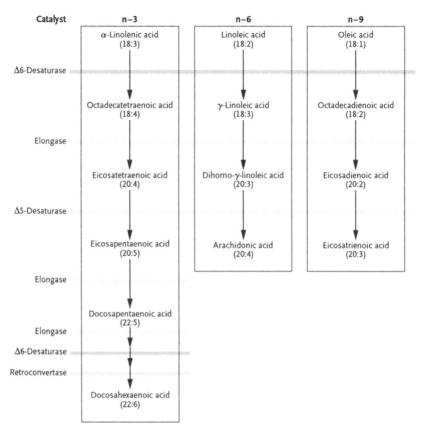

Fig. 6. An overview of the n-3, n-6, and n-9 biosynthetic pathways. (*Reprinted from* Freedman SD, Blanco PG, Zaman MM, et al. Association of cystic fibrosis with abnormalities in fatty acid metabolism. N Engl J Med 2004;350:562; with permission.)

this extrapolation are autopsy data that show abnormal DHA and AA content in the brain of preterm infants maintained on prolonged parenteral nutrition or high n-6/n-3 diets.[11]

EVIDENCE SUPPORTING THE ROLE OF LCPUFAS IN OPTIMIZING HEALTH IN PRETERM INFANTS

LCPUFAs play a critical role in cellular structure and function, including the regulation of membrane fluidity, cell signaling, and protein expression. It is through these intracellular pathways that LCPUFAs modulate immune and inflammatory responses as well as organogenesis (**Fig. 7**). Accruing animal studies and data from small human clinical trials support the role of LCPUFA supplementation to optimize the health of preterm infants. Examples are presented in the following sections for CLD, necrotizing enterocolitis (NEC), retinopathy of prematurity (ROP), and neurodevelopment.

CLD

As discussed previously, in a cohort study of preterm infants of less than 30 weeks of gestation, for every 1 mol% decline in DHA, there was a 2.5-fold increase in the odds of developing CLD.[16] By the first postnatal week, infants who developed CLD had

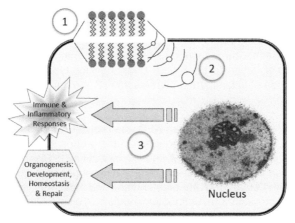

Fig. 7. Role of fatty acids in cellular mechanisms. (1) Formation of phospholipid bilayer of the cell membrane, (2) cell signaling, (3) regulation of protein expression responsible for immune and inflammatory responses and organogenesis.

lower mean whole blood DHA levels compared with infants who did not develop CLD (**Fig. 8**). The differences between these 2 groups persisted throughout the first postnatal month. Supporting these observational data is the reduction of CLD in breast milk–fed infants less than 1250 g whose mothers were supplemented with a high-DHA diet compared with infants whose mothers were not supplemented (34.5% vs 47%, respectively).[30] In addition, in a small clinical trial comparing delivery of IntraLipid versus SMOFlipid (15% fish oil) in preterm infants, the subgroup of infants less

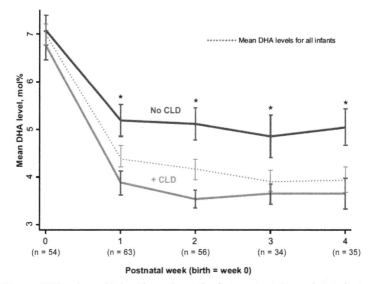

Fig. 8. Mean DHA levels are higher throughout the first postnatal month in infants without CLD compared with infants with CLD. *All P values <.02 comparing the mean DHA level in each postnatal week in infants with and without CLD. Bars represent standard error of the mean. (*Reprinted from* Martin CR, Dasilva DA, Cluette-Brown JE, et al. Decreased postnatal docosahexaenoic and arachidonic acid blood levels in premature infants are associated with neonatal morbidities. J Pediatr 2011;159:746; with permission.)

than 1500 g who received SMOFlipid were less likely to develop CLD.[31] Animal data provide further biological plausibility for the role of LCPUFAs in ameliorating neonatal lung injury. In a murine model of neonatal hyperoxia-induced lung injury, increased exposure to DHA, either through increased maternal content in dam milk or directly through oral administration to the mouse pups, ameliorated the expression of lung injury with reduction of inflammatory biomarkers[32,33] and improved alveolarization.[32]

NEC

In a rat model of NEC, the incidence of NEC was reduced with enteral supplementation of LCPUFAs, with the greatest reduction in the groups supplemented with DHA (50% reduction) or both DHA and AA (30% reduction).[34] Mechanisms proposed include a decrease in platelet-activating factor messenger RNA (mRNA) expression in response to both DHA and AA supplementation and a decrease in toll-like receptor 4 (TLR4) mRNA expression with AA supplementation. Clinical trials of LCPUFA supplementation in preterm infants have not shown a reduction in NEC. However, the few trials of LCPUFA supplementation in preterm infants were not designed to study NEC as a primary aim nor were they adequately powered to look at NEC even as a secondary outcome. The best supporting evidence for the potential role of LCPUFAs in preventing NEC comes from the scientific literature in inflammatory bowel disease, an intestinal disease process that may share similar mechanisms with NEC.[35,36] The current scientific literature supports an immunomodulatory role of LCPUFAs at the level of the enterocyte, including inhibition of TLR4 expression; downregulation of nuclear factor B (NF-B) signaling of inflammatory biomarkers through interaction with the nuclear receptor, peroxisome proliferator activated receptor (PPAR), or through the production of antiinflammatory terminal metabolites of DHA, such as the resolvin D series; and, through modulation of other fatty acid–derived proinflammatory cytokines such as eicosanoids (**Fig. 9**).[35]

ROP

In preterm infants of less than 32 weeks of gestation and less than 1250 g given either a standard lipid emulsion without fish oil or a standard lipid emulsion blended with 100% fish oil (Omegaven), the infants receiving fish oil had a trend toward a reduced incidence of ROP requiring laser therapy.[37] Supporting this clinical finding are results from a murine model of ROP. Pups born to mothers with an n-3–dominant diet versus an n-6–dominant diet showed less retinal vaso-obliteration and neovascularization secondary to hyperoxia exposure.[38] In addition, the same protective effect against retinal injury with hyperoxia was found in pups in the n-6–dominant diet group when concurrently provided resolvin D1, resolvin E1 or neuroprotectin D1, all terminal anti-inflammatory, bioactive metabolites of the n-3 fatty acids, DHA and eicosapentaenoic acid (EPA). The protective effect of the n-3 fatty acid diet seems to be partially mediated through a downregulation of tumor necrosis factor mRNA expression in the retina.

Neurodevelopment

Overall, the data for long-term neurodevelopmental benefits of LCPUFA supplementation in preterm infants are mixed.[39] Some of the potential reasons for this finding are discussed in more detail later and include considerations such as dosing, timing of delivery, and bioavailability with enteral consumption. However, intriguing data are accumulating regarding the role of LCPUFAs in upregulating signaling pathways important for brain development, reducing lipopolysaccharide (LPS)-induced neuronal injury and attenuating the sequelae of traumatic brain injury. It was previously discussed that, compared with term newborns, preterm infants have lower levels of

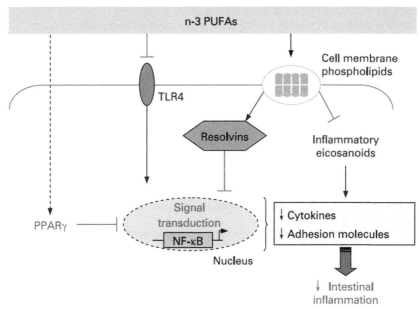

Fig. 9. Mechanisms of action of n-3 polyunsaturated fatty acids (PUFAs) in intestinal inflammation. The n-3 PUFAs activate peroxisome proliferator activated receptor c (PPARc), which inhibits the NF-κB signaling pathway. The effects of n-3 PUFAs may also inhibit TLR4. The n-3 PUFAs could also modulate fatty acid composition in cell membrane phospholipids, leading to a decrease of inflammatory eicosanoids derived from AA and to an increased production of antiinflammatory compounds such as resolvins. These regulatory pathways lead to decreased generation of proinflammatory cytokines and decreased expression of adhesion molecules, resulting in an inhibition of intestinal inflammation. (*Reprinted from* Marion-Letellier R, Dechelotte P, Iacucci M, et al. Dietary modulation of peroxisome proliferator-activated receptor gamma. Gut 2009;58:588; with permission.)

BDNF,[28] which can be further compromised with n-3 fatty acid deprivation.[25] The investigators of the latter study also reported that BDNF protein levels can be restored with DHA supplementation. Adequate levels of BDNF allow for downstream activation of the Akt, CREB, and mTOR pathways, all critical pathways in the regulation of proteins involved in brain organogenesis, homeostasis, and repair.

Neonatal sepsis is an independent risk factor for poor neurocognitive outcomes.[40] It is hypothesized that systemic inflammation leads to microglial activation and subsequent oxidative injury and cell death. In vitro studies of cultured LPS-activated glial cells show a DHA dose-dependent effect in reducing oxidative injury and attenuating the production of proinflammatory biomarkers.[41] Furthermore, in a neonatal murine model of cerebral hypoxic ischemic injury, provision of DHA after the brain insult decreased the total infarction volume and thus brain injury.[42] Although, not specifically evaluated, it was speculated that the protective effect of DHA was imparted by reducing oxidative injury and subsequent cell death.

CHALLENGES IN DELIVERING LCPUFAS TO PRETERM INFANTS

Nutritional delivery to the preterm infant largely consists of 2 phases: the parenteral phase, in which much of the nutritional content is delivered intravenously, and the enteral phase, in which most of the nutritional intake is given through the gut. As a result, delivering LCPUFAs to meet fetal accretion rates and to prevent the early alterations in postnatal changes in fatty acid levels must consider both phases.

Parenteral

As described earlier, the commonly used lipid emulsion in the United States, IntraLipid, fails to meet the fatty acid requirements of the preterm infant. Other lipid emulsions are commercially available but have not received FDA approval. However, it is not clear that even these emulsions fully meet the specific needs of the preterm infant. Ideally, any lipid emulsion uniquely tailored for the preterm infant should meet intrauterine fetal accretion rates of critical LCPUFAs, which, in addition, would maintain birth levels of these fatty acids (ie, prevent the early decline of DHA and AA and minimize the increase in LA). Small trials comparing various lipid emulsions in the preterm population indicate that currently available preparations are unable to preserve critical LCPUFA levels and, furthermore, may lead to changes in other fatty acids, which may pose different risks.

Forty-eight preterm infants with birth weights between 500 g and 1249 g were randomized to receive a standard lipid emulsion (50:50 medium-chain triglyceride [MCT]/soybean oil) or a study lipid emulsion containing 10% fish oil, 50% MCT, and 40% soybean oil. Plasma phospholipid levels of AA, DHA, and EPA were determined at birth, postnatal day 7, and postnatal day 14 (**Fig. 10**).[43] Compared with the standard lipid

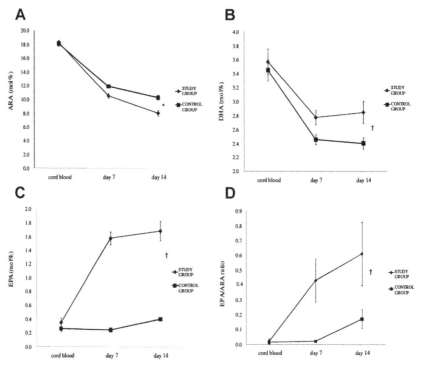

Fig. 10. (*A*) AA; (*B*) DHA; (*C*) EPA content, as mol%; and (*D*) EPA/AA ratio in plasma phospholipids (mean ± standard error of the mean) at day 0 (cord blood), day 7, and day 14. *$P = .02$. †$P<.01$. (*Reprinted from* D'Ascenzo R, D'Egidio S, Angelini L, et al. Parenteral nutrition of preterm infants with a lipid emulsion containing 10% fish oil: effect on plasma lipids and long-chain polyunsaturated fatty acids. J Pediatr 2011;159:36; with permission.)

emulsion group, receipt of the study lipid emulsion with 10% fish oil did not change the overall postnatal decline in DHA and AA levels. DHA plasma phospholipid levels were only slightly greater in the fish oil group compared with the standard lipid emulsion group, and AA levels decreased in the fish oil group versus the standard lipid group. There was a substantial, almost 5-fold increase in EPA (20:5 n-3) levels in the fish oil group versus standard lipid group.

Although other small clinical trials of lipid emulsions containing fish oil have been conducted, few have adequately described the changes in systemic fatty acid profiles with parenteral administration of fish oil. Considering the data described earlier, increasing the fish oil content of the lipid emulsion from 10% (Lipoplus) to 15% (SMO-Flipid) to 100% (Omegaven) may lead to more exaggerated fatty acid profiles compared with those described in the preceding paragraph. Thus, providing enriched DHA and EPA substantially increases DHA and EPA levels, but because of lower delivery of LA and substrate competition between n-3 and n-6 fatty acids, systemic levels of AA would decrease further. Supporting this premise are data from older, parenteral nutrition–dependent preterm infants who were switched from a predominantly soybean lipid emulsion to one containing a high concentration of fish oil.[44] Over time, plasma fatty acid patterns showed an 8-fold increase in DHA, a more than 20-fold increase in EPA, and a substantial decrease in LA and AA levels.

Although increasing levels of DHA may be clinically desirable, a concomitant increase in EPA may produce unknown but potential, adverse effects in the preterm population. Prolific literature on the role of n-3 fatty acids in adult cardiovascular health show biological effects of these fatty acids in inhibiting platelet-activating factor, decreasing platelet aggregation, and increasing bleeding time.[45] In addition, n-3 fatty acids reduce plasma triglyceride levels and the delivery of cholesterol to tissues. Unique to EPA is the decrease in natural killer cell activity and in T-lymphocyte function with increasing levels. All of these effects may be beneficial in an adult with cardiovascular disease; however, these effects may be problematic in the preterm infant, in whom there is a developmental bleeding diathesis and risk for intracranial hemorrhage, immune dysfunction, and a nutritional need for triglyceride and cholesterol production for organ development. The decrease in AA levels seen in parallel with enriched DHA/EPA delivery may be of concern given the critical functions that AA serves in brain and eye development as well as overall growth. Different lipid emulsions need to be developed and studied to meet the unique LCPUFA needs of the preterm infant. It is imperative to carefully quantify the changes in systemic fatty acid profiles with novel lipid emulsions and document potential side effects of the changing fatty acid profiles in addition to its potential clinical benefits.

Enteral

Despite the presence of LCPUFAs in human milk as well as DHA and AA supplementation in formulas, dietary provision of breast milk or formula fails to meet the fatty acid requirements in preterm infants[22] or fully attain the potential neurocognitive and visual benefits of fatty acid supplementation.[39] Although some clinical trials of LCPUFA supplementation have shown short-term benefits in neurocognitive outcomes and visual motor function, these benefits are not sustained nor shown consistently in all studies. The lack of a clear benefit of LCPUFA supplementation likely reflects inadequate LCPUFA timing and delivery rather than a failure of clinical benefit from the fatty acid itself. Many enteral supplementation studies have started the supplementation after the infant has begun on enteral feedings or after the infant has achieved a substantial daily intake by the enteral route, both of these time points well after the time when deficits in systemic DHA and AA levels have already occurred in the preterm infant.

Another factor complicating the enteral delivery of LCPUFAs is the ability of the preterm infant to hydrolyze dietary triglycerides to allow absorption of the resultant monoglycerides and free fatty acids. A measure of efficient fat hydrolysis and absorption is the coefficient of fat absorption (CFA), which is expressed as the fraction (percent) of the difference between total fat intake and total fecal fat losses over total fat intake. A perfect rate of hydrolysis and absorption is 100%, with normal values being greater than 90%. Thus, the higher the CFA value, the more efficient the hydrolysis and absorption. This value can be calculated for total fat as well as for individual fatty acids. Total CFA and specific fatty acid CFAs for DHA and AA all show values in the 70% to 80% range in preterm infants fed formula or pasteurized human milk.[46] The lower DHA and AA CFA values in infants fed formula and pasteurized human milk may be accounted for by developmental pancreatic insufficiency and decreased production of lipase as well as a reduction in bile acid pools. Preterm infants fed mother's own milk (nonpasteurized) show higher CFA levels, likely because of the presence of bile salt–stimulated lipase in the milk, which is absent in formula and degraded in pasteurized human milk.

Increasing the total content of DHA and AA in formulas to overcome the limitations in lipid hydrolysis and intestinal absorption may be of limited value. In a lipase-deficient murine model, enteral delivery of fats led to lipid-laden fat accumulation in the intestinal enterocytes and intestinal injury.[47] Thus, the effects of surpassing the capacity of the preterm infant's ability to hydrolyze and absorb dietary fatty acids are unknown but may be potentially harmful to the developing gut.

Enteral delivery of nutrients is preferred over parenteral administration. However, adequate delivery of enteral fatty acids that translates to improved systemic fatty acid profiles needs to consider and overcome the inadequacy of the current dosing of DHA and AA in formula and breast milk to meet the fatty acid requirements of the preterm infant. This necessity is especially important during the early postnatal period, when the relative decrease in lipase production and bile acid pools to efficiently hydrolyze and absorb enterally administered fatty acids is at play.

Maternal

Another potential route to increase LCPUFA levels in the preterm infant is through maternal strategies. An increase in the intake of maternal LCPUFAs can increase the breast milk content of LCPUFAs, allowing for more efficient delivery to the preterm infant. Although this strategy can lead to higher LCPUFA levels in the preterm infant and is important in maintaining LCPUFA levels during the enteral phase of nutrition,[48] it is unlikely that this strategy alone ameliorates the deficits in LCPUFA levels that become evident in the early postnatal period.

FUTURE DIRECTIONS

The premise that LCPUFAs are essential for neonatal health is validated given:

- The presence of specialized mechanisms to enhance placental transfer from the mother to the developing fetus
- Their biological roles in fetal development, ongoing organogenesis, and regulation of inflammation
- Accruing promising data supporting their immunomodulatory capabilities in ameliorating neonatal disease pathogenesis and optimizing normal development

However, before implementing new practices, either adopting new lipid emulsions or administering new enteral formulations, careful research needs to be conducted

to understand the balance of what is required, for what therapeutic goal, and to minimize potential harm.
Questions and concepts that need to be thoroughly considered include:

- What is our therapeutic goal? Is it to fully emulate our current understanding of fetal accretion rates? Is it to provide doses that support maintenance requirements to maintain birth levels of fatty acids and ongoing development? Or is it to provide doses that target specific disease processes or inflammatory states?
- What are the target levels (whole blood, plasma, tissue, or even cellular) and fatty acid ratios that need to be attained to achieve the therapeutic goal? How are these target levels modified, given the acuity and metabolic state of the infant?
- What are the unique challenges with parenteral delivery of fatty acids versus enteral delivery? What is the ideal formulation, including the biochemical structure, that supports fatty acid hydrolysis, absorption, and incorporation into the target tissue?
- What are biochemical assays and clinical parameters that need to collected and evaluated to ensure the optimal balance between clinical benefit and potential harm?

SUMMARY

The preterm infant presents a unique challenge but an exciting opportunity to define the role of LCPUFAs in both maintenance of health and prevention of disease. Through understanding of basic mechanisms and the pathophysiologic consequences of altered fatty acid levels, the provision of critical fatty acids through parenteral or enteral routes can mitigate the risk of diseases such as CLD, nosocomial sepsis, NEC, ROP, and neurocognitive impairment. The challenge is to understand the changing nutritional and therapeutic goals along a developmental timeline with superimposed exposures to disease risks. The result is an effect on immunomodulatory functions, organ development, and neuroprotection. Diligent research efforts to further define fetal accretion requirements, mechanisms of intestinal fatty acid lipolysis and absorption, and fatty acid metabolism and tissue incorporation will provide a rational approach to novel therapeutic strategies.

REFERENCES

1. Gil-Sanchez A, Demmelmair H, Parrilla JJ, et al. Mechanisms involved in the selective transfer of long chain polyunsaturated fatty acids to the fetus. Front Genet 2011;2:57.
2. Larque E, Demmelmair H, Gil-Sanchez A, et al. Placental transfer of fatty acids and fetal implications. Am J Clin Nutr 2011;94:1908S–13S.
3. Pagan A, Prieto-Sanchez MT, Blanco-Carnero JE, et al. Materno-fetal transfer of docosahexaenoic acid is impaired by gestational diabetes mellitus. Am J Physiol Endocrinol Metab 2013;305:E826–33.
4. Haggarty P. Fatty acid supply to the human fetus. Annu Rev Nutr 2010;30: 237–55.
5. Hanebutt FL, Demmelmair H, Schiessl B, et al. Long-chain polyunsaturated fatty acid (LC-PUFA) transfer across the placenta. Clin Nutr 2008;27:685–93.
6. Larque E, Krauss-Etschmann S, Campoy C, et al. Docosahexaenoic acid supply in pregnancy affects placental expression of fatty acid transport proteins. Am J Clin Nutr 2006;84:853–61.

7. Gil-Sanchez A, Larque E, Demmelmair H, et al. Maternal-fetal in vivo transfer of [13C]docosahexaenoic and other fatty acids across the human placenta 12 h after maternal oral intake. Am J Clin Nutr 2010;92:115–22.

8. Lapillonne A, Jensen CL. Reevaluation of the DHA requirement for the premature infant. Prostaglandins Leukot Essent Fatty Acids 2009;81:143–50.

9. O'Brien JS, Sampson EL. Lipid composition of the normal human brain: gray matter, white matter, and myelin. J Lipid Res 1965;6:537–44.

10. Lauritzen L, Hansen HS, Jorgensen MH, et al. The essentiality of long chain n-3 fatty acids in relation to development and function of the brain and retina. Prog Lipid Res 2001;40:1–94.

11. Martinez M. Tissue levels of polyunsaturated fatty acids during early human development. J Pediatr 1992;120:S129–38.

12. Su HM, Corso TN, Nathanielsz PW, et al. Linoleic acid kinetics and conversion to arachidonic acid in the pregnant and fetal baboon. J Lipid Res 1999;40:1304–12.

13. Carlson SE, Werkman SH, Peeples JM, et al. Arachidonic acid status correlates with first year growth in preterm infants. Proc Natl Acad Sci U S A 1993;90: 1073–7.

14. Koletzko B, Braun M. Arachidonic acid and early human growth: is there a relation? Ann Nutr Metab 1991;35:128–31.

15. Leaf AA, Leighfield MJ, Costeloe KL, et al. Factors affecting long-chain polyunsaturated fatty acid composition of plasma choline phosphoglycerides in preterm infants. J Pediatr Gastroenterol Nutr 1992;14:300–8.

16. Martin CR, Dasilva DA, Cluette-Brown JE, et al. Decreased postnatal docosahexaenoic and arachidonic acid blood levels in premature infants are associated with neonatal morbidities. J Pediatr 2011;159:743–9.e2.

17. Vanek VW, Seidner DL, Allen P, et al. ASPEN position paper: clinical role for alternative intravenous fat emulsions. Nutr Clin Pract 2012;27:150–92.

18. Freedman SD, Blanco PG, Zaman MM, et al. Association of cystic fibrosis with abnormalities in fatty acid metabolism. N Engl J Med 2004;350:560–9.

19. Carnielli VP, Wattimena DJ, Luijendijk IH, et al. The very low birth weight premature infant is capable of synthesizing arachidonic and docosahexaenoic acids from linoleic and linolenic acids. Pediatr Res 1996;40:169–74.

20. Larque E, Demmelmair H, Koletzko B. Perinatal supply and metabolism of long-chain polyunsaturated fatty acids: importance for the early development of the nervous system. Ann N Y Acad Sci 2002;967:299–310.

21. Szitanyi P, Koletzko B, Mydlilova A, et al. Metabolism of 13C-labeled linoleic acid in newborn infants during the first week of life. Pediatr Res 1999;45:669–73.

22. Lapillonne A, Eleni dit Trolli S, Kermorvant-Duchemin E. Postnatal docosahexaenoic acid deficiency is an inevitable consequence of current recommendations and practice in preterm infants. Neonatology 2010;98:397–403.

23. Cruz-Hernandez C, Goeuriot S, Giuffrida F, et al. Direct quantification of fatty acids in human milk by gas chromatography. J Chromatogr A 2013;1284:174–9.

24. Valentine CJ, Morrow G, Fernandez S, et al. Docosahexaenoic acid and amino acid contents in pasteurized donor milk are low for preterm infants. J Pediatr 2010;157:906–10.

25. Rao JS, Ertley RN, DeMar JC Jr, et al. Dietary n-3 PUFA deprivation alters expression of enzymes of the arachidonic and docosahexaenoic acid cascades in rat frontal cortex. Mol Psychiatry 2007;12:151–7.

26. Fretham SJ, Carlson ES, Georgieff MK. Neuronal-specific iron deficiency dysregulates mammalian target of rapamycin signaling during hippocampal development in nonanemic genetic mouse models. J Nutr 2013;143:260–6.

27. Lonze BE, Ginty DD. Function and regulation of CREB family transcription factors in the nervous system. Neuron 2002;35:605–23.

28. Malamitsi-Puchner A, Economou E, Rigopoulou O, et al. Perinatal changes of brain-derived neurotrophic factor in pre- and fullterm neonates. Early Hum Dev 2004;76:17–22.

29. Sarkadi-Nagy E, Wijendran V, Diau GY, et al. The influence of prematurity and long chain polyunsaturate supplementation in 4-week adjusted age baboon neonate brain and related tissues. Pediatr Res 2003;54:244–52.

30. Manley BJ, Makrides M, Collins CT, et al. High-dose docosahexaenoic acid supplementation of preterm infants: respiratory and allergy outcomes. Pediatrics 2011;128:e71–7.

31. Skouroliakou M, Konstantinou D, Agakidis C, et al. Cholestasis, bronchopulmonary dysplasia, and lipid profile in preterm infants receiving MCT/omega-3-PUFA-containing or soybean-based lipid emulsions. Nutr Clin Pract 2012;27:817–24.

32. Ma L, Li N, Liu X, et al. Arginyl-glutamine dipeptide or docosahexaenoic acid attenuate hyperoxia-induced lung injury in neonatal mice. Nutrition 2012;28: 1186–91.

33. Rogers LK, Valentine CJ, Pennell M, et al. Maternal docosahexaenoic acid supplementation decreases lung inflammation in hyperoxia-exposed newborn mice. J Nutr 2011;141:214–22.

34. Lu J, Jilling T, Li D, et al. Polyunsaturated fatty acid supplementation alters proinflammatory gene expression and reduces the incidence of necrotizing enterocolitis in a neonatal rat model. Pediatr Res 2007;61:427–32.

35. Marion-Letellier R, Dechelotte P, Iacucci M, et al. Dietary modulation of peroxisome proliferator-activated receptor gamma. Gut 2009;58:586–93.

36. Marion-Letellier R, Savoye G, Beck PL, et al. Polyunsaturated fatty acids in inflammatory bowel diseases: a reappraisal of effects and therapeutic approaches. Inflamm Bowel Dis 2013;19:650–61.

37. Pawlik D, Lauterbach R, Walczak M, et al. Fish-oil fat emulsion supplementation reduces the risk of retinopathy in very low birth weight infants: a prospective, randomized study. JPEN J Parenter Enteral Nutr 2013. [Epub ahead of print].

38. Connor KM, SanGiovanni JP, Lofqvist C, et al. Increased dietary intake of omega-3-polyunsaturated fatty acids reduces pathological retinal angiogenesis. Nat Med 2007;13:868–73.

39. Schulzke SM, Patole SK, Simmer K. Longchain polyunsaturated fatty acid supplementation in preterm infants. Cochrane Database Syst Rev 2011;(2):CD000375.

40. Stoll BJ, Hansen NI, Adams-Chapman I, et al. Neurodevelopmental and growth impairment among extremely low-birth-weight infants with neonatal infection. JAMA 2004;292:2357–65.

41. Antonietta Ajmone-Cat M, Lavinia Salvatori M, De Simone R, et al. Docosahexaenoic acid modulates inflammatory and antineurogenic functions of activated microglial cells. J Neurosci Res 2012;90:575–87.

42. Williams JJ, Mayurasakorn K, Vannucci SJ, et al. N-3 fatty acid rich triglyceride emulsions are neuroprotective after cerebral hypoxic-ischemic injury in neonatal mice. PLoS One 2013;8:e56233.

43. D'Ascenzo R, D'Egidio S, Angelini L, et al. Parenteral nutrition of preterm infants with a lipid emulsion containing 10% fish oil: effect on plasma lipids and long-chain polyunsaturated fatty acids. J Pediatr 2011;159:33–8.e1.

44. Klein CJ, Havranek TG, Revenis ME, et al. Plasma fatty acids in premature infants with hyperbilirubinemia: before-and-after nutrition support with fish oil emulsion. Nutr Clin Pract 2013;28:87–94.

45. Torrejon C, Jung UJ, Deckelbaum RJ. n-3 Fatty acids and cardiovascular disease: actions and molecular mechanisms. Prostaglandins Leukot Essent Fatty Acids 2007;77:319–26.
46. Lapillonne A, Groh-Wargo S, Gonzalez CH, et al. Lipid needs of preterm infants: updated recommendations. J Pediatr 2013;162:S37–47.
47. Howles PN, Stemmerman GN, Fenoglio-Preiser CM, et al. Carboxyl ester lipase activity in milk prevents fat-derived intestinal injury in neonatal mice. Am J Physiol 1999;277:G653–61.
48. Makrides M. DHA supplementation during the perinatal period and neurodevelopment: do some babies benefit more than others? Prostaglandins Leukot Essent Fatty Acids 2013;88:87–90.

Pediatric Lipid Management
An Earlier Approach

Justin P. Zachariah, MD, MPH[a,b,*], Philip K. Johnson, BS[a,b]

KEYWORDS

- Pediatrics • Lipids • Atherosclerosis • Dyslipidemia

KEY POINTS

- Numerous long-term observational cohort studies show that subclinical atherosclerosis is a progressive disease that arises in childhood and continues through the adulthood.
- Deficiencies in targeted lipid screening to identify high-risk individuals led the 2011 National Heart, Lung and Blood Institute Expert Panel for Pediatric Cardiovascular Disease (CVD) Risk Reduction to recommend universal screening.
- Amid concerns that extended screening may induce inappropriate treatment, pharmacotherapy is restricted to patients with genetic dyslipidemias and multiple high-risk CVD factors.
- This article summarizes the current guidelines, enumerates challenges to the guidelines, and suggests future directions.

INTRODUCTION

Although adult cardiovascular disease (CVD) mortality has been curtailed primarily from improvements in atherosclerotic risk factor treatment, an alarming countervailing trend dominates the present and future of CVD: obesity, obesity-related dyslipidemia, and type 2 diabetes.[1–6] Children offer a prime opportunity to continue CVD risk factor reduction and address emerging trends, especially dyslipidemia.

There are 4 general classes of pediatric dyslipidemias:

- Medication-related dyslipidemia
- Dyslipidemia related to lifestyle factors

This article originally appeared in Endocrinology and Metabolism Clinics, Volume 43, Issue 4, December 2014.

Disclosures: The authors have no financial conflicts of interest. This work was supported by NHLBI Career Development Award K23 HL111335 (J.P. Zachariah). No funding sources had any role in the design, writing, editing, or decision to publish any part of this work.

[a] Department of Cardiology, Boston Children's Hospital, 300 Longwood Avenue, Boston, MA 02115, USA; [b] Department of Pediatrics, Harvard Medical School, 300 Longwood Avenue, Boston, MA 02115, USA

* Corresponding author. Department of Cardiology, Boston Children's Hospital, 300 Longwood Avenue, Boston, MA 02115.

E-mail address: justin.zachariah@childrens.harvard.edu

Clinics Collections 5 (2015) 355–366
http://dx.doi.org/10.1016/j.ccol.2015.05.021
2352-7986/15/$ – see front matter © 2015 Elsevier Inc. All rights reserved.

- Genetic dyslipidemia
- Dyslipidemia secondary to a medical condition.

There are 3 chief genetic dyslipidemias (**Table 1**).

- Familial hypercholesterolemia (FH). FH is an autosomal dominant disorder that interferes with either apolipoprotein B (ApoB) assembly or the receptor-mediated clearance of low-density lipoprotein cholesterol (LDL-C) in roughly 1 in 500 persons with heterozygosity or 1 in a million homozygotes.[7–10] However, homozygotes frequently develop xanthelasmas of the canthi, xanthomas on the extensor surfaces of limb joints, arcus senilis of the eye, and internal conse-quences, including myocardial infarction and ischemic cardiomyopathy, often in the first 2 decades of life. The heterozygous phenotype predisposes to early atherosclerosis and is more common than, and as treatable as, any disorder within national newborn screening programs.
- Familial combined hyperlipidemia. Familial combined hyperlipidemia is another genetic dyslipidemia with high LDL-C and triglycerides (TGs), but lacks the de-gree of TG increase necessary to trigger pancreatitis. It confers CVD risks nearly as high as FH and may be as prevalent as 1% of the population.[11,12]
- Familial severe hypertriglyceridemia (HTG). Although 1 in 600 individuals have se-vere HTG (defined as TG>10 mmol/L or 885 mg/dL),[13] much of this is caused by environment and lifestyle. Genetic or familial HTG has many implicated genes, but the most common is homozygous autosomal recessive loss of function mu-tations in lipoprotein lipase or apolipoprotein C2 and occurs in 1 in 1 × 10^5 indi-viduals.[13,14] Hindered degradation of TG leads to significantly increased serum TG.[15,16] At levels of more than 1000 mg/dL, the risk of acutely life-threatening pancreatitis increases. However, risk stratification by TG level is inadequate because many lipid providers follow persons with TG greater than 2000 mg/dL who have never had pancreatitis. Despite this uncertainty, prompt treatment is recommended.[17]

Suggested responses to pediatric dyslipidemias include, but are not limited to, removing a causative agent, lifestyle modification, treating an underlying medical con-dition, and in severe cases pharmacotherapy. Each of these therapeutic maneuvers is intended to accomplish 2 important goals: preventing acute pancreatitis in individuals with very increased TGs levels and preventing atherosclerotic CVD later in life.

Table 1
Prominent genetic dyslipidemias in children

Dyslipidemia	Abnormal Lipid Fraction	Prevalence Estimate	Predominant Mechanism
Familial hypercholesterolemia	High LDL-C	Heterozygotes, 1 in 500 Homozygotes, 1 in million	Decreased LDL-C clearance
Familial combined hypercholesterolemia	High LDL-C and high triglycerides/ VLDL	1 in 100[11]	Increased ApoB production
Familial severe hypertriglyceridemia	High triglycerides/ VLDL	1 in 100,000[13]	Decreased triglyceride/ VLDL degradation

Abbreviations: ApoB, apolipoprotein B; LDL-C, low-density lipoprotein cholesterol; VLDL, very low-density lipoprotein.

Childhood is also a key period for progress because children are susceptible to deleterious lifestyle influences; are directly affected by CVD risk factors; already accumulate atherosclerotic phenotypic changes; are more malleable to lifestyle habit alterations to avoid CVD risk factors; and, through internal motivation and/or support form guardians or peers, have the capacity to treat CVD risk factors through lifestyle modification alone. The clinical encounter offers an opportunity to leverage abnormal laboratory results into a multifaceted cardiometabolic remedy. In a recent study of medical providers caring for children, 74% thought that lipid screening and treatment would reduce future CVD outcomes. Despite this belief, only 16% universally screened their patients, 54% selectively screened, and 34% did not screen at all.[18] These data underscore the need to engage providers.

The National Heart, Lung and Blood Institute (NHLBI) Expert Panel on Integrated Guidelines for Cardiovascular Disease Health and Risk Reduction in Children and Adolescents released their guidelines in November 2011, unifying previously disjointed aspects of CVD prevention, including physical activity, nutrition, obesity, blood pressure, lipids, and tobacco use, under a singular aegis and updated these domains with a comprehensive review of relevant data.[19] In compiling these revised recommendations, the NHLBI guidelines lengthen the reach of CVD prevention to an earlier, more plastic stage of life.

THE GUIDELINES: FRAMEWORK AND SYNOPSIS

CVD risk factor modification can be subdivided into primary, secondary, and primordial prevention.[20] Primary prevention is the treatment of risk factors to avoid the first event, secondary prevention is the evasion of recurrent cardiovascular events in patients with a history of CVD, and primordial prevention is intervention to prevent CVD risk factors from arising at all.[21] In order to inhibit the development of CVD risk factors, the NHLBI Integrated Guidelines make precise, developmentally appropriate suggestions interweaving CVD risk factor prevention within general pediatric practice. The screening and treatment sections focus on the premise that CVD risk factors must be centered on the child's aggregate combination of cardiac risks, rather than any particular risk factor.

It is well recognized that atherosclerotic abnormalities arise in childhood, that these changes are related to the presence of CVD risk factors, and that risk factors in adults are directly related to cardiac events in a continuous fashion.[22–26] However, when the population is "sick", as Geoffrey Rose[27] described, what is to be done? Nationally representative pediatric data show that overweight and obesity increase the relative risk of increased LDL cholesterol (LDL-C); however, approximately 45% of all adolescents with high LDL-C are of normal weight, suggesting that CVD risk factors are widespread. It is therefore essential that the proposed suggestions be scaled to the population level because fixating on excess weight misses almost half the problem.[28]

It is also clear that population-wide interventions can be successful, as shown by tobacco use reduction. Tobacco use reduction has been achieved through mobilizing public sentiment; initiating economic disincentives; and placing restrictions on the procurement, advertisement, and use of tobacco products. Similar efforts to reduce the causes of hyperlipidemia, hypertension, or obesity meet entrenched resistance from the lack of data supporting secondhand harm from lifestyle behaviors and trepidation about the freedom of personal choice. Protecting children from circumstances that ultimately lead to CVD risk factors may be more readily accepted because their lifestyle choices are appropriately constrained by caregivers since they are less proficient in making their own healthy choices. Therefore the guidelines make primordial prevention recommendations for all children and primary prevention recommendations for affected children, including those with dyslipidemia.

Primordial Prevention Recommendations

1. The Integrated Guidelines seek to perform population-level prevention through each child. Nutrition recommendations include:
   - Breastfeeding for the first 12 months
   - Restricting calories derived from milk fat and fruit juice
   - After age 2 years, adherence to the Cardiovascular Health Integrated Lifestyle Diet (CHILD-1) diet[19]
2. Tobacco abolition is recommended from infancy through childhood and adolescence
3. Universal recommendations with respect to activity and inactivity consist of:
   - Consistent active play in toddlerhood
   - One hour per day of moderate to vigorous exercise in older children and adolescents
   - Inactive screen time is fully discouraged before age 2 years
   - Screen time is restricted to less than 2 hours per day in older children

The guidelines advance, endorse, and stress this population-level approach to CVD risk factor mitigation as the new norm for US children. It is thought that this combination of interventions will simultaneously protect against incident dyslipidemia, diabetes, hypertension, and obesity.

Primary Prevention Recommendations

The Integrated Guidelines refine, extend, and combine previous guidelines from the American Academy of Pediatrics (AAP) 2008 guidelines on dyslipidemia detection.[29,30] These prior efforts advocated for screening for lipid disorders in patients with high-risk medical conditions and/or abnormal family histories and pharmacologic management of severe pediatric lipid disorders. The 2011 NHLBI guidelines expand the AAP cholesterol guidelines by recommending universal screening to enhance the detection of young patients with FH who are subject to atherosclerotic events in early adulthood.

1. Universal screening can be initiated with either:
   a. A calculated nonfasting non–high-density lipoprotein cholesterol (HDL-C) level, and HDL-C level, or
   b. A fasting lipid panel
2. Abnormal levels should be confirmed with a repeated fasting test, especially for TG irregularities
3. Targeted lipid screening can occur
   a. At any time after age 2 years for children at high atherosclerotic risk (**Box 1**)[19]
   b. At the provider's preference, or
   c. At the family's discretion
4. Very high levels of TG or LDL-C ($\geq$500 mg/dL and $\geq$250 mg/dL, respectively) trigger a referral to a lipid specialist in order to manage genetic dyslipidemias

The NHLBI guidelines are designed to set thresholds to reflect the well-documented age-specific distribution of lipid levels in the hope of increasing the number of children eligible for attention but constraining the number eligible for medication. They also mirror the 3 category groupings of the Adult Treatment Panel III/National Cholesterol Education Program in defining acceptable lipid values (**Table 2**).

Box 1
Risk factor definitions for dyslipidemia algorithms

Family history

In parent, grandparent, aunt, or uncle a history of myocardial infarction, angina, coronary artery bypass graft/stent/angioplasty, or sudden cardiac death before age 55 years in men or 65 years in women

High-level risk factors

Hypertension requiring therapy

Current cigarette smoker

Body mass index (BMI) greater than 97%

High-risk conditions

   Diabetes mellitus, type 1 or 2

   After heart transplant

   Chronic kidney disease

   End-stage renal disease

   After renal transplant

   Kawasaki disease with coronary aneurysms

Moderate-level risk factors

Hypertension not requiring medication

BMI greater than 95% but less than or equal to 97%

HDL-C less than 40 mg/dL

Moderate-risk condition

   Chronic inflammatory disease

   Human immunodeficiency virus infection

   Nephrotic syndrome

   Kawasaki disease without coronary aneurysm

Data from Expert panel on integrated guidelines for cardiovascular health and risk reduction in children and adolescents: summary report. Pediatrics 2011;128(Suppl 5):S237.

Treatment of CVD risk factors is an essential part of the NHLBI guidelines. It is also clear that CVD risk factors are modifiable. Adult cohort studies show that 90% of coronary heart disease (CHD) and incident stroke and were attributable to modifiable risk factors.[31–34] Temporal trends show that smoking rates have decreased in adults, and, in American children, cholesterol levels seem to be declining as well.[35,36] According to recent randomized controlled trials in adults with type 2 diabetes, coronary disease with systolic heart failure, and chronic stable angina, aggressive CVD risk factor modification was as effective as invasive revascularization in averting CVD events.[37–39] In contrast, 30-year global trends show that obesity prevalence is increasing and cholesterol levels are worsening.[40,41] Therefore, clinicians can be confident that CVD risk factors are modifiable in both the positive and negative directions. Therapy in children is justified by direct links between risk factors in adolescence and atherosclerotic disorders, CVD risk factor stability from childhood to adulthood, and the ability of pediatric risk factors to predict adverse vascular changes and CVD events, even after adult CVD risk factor level adjustment.[24,25,42–46]

Table 2
Lipid parameter classification

Category	Acceptable	Borderline	High
Total cholesterol	<170	170–199	≥200
LDL-C	<110	110–129	≥130
TG			
0–9 y	<75	75–99	≥100
10–19 y	<90	90–129	≥130
Non–HDL-C	<120	120–144	≥145
ApoB	<90	90–109	≥110

Category	Acceptable	Borderline	Low
HDL-C	>45	40–45	<40
ApoA-I	>120	115–120	<115

Abbreviation: ApoA-I, apolipoprotein A-I.
Data from Expert panel on integrated guidelines for cardiovascular health and risk reduction in children and adolescents: summary report. Pediatrics 2011;128(Suppl 5):S240.

The Expert Panel recommends that children with lipid disorders partake of dyslipidemia-determined special diets for at least 6 months and diminish obesity if appropriate. After 6 months of lifestyle modification, triggers referral to lipid specialists to consider statin initiation. The presence of multiple risks or higher intensity risks progressively decreases the LDL-C threshold to initiate statin pharmacotherapy, and decreases the goal LDL-C concentration on treatment.[47–51] The key components of TG treatment center on simple carbohydrate intake reduction, increased omega-3 intake through fish consumption or omega-3 supplements, or severe reduction in fat intake as appropriate. If these maneuvers are ineffective in reducing TG levels sufficiently to mitigate the risk of pancreatitis, referral to a lipid specialist for non-HDL reduction through lipid pharmacotherapy is advised.

CHALLENGES TO THE LIPID MANAGEMENT GUIDELINES
Universal Screening

The most controversial topic raised by the integrated panel has been a call for universal lipid screening, which is intended to improve identification of genetic dyslipidemias like heterozygous FH. FH seems to fulfill 1968 World Health Organization criteria: it occurs in 1 in 500 births, silently leads to highly increased LDL-C over a person's life, manifests as CVD mortality events in young adulthood, and the combination of lipid-lowering drugs and lifestyle modification seems to attenuate the excess risk.[52] Approximately 20% of girls and 50% of boys with FH heterozygosity will have a coronary event before age 50 years.[7,8,53] Although previous guidelines restricted screening to only those children with an increased risk of dyslipidemia based on personal health features or family history, studies show that reliance on family history of CVD events or high lipid levels may miss 30% to 60% of afflicted children because of a lack of knowledge about family history, lack of understanding about lipid levels, the ability of medications presently available to profoundly reduce or prevent CVD events in affected adults, or a parent's refusal to be tested for cholesterol level.[9,54–57] Focusing on children treats them as individuals worthy of care independent of the dependability of their parents and, in a reverse cascade, may boost identification of family members with FH who might not have been detected otherwise.

The disadvantages of universal screening should not be glossed over.[58–60] Children could be incorrectly labeled as abnormal from a nonfasting lipid screening, because CVD risk factors fluctuate throughout childhood and adulthood. However, also similar to adults, isolated lipid measurements in childhood predict atherosclerosis in adulthood.[24,25,42] The guidelines recommend using high thresholds to designate abnormal levels in conjunction with taking the average of multiple lipid values to help avoid misclassification and errors from regression to the mean. It is highly likely that a small number will be inappropriately labeled as FH despite following the guidelines in obtaining 2 more fasting lipid panels. More data must be gathered to assess the negative and positive biological, social, and psychological effects of this screening approach.

Lifestyle Dyslipidemias

The panel acknowledges the probability of discovering lifestyle-driven dyslipidemias and advocates that such children should receive medical attention. Critics note that lipid values fluctuate during childhood and that obesity increases an individual's risk for having abnormal lipid values. With this information they object to classifying a multitude of children, who are already psychologically vulnerable from an abnormal weight label, with an abnormal cholesterol label. If the goal is to lose weight, failure is common and makes the child feel even worse.[58–60]

Although obesity increases the risk of accruing lifestyle-induced dyslipidemias, note that a large proportion of dyslipidemic children are of normal weight, and the most patients who are of abnormal weight are not dyslipidemic.[28] In a related analysis that may parallel efforts in lipid management, detecting and treating abnormal weight with the goal of modifying blood pressure–related CVD did not seem to be a cost-effective way to prevent CVD outcomes.[61] Although the origins of both derive from suboptimal diets and activity levels, dyslipidemia and excess weight are not synonymous. Specific lifestyle modification can modify dyslipidemia without affecting weight immediately.[62–65] As described in the guidelines, for example, the avoidance of simple carbohydrates is not expected to significantly alter LDL-C, but may be useful in hindering insulin resistance mediated by high TG. These dyslipidemia-specific dietary instructions are effective but onerous for families and so should not be applied to the entire population. On the contrary, recent adult meta-analytical data on the effects of dietary saturated fat on CVD and CHD risk outcomes in prospective adult cohort studies suggested that dietary saturated fat was not associated with increased CVD or CHD risk.[11] However, a broad-based adult cohort is not equivalent to a population presenting early in life with markedly abnormal lipid values, and thus the data cannot be generalized to pediatric dyslipidemia. In addition, the CHILD-1 diet recommended for all children without dyslipidemias safely encourages moderation in simple carbohydrates, processed foods, and saturated fat, as well as encouraging consumption of vegetables and lean proteins, which is widely accepted as a sensible approach.[19] In addition, when motivated to avoid medication, youth and families may become more engaged.

By extension, critics are concerned about lifestyle dyslipidemic patients being loosely prescribed statins. The NHLBI panel instead mandates lifestyle alterations as the primary response. Only after this has been assiduously exhausted and additional CVD risks are also present can pharmacotherapy be considered, preferably under a lipid specialist's guidance. This advice is distinctly at odds with treatment patterns among adult providers. The most recent evidence on lipid-lowering therapy indicates that the number of children being treated is grossly inadequate.[66,67] Contrary to popular fears, the guidelines advocate against the indiscriminate distribution of statin drugs to obese children.

Lipid-lowering Treatment

The main criticisms of pediatric lipid pharmacotherapy in general are:

- Invocation of 10-year CVD risk calculators to show that children are inherently low risk
- Lack of data on the benefits of childhood treatment
- Lack of long-term safety data

It is important to recall that the primary intended pediatric recipients of lipid-lowering medications are those with FH. It is improper to use the Framingham 10-year risk calculator on those with genetic dyslipidemia. The Framingham calculator is intended for and derived from a general population cohort, not a high-risk diagnosis such as FH. For example, inputting a cholesterol value of more than 320 mg/dL into the online calculator results in an error message requesting a smaller value. A more suitable risk assessment is family history data in patients with FH showing 50% and 20% risk of coronary events in men and women less than 50 years of age, respectively.[7,8,68]

The criticism regarding lack of long-term data is well taken. The guidelines outline existing data regarding the efficacy and tolerability of statins in reducing LDL-C. However, there are neither studies on the ability of statin therapy started in youth to reduce CVD events nor long-term safety studies, because the logistical complexity and cost of clinical trials following large numbers of patients over several decades are impractical. A recent meta-analysis of placebo adult randomized controlled trials compared the effect of short-term lipid-lowering agents versus naturally occurring LDL-C–lowering genetic mutations on CVD events.[51] This elegant study revealed that CVD prevention per unit LDL-C decrease was several times more effective by genetic polymorphism than by pharmacologic intervention, implying that the amount of time spent at a reduced LDL-C concentration was the leading feature of additional CVD protection. Furthermore, sequence variations in the *PCSK9* gene, which is known to reduce LDL-C, caused 88% and 47% reductions in cardiac disease in African American and white populations.[18] These findings are also in accord with anthropologic epidemiology, which shows lower rates of CVD in cultures with habitually low LDL-C on a population basis.[69,70]

Critics of the guidelines cite unforeseen side effects from other medicines in the past as a reason to avoid a hypothetical pediatric-specific adverse event for lipid-lowering medicine. In contrast, the volume of patient data from statin therapy in adults and children is overwhelming and argues against additional adverse events beyond the well-described myotoxicity, emerging risks regarding incident diabetes mellitus, and possible risk of hepatoxicity.[47–49,71] When family history involves early and severe CVD in a parent, the discussion about treatment takes on a greater sense of urgency. Although the described risks are important to consider, the preponderance of data support the use of lipid-lowering medication in children affected by FH. However, the decision to treat an affected child is always a collaborative one between provider, parent, and child.

SUMMARY

The NHLBI Expert Panel Integrated Guidelines promote the prevention of CVD events by encouraging healthy behaviors in all children, screening and treatment of children with genetic dyslipidemias, usage of specific lifestyle modifications, and limited administration of lipid pharmacotherapy in children with the highest CVD risk. These recommendations place children in the center of the fight against future CVD.

Pediatric providers may be in a position to shift the focus of CVD prevention from trimming multiple risk factors to attacking the roots of CVD.

ADDITIONAL RESOURCES

Centers for Disease Control resources on obesity. Available at:http://www.cdc.gov/obesity/resources/index.html.

2011 NHLBI integrated guidelines for cardiovascular health and risk reduction in children and adolescents. Available at: http://www.nhlbi.nih.gov/health-pro/guidelines/current/cardiovascular-health-pediatric-guidelines/index.htm.

REFERENCES

1. Bandosz P, O'Flaherty M, Drygas W, et al. Decline in mortality from coronary heart disease in Poland after socioeconomic transformation: modelling study. BMJ 2012;344:d8136.
2. Ford ES, Ajani UA, Croft JB, et al. Explaining the decrease in U.S. deaths from coronary disease, 1980-2000. N Engl J Med 2007;356:2388–98.
3. O'Flaherty M, Ford E, Allender S, et al. Coronary heart disease trends in England and Wales from 1984 to 2004: concealed levelling of mortality rates among young adults. Heart 2008;94:178–81.
4. Roger VL, Go AS, Lloyd-Jones DM, et al. Executive summary: heart disease and stroke statistics–2012 update: a report from the American Heart Association. Circulation 2012;125:188–97.
5. Vaartjes I, O'Flaherty M, Grobbee DE, et al. Coronary heart disease mortality trends in the Netherlands 1972-2007. Heart 2011;97:569–73.
6. Bajekal M, Scholes S, Love H, et al. Analysing recent socioeconomic trends in coronary heart disease mortality in England, 2000-2007: a population modelling study. PLoS Med 2012;9:e1001237.
7. Mortality in treated heterozygous familial hypercholesterolaemia: implications for clinical management. Scientific Steering Committee on behalf of the Simon Broome Register Group. Atherosclerosis 1999;142:105–12.
8. Risk of fatal coronary heart disease in familial hypercholesterolaemia. Scientific Steering Committee on behalf of the Simon Broome Register Group. BMJ 1991; 303:893–6.
9. Marks D, Wonderling D, Thorogood M, et al. Screening for hypercholesterolaemia versus case finding for familial hypercholesterolaemia: a systematic review and cost-effectiveness analysis. Health Technol Assess 2000;4:1–123.
10. Brown MS, Goldstein JL. Familial hypercholesterolemia: a genetic defect in the low-density lipoprotein receptor. N Engl J Med 1976;294:1386–90.
11. Talmud PJ, Futema M, Humphries SE. The genetic architecture of the familial hyperlipidaemia syndromes: rare mutations and common variants in multiple genes. Curr Opin Lipidol 2014;25:274–81.
12. Cortner JA, Coates PM, Gallagher PR. Prevalence and expression of familial combined hyperlipidemia in childhood. J Pediatr 1990;116:514–9.
13. Johansen CT, Hegele RA. Genetic bases of hypertriglyceridemic phenotypes. Curr Opin Lipidol 2011;22:247–53.
14. Johansen CT, Kathiresan S, Hegele RA. Genetic determinants of plasma triglycerides. J Lipid Res 2011;52:189–206.
15. Brunzell JD, Iverius PH, Scheibel MS, et al. Primary lipoprotein lipase deficiency. Adv Exp Med Biol 1986;201:227–39.

16. Evans V, Kastelein JJ. Lipoprotein lipase deficiency–rare or common? Cardiovasc Drugs Ther 2002;16:283–7.

17. Miller M, Stone NJ, Ballantyne C, et al. Triglycerides and cardiovascular disease: a scientific statement from the American Heart Association. Circulation 2011;123:2292–333.

18. Cohen JC, Boerwinkle E, Mosley TH Jr, et al. Sequence variations in PCSK9, low LDL, and protection against coronary heart disease. N Engl J Med 2006;354: 1264–72.

19. Expert panel on integrated guidelines for cardiovascular health and risk reduction in children and adolescents: summary report. Pediatrics 2011;128(Suppl 5): S213–56.

20. Weintraub WS, Daniels SR, Burke LE, et al. Value of primordial and primary prevention for cardiovascular disease: a policy statement from the American Heart Association. Circulation 2011;124:967–90.

21. Strasser T. Reflections on cardiovascular diseases. Interdiscip Sci Rev 1978;3: 225–30.

22. Lewington S, Clarke R, Qizilbash N, et al. Age-specific relevance of usual blood pressure to vascular mortality: a meta-analysis of individual data for one million adults in 61 prospective studies. Lancet 2002;360:1903–13.

23. Di Angelantonio E, Sarwar N, Perry P, et al. Major lipids, apolipoproteins, and risk of vascular disease. JAMA 2009;302:1993–2000.

24. Berenson GS, Srinivasan SR, Bao W, et al. Association between multiple cardiovascular risk factors and atherosclerosis in children and young adults. The Bogalusa Heart Study. N Engl J Med 1998;338:1650–6.

25. Newman WP 3rd, Freedman DS, Voors AW, et al. Relation of serum lipoprotein levels and systolic blood pressure to early atherosclerosis. The Bogalusa Heart Study. N Engl J Med 1986;314:138–44.

26. Natural history of aortic and coronary atherosclerotic lesions in youth. Findings from the PDAY Study. Pathobiological Determinants of Atherosclerosis in Youth (PDAY) Research Group. Arterioscler Thromb 1993;13: 1291–8.

27. Rose G. Sick individuals and sick populations. Int J Epidemiol 1985;14:32–8.

28. May AL, Kuklina EV, Yoon PW. Prevalence of cardiovascular disease risk factors among US adolescents, 1999-2008. Pediatrics 2012;129(6):1035–41.

29. The fourth report on the diagnosis, evaluation, and treatment of high blood pressure in children and adolescents. Pediatrics 2004;114:555–76.

30. Daniels SR, Greer FR. Lipid screening and cardiovascular health in childhood. Pediatrics 2008;122:198–208.

31. Dobson AJ, Evans A, Ferrario M, et al. Changes in estimated coronary risk in the 1980s: data from 38 populations in the WHO MONICA project. World Health Organization. Monitoring trends and determinants in cardiovascular diseases. Ann Med 1998;30:199–205.

32. Kuulasmaa K, Tunstall-Pedoe H, Dobson A, et al. Estimation of contribution of changes in classic risk factors to trends in coronary-event rates across the WHO MONICA Project populations. Lancet 2000;355:675–87.

33. Yusuf S, Hawken S, Ounpuu S, et al. Effect of potentially modifiable risk factors associated with myocardial infarction in 52 countries (the INTERHEART study): case-control study. Lancet 2004;364:937–52.

34. O'Donnell MJ, Xavier D, Liu L, et al. Risk factors for ischaemic and intracerebral haemorrhagic stroke in 22 countries (the INTERSTROKE study): a case-control study. Lancet 2010;376:112–23.

35. Gregg EW, Cheng YJ, Cadwell BL, et al. Secular trends in cardiovascular disease risk factors according to body mass index in US adults. JAMA 2005; 293:1868–74.
36. Kit BK, Carroll MD, Lacher DA, et al. Trends in serum lipids among US youths aged 6 to 19 years, 1988-2010. JAMA 2012;308:591–600.
37. Boden WE, O'Rourke RA, Teo KK, et al. Optimal medical therapy with or without PCI for stable coronary disease. N Engl J Med 2007;356:1503–16.
38. Frye RL, August P, Brooks MM, et al. A randomized trial of therapies for type 2 diabetes and coronary artery disease. N Engl J Med 2009;360:2503–15.
39. Velazquez EJ, Lee KL, Deja MA, et al. Coronary-artery bypass surgery in patients with left ventricular dysfunction. N Engl J Med 2011;364:1607–16.
40. Finucane MM, Stevens GA, Cowan MJ, et al. National, regional, and global trends in body-mass index since 1980: systematic analysis of health examination surveys and epidemiological studies with 960 country-years and 9.1 million participants. Lancet 2011;377:557–67.
41. Farzadfar F, Finucane MM, Danaei G, et al. National, regional, and global trends in serum total cholesterol since 1980: systematic analysis of health examination surveys and epidemiological studies with 321 country-years and 3.0 million participants. Lancet 2011;377:578–86.
42. Magnussen CG, Koskinen J, Chen W, et al. Pediatric metabolic syndrome predicts adulthood metabolic syndrome, subclinical atherosclerosis, and type 2 diabetes mellitus but is no better than body mass index alone: the Bogalusa Heart Study and the Cardiovascular Risk in Young Finns Study. Circulation 2010;122:1604–11.
43. Magnussen CG, Raitakari OT, Thomson R, et al. Utility of currently recommended pediatric dyslipidemia classifications in predicting dyslipidemia in adulthood: evidence from the Childhood Determinants of Adult Health (CDAH) study, Cardiovascular Risk in Young Finns study, and Bogalusa Heart Study. Circulation 2008;117:32–42.
44. Gray L, Lee IM, Sesso HD, et al. Blood pressure in early adulthood, hypertension in middle age, and future cardiovascular disease mortality: HAHS (Harvard Alumni Health Study). J Am Coll Cardiol 2011;58:2396–403.
45. Franks PW, Hanson RL, Knowler WC, et al. Childhood obesity, other cardiovascular risk factors, and premature death. N Engl J Med 2010;362:485–93.
46. Koivistoinen T, Hutri-Kahonen N, Juonala M, et al. Metabolic syndrome in childhood and increased arterial stiffness in adulthood: the Cardiovascular Risk in Young Finns study. Ann Med 2011;43:312–9.
47. Avis HJ, Vissers MN, Stein EA, et al. A systematic review and meta-analysis of statin therapy in children with familial hypercholesterolemia. Arterioscler Thromb Vasc Biol 2007;27:1803–10.
48. Carreau V, Girardet JP, Bruckert E. Long-term follow-up of statin treatment in a cohort of children with familial hypercholesterolemia: efficacy and tolerability. Paediatr Drugs 2011;13:267–75.
49. O'Gorman CS, Higgins MF, O'Neill MB. Systematic review and metaanalysis of statins for heterozygous familial hypercholesterolemia in children: evaluation of cholesterol changes and side effects. Pediatr Cardiol 2009;30:482–9.
50. Vuorio A, Kuoppala J, Kovanen PT, et al. Statins for children with familial hypercholesterolemia. Cochrane Database Syst Rev 2010;7:CD006401.
51. Ference BA, Yoo W, Alesh I, et al. Effect of long-term exposure to lower low-density lipoprotein cholesterol beginning early in life on the risk of coronary heart disease: a mendelian randomization analysis. J Am Coll Cardiol 2012;60:2631–9.

52. Wilson JG, Junger G. Principles and practice of screening for disease. In: WHO public health papers no 34. Geneva (Switzerland): World Health Organization; 1968.
53. Stone NJ, Levy RI, Fredrickson DS, et al. Coronary artery disease in 116 kindred with familial type II hyperlipoproteinemia. Circulation 1974;49:476–88.
54. Claassen L, Henneman L, Kindt I, et al. Perceived risk and representations of cardiovascular disease and preventive behaviour in people diagnosed with familial hypercholesterolemia: a cross-sectional questionnaire study. J Health Psychol 2010;15:33–43.
55. Resnicow K, Cross D. Are parents' self-reported total cholesterol levels useful in identifying children with hyperlipidemia? An examination of current guidelines. Pediatrics 1993;92:347–53.
56. Wald DS, Bestwick JP, Wald NJ. Child-parent screening for familial hypercholesterolaemia: screening strategy based on a meta-analysis. BMJ 2007;335:599.
57. Wald DS, Kasturiratne A, Godoy A, et al. Child-parent screening for familial hypercholesterolemia. J Pediatr 2011;159:865–7.
58. Gillman MW, Daniels SR. Is universal pediatric lipid screening justified? JAMA 2012;307:259–60.
59. Klass P. Screening children for cholesterol. In: The New York Times. New York: The New York Times Company; 2012.
60. Newman TB, Pletcher MJ, Hulley SB. Overly aggressive new guidelines for lipid screening in children: evidence of a broken process. Pediatrics 2012;130:349–52.
61. Wang YC, Cheung AM, Bibbins-Domingo K, et al. Effectiveness and cost-effectiveness of blood pressure screening in adolescents in the United States. J Pediatr 2011;158:257–64.e1–7.
62. Ebbeling CB, Leidig MM, Feldman HA, et al. Effects of a low-glycemic load vs low-fat diet in obese young adults: a randomized trial. JAMA 2007;297:2092–102.
63. Jacobson MS, Tomopoulos S, Williams CL, et al. Normal growth in high-risk hyperlipidemic children and adolescents with dietary intervention. Prev Med 1998; 27:775–80.
64. Starc TJ, Shea S, Cohn LC, et al. Greater dietary intake of simple carbohydrate is associated with lower concentrations of high-density-lipoprotein cholesterol in hypercholesterolemic children. Am J Clin Nutr 1998;67:1147–54.
65. Van Horn L, Obarzanek E, Barton BA, et al. A summary of results of the Dietary Intervention Study in Children (DISC): lessons learned. Prog Cardiovasc Nurs 2003;18:28–41.
66. Lasky T. Statin use in children in the United States. Pediatrics 2008;122:1406–8.
67. Liberman JN, Berger JE, Lewis M. Prevalence of antihypertensive, antidiabetic, and dyslipidemic prescription medication use among children and adolescents. Arch Pediatr Adolesc Med 2009;163:357–64.
68. Williams RR, Hasstedt SJ, Wilson DE, et al. Evidence that men with familial hypercholesterolemia can avoid early coronary death. An analysis of 77 gene carriers in four Utah pedigrees. JAMA 1986;255:219–24.
69. Keys A, Menotti A, Aravanis C, et al. The seven countries study: 2,289 deaths in 15 years. Prev Med 1984;13:141–54.
70. O'Keefe JH Jr, Cordain L, Harris WH, et al. Optimal low-density lipoprotein is 50 to 70 mg/dl: lower is better and physiologically normal. J Am Coll Cardiol 2004; 43:2142–6.
71. Bulbulia R, Bowman L, Wallendszus K, et al. Effects on 11-year mortality and morbidity of lowering LDL cholesterol with simvastatin for about 5 years in 20,536 high-risk individuals: a randomised controlled trial. Lancet 2011;378: 2013–20.

Dyslipidemia in Pregnancy

Robert Wild, MD, MPH, PhD[a], Elizabeth A. Weedin, DO[a],*,
Don Wilson, MD, FNLA[b]

KEYWORDS

- Dyslipidemia • Hyperlipidemia • Pregnancy • Fetal metabolism
- Metabolic syndrome

KEY POINTS

- Exposure of the fetus to elevated levels of cholesterol and oxidative byproducts of cholesterol metabolism has been shown to result in programming of fetal arterial cells with a predisposition to atherosclerosis later in life.
- For many women, the reproductive years span 2 decades, representing an optimal time to reduce cardiovascular disease risk factors before conception.
- Recent discoveries highlight the importance of preventing or optimizing maternal dyslipidemia for the benefit of the mother and the child.
- Currently no reference standards are defined for lipid parameters during pregnancy, although it is well-known that pregnancy is a state of insulin resistance and that lipoprotein lipid profiles reflect this process.
- Overweight and obese women are significantly more likely to exceed the pregnancy-related weight gain recommendations.

INTRODUCTION

Historically dyslipidemia in pregnancy has been considered physiologic with little clinical relevance. Lipids and lipoproteins have not been routinely measured at any time point during pregnancy, irrespective of their role in cardiovascular disease (CVD) or pregnancy outcomes. Recent evidence describing fatty streaks in the aortas of 6-month-old fetuses of mothers who were hypercholesterolemic[1] and studies in animal models have challenged the assumption that maternal cholesterol does not cross the placental barrier. Poorly controlled cholesterol, triglycerides, and their metabolites

This article originally appeared in Cardiology Clinics, Volume 33, Issue 2, May 2015.
Financial Disclosures: None.
[a] Section of Reproductive Endocrinology and Infertility, Department of Obstetrics and Gynecology, University of Oklahoma Health Sciences Center, 1100 N Lindsay Ave, Oklahoma City, OK 73104, USA; [b] Department of Pediatric Endocrinology, Cook Children's Medical Center, 1500 Cooper Street, Fort Worth, TX 76104, USA
* Corresponding author. 920 S.L. Young Boulevard, WP2410, Oklahoma City, OK 73104.
E-mail address: Elizabeth-weedin@ouhsc.edu

Clinics Collections 5 (2015) 367–375
http://dx.doi.org/10.1016/j.ccol.2015.05.022
2352-7986/15/$ – see front matter Published by Elsevier Inc.

associated with cardiometabolic dysfunction seem to have significant detrimental maternal and fetal vascular consequences. Maternal cardiometabolic dysfunction may not only contribute to long-term effects of the mother and child's vascular health but also potentially create CVD risk for generational offspring.

In providing an update on this rapidly expanding and multifaceted topic, this article first outlines the basic understanding of the importance of cholesterol in fetal development. New insight is then reviewed regarding why this new recognition of disordered maternal cholesterol and triglyceride metabolism is likely to have a long-term effect for future generations. Diagnosing and treating dyslipidemia before, during, and after pregnancy in an effort to provide the best opportunity to reduce the increasing atherosclerotic burden of the rapidly expanding population.

CHOLESTEROL AND FETAL DEVELOPMENT

Cholesterol is required for normal fetal development. It plays a key role in the formation of cell membranes, membrane integrity, and maintaining cholesterol-rich domains that are essential for most membrane-associated signaling cascades, including sonic hedgehog signaling.[2] Cholesterol is also a precursor of hormones, such as steroids, vitamin D, and bile acids. Sources of fetal cholesterol seem to include endogenous production, the maternal circulation, and synthesis within the yolk sac or placenta.

Because of its critical role in fetal development, it was previously thought that most cholesterol is synthesized de novo by the fetus. Emerging evidence, however, suggests that maternal cholesterol and the placenta may also play a meaningful role. For exogenous cholesterol to be available for fetal use, the yoke sac and placenta must take up maternal cholesterol via receptor-mediated or receptor-independent transport processes, transport lipids across cellular barriers, and/or secrete the maternally derived or newly synthesized cholesterol into the fetal circulation.[3,4] Cultured trophoblast cells have been shown to express low-density lipoprotein (LDL) receptors (LDLRs), LDLR-related proteins, scavenger receptors A, and high-density lipoprotein (HDL)–binding scavenger receptors B1 (SR-B1s) on their apical side. Cholesterol taken up by internalization of receptor-bound ApoB- or ApoE-carrying lipoproteins and oxidized LDL, and from SR-B1–bound HDL, is then released on the basolateral side.[4] Although the uptake of cholesterol by endothelial cells is well understood, knowledge about the mechanisms through which placental endothelial cells transport cholesterol to the fetal microcirculation, the regulation of efflux, and their ability to deliver substantial quantities of cholesterol is incomplete.

Maternal cholesterol has been shown to cross the placental and enter the fetal circulation, contributing substantially to the fetal cholesterol pool in animals and humans.[4,5] Vuorio and colleagues[6] found that plant stanol concentrations in cord blood of healthy newborns were 40% to 50% of maternal levels, demonstrating active maternal-fetal sterol transport. Compared with the umbilical arteries, the umbilical vein has been found to have a greater concentration of cholesterol.[7]

Maternal hypercholesterolemia, as seen in a woman with familial hypercholesterolemia (FH), may pose a significant risk to the fetus.[8] A substantial increase in maternal cholesterol has been shown to significantly increase cholesterol transfer from the mother to the fetus, without upregulation of liver X receptors.[9] Fetal cholesterol levels in mid-pregnancy are much higher than they are at term, and these levels correlate with maternal cholesterol before the sixth month of gestation.[9] This finding suggests maternal hypercholesterolemia does not, a priori, result in upregulation of cholesterol transport. However, exposure of the fetus to very high levels of cholesterol and oxidative products of cholesterol has been shown to result in programming of arterial cells with a predisposition to atherosclerosis later in life.[1] Similar findings have been observed in pregnant women who are obese, have the metabolic syndrome, and/or have diabetes.[10] Napoli and colleagues[1] have shown a direct correlation between the concentration of maternal cholesterol and the presence of fatty streaks in the fetus; effects more strongly correlated earlier in gestation.

Studies have also shown adverse fetal effects as a consequence of decreased exogenous cholesterol. Women with lower plasma cholesterol levels, for example, were found to have smaller newborns; a correlation has been reported between low plasma cholesterol and microcephaly.[11] Ultimately, however, the mechanisms underlying fetal effects related to maternal hypercholesterolemia remain incompletely understood.[9]

PREVALENCE OF CARDIOVASCULAR DISEASE RISK FACTORS

According to the National Health and Nutrition Examination Survey 1999–2008 data, among women aged 18 to 44 years in the United States, 2.4% have diabetes, 7.7% are estimated to have hypertension, 25.4% use tobacco, 2.9% have chronic kidney disease, and 57.6% are either overweight or obese. Prepregnancy cardiometabolic and inflammatory risk factors predict the risk of hypertensive disorders of pregnancy. An increased risk of hypertension is seen in women who are obese. The odds of hypertension during pregnancy are 1.8 times greater for individuals who are normotensive yet obese before pregnancy. The odds of a hypertension-related complication during pregnancy are 3.5 times higher in women who are overweight and hypertensive before pregnancy.[12]

Approximately 50% of pregnancies are unplanned, limiting the ability to identify women with CVD risk factors before pregnancy. A Kaiser Family Foundation national survey recently noted that the rate of CVD screening for women aged 18 to 44 years was 58%, compared with 78% for women aged 45 to 64 years.[13] This proportion is even lower compared with blood pressure screening in 18- to 44-year olds. Another national survey found that among women aged 18 to 64 years, 15% were seen by general medicine physicians, 62% by gynecologists alone, and 23% by both. Those seen by gynecologists received more counseling and preventive services.[14] In an evaluation of 2 different health care plans servicing nearly 3.6 million members, hypertension was recognized in fewer than one-third of women during the course of their care. Furthermore, irrespective of which specialty provided the care, less than 70% of women received lipid screening, nutrition, or weight counseling. The survey also illustrated that limited knowledge about preeclampsia and future risk in reproductive age women was common among all specialties.

The most recent National Vital Statistics report illustrates that pregnancy rates for women aged 25 to 29 years have changed very little since 1990.[15] Rates for women in their 30s and 40s, however, have increased. Additionally, in the past 45 years, women aged 35 to 44 years in the United States have experienced the greatest increase in prevalence of obesity. With the known association between obesity and dyslipidemia, the implications of this trend are profound. Currently, 45% of women begin pregnancy either overweight or obese, a statistic that has almost doubled in the past 30 years. Furthermore, approximately 43% of pregnant women gain more weight than recommended during the course of their pregnancy. It is well understood that maternal obesity contributes to other high-risk conditions, such as gestational diabetes, hypertensive disorders, newborn macrosomia, and perinatal complications.[16] For many women, the reproductive years can span 2 decades, representing an optimal time to reduce CVD risk factors before conception, for the benefit of both the mother and her future offspring.

FETAL CONSIDERATIONS

Because gestational dyslipidemia has historically been considered physiologic, with little clinical significance, lipid and lipoproteins have not been measured routinely during pregnancy. However, the recent discoveries of fatty streaks in the aortas of 6-month-old fetuses of mothers with hypercholesterolemia, and the identification of aortic atherosclerosis at autopsy of deceased children with normal levels cholesterol born to mothers with hypercholesterolemia, highlight the importance of correcting maternal dyslipidemia.[1,17] In New Zealand white rabbits, diet-induced maternal dyslipidemia causes a dose-dependent fetal and postnatal atherogenesis, which was reduced by lowering maternal cholesterol with cholestyramine.[18] Similar data have been obtained in a murine model.[19]

A large body of literature suggests that an unhealthy uterine environment can lead to maladaptations in postuterine life, many of which are suspected to be the origin of chronic, noncommunicable diseases. Atherosclerosis is among the first of several conditions for which a role of developmental programming was described.[20] Several factors have been suggested that may play a role in developmental programming of the fetus.[21] Genetic factors, metabolic or environmental disturbances of the mother, and the father's lifestyle and genetics are important prepregnancy components that may contribute to fetal programming. During pregnancy, maternal malnutrition (either underfeeding or overfeeding), maternal stress, chemical exposure, preeclampsia, hypertension, gestational diabetes, maternal smoking, secondhand smoke exposure, metabolic syndrome, hyperlipidemia, obesity, intrauterine growth retardation, placental function, and hypoxia may be important influences. At the cellular level, adaptation occurs through DNA methylation, genetics, lifestyle choices during childhood, and altered immune responses, ultimately contributing to childhood atherosclerosis. Recent animal studies have revealed that changes in DNA methylation and chromatin modification may be responsible for the epigenetic programming and increased atherosclerotic susceptibility.[22] However, the exact mechanisms underlying the effects of maternal hypercholesterolemia in the offspring are still unclear.

Despite this lack of clarity, increasing evidence shows that epigenetic programming of metabolism during embryonic or fetal development might be involved.[23] Epigenetic phenomena occur at the interface between the genome and the environment. The environment can influence epigenetic information that is superimposed on the DNA, which may have long-term consequences for the transcription of specific regions of the genome. Results of animal studies show that permanent changes in either DNA methylation or chromatin modification, or both, may be responsible for the epigenetic programming of increased atherosclerotic susceptibility.[24] For instance, maternal hypercholesterolemia in ApoE-deficient mice leads to the activation of genes involved in cholesterol synthesis and LDLR activity in adult offspring.[17,24] Other animal studies have shown that the genes involved in immune pathways and fatty acid metabolism are upregulated in the offspring of hypercholesterolemic dams.[25] These findings indicate that an adverse maternal environment may alter basic cellular programming of the fetus.[24] Further research is needed to unravel the exact mechanisms through which maternal hypercholesterolemia influences this process.

Depending on what deleterious influences occur in utero and during childhood, the adult phenotype of insulin resistance and obesity that results in cardiometabolic disease is expressed at different genetic set points.[19]

In utero, the fetus handles lipid metabolism in a dynamic fashion. Pregnancy is associated with increased permeability of the vascular endothelium by small molecules, which can lead to vascular inflammation. This permeability is further increased in the presences of diabetes. Additionally, it is now known that there is active transport of lipids to the fetus. This transport seems to vary at different stages of pregnancy. Early in gestation, the fetus seems to preferentially use lipids for the purposes of adequate membrane development and possibly for protection. Excess fat may, thereafter, be deposited in the liver, depending on gestational age and hepatic maturity. Additionally, fetal epicardial fat can be identified early in gestation. Presumably these mechanisms occur in an attempt to protect the fetal brain.[9]

The offspring of obese mothers have an increased risk of mortality in later life.[26] Minimal mortality is found in offspring of mothers with a normal body mass index (BMI).[26] Long-term studies have shown that offspring of mothers with a greater BMI and waist circumference have higher triglycerides and increased blood pressure and insulin resistance.[27]

MATERNAL CONSIDERATIONS

Lipid and lipoprotein levels have been tracked throughout pregnancy in groups of women with uncomplicated and complicated pregnancies. Nonetheless, no reference standards for lipid or lipoproteins during pregnancy currently exist.[9] Pregnancy is a state of insulin resistance reflected by the lipid and lipoprotein profiles of the mother. Within 6 weeks of gestation, lipid levels drop slightly, followed by an increase during each trimester of pregnancy. Triglyceride levels increase sharply during pregnancy, as do cholesterol levels. LDL increases in a similar pattern as that of total cholesterol. On average, cholesterol and triglyceride levels do not exceed 250 mg/dL. However, when abnormal pregnancies are included, levels can exceed 300 mg/dL.[28] Abnormally high triglyceride levels in the first trimester are significantly associated with gestational hypertension, preeclampsia, induced preterm birth, and fetuses considered large for gestational age.[29] Estrogens increase triglyceride levels through stimulating hepatic production of very-low-density lipoprotein (VLDL) and inhibiting hepatic and adipose lipoprotein lipase. Progesterone opposes these actions, whereas cytokines and inflammatory factors are important contributors of insulin resistance. However, this physiologic increase in lipids and lipoproteins is a mechanism aimed at accommodating fetal demands for normal growth and development.[23]

Preeclampsia is characterized by endothelial dysfunction prompted by an increase in triglyceride and free fatty acid levels. Triglyceride levels and ApoB and small LDL particles are all increased in preeclampsia, vascular cell adhesion molecule specifically is increased and serves as an indicator of endothelial dysfunction. Whether ApoB or small LDL particles cause this endothelial disruption is currently unclear.[30] Additionally, some indication exists that endothelial dysfunction may be caused partly by oxidative stress and decreased prostacyclin. Metabolic syndrome and gestational diabetes are conditions that predispose women to preeclampsia and overt diabetes.[29] Women with polycystic ovarian syndrome, for example, are more likely to have adverse pregnancy outcomes even if they are not obese.[31] This finding is particularly important because these women have insulin resistance and are prone to metabolic syndrome and diabetes.

Medical conditions that cause abnormal lipids and lipoproteins should be investigated and, if present, treated appropriately. Hypothyroidism, alcohol consumption, low-molecular-weight heparin, glucocorticoids, psychotropic medications, kidney disease, and lipodystrophy have all been associated with dyslipidemia; however, their effects during pregnancy are poorly characterized. The observed dyslipidemia is independent of diabetes, which is the most common reason for the disturbed lipid metabolism in general.[32] One of the more common reasons for high triglyceride levels during pregnancy is the use of medications. Alcohol, estrogen, oral contraceptives, glucocorticoids, ß-blockers, valproate, sertraline, retinoic acids, cyclosporine, and tacrolimus are a few examples of potential causes. Cocaine use can also cause dyslipidemia. Offending agents should be identified and discontinued, ideally before conception.

Elevated VLDL and chylomicrons levels may occur and are thought to be secondary to a genetic predisposition. Triglyceride levels are typically very high, greater than 2000 mg/dL, increasing the risk of pancreatitis. Clinical features of severe hypertriglyceridemia include eruptive xanthoma, hepatosplenomegaly, abdominal pain, dyspnea, peripheral neuropathy, memory loss, and dementia. These neurologic symptoms need be addressed in pregnant women just as in nonpregnant persons. With severe hypertriglyceridemia, a reduction in fat calories to 15% to 20% daily is usually necessary. Insulin therapy may be used even in the absence of overt diabetes. Fish oil capsules are often used when triglyceride levels are greater than 500 mg/dL. Gemfibrozil or fenofibrate are widely used despite their classification as class C medications. The ultimate goal is to reduce triglyceride levels to less than 400 mg/dL in an effort to reduce the risk of pancreatitis. Other acute therapies reported in case studies include medium-chain triglycerides, niacin, sunflower oil, gene therapy, and plasmapherisis.[33]

All lipid-lowering medications, aside from bile sequestrate and omega-3-fatty acids, should be stopped before conception or immediately when pregnancy occurs unexpected. Lifestyle changes and glycemic control should be instituted where needed. During pregnancy, elevated cholesterol levels can be treated safely with a bile acid sequestrant. Severe hypertriglyceridemia associated with pancreatitis can be treated with omega-3 fatty acids, parenteral nutrition, plasmapheresis, and other lipid-lowering agents in the last trimester of pregnancy, notably gemfibrozil. Monitoring is recommended, at a minimum, every trimester or within 6 weeks of initiating treatment. Close follow-up of the mother with FH or with dysmetabolic issues of pregnancy is strongly recommended.

Women with gestational diabetes and/or preeclampsia are also at increased risk for elevated triglyceride levels, development of chronic hypertension, recurrent gestation diabetes and/or overt diabetes, recurrent preeclampsia, and development of albuminuria later in life. Two registered clinical trials are currently evaluating the effects of lipophilic statins to prevent preeclampsia in pregnancy. The true risk of congenital anomalies caused by statins in pregnancy is not well substantiated in humans. However, because statins are category X, statin use in pregnancy should be conducted only in a research setting until more information is available.[33]

A lipid profile should be obtained before conception and every trimester in women with FH who become pregnant. In these women, N-terminal pro-brain natriuretic peptide has been suggested as a useful marker for possible cardiac ischemia. FH can be treated with lifestyle and bile acid sequestrates, preferably colesevelam. Lastly, mipomersen (class B) and LDL apheresis may be necessary in pregnancy. Evaluation and treatment in a specialized center where facilities are available is recommended.

A thorough understanding of pregnancy and lactation-safe medications is imperative to ensure maternal and fetal safety. Class A and B medications are widely used as needed. Class C medications are often used when the benefit outweighs the risk. The chance for fetal harm is greatest during the first trimester. Category D medications have shown definitive evidence of human fetal risk, although potential benefits may warrant use. For category X medications, however, which have investigational or marketing data showing fetal abnormalities, the risks clearly outweigh the benefit. Class N medications have not been classified. Statins are currently classified as category X, whereas fibrates, ezetimibe, niacin, cholestyramine, and omega-3 are category C. Colesevelam and mipomersen are class B.

POSTPARTUM CONSIDERATIONS

Postpartum follow-up of women with dyslipidemia during pregnancy includes close observation, specifically for those who experienced preeclampsia and/or diabetes. Compared with women who underwent an uncomplicated pregnancy, women who had preeclampsia were found to have worse cardiometabolic profiles at 1-year postpartum. Given the variety of providers who may participate in a women's antepartum, intrapartum, postpartum, and postpuerperal care, there is often loss of continuity and appropriate follow-up of pregnancy-related conditions. Women often do not lose the weight gained during pregnancy, which frequently goes unrecognized or may not be properly addressed. Overweight and obese women are 6 times more likely to exceed the pregnancy-related weight gain recommendations. These women are predisposed to higher postpartum weight gain and retention after pregnancy, with 13% to 20% of women being 5 kg or more above their preconception weight by 1-year postpartum.[16] The Health, Aging, and Body Composition Study found that the odds ratio for developing CVD was 3.31 for women and infants that were both <2500 gm and preterm compared with women having normal weight infants at term.[34] Weight gain and overweight status during midlife were strong independent predictors of the development of metabolic syndrome, type II diabetes mellitus, and early mortality.[35,36] Additionally, a positive obstetric history for preeclampsia doubles the long-term risk of CVD in the mother.[35] An obstetric history that includes gestational diabetes increases the 10-year risk for developing overt type II diabetes to approximately 40%. The prevalence of a significant and treatable dyslipidemia is approximately one-third in these populations.[36]

Although understanding of maternal dyslipidemia and its impact on the future health and well-being of the mother and her offspring is incomplete, increasing evidence suggests that providers must be more vigilant in assessing and treating CVD risk factors during pregnancy.[36,37] Additional assessments and studies addressing individual and public health consequences of the obesity epidemic are also urgently needed.

REFERENCES

1. Napoli C, D'Armiento FP, Mancini FP, et al. Fatty streak formation occurs in human fetal aortas and is greatly enhanced by maternal hypercholesterolemia. Intimal accumulation of low density lipoprotein and its oxidation precede monocyte recruitment into early atherosclerotic lesions. J Clin Invest 1997;100(11):2680–90.
2. Woollett LA. Where does fetal and embryonic cholesterol originate and what does it do? Annu Rev Nutr 2008;28:97–114.
3. Woollett LA. Fetal lipid metabolism. Front Biosci 2001;6:D536–45.
4. Woollett LA. Maternal cholesterol in fetal development: transport of cholesterol from the maternal to the fetal circulation. Am J Clin Nutr 2005;82(6):1155–61.
5. Yoshida S, Wada Y. Transfer of maternal cholesterol to embryo and fetus in pregnant mice. J Lipid Res 2005;46(10):2168–74.
6. Vuorio AF, Miettinen TA, Turtola H, et al. Cholesterol metabolism in normal and heterozygous familial hypercholesterolemic newborns. J Lab Clin Med 2002; 140(1):35–42.
7. Spellacy WN, Ashbacher LV, Harris GK, et al. Total cholesterol content in maternal and umbilical vessels in term pregnancies. Obstet Gynecol 1974;44(5):661–5.

8. Narverud I, Iversen PO, Aukrust P, et al. Maternal familial hypercholesterolaemia (FH) confers altered haemostatic profile in offspring with and without FH. Thromb Res 2013;131(2):178–82.
9. Palinski W. Maternal-fetal cholesterol transport in the placenta: good, bad, and target for modulation. Circ Res 2009;104(5):569–71.
10. Palinski W, Napoli C. Impaired fetal growth, cardiovascular disease, and the need to move on. Circulation 2008;117(3):341–3.
11. Edison RJ, Berg K, Remaley A, et al. Adverse birth outcome among mothers with low serum cholesterol. Pediatrics 2007;120(4):723–33.
12. Hedderson MM, Darbinian JA, Sridhar SB, et al. Prepregnancy cardiometabolic and inflammatory risk factors and subsequent risk of hypertensive disorders of pregnancy. Am J Obstet Gynecol 2012;207(1):68–9.
13. Salganicoff A, Ranji U, Beamesderfer A, et al. Women and Health Care in the Early Years of the ACA: Key Findings from the 2013 Kaiser Women's Health Survey – Preventive Services – 8590. May 14, 2014. Available at: http://kff.org/report-section/women-and-health-care-in-the-early-years-of-the-aca-key-findings-from-the-2013-kaiser-womens-health-survey-preventive-services/. Accessed March 25, 2015.
14. Ehrenthal DB, Catov JM. Importance of engaging obstetrician/gynecologists in cardiovascular disease prevention. Curr Opin Cardiol 2013;28(5):547–53.
15. Ventura SJ, Curtin SC, Abma JC, et al. Estimated pregnancy rates and rates of pregnancy outcomes for the United States, 1990-2008. National vital statistics reports, vol. 60 no. 7. Hyattsville, MD: National Center for Health Statistics. 2012.
16. Gunderson EP. Childbearing and obesity in women: weight before, during, and after pregnancy. Obstet Gynecol Clin North Am 2009;36(2):317–32, ix.
17. Napoli C, Glass CK, Witztum JL, et al. Influence of maternal hypercholesterolaemia during pregnancy on progression of early atherosclerotic lesions in childhood: Fate of Early Lesions in Children (FELIC) study. Lancet 1999;354(9186):1234–41.
18. Napoli C, Witztum JL, Calara F, et al. Maternal hypercholesterolemia enhances atherogenesis in normocholesterolemic rabbits, which is inhibited by antioxidant or lipid-lowering intervention during pregnancy: an experimental model of atherogenic mechanisms in human fetuses. Circ Res 2000;87(10):946–52.
19. Palinski W. Effect of maternal cardiovascular conditions and risk factors on offspring cardiovascular disease. Circulation 2014;129(20):2066–77.
20. Goharkhay N, Tamayo EH, Yin H, et al. Maternal hypercholesterolemia leads to activation of endogenous cholesterol synthesis in the offspring. American Journal of Obstetrics and Gynecology 2008;199(3). http://dx.doi.org/10.1016/j.ajog.2008.06.064. 273.e1–273.e6.
21. Hanson M, Godfrey KM, Lillycrop KA, et al. Developmental plasticity and developmental origins of non-communicable disease: theoretical considerations and epigenetic mechanisms. Prog Biophys Mol Biol 2011;106(1):272–80.
22. Deruiter M, Alkemade F, Groot A, et al. Maternal transmission of risk for atherosclerosis. Current Opinion in Lipidology 2008;4:333–7.
23. Herrera E. Metabolic adaptations in pregnancy and their implications for the availability of substrates to the fetus. Eur J Clin Nutr 2000;54(Suppl 1):S47–51.
24. DeRuiter MC, Alkemade FE, Gittenberger-de Groot AC, et al. Maternal transmission of risk for atherosclerosis. Curr Opin Lipidol 2008;19(4):333–7.
25. Reymer PW, Groenemeyer BE, van de Burg R, et al. Apolipoprotein E genotyping on agarose gels. Clin Chem 1995;41(7):1046–7.
26. Reynolds RM, Allan KM, Raja EA, et al. Maternal obesity during pregnancy and premature mortality from cardiovascular event in adult offspring: follow-up of 1 323 275 person years. BMJ 2013;347:f4539.

27. Hochner H, Friedlander Y, Calderon-Margalit R, et al. Associations of maternal prepregnancy body mass index and gestational weight gain with adult offspring cardiometabolic risk factors: the Jerusalem Perinatal Family Follow-up Study. Circulation 2012;125(11):1381–9.
28. Potter JM, Nestel PJ. The hyperlipidemia of pregnancy in normal and complicated pregnancies. Am J Obstet Gynecol 1979;133(2):165–70.
29. Wiznitzer A, Mayer A, Novack V, et al. Association of lipid levels during gestation with preeclampsia and gestational diabetes mellitus: a population-based study. Am J Obstet Gynecol 2009;201(5):482–8.
30. Hubel CA, Roberts JM, Taylor RN, et al. Lipid peroxidation in pregnancy: new perspectives on preeclampsia. Am J Obstet Gynecol 1989;161(4):1025–34.
31. Palomba S, Falbo A, Chiossi G, et al. Lipid profile in nonobese pregnant women with polycystic ovary syndrome: a prospective controlled clinical study. Steroids 2014;88:36–43.
32. Toescu V, Nuttall SL, Martin U, et al. Changes in plasma lipids and markers of oxidative stress in normal pregnancy and pregnancies complicated by diabetes. Clin Sci (Lond) 2004;106(1):93–8.
33. Cleary KL, Roney K, Costantine M. Challenges of studying drugs in pregnancy for off-label indications: pravastatin for preeclampsia prevention. Semin Perinatol 2014;38(8):523–7.
34. Catov JM, Newman AB, Roberts JM, et al. Preterm delivery and later maternal cardiovascular disease risk. Epidemiology 2007;18(6):733–9.
35. Brown MC, Best KE, Pearce MS, et al. Cardiovascular disease risk in women with pre-eclampsia: systematic review and meta-analysis. Eur J Epidemiol 2013;28(1): 1–19.
36. Nerenberg K, Daskalopoulou SS, Dasgupta K. Gestational diabetes and hypertensive disorders of pregnancy as vascular risk signals: an overview and grading of the evidence. Can J Cardiol 2014;30(7):765–73.
37. Sattar N, Greer IA. Pregnancy complications and maternal cardiovascular risk: opportunities for intervention and screening? BMJ 2002;325(7356):157–60.

Women's Health Considerations for Lipid Management

Robert Wild, MD, MPH, PhD[a],*, Elizabeth A. Weedin, DO[b],
Edward A. Gill, MD, FASE, FAHA, FACC, FACP, FNLA[c]

KEYWORDS

- Women's health • Lipids • Dyslipidemia • Hypertriglyceridemia

KEY POINTS

- Understanding opportunities to reduce dyslipidemia before, during, and after pregnancy has major implications for cardiovascular disease risk prevention for the entire population.
- The best time to screen for dyslipidemia is before pregnancy or in the early antenatal period after pregnancy is diagnosed.
- The differential diagnosis of hypertriglyceridemia in pregnancy is the same as in nonpregnant women with the exception that clinical lipidologists need to be aware of the potential obstetric complications associated with hypertriglyceridemia.
- Dyslipidemia discovered during pregnancy should be treated with diet and exercise intervention, as well as glycemic control if indicated.
- A complete lipid profile assessment during each trimester of pregnancy is recommended.

INTRODUCTION

Although, in general, reducing atherosclerosis and preventing cardiovascular disease (CVD) require the practice and prevention of universal principles common to both genders, the diagnosis and treatment of lipid disorders in women pose unique challenges. Dyslipidemia and sequelae such as atherosclerosis are disease processes that can also affect offspring during a pregnancy and produce long-term comorbidities for both the mother and the child.[1] Acknowledging the principle that lipid awareness is

This article originally appeared in Cardiology Clinics, Volume 33, Issue 2, May 2015.
[a] Section of Reproductive Endocrinology and Infertility, Department of Obstetrics and Gynecology, University of Oklahoma Health Sciences Center, 1100 N Lindsay Ave, Oklahoma City, OK 73104, USA; [b] Section of General Obstetrics and Gynecology, Department of Obstetrics and Gynecology, University of Oklahoma Health Sciences Center, 1100 N Lindsay Ave, Oklahoma City, OK 73104, USA; [c] Division of Cardiology, UW Department of Medicine, Harborview Medical Center Echocardiography, University of Washington School of Medicine, Seattle University, 325 Ninth Avenue, Box 359748, Seattle, WA 98104-2499, USA
* Corresponding author.
E-mail address: robert-wild@ouhsc.edu

critical throughout the life of the individual is paramount for modern clinical lipidologists. This article discusses some unique women's health issues that are important in lipid management because of the epidemic of obesity in society. Practitioners caring for women of reproductive age are in ideally placed to work toward improving atherosclerosis development for the entire population through examining and controlling lipid levels during gestation.[1]

CVD caused by atherosclerosis of the vessel wall is caused by multiple interrelating factors. Some of the factors relate to lifestyle and are modifiable; others are nonmodifiable. In most women, CVD is recognized an average of 10 years later than in their male counterparts, which leads to an inadvertently decreased emphasis on atherosclerosis prevention in women. Given that most women's health care is practiced by primary care physicians, clinical lipidologists must have a working knowledge of issues important for managing dyslipidemia for women. Recognition of high-risk areas and how lipids are affected by major reproductive issues affecting women's health should be areas of high priority for these physicians.

Understanding opportunities to reduce dyslipidemia before, during, and after pregnancy all have major implication for CVD risk prevention for the entire population. Understanding how contraceptive and hormone choices affect clinical lipid management for women is also essential.

DETECTION, MANAGEMENT, AND TREATMENT OF DYSLIPIDEMIA IN PREGNANCY
Lipid Values in Normal and Abnormal Pregnancies

Fig. 1 shows the average circulating values of total cholesterol, low-density lipoprotein cholesterol (LDL-C), high-density lipoprotein cholesterol (HDL-C), and triglycerides (TG) measured in normal women followed before, during, and after pregnancy in a large cohort of women proceeding through normal pregnancy and delivery. Most of the women are of young reproductive age and as such their values before pregnancy are in the normal range for nonpregnant women. Clinical lipidologists need to

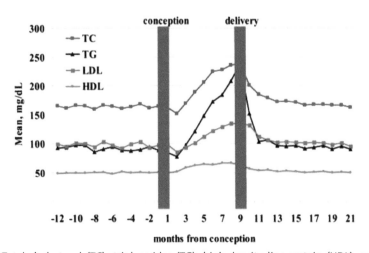

Fig. 1. Total cholesterol (TC), triglycerides (TG), high-density lipoprotein (HDL), and low-density lipoprotein (LDL) 1 year before, during, and after pregnancy. (*From* Wiznitzer A, Mayer A, Novack V, et al. Association of lipid levels during gestation with preeclampsia and gestational diabetes mellitus: a population-based study. Am J Obstet Gynecol 2009;201(5):482.e1–8; with permission.)

understand the pattern throughout pregnancy. Note that in the first trimester, depicted as months since conception, early in gestation there is a noticeable decrease in levels in the first 6 weeks and then a noticeable increase easily discerned by the third month or the end of the first trimester. There begins a steady increase throughout pregnancy in the major lipoprotein lipids. By the third trimester of pregnancy, levels peak to maximize near term.[2] Lipid metabolism favors proper fuel for the fetus and the natural increase reflects the increasing insulin resistance for the mother as pregnancy progresses through term. Also note that the values noted here do not exceed 250 mg/dL at any time during pregnancy.

Contrast the sequential average fasting lipid and lipoproteins measured in the different population shown in **Fig. 2**.

Fig. 2 shows the increase in mean lipid levels referred to in **Fig. 1**; however, these measurements also include persons who have complicated pregnancies. Also displayed are the values of triglycerides and total cholesterol seen increasing to term as well; however, average values exceed 300 mg/dL.[3] There is a significant increase in triglyceride content in all circulating lipoprotein fractions in pregnancy.[4]

Assessment of normal values should include specifics of the relevant trimester of pregnancy. When values exceed 250 mg/dL this should alert the clinical lipidologist that an abnormal or complicated pregnancy is underway.

Fig. 3 shows first trimester maternal triglyceride relationships.

Triglyceride levels exceeding 250 mg/dL during pregnancy are associated with complications of pregnancy-induced hypertension, preeclampsia, gestational diabetes, and large-for-gestational-age babies.[5]

Optimum Strategies for Detection and Treatment of Dyslipidemia in Pregnancy

Many women have significant undiscovered dyslipidemia before pregnancy. The dyslipidemia is often associated with conditions that make them at risk for obstetric and fetal complications should they become pregnant. Uncontrolled diabetes mellitus, polycystic ovarian syndrome (PCOS), and genetic lipid disorders can all be associated

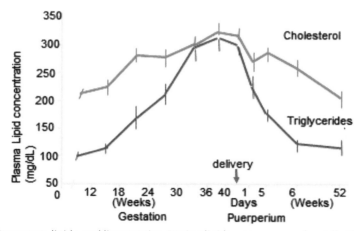

Fig. 2. Pregnancy, lipids, and lipoproteins. Fasting lipids were measured serially throughout pregnancy, at delivery, and in the puerperium and at 12 months. Results are ± standard error of the mean and include normal and complicated pregnancies. (*Adapted from* Potter JM, Nestel PJ. The hyperlipidemia of pregnancy in normal and complicated pregnancies. Am J Obstet Gynecol 1979;133(2):165–70; with permission.)

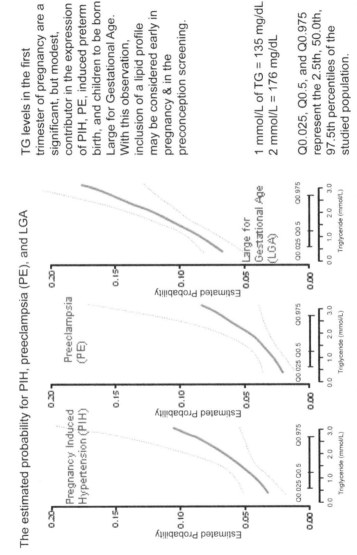

The estimated probability for PIH, preeclampsia (PE), and LGA

TG levels in the first trimester of pregnancy are a significant, but modest, contributor in the expression of PIH, PE, induced preterm birth, and children to be born Large for Gestational Age. With this observation, inclusion of a lipid profile may be considered early in pregnancy & in the preconception screening.

1 mmol/L of TG = 135 mg/dL
2 mmol/L = 176 mg/dL

Q0.025, Q0.5, and Q0.975 represent the 2.5th, 50.0th, 97.5th percentiles of the studied population.

Fig. 3. First trimester maternal triglyceride relationships. (*Adapted from* Vrijkotte TG, Krukziener N, Hutten BA, et al. Maternal lipid profile during early pregnancy and pregnancy complications and outcomes: the ABCD study. J Clin Endocrinol Metab 2012;97(11):3917–25.)

with problems for the mother, for the child, and for possible future generations should she conceive. In recent surveys, about one-third of women presenting to obstetrics and Gynecology practices had CVD risk factors that should be diagnosed and reversed if possible. Familial hyperlipidemia (FH) is more common than any of the genetic diseases that are routinely screened for in pregnancy[6] but there are currently no obstetric recommendations in place to screen for FH. Severe hypertriglyceridemia is sometimes encountered because of genetic or acquired conditions. Ultimately, pregnancy can serve as a cardiometabolic stress test for some individuals. Maternal and fetal complications can be affected by proper screening and management and taking a detailed metabolic/pregnancy history can provide insight as to the cardiometabolic future risk of mother and child.

The best time to screen for dyslipidemia is before pregnancy or in the early antenatal period after pregnancy is diagnosed. Screening should be performed routinely after the pregnancy is concluded, usually at a minimum by the 6-week routine postpartum visit. Women who experience complications of pregnancy or who gain excessive weight before or during pregnancy are more like to have abnormal cardiometabolic profiles.[7] In patients whose primary provider changes based on development of pregnancy-related complications, continuity and attention to long-term assessment of hyperlipidemia during the puerperal period and beyond is prudent. This potential factor alone can contribute to lack of continuity in proper screening, detection, and management of dyslipidemia in the long term.

Differential Diagnosis and Evaluation of Hypertriglyceridemia in Pregnancy

The differential diagnosis of hypertriglyceridemia in pregnancy is the same as in a nonpregnant woman with the exception that clinical lipidologists need to be aware of the potential obstetric complications associated with hypertriglyceridemia. Evaluation of hypertriglyceridemia in women preparing for pregnancy or in pregnant women is not different from that in nonpregnant women, with the realization that a 2-fold to 3-fold triglyceride level increase by the third trimester is expected. Furthermore, women with gestational diabetes and preeclampsia often have abnormal triglyceride levels greater than and additive to hypertriglyceridemia associated with obesity before pregnancy. Average values in persons with these disorders exceed 300 mg/dL and levels escalate as pregnancy progresses. What is considered abnormal depends on the trimester in which the triglycerides are measured, with the maximum values usually seen at term. The most common reason for hypertriglyceridemia is poorly controlled or undiscovered diabetes mellitus. Common nondiabetic reasons for increased triglyceride levels are medications that aggravate triglyceride metabolism, particular psychiatric and/or human immunodeficiency virus medications, illicit drugs, and/or alcohol. Hypothyroidism and/or genetic dyslipidemias can also initially be uncovered during pregnancy. Each woman with hypertriglyceridemia needs a careful analysis of family history for hypertriglyceridemia, pancreatitis, diabetes, hypertension, smoking status, cardiometabolic disease, illicit drugs, or lifestyle issues (including carbohydrate and alcohol intake), as well as use of prescription medicines and supplements. Glycemic, thyroid, hepatic, and renal evaluations are also indicated in this scenario.

Treatment and Monitoring of Dyslipidemia Associated with Pregnancy

For women with the diagnosis of dyslipidemia before pregnancy, any lipid level–lowering medications aside from bile acid sequestrates and omega-3 fatty acids should be stopped. Recommendations for stopping statins range from 3 months to 1 month before conception. These recommendations are based on expert opinion alone, without definitive evidence. At present, there are 2 ongoing randomized clinical trials to determine whether hydrophilic statins can reduce preeclampsia in pregnancy. Despite this, because of animal data showing that very large doses of lipophilic statins caused birth defects, the US Food and Drug Administration (FDA) has categorized stains as category X. **Box 1** shows the current FDA classification system for medication use in pregnancy. All medication recommendations aside, it is always important to emphasize proper diet and exercise in the given patient scenario.

Even when a medication is labeled as class D, the FDA does not prohibit use but is pointing out that potential benefits may warrant use of the drug in pregnant women despite the risks.

Table 1 provides the pregnancy classification of widely used lipid level–lowering agents.

Dyslipidemia discovered during pregnancy should be treated with diet and exercise intervention, as well as glycemic control if indicated. Diabetes types I and II during pregnancy can be associated with hypertriglyceridemia. Essential to managing the

---

Box 1
FDA pregnancy drug classifications

Category A

Adequate and well-controlled studies have failed to show a risk to the fetus in the first trimester of pregnancy and there is no evidence of risk in later trimesters.

Examples of drugs or substances: levothyroxine, folic acid, magnesium sulfate, liothyronine.

Category B

Animal reproduction studies have failed to show a risk to the fetus and there are no adequate and well-controlled studies in pregnant women.

Examples of drugs: metformin, hydrochlorothiazide, cyclobenzaprine, amoxicillin, pantoprazole.

Category C

Animal reproduction studies have shown an adverse effect on the fetus and there are no adequate and well-controlled studies in humans, but potential benefits may warrant use of the drug in pregnant women despite potential risks.

Examples of drugs: tramadol, gabapentin, amlodipine, trazodone, prednisone.

Category D

There is positive evidence of human fetal risk based on adverse reaction data from investigational or marketing experience or studies in humans, but potential benefits may warrant use of the drug in pregnant women despite potential risks.

Examples of drugs: lisinopril, alprazolam, losartan, clonazepam, lorazepam.

Category X

Studies in animals or humans have shown fetal abnormalities and/or there is positive evidence of human fetal risk based on adverse reaction data from investigational or marketing experience, and the risks involved in use of the drug in pregnant women clearly outweigh potential benefits.

Examples of drugs: atorvastatin, simvastatin, warfarin, methotrexate, finasteride.

Category N

FDA has not classified the drug.

Examples of drugs: aspirin, oxycodone, hydroxyzine, acetaminophen, diazepam.

Table 1	
Lipid level–lowering agents and pregnancy classification	
Lipid Level–lowering Agent	Pregnancy Class
Statins	X
Fibrates	C
Ezetimibe	C
Niacin	C
Cholestyramine	C
Colesevelam	B
Mipomersen	B

triglyceride level increases is first to control the diabetes. Common agents used are glyburide and metformin as well as insulin to control blood glucose. Routine glucose screening is an essential component of obstetric care. Hypercholesterolemia can be treated with bile acid sequestrates, notably colesevelam, which is preferred because it is category B.

Severe hypertriglyceridemia (including at levels associated with pancreatitis) can be treated with omega-3 fatty acids, parenteral nutrition, plasmapheresis, or historically with gemfibrozil in the mid to late trimesters (class C medication).[8] It is recommended that lipids be monitored every trimester or within 6 weeks of an intervention to evaluate for compliance, response, and adjustment if needed. Close postpartum follow-up of mothers and children with FH or dysmetabolic issues of pregnancy is required. States of severe hypertriglyceridemia, hypertension of pregnancy, preeclampsia, gestational diabetes, and/or albuminuria need to be evaluated for residual cardiometabolic risk.

Familial Hyperlipidemia Monitoring and Treatment

A complete lipid profile assessment during each trimester of pregnancy is recommended. For women with FH, following brain natriuretic peptide, or B-type natriuretic peptide, as a useful monitor for potential coronary ischemia has been suggested.[9] FH can be treated with lifestyle interventions, bile acid sequestrants (preferably colesevelam, as noted earlier), with monitoring of potential triglyceride level increase in response. If adequate control is not obtained with these regimens, mipomersen (class B medication) and/or low-density lipoprotein (LDL) apheresis may be necessary.[10] Given the complex nature of treatment in such cases, patients with FH are best followed in tertiary care centers with experience in treating these disorders.

Recommendations for Women with Dyslipidemia Who Are Breastfeeding

Diet and exercise are indicated and tailored to the specific patient scenario. Nutritional consultation is advised. Patients with FH may receive bile acid sequestrates. Lactation may attenuate unfavorable metabolic risk factor changes that occur with pregnancy, with effects apparent after weaning. As a modifiable behavior, lactation may affect women's future risk of cardiovascular and metabolic diseases.[11] For disorders with high triglyceride levels it is advisable to avoid estrogenic oral contraception even with late breastfeeding. However, breastfeeding does not guarantee lactational anovulation and thereby contraception. Approximately 1 in 3 women ovulate during prolonged breast feeding, highlighting the need to advise patients regarding the best contraceptives despite breastfeeding.

LONG-TERM IMPLICATIONS OF COMPLICATIONS IN PREGNANCY

Recent studies indicate that the endothelial dysfunction incurred during preeclampsia pregnancies may increase the risk of CVD later in life.[12] Contributions of dyslipidemia, obesity, the presence of the metabolic syndrome or insulin-resistance states before pregnancy,[12,13] as well as hypertensive disorders of pregnancy also host important future CVD risk scenarios. The accumulated weight gain during pregnancies and the inability to effect adequate weight loss during middle age is a well-known risk factor for CVD.[14,15] The increase in lipid components during pregnancy, notably triglycerides and their metabolically dangerous atherogenic particle metabolites, may not be corrected postpartum. Strategies to control blood pressure are well established in the nonpregnant population, and previous preeclampsia and gestational hypertension should be considered as important historical risk factors for stratification of cardiovascular risk and determining the aggressiveness of therapy. Yet to be determined is whether or not blood pressure control in pregnancy has any identifiable long-term benefit.

Polycystic Ovary Syndrome

PCOS affects 7% to 22% of reproductive-aged women, so an understanding of the diagnosis and therapeutic options for this condition is paramount for lipidologists.[16] Women with PCOS are at increased risk for metabolic syndrome, diabetes mellitus, complications of pregnancy, and endometrial cancer.[13,17] Most individuals with PCOS show insulin resistance, which is intensified by obesity and often the pregnant state, potentially leading to attendant complications. The most common high-risk condition of pregnancy is obesity because it is a foundation for the development of diabetes, preeclampsia, large-for-gestational-age infants, complications of delivery, and neonatal intensive care unit admissions. In addition, women with PCOS are at greater risk for obstetric complications irrespective of whether or not they have developed overt metabolic syndrome.[13]

The most widely used criteria to diagnose PCOS are the Rotterdam criteria, as shown in **Table 2**. However, different criteria have evolved in attempts to capture

Table 2 Criteria recognized to diagnose PCOS			
	Diagnostic Criteria of PCOS		
Criteria	NIH 1990 Classic	Rotterdam 2003	Androgen Excess PCOS
Oligomenorrhea[a]	+	+/−	+/−
Clinical or biochemical hyperandrogenism[b]	+	+/−	+/−
Polycystic ovaries on ultrasonography[c]	+/−	+/−	+/−

NIH criteria include both oligomenorrhea and clinical/biochemical hyperandrogenism; Rotterdam criteria include any 2 of the Androgen Excess and Polycystic Ovarian Syndrome Society criteria, presence of clinical/biochemical hyperandrogenism, and 1 other criterion.
[a] Eight or fewer menses per year.
[b] Acne, or hirsutism, or androgenic alopecia.
[c] Ovarian volume greater than 10 mL and/or greater than 12 follicles less than 9 mm in at least 1 ovary.
Adapted from Wild RA, Carmina E, Diamanti-Kandarakis E, et al. Assessment of cardiovascular risk and prevention of cardiovascular disease in women with the polycystic ovary syndrome: a consensus statement by the Androgen Excess and Polycystic Ovary Syndrome (AE-PCOS) Society. J Clin Endocrinol Metab 2010;95(5):2038–49.

the heterogeneous nature of the condition. The term PCOS originates from the characteristic morphology of the ovary (polycystic ovary), which is derived from the ultrasonographic pathognomonic string-of-pearls sign. This sign results from multiple follicles suspended in similar stages of development. The follicles most often are seen around the periphery as they surround a very endocrinologically active, androgen-secreting inner stroma (**Fig. 4**).

The criteria are based on the presence of at least 2 of the following: androgen excess (clinically in the form of hirsutism, acne, and/or androgenic alopecia, or measured in the blood), ovulatory dysfunction, or the presence of polycystic ovaries (usually assessed by vaginal ultrasonography). The Androgen Excess Society insists that some form of androgen excess is necessary for the diagnosis. The spectrum of the condition can include persons mildly affected to severely affected with androgen excess bordering on severe virilization.

Women with PCOS frequently develop dyslipidemia and/or metabolic syndrome at any age, including at the onset of menses and continuing throughout the adolescent years. Diagnosing PCOS can be difficult at times of physiologic oligomenorrhea commonly observed around menarche as well as menopausal transition. Diagnosing PCOS can be difficult at times of physiologic oligomenorrhea commonly observed around menarche as well as menopausal transition.

SCREENING FOR ASSOCIATED DYSLIPIDEMIA IN POLYCYSTIC OVARIAN SYNDROME

We recommend that all patients with PCOS, regardless of age, should undergo lipid and diabetes screening given the increased prevalence of dyslipidemia and insulin resistance in this population.[18] We also recommend increased frequency of

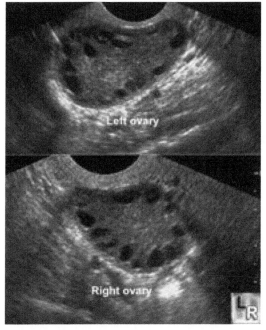

Fig. 4. Characteristic ovarian morphology of PCOS revealing the source of the name for the syndrome.

monitoring for such clinical changes compared with the general population even if initial values are normal because risk of developing these conditions increases with age. Two-year screening intervals have been suggested by some experts. Given that normalizing dyslipidemia and glucose intolerance can reduce atherogenesis, clinical lipidologists need to be familiar with the principles of management for such conditions throughout the reproductive period. We recommend similar, if not tighter, lipid level goals in dyslipidemia as those used in metabolic syndrome. The Androgen Excess Society consensus document recommends the target values shown in **Table 3** in lipid management of women with PCOS.

TREATMENT OF DYSLIPIDEMIA IN POLYCYSTIC OVARIAN SYNDROME

Diet and exercise are the foundation of intervention. Use of medication to control lipids has special considerations for women with PCOS. Therapy should be focused on reversing all components of the metabolic syndrome through diet, exercise, and medication only if needed.[19] In general, metformin is widely used because of low cost, long-term safety data, and low side effect profile. Unlike the glitazones, metformin is not associated with weight gain or fluid retention and this feature alone leads to wide acceptance. It is often used for its weight loss properties; however, it is not a successful medication for acute weight loss or for reduction of hirsutism. Although diet and exercise have been shown to be superior to metformin in reducing the onset of diabetes,[19] metformin is often used because of ease of improved compliance with the initially once-daily dosing. This dosing profile assists with avoidance of gastrointestinal side effects. In addition, glitazones and metformin are associated with improved ovulation, which may or may not be useful depending on the setting. Ovulation is more likely monofollicular with these agents in women with PCOS, although these medications are not first-line therapy for ovulation induction in women with

Table 3 PCOS risk categories and lipid target values			
	Risk	LDL Target Values; mg/dL (mmol/L)[a]	Non-HDL Target Values; mg/dL (mmol/L)[a]
PCOS	At optimal	≤130 (3.37)	≤160 (4.14)
PCOS (obesity, hypertension, dyslipidemia, cigarette smoking, IGT, subvascular disease	At risk	≤130 (3.37)	≤160 (4.14)
PCOS with MetS	High risk	≤100 (2.59)	≤130 (3.37)
PCOS[b] with MetS and T2DM, overt renal disease, or other vascular disease	—	≤70 (1.81)	≤100 (2.59)

Values are based on 12 h fast.
Abbreviations: IGT, impaired glucose tolerance; MetS, metabolic syndrome; T2DM, type 2 diabetes mellitus.
[a] To convert mg/dL to mmol/L, divide by 39.
[b] Odds for CVD increase with number of MetS components and with other risk factors, smoking, poor diet, inactivity, obesity, family history of premature CVD (men <55 years old or women <65 years old), and subclinical vascular disease.
Adapted from Wild RA, Carmina E, Diamanti-Kandarakis E, et al. Assessment of cardiovascular risk and prevention of cardiovascular disease in women with the polycystic ovary syndrome: a consensus statement by the Androgen Excess and Polycystic Ovary Syndrome (AE-PCOS) Society. J Clin Endocrinol Metab 2010;95(5);2038–49.

PCOS who desire pregnancy. Alternatively, because of improved reproductive function states with these medicines and associated risk of pregnancy in women who require contraception, this fact should always be considered by the primary care provider. As alluded to earlier, glitazones and metformin improve insulin resistance and menstrual irregularity, but they are not first-line agents to enhance fertility.[20]

Of the numerous diet interventions available, Heart Healthy, Mediterranean, and the Dietary Approaches to Stop Hypertension (DASH) diets have shown short-term improved lipid and other biomarker effects for women with PCOS.[21] High-carbohydrate diets tend to aggravate insulin resistance and severely restricting low-carbohydrate diets acutely offer weight loss; however, this is not sustainable with long-term lipid reduction and normalization. Weight loss should be targeted in all overweight women with PCOS through reducing caloric intake in the setting of adequate nutritional intake and healthy food choices, irrespective of diet composition.[22]

Statins are used in women with PCOS to treat their metabolic syndrome as well as to reduce testosterone and androstenedione levels. Statins reduce LDL-C and non–HDL-C levels in women with PCOS. In a high alpha and beta short-term clinical trial, atorvastatin therapy improved chronic inflammation and lipid profile and also reduced the testosterone level in women with PCOS. However, it has also been found to impair insulin sensitivity. Because women with PCOS have an increased risk of developing type 2 diabetes mellitus, the results suggest that statin therapy should be initiated from generally accepted criteria and individual risk assessment of CVD, and not solely in the setting of a PCOS diagnosis.[23] Another challenge with statin use is the pregnancy categorization of X. Although the reliability of the data behind this X recommendation has recently been questioned, the potential teratogenic risk of statin use in women who are pregnant or who are at risk of becoming pregnant must be clearly explained to any person of reproductive age.[24] Reliable forms of contraception and avoidance of statin use in a person who is pregnant are prudent. However, rosuvastatin and pravastatin are water soluble and thus these agents have been suggested to be less likely to cause teratogenic effects. Ongoing multicenter clinical trials are assessing whether such water-soluble statins can reduce preeclampsia when given in the midtrimester of pregnancy. In addition, stains can be useful in treating fatty liver, which is common in women with PCOS who have the metabolic syndrome.[25]

When effectiveness alone is considered, other lipid level–lowering medications have been used successfully in women with PCOS as well. However, given the predominance of women in the reproductive age range when PCOS is diagnosed, teratogenic risks in the scenario of unplanned pregnancy must be acknowledged, which limits the selection of lipid level–lowering agents. This acknowledgment also highlights the importance of contraceptive counseling.

DYSLIPIDEMIA TREATMENT AND UNIQUE CHALLENGES FOR WOMEN WITH POLYCYSTIC OVARIAN SYNDROME

Therapy for PCOS is complex given the multiorigin cause of the syndrome as well as differing patient concerns. In general, areas to consider are cosmetic (considerations to reduce unwanted hair growth), menstrual regulation (to improve fertility and/or to reduce endometrial cancer risk), as well as metabolic (to control or to prevent diabetes and associated atherogenesis and CVD).

The standard medication used to control menses, to reduce endometrial and ovarian cancer risk, and to reduce hirsutism is the combined oral contraceptive (COC). Acne can accompany the androgen excess, although the true cause is multifactorial, which can also be improved by COC use. In general, the more estrogenic an oral contraceptive compound, the more effective the hirsutism control that will be obtained. In addition, spironolactone is used concomitantly, primarily because of its ability to reduce 5-alpha reductase, the primary enzyme responsible for converting circulating testosterone into the more potent, locally active metabolite, dihydrotestosterone. The topic of contraceptive counseling is also important to review given that 5-alpha reductase inhibitors can cross the placenta and cause ambiguous genitalia in the newborn if used during pregnancy.

Endometrial hyperplasia and ultimately cancer can occur as a result of years of unopposed estrogen. This cycle can begin as early as the teen years in adolescents with PCOS. Given this, the use of oral contraceptives has to be weighed for its contraceptive benefits as well as its cancer prevention abilities even in the adolescent population. The major risk associated with COC use is thrombotic risk and combined oral contraceptives should not be used in women 35 years or older who smoke because of additive stroke and heart attack risk.

In general, the dyslipidemia associated with PCOS reflects the effects of insulin resistance. However, there are other consequences of insulin resistance. The androgen excess seems to occur from effects of insulin on the ovary and/or adrenal glands. Concomitantly, the HDL-C level is often reduced, triglyceride production increases, and circulating atherogenic small LDL particles increase, all of which are further aggravated when women with PCOS become obese. Depending on which COC is chosen for which clinical manifestation of PCOS, triglyceride levels may increase, HDL-C levels may increase, and LDL-C levels may decrease when COCs are given to women with PCOS who have associated dyslipidemia.

Rarely, a genetic lipid disorder is uncovered when screening for dyslipidemia in women with PCOS. Very high triglyceride levels (ie, >500 mg/dL) are rarely caused by PCOS. Using an oral contraceptive can further aggravate hypertriglyceridemia of this magnitude and can precipitate pancreatitis.

Treatment considerations should include sensitivity to all 3 foci of patient concern. Clinical lipidologists need to understand that the choices for lipid control beyond heart-healthy diets and exercise advice depend on all of these considerations.

Contraception

As outlined earlier, the best time to detect and treat dyslipidemia as it relates to pregnancy is before conception. Understanding the effects of pregnancy on a woman who is or becomes dyslipidemic during pregnancy is relevant for considerations for contraception because family planning in the long run is the best way to optimize pregnancy and maternal outcomes. Avoiding closely timed pregnancies is important to allow return of the body to its baseline metabolic state without prolonged periods of stress-induced hyperlipidemia. Clinical lipidologists need insight into the effects of contraceptive types on lipid metabolism and the effects of lipid management on contraceptive choice, keeping in mind the risk of pregnancy if contraception is not used.

Most surveys show that approximately 50% of pregnancies are unexpected or unwanted.[26] Contraceptive education is important for prevention and the choice of contraceptive method has implications for lipid management. No contraceptive method fits everyone. Each method may have an impact on lipid metabolism and resultant factors relevant to lipid management. The risk of complications associated with pregnancy given the contraceptive choice made include its efficacy in preventing pregnancy (which most often carries greater risk to the mother if the contraceptive is not used or fails) as well as the cardiometabolic impact of the method chosen.

Screening for lipid levels must be kept up to date according to childhood, adolescent, and adult guidelines for population screening (see the National Lipid Association guidelines). Special thought must be used to identify persons with FH, hypertriglyceridemia, or rare genetic forms of hyperlipidemia on routine screening and/or family history. A detailed metabolic/pregnancy history provides insight as to the cardiometabolic future risk of the mother and her children.

LIPID CHANGES WITH DIFFERENT FORMS OF CONTRACEPTION
Combined Oral Contraceptives

In order to effect contraception through ovulation inhibition while concomitantly reducing cardiovascular side effects such as myocardial infarction or cardiovascular accident from sex steroids, various formulations of COC have been developed over the years. First-generation COCs were developed exclusively to avoid pregnancy. If used properly, they were effective at pregnancy prevention. Both minor and major side effects were discovered predominantly through population studies. If used perfectly, the first-generation COCs are 99.9% effective in preventing pregnancy, but they are associated with greater risk of thrombotic events. However, when sex steroid content is reduced, efficacy for preventing pregnancy is reduced either through a lower threshold of ovulation inhibition when used perfectly or through the usual use issues with compliance.

Second-generation COCs were primarily designed to reduce heavy or abnormal menstrual bleeding, which is a significant issue for many women. The increased androgen content in second-generation COCs allows improved bleeding control. However, androgenic side effects lead to worse compliance, usually because of side effects such as acne, hair growth, or perceived weight gain. Complaints among women regarding these side effects prompted the creation of third-generations COCs, which are slightly less androgenic.

COCs have multiple tissue effects, including estrogenic, progestational, androgenic, antiestrogenic, and antiandrogenic effects. All forms reduce risk for endometrial and ovarian cancers. The major risk associated with all COCs is thromboembolic disease. Women with various medical comorbidities, older age, and tobacco users are at increased risk for the cardiovascular events. There are 2 types of estrogen (ethinyl-estradiol and mestranol) used in the United States. Various doses of estrogen within COCs are available. Higher doses carry greater risk of thromboembolic events. Few 50-μg estrogen-containing pills are available on the market today for this reason. At present, most COCs contain 35-μg of ethinyl-estradiol or less and there are multiple types of progestins used in the COCs that are marketed today.

The estrogenic effect of COCs increases levels of TGs and HDL-C, and lowers levels of LDL-C. Androgenic progestins (such as norgestrel and levonorgestrel) can increase LDL-C levels and reduce HDL-C levels. The progestational effect is lipid neutral. For example, desogestrel, a third-generation COC that uses low-dose norethindrone, reduces LDL-C levels and increases HDL-C levels. In addition, the more overall estrogenic a COC is, the more it seems to increase triglyceride and high-density lipoprotein (HDL) levels. This effect carries a greater risk of precipitating pancreatitis in scenarios in which baseline triglyceride levels are increased and increase further with estrogenic COC use. However, transdermal or vaginal combination contraceptives (estrogenic plus progestin) do not reduce the risk of a thrombotic event compared with COCs.

There are several medical conditions that require a thorough evaluation of risks, benefits, and alternatives in choosing a contraceptive agent. One example of such a condition is factor V Leiden thrombophilia, an inheritable hypercoagulable state. Detailing each of these conditions is beyond the scope of this article. For each condition of interest the reader is encouraged to access the US Centers for Disease Control and Prevention compendium for medical conditions, which provides recommendations for contraceptive choice for specific comorbidities. **Box 2** shows an example of a recommendation.

NON–COMBINED ORAL CONTRACEPTIVE METHODS
Intrauterine Devices

Use of a contraceptive should always include a discussion of risks, benefits, and alternatives, as well as a clear review of proper use. Persons with known hyperlipidemia can be given a progestin-impregnated intrauterine device (IUD) (level 2 recommendation). Less overall bleeding is noted with this method, but breakthrough bleeding is commonly observed. A nonhormonal option is the copper IUD, which can be used for up to 10 years per device. Although this is a lipid-neutral option, most women complain of increased menstrual bleeding with the device.

Progestin Only

Implantable or injectable progestins are widely used, especially for persons at risk of noncompliance. In general, progestin-only methods are lipid neutral. There is some evidence that injectable Provera is associated with weight gain. Persons at risk for weight gain (eg, persons with PCOS) seem to be at greater risk for this adverse effect. Weight gain is associated with creating or aggravating a current metabolic syndrome with associated risk of diabetes and mixed dyslipidemia. Despite this, implantable and injectable progestin forms of contraception are extremely efficacious for preventing pregnancy. Progestin-only oral contraceptives are available and are often used when estrogenic preparations are contraindicated or when the risk/benefit ratio is a concern with a COC. However, progestin-only formulations are associated with increased breakthrough bleeding and are of decreased contraceptive efficacy.

Permanent Sterilization

Male and female permanent sterilization procedures are widely used and highly effective forms of contraception. Although nonhormonal and thus lipid neutral, permanent sterilization can unfortunately lead to loss of general-care follow-up as patients are no longer seeking medical care for pregnancy. As primary care providers offering such contraceptive options, it is prudent to recognize the importance of continuing screening for CVD risk factors.

Box 2
Classification for clinical recommendations for intrauterine device use are provided in a Likert scale; this scale can be modified for ease of use

1. A condition for which there is no restriction for use.

2. A condition for which advantages of using the method usually outweigh the theoretic or proven risk.

3. A condition for which the theoretic risk or proven risks usually outweigh the advantages of using the method.

4. A condition posing an unacceptable health risk if the method is used.

MENOPAUSE TRANSITION
Lipid Changes During Menopause

With the onset of waning of ovarian function, lipid changes are noticeable on both a population and an individual basis. The changes tend to occur primarily during the later phases of menopause transition. The magnitude of change toward dyslipidemia is similar to the changes that occur with aging. The relative odds of having an LDL-C level of 130 mg/dL before to after menopause has been reported to be 2.1 (confidence interval [CI], 1.5–2.9).[27]

The changes that occur are presumably related to declining ovarian estradiol production as follicles diminish and secrete less estradiol. Changes in body fat distribution are also observed during this transitional time.[28] In addition, there is a link to an increased prevalence of metabolic syndrome.[29] With expert treatment, it has been shown that carotid atherosclerosis is observed more frequently beginning in the menopause transition, and a significant number of women also possess coronary calcium deposition before this.[30,31]

The absolute risk for CVD increases substantially in midlife for women. Rates associated with a particular adverse effect on lipid metabolism increase at the time of menopause. Those persons with significant risk factors before menopause are additionally affected. It is important for primary care physicians to identify these individuals early to plan for best control of these same risk factors during the menopause transition.[27,32]

Fig. 5 shows natural changes of the major lipid and apolipoprotein lipid levels using cross-sectional panel design analysis as these women transitioned through the menopause years, studied in the multiethnic Study of Women's Health Across the Nation (SWAN) data set. Note that levels are assessed and measured as annual mean data comparing years before and after the final menstrual period. Menopause is defined in retrospect as 1 year with nonmenses during this transition. Day 0 in the graphs is labeled and standardized as the final menstrual period. Importantly, apolipoprotein (Apo) B levels increase noticeably.

Annual rates of change in carotid intima-media thickness and adventitial diameter have been reported, as noted in **Fig. 6**. The rate of change at the late perimenopausal stage significantly differs from that at the premenopausal stage. The rate of change at the late perimenopausal stage significantly differs from that at the early perimenopausal stage. The rate of change at the postmenopausal stage significantly differs from that at the premenopausal stage ($P<.05$).

CURRENT RECOMMENDATIONS FOR HORMONE THERAPY

Menopausal hormone replacement therapy is primarily indicated to control menopause-related quality-of-life issues. Replacement therapy should not be prescribed for cardiovascular purposes (ie, for prevention or treatment of vascular diseases). There is a black box warning by the FDA for women with known coronary artery disease, thromboembolic disorders, or who have had a cerebrovascular accident because these preparations carry thrombotic risk and critical events in persons with these disorders involving thrombotic pathophysiology.

Identifying appropriate candidates for menopausal hormone therapy (HT) is challenging given the complex profile of risks and benefits associated with treatment.[33] Most professional societies agree that HT should not be used for chronic disease prevention.

Recent findings from the Women's Health Initiative and other randomized trials suggest that a woman's age, proximity to menopause, underlying cardiovascular risk

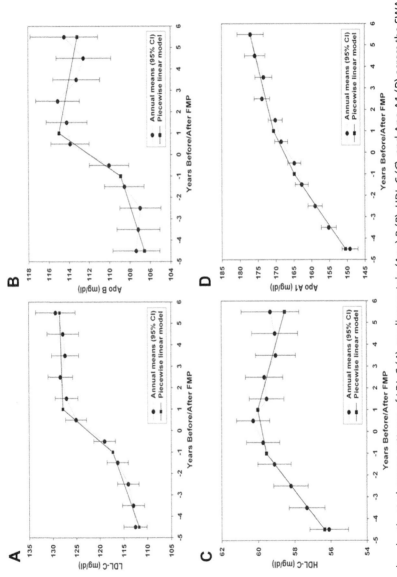

Fig. 5. Lipids annual and estimated means patterns of LDL-C (*A*), apolipoprotein (Apo) B (*B*), HDL-C (*C*), and Apo A1 (*D*) across the SWAN study follow-up period. FMP, final menstrual period. (*From* Matthews KA. Are changes in cardiovascular disease risk factors in midlife women due to chronological aging or to the menopausal transition? J Am Coll Cardiol 2009;54(25):2366–73; with permission.)

A

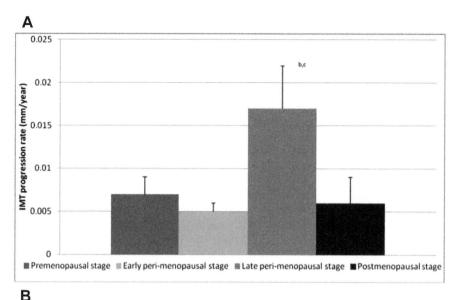

B

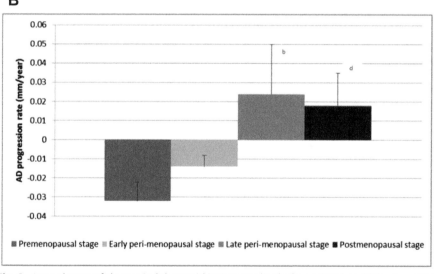

Fig. 6. Annual rates of change in (*A*) carotid intima-media thickness (IMT) and (*B*) adventitial diameter (AD). (*From* El Khoudary SR, Wildman RP, Matthews K, et al. Progression rates of carotid intima-media thickness and adventitial diameter during the menopausal transition. Menopause 2013;20(1):8–14; with permission.)

factor status, and various biological characteristics may modify health outcomes with HT. An emerging body of evidence suggests that it may be possible to assess individual risk and therefore better predict who is likely to have favorable outcomes versus adverse effects when taking HT. Thus, once a woman is identified as a potential candidate for HT for quality-of-life improvement because of moderate to severe menopausal symptoms or other indications, risk stratification may be an important tool for minimizing patient risk.[33]

This individualized approach holds great promise for improving the safety of HT. Patient-centered outcomes including quality of life and sense of well-being should also be incorporated and will directly affect the risk/benefit ratio as well as compliance. Additional research on hormone dose, formulation, and route of delivery will be important for improving this decision model.

Ultimately, a treatment decision to provide symptom relief should be made with a patient's full understanding of potential risks and benefits, and taking into account her personal preferences. To better integrate patient values, practical considerations, and emerging clinical experience, recent research from observational studies and randomized clinical trials on HT should be considered. Note the results from an analysis of the Women's Health Initiative in which oral estrogen plus progestin and estrogen alone were used in the randomized clinical trial (**Table 4**).

This analysis suggests that persons at higher risk for CVD events (increased dyslipidemia or presence of metabolic syndrome) are more likely to have this risk aggravated by administration of oral hormone replacement therapy. The message is clear: assessing CVD risk before HT is given for menopausal symptoms is prudent to identify persons who may be at increased adverse event risk with oral HT.

There are several biomarkers under study to determine whether they provide incremental risk prediction for CVD in women taking HT. However, thus far none have been shown to provide added risk prediction and currently they are not recommended for clinical use.

Using the lowest effective dose of HT is recommended, regardless of clinical scenario. In general, doses lower than 0.3 mg of oral conjugated estrogen daily do not control hot flashes for most women. However, this dose is protective against bone loss from estrogen deficiency osteopenia.[34] Delivering the medication transdermally may be associated with fewer adverse events than when given by the oral route.[35] Tissue effects may differ depending on whether there is a first-pass hepatic effect, as is the case with oral estrogen.

With vaginal and transdermal preparations there is less effect on clotting factors, lipid metabolism, inflammatory biomarkers, and sex hormone–binding globulin

Table 4
CHD risk in the Women's Health Initiative HT trials (estrogen and progestin and estrogen alone) according to baseline levels of biomarkers

Biomarker P Value for Interaction	Odds Ratio (95% CI) for HT Treatment Effect	P for Interaction
LDL-C (mg/dL)		
<130	0.66 (0.34–1.27)	0.03
≥130		
LDL-C/HDL-C Ratio		
<2.5	0.66 (0.34–1.27)	0.002
≥2.5	1.73 (1.18–2.53)	
Hs-CRP(mg/dL)		
<2.0	1.01 (0.63–1.62)	0.16
≥2.0	1.58 (1.05–2.39)	
MetS	2.26 (1.26–4.07)	0.03
No MetS	0.97 (0.58–1.61)	—

Abbreviation: hs-CRP, high-sensitivity C-reactive protein.
Adapted from Wild RA, Manson JE. Insights from the Women's Health Initiative: individualizing risk assessment for hormone therapy decisions. Semin Reprod Med 2014;32(6):433–37.

synthesis. Differences in dose, route, and formulations, in conjunction with genetic metabolic differences, may lead to different outcomes.

Observational studies, although limited in number, suggest that transdermal delivery may be associated with less risk of venous thromboembolism and stroke than with oral estrogen administration; however, these studies do not prove a cause-effect relationship.[36] Randomized clinical trial evidence is needed to answer this question more definitively.

REFERENCES

1. Palinski W, D'Armiento FP, Witztum JL, et al. Maternal hypercholesterolemia and treatment during pregnancy influence the long-term progression of atherosclerosis in offspring of rabbits. Circ Res 2001;89(11):991–6.
2. Wiznitzer A, Mayer A, Novack V, et al. Association of lipid levels during gestation with preeclampsia and gestational diabetes mellitus: a population-based study. Am J Obstet Gynecol 2009;201(5):482–8.
3. Potter JM, Macdonald WB. Primary type I hyperlipoproteinaemia–a metabolic and family study. Aust N Z J Med 1979;9(6):688–93.
4. Herrera E. Metabolic adaptations in pregnancy and their implications for the availability of substrates to the fetus. Eur J Clin Nutr 2000;54(Suppl 1):S47–51.
5. Vrijkotte TG, Krukziener N, Hutten BA, et al. Maternal lipid profile during early pregnancy and pregnancy complications and outcomes: the ABCD study. J Clin Endocrinol Metab 2012;97(11):3917–25.
6. Nordestgaard BG, Chapman MJ, Humphries SE, et al. Familial hypercholesterolaemia is underdiagnosed and undertreated in the general population: guidance for clinicians to prevent coronary heart disease: consensus statement of the European Atherosclerosis Society. Eur Heart J 2013;34(45): 3478–3490a.
7. Smith GN, Walker MC, Liu A, et al. A history of preeclampsia identifies women who have underlying cardiovascular risk factors. Am J Obstet Gynecol 2009; 200(1):58.e1–8.
8. Goldberg AS, Hegele RA. Severe hypertriglyceridemia in pregnancy. J Clin Endocrinol Metab 2012;97(8):2589–96.
9. Tanous D, Siu SC, Mason J, et al. B-type natriuretic peptide in pregnant women with heart disease. J Am Coll Cardiol 2010;56(15):1247–53.
10. Kusters DM, Homsma SJ, Hutten BA, et al. Dilemmas in treatment of women with familial hypercholesterolaemia during pregnancy. Neth J Med 2010;68(1): 299–303.
11. Zarrati M, Shidfar F, Moradof M, et al. Relationship between breast feeding and obesity in children with low birth weight. Iran Red Crescent Med J 2013;15(8): 676–82.
12. Charlton F, Tooher J, Rye KA, et al. Cardiovascular risk, lipids and pregnancy: preeclampsia and the risk of later life cardiovascular disease. Heart Lung Circ 2014;23(3):203–12.
13. Kjerulff LE, Sanchez-Ramos L, Duffy D. Pregnancy outcomes in women with polycystic ovary syndrome: a metaanalysis. Am J Obstet Gynecol 2011;204(6): 558.e1–6.
14. Gunderson EP. Childbearing and obesity in women: weight before, during, and after pregnancy. Obstet Gynecol Clin North Am 2009;36(2):317–32, ix.
15. Manson JE, Willett WC, Stampfer MJ, et al. Body weight and mortality among women. N Engl J Med 1995;333(11):677–85.

16. Wild RA, Carmina E, Diamanti-Kandarakis E, et al. Assessment of cardiovascular risk and prevention of cardiovascular disease in women with the polycystic ovary syndrome: a consensus statement by the Androgen Excess and Polycystic Ovary Syndrome (AE-PCOS) Society. J Clin Endocrinol Metab 2010;95(5): 2038–49.

17. Barry JA, Azizia MM, Hardiman PJ. Risk of endometrial, ovarian and breast cancer in women with polycystic ovary syndrome: a systematic review and meta-analysis. Hum Reprod Update 2014;20(5):748–58.

18. Moran LJ, Misso ML, Wild RA, et al. Impaired glucose tolerance, type 2 diabetes and metabolic syndrome in polycystic ovary syndrome: a systematic review and meta-analysis. Hum Reprod Update 2010;16(4):347–63.

19. Diabetes Prevention Program Research Group, Knowler WC, Fowler SE, et al. 10-year follow-up of diabetes incidence and weight loss in the Diabetes Prevention Program Outcomes Study. Lancet 2009;374(9702):1677–86.

20. Legro RS, Arslanian SA, Ehrmann DA, et al. Diagnosis and treatment of polycystic ovary syndrome: an Endocrine Society clinical practice guideline. J Clin Endocrinol Metab 2013;98(12):4565–92.

21. Asemi Z, Esmaillzadeh A. DASH diet, insulin resistance, and serum hs-CRP in polycystic ovary syndrome: a randomized controlled clinical trial. Horm Metab Res 2014;47(3):232–8.

22. Moran LJ, Ko H, Misso M, et al. Dietary composition in the treatment of polycystic ovary syndrome: a systematic review to inform evidence-based guidelines. J Acad Nutr Diet 2013;113(4):520–45.

23. Puurunen J, Piltonen T, Puukka K, et al. Statin therapy worsens insulin sensitivity in women with polycystic ovary syndrome (PCOS): a prospective, randomized, double-blind, placebo-controlled study. J Clin Endocrinol Metab 2013;98(12): 4798–807.

24. Zarek J, Koren G. The fetal safety of statins: a systematic review and meta-analysis. J Obstet Gynaecol Can 2014;36(6):506–9.

25. Setji TL, Brown AJ. Polycystic ovary syndrome: update on diagnosis and treatment. Am J Med 2014;127(10):912–9.

26. Sanga K, Mola G, Wattimena J, et al. Unintended pregnancy amongst women attending antenatal clinics at the Port Moresby General Hospital. Aust N Z J Obstet Gynaecol 2014;54(4):360–5.

27. Derby CA, Crawford SL, Pasternak RC, et al. Lipid changes during the menopause transition in relation to age and weight: the Study of Women's Health Across the Nation. Am J Epidemiol 2009;169(11):1352–61.

28. Park JK, Lim YH, Kim KS, et al. Changes in body fat distribution through menopause increase blood pressure independently of total body fat in middle-aged women: the Korean National Health and Nutrition Examination Survey 2007-2010. Hypertens Res 2013;36(5):444–9.

29. Mendes KG, Theodoro H, Rodrigues AD, et al. Prevalence of metabolic syndrome and its components in the menopausal transition: a systematic review. Cad Saude Publica 2012;28(8):1423–37 [in Portuguese].

30. El Khoudary SR, Wildman RP, Matthews K, et al. Progression rates of carotid intima-media thickness and adventitial diameter during the menopausal transition. Menopause 2013;20(1):8–14.

31. Kuller LH, Matthews KA, Sutton-Tyrrell K, et al. Coronary and aortic calcification among women 8 years after menopause and their premenopausal risk factors: the Healthy Women Study. Arterioscler Thromb Vasc Biol 1999;19(9):2189–98.

32. Matthews KA, Gibson CJ, El Khoudary SR, et al. Changes in cardiovascular risk factors by hysterectomy status with and without oophorectomy: Study of Women's Health Across the Nation. J Am Coll Cardiol 2013;62(3):191–200.
33. Wild RA, Manson JE. Insights from the Women's Health Initiative: individualizing risk assessment for hormone therapy decisions. Semin Reprod Med 2014; 32(6):433–7.
34. Mizunuma H, Shiraki M, Shintani M, et al. Randomized trial comparing low-dose hormone replacement therapy and HRT plus 1alpha-OH-vitamin D3 (alfacalcidol) for treatment of postmenopausal bone loss. J Bone Miner Metab 2006;24(1): 11–5.
35. North American Menopause Society. The 2012 hormone therapy position statement of: The North American Menopause Society. Menopause 2012;19(3): 257–71.
36. Canonico M, Oger E, Plu-Bureau G, et al. Hormone therapy and venous thromboembolism among postmenopausal women: impact of the route of estrogen administration and progestogens: the ESTHER study. Circulation 2007;115(7): 840–5.

Dyslipidemia and Cardiovascular Risk in Human Immunodeficiency Virus Infection

Theodoros Kelesidis, MD, PhD, Judith S. Currier, MD, MSc*

KEYWORDS

- Dyslipidemia • Cardiovascular risk • Human immunodeficiency virus
- Antiretroviral therapy

KEY POINTS

- Since the advent of effective antiretroviral therapy, cardiovascular disease has become a major cause of morbidity and mortality in the population with human immunodeficiency virus.
- The pathogenesis of atherosclerosis in human immunodeficiency virus–infected individuals is complex, and proatherogenic quantitative and qualitative changes in lipids have a major role in this process.
- HIV replication, chronic inflammation and immune activation, and exposure to antiretroviral drugs (either directly or through metabolic abnormalities) may contribute to development of dyslipidemia in human immunodeficiency virus infection.
- As we gain a better understanding of lipid abnormalities in human immunodeficiency virus–infected patients and their role in immune activation and cardiovascular disease, these findings must translate into interventions for clinical care.

INTRODUCTION

In the setting of highly active antiretroviral therapy (ART), cardiovascular disease (CVD), particularly coronary artery disease, is among the leading causes of mortality among human immunodeficiency virus (HIV)-infected subjects.[1] Several studies suggest that adults and children with HIV have an increased risk of CVD.[2–4] The full details of the pathogenesis of atherogenesis in HIV infection remain to be elucidated. Traditional risk prediction models to estimate cardiovascular risk do not include emerging

This article originally appeared in Endocrinology and Metabolism Clinics, Volume 43, Issue 3, September 2014.

Disclosures: J.S. Currier: Received grant funds to UCLA from Merck. T. Kelesidis: None.

Division of Infectious Diseases, Department of Medicine, David Geffen School of Medicine, UCLA, 9911 W. Pico Boulevard, Suite 980, Los Angeles, CA 90035, USA

* Corresponding author. Center for Clinical AIDS Research and Education, David Geffen School of Medicine, UCLA, 9911 W. Pico Boulevard, Suite 980, Los Angeles, CA 90035.

E-mail address: jscurrier@mednet.ucla.edu

Clinics Collections 5 (2015) 399–418

http://dx.doi.org/10.1016/j.ccol.2015.05.024

cardiovascular risk factors such as inflammation, coagulation disorders, immune activation, kidney disease, and HIV-1 RNA levels.[4–6] Understanding the pathophysiology of increased CVD in HIV infection will help us develop strategies to prevent and treat this leading cause of morbidity and mortality in HIV-infected subjects.

The prevalence of several traditional risk factors for CVD is higher in HIV-infected individuals than among age-matched controls.[2] Lipid changes may promote atherogenesis and may contribute to increased risk of CVD in HIV-infected subjects.[7] The patterns of dyslipidemia change during the course of HIV disease. In untreated disease, elevations in triglycerides and low high-density lipoprotein cholesterol (HDL-c) predominate. Dyslipidemia that occurs during treatment for HIV disease is characterized by a range of values of serum concentrations of total cholesterol (TC); triglycerides, depending on the ART used; very low-density lipoprotein (VLDL); low-density lipoprotein cholesterol (LDL-c); apolipoprotein B (apoB); and low levels of HDL-c.[7] In view of the high prevalence of dyslipidemia and the increased risk for CVD among patients with HIV, which is concerning for public health, this review aims to describe the changes in the lipid profile of HIV-infected patients and how these changes directly or indirectly contribute to the pathogenesis of atherosclerosis in HIV-infected subjects.[8] Although the exact mechanisms are incompletely understood,[9] we describe how host factors, HIV per se and ART, may contribute to lipid changes and how these atherogenic lipids may have a role in the development of atherosclerosis in HIV-infected patients.

FACTORS OTHER THAN DYSLIPIDEMIA MAY CONTRIBUTE TO ACCELERATED ATHEROSCLEROSIS IN HIV INFECTION

Cardiovascular risk factors have a major role in development of CVD disease. HIV-infected subjects have higher prevalence of established CVD risk factors, such as smoking, hypertension, insulin resistance, and dyslipidemia, compared with age-matched individuals.[9] Cocaine use, which is relatively common among some groups of HIV-infected patients, renal function, and albuminuria have also been associated with the risk for coronary artery disease in HIV-infected patients.[9,10] All of these risk factors are synergistic, and it is difficult to analyze the specific role of each. Recently, the Data Collection on Adverse Events of Anti-HIV Drugs (D:A:D) Study Group developed a risk assessment tool tailored to HIV-infected patients.[11]

HIV replication can directly promote atherogenesis. HIV replication increases chronic inflammation as a part of the immune response to the virus. These changes may, in turn, contribute to an increased risk for death.[4] HIV replication is associated with increased biomarkers of inflammation, including C-reactive protein (CRP). Elevated levels of CRP have been found to independently be associated with the risk of risk of myocardial infarction (MI) in adults, including those with HIV.[4] In HIV infection, high CRP levels predict HIV disease progression.[4] Increased concentrations of CRP, interleukin 6, and d-dimer have also been independently associated with CVD events in patients with HIV.[12] Identifying biomarkers of inflammation and cardiovascular disease in HIV-infected subjects on ART with suppressed viremia may help us develop new targets for therapeutic interventions.[13] The HIV virus can also cause increased endothelial injury caused by adhesion molecules and HIV Tat protein and may stimulate proliferation of vascular smooth muscle cells and induce coagulation disorders.[14] Collectively, these HIV-induced effects may directly increase atherogenesis.

Immune activation may promote atherosclerosis in the absence of residual viral replication. Several studies suggest that increased activation of innate immunity is associated with the presence of subclinical atherosclerosis in patients with HIV.[15–18] One potential mechanism that might trigger monocyte activation in HIV infection is microbial translocation across the gastrointestinal tract, which has been found to persist in treated HIV infection.[4,19] Markers of monocyte activation, such as high soluble CD14 and CD163, and bacterial translocation, such as endotoxin and soluble CD14, were independently associated with a faster rate of progression of subclinical atherosclerosis in several independent studies.[15–18] Collectively, these studies suggest that chronic monocyte activation could be an important marker of or target for future interventions to reduce CVD risk in treated patients with HIV. Further work is needed to determine contributing factors to immune activation and CVD and, importantly, whether atherogenic lipids may drive both immune activation and CVD in HIV infection.

DYSLIPIDEMIA AND CVD IN HIV INFECTION

Host Factors in HIV-Infected Subjects May Contribute to Dyslipidemia Development

HIV-infected subjects have increased prevalence of dyslipidemia; however, it is unclear to what extent this is associated with specific host factors. In the D:A:D study, 33.8% and 22.2% of a group of treated HIV-infected individuals had elevated levels of triglyceride and TC, respectively.[20] Longitudinal and cross-sectional studies have assessed the role of single-nucleotide polymorphisms on the incidence of dyslipidemia in HIV patients.[21] The Multicenter AIDS Cohort Study showed that biogeographical ancestry may contribute to development of ART-induced lipid changes.[22] In a study of the metabolome in HIV-infected patients on suppressive ART, the observed patterns of metabolites suggested decreased lipolysis and dysregulation of receptors controlling inflammation and lipid metabolism.[23] Overall, these data suggest that genetic and nongenetic host factors may contribute to the dyslipidemia in HIV-infected subjects.

The HIV Virus May Directly Induce Dyslipidemia

Mechanisms such as altered cytokine profile, decreased lipid clearance, and increased hepatic synthesis of VLDL, may explain how HIV infection, per se, might induce dyslipidemia and accelerate atherosclerosis based on data from in vitro, animal, and clinical studies.[6,9,24,25] The SMART (Strategies for Management of Antiretroviral Therapy) study compared the outcomes of HIV-infected patients who were randomly assigned to receive continuous or intermittent ART. This study confirmed an increased risk of CVD among patients who discontinued ART[6] and allowed comparison of lipid profiles between the treatment-interruption group and the continuous treatment group.[8] These findings suggested that HIV viremia may have a role in accelerated atherogenesis. More recently, data from a large cohort study of 27,000 HIV-infected adults in care suggested that immunodeficiency and ongoing viral replication both independently contributed to the risk of MI, further confirming the putative role of HIV in the pathogenesis of CVD.[26]

HIV viremia is associated with quantitative lipid abnormalities, including elevated serum concentrations of triglycerides and low levels of cholesterol. Several studies found the associations between uncontrolled HIV viremia and dyslipidemia and increased CVD risk. The impact of HIV infection on lipids was studied within the Multicenter AIDS Cohort Study, in which a significant reduction in TC, LDL, and HDL was found in a group of 50 HIV seroconverters comparing pre-HIV with post-HIV infection lipid levels.[27] In other studies, the levels of triglycerides were higher, and the levels of TC, LDL, and HDL were lower in HIV-infected patients receiving no ART when compared with uninfected controls.[28] Elevations in triglyceride levels during untreated HIV infection are thought to be caused by an increase in the levels of inflammatory cytokines (tumor necrosis factor–α, interleukins, interferon-α)[24] and steroid hormones.[28] HDL levels are also found to be low in both untreated and treated HIV-infected patients, regardless of the CD4+ T cell count.[27] The SMART study found that declines in HDL levels after stopping nonnucleoside reverse transcriptase inhibitor (NNRTI) treatment were associated with an increased risk of CVD, suggesting that the HDL-raising effects of this therapy had been cardioprotective.[29] Enkhmaa and colleagues[30] found that allele-specific apolipoprotein A (apoa) levels, which determine the amount of atherogenic small apoa related to a defined apoa allele size, were higher in individuals with low HIV viremia and high CD4 cell counts, indicating that HIV replication reduced allele-specific apoa levels. Therefore, HIV-infected individuals with immune reconstitution may have higher allele-specific apoa levels, which are related to progression of atherosclerosis.[30] Overall, these data suggest mechanisms that explain how the HIV virus, per se, may induce dyslipidemia.

HIV may induce qualitative changes in lipids such as HDL through effects on metabolism and function that lead to increased atherogenesis. HDL is generally accepted to have anti-inflammatory/antioxidant effects.[31] HIV may directly affect HDL metabolism by up-regulating the cholesteryl ester transfer protein activity, which enhances transfer of cholesterol to apoB lipoproteins that promote atherogenesis.[32] These effects on HDL metabolism in combination with HIV-related hypertriglyceridemia,[25] lead to an increased delivery of cholesterol to the arterial wall, where it is then taken up by macrophages, and atherogenic foam cells are formed. The capacity of HDL to increase cholesterol efflux from macrophages is an important function of HDL and may predict development of atherosclerosis.[33] The HIV Nef protein (which is abundant during untreated HIV) inhibits transporters important to cholesterol efflux in macrophages, and this may initiate atherogenesis in the arterial wall.[34] Intracellular cholesterol in monocytes in HIV-infected subjects is inversely associated with HDL-c levels; in contrast, in HIV-negative controls, cholesterol content in macrophages is correlated with LDL-c levels rather than with HDL-c.[35] In the SMART study, HDL-c, lipoprotein particle concentrations, and the apolipoproteins were better indices of CVD risk than LDL-c levels.[29] Consistent with these data, reduction in large lipoprotein particle concentrations after treatment with ART may indicate increased efflux of cholesterol from macrophages into smaller HDL particles.[8] Thus, HIV induces effects on HDL function and cholesterol transport that may contribute to increased rates of CVD in HIV- infected patients.

HIV replication may also modify HDL indirectly through increases in systemic inflammation. The inflammatory response observed during HIV infection may reduce HDL levels and compromise cholesterol efflux from macrophages.[31] Infections may induce nonspecific systemic inflammation that may at least partially modify HDL.[36] In the SMART trial, levels of biomarkers of inflammation were associated with changes in HDL levels independently of HIV RNA levels.[5,8] Finally, cytokines such as tumor necrosis factor-α and interleukin-6 appear to promote lipid peroxidation, and the production of reactive oxygen species,[37] and this may further contribute to formation of oxidized, modified lipoproteins such as oxidized HDL. However, it is unclear whether HIV-infected subjects have increased levels of oxidized LDL, a marker of oxidative stress associated with lipoproteins and an emerging CVD risk factor,[38] compared with uninfected subjects. The role of modified lipoproteins in CVD in HIV-infected subjects remains incompletely understood.

ART and Dyslipidemia

The introduction of ART led to substantial improvement in the prognosis of HIV patients,[39] but several of the drugs in the first generation of effective combination ART were associated with changes in lipid metabolism, abnormalities in fat (both lipohypertrophy and subcutaneous fat loss), insulin resistance, dyslipidemia, osteopenia, and lactic acidosis.[39] ART-associated dyslipidemia usually occurs within 3 months of starting treatment[9] and was first described in patients who used first-generation protease inhibitors (PIs) but was also observed in patients who received regimens consisting of nucleoside reverse-transcriptase inhibitors (NRTI) and NNRTIs. Studies with HIV-infected children and adolescents and HIV-infected older adults receiving effective ART found high rates of fat changes and dyslipidemia, therefore, high risk for cardiovascular diseases in all age groups of HIV-infected subjects.[9,39] A component of the initial changes in lipids has been ascribed to a return to health among patients with a chronic untreated illness who are undergoing effective treatment.[27]

Several studies investigated the potential effects of ART on risk of CVD and dyslipidemia. The specific effects of ART on dyslipidemia vary both within and across drug classes. Several randomized clinical trials have characterized changes in lipids after the initiation of ART. The AIDS Clinical Trials Group (ACTG) 5142 trial found important differences in metabolic outcomes in treatment-naive patients after the initiation of an NNRTI-sparing regimen (the boosted PI, lopinavir/ritonavir plus 2 NRTIs), PI-sparing regimen (NNRTI efavirenz [EFV] plus 2 NRTIs), or an NRTI-sparing regimen (lopinavir/ritonavir plus EFV).[40] Although the NRTI-sparing regimen (a combination that included lopinavir/ritonavir and EFV) had the lowest risk of lipoatrophy, it also had the greatest likelihood of lipid elevations and subsequent use of lipid-lowering agents. The SMART study helped put these changes into perspective by showing that interrupting therapy through a structured treatment interruption was associated with worse outcomes than remaining on treatment.[6] The D:A:D study, one of the most comprehensive surveys of CVD adverse events associated with ART, found a strong association between dyslipidemia and ART.[11,20] These studies highlighted common (owing to viral suppression) and differential (owing to ART) lipid effects on starting ART in ART-naive HIV-infected patients.

HIV-infected patients on ART have low levels HDL and modified lipoproteins compared with normolipemic subjects. HIV patients with dyslipidemia on ART have impaired plasma lipolytic activity that may lead to low HDL-c plasma concentration and triglyceride-rich LDL and HDL, which become less stable than HDL particles in normolipemic patients.[34] In addition, systemic inflammation may contribute to modification of HDL to a dysfunctional form that may increase the risk of CVD.[41] We previously found that HIV-infected subjects with suppressed viremia on ART have dysfunctional HDL.[42,43] In small study of HIV patients with low CVD risk profile, HDL function changed over time and was independently associated with obesity but not with subclinical atherosclerosis.[44] In another study, HIV-infected subjects had dysfunctional HDL compared with matched uninfected subjects with comparable HDL levels, and this modified HDL was associated with macrophage activation and with presence of noncalcified coronary plaque.[45] The role of HDL function in CVD in HIV-infected subjects with suppressed viremia remains to be determined.

Dyslipidemic effects of PIs

Patients, including children and pregnant women, with prolonged use of PIs often have hypertriglyceridemia, low levels of HDL-c and high levels of LDL-c, and apolipoproteins E and CIII; however, the effects vary by drugs within this class.[9,39] **Fig. 1** summarizes the mechanisms through which PIs may cause dyslipidemia.[46] **Table 1** summarizes the lipid effects of different drugs within the PI class.[20,47–51] Newer agents

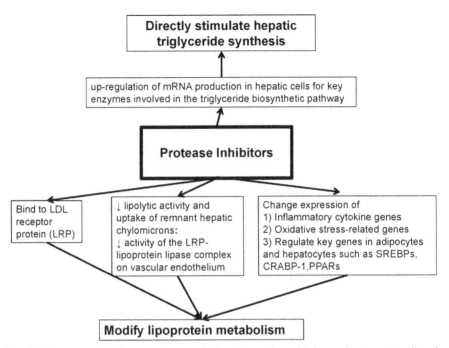

Fig. 1. PIs may modify lipoprotein metabolism through multiple mechanisms. PIs directly stimulate the biosynthesis of triglycerides in hepatic cells and may also directly modify the metabolism of lipoproteins by binding to cellular receptors, reducing lipolysis and by regulating expression of key genes involved in the regulation of metabolic pathways in adipocytes and hepatocytes. CRABP-1, cellular retinoic acid-binding protein 1; LRP, low-density lipoprotein receptor protein; PPARs, peroxisome proliferator-activated receptors; SREBPs, sterol regulatory element-binding proteins.

have less significant effects on lipids than the first drugs to be available within this class.[9,39,46] In the Data Collection on Adverse Events of Anti-HIV Drugs studies, within the PI class only cumulative exposure to lopinavir/ritonavir and indinavir were associated with increased risk of CVD, independently of lipid concentrations.[52] Overall, ritonavir-boosted atazanavir and darunavir have more favorable lipid effects and tolerability compared with other PIs (see **Table 1**). In view of the differences in metabolic effects of drugs within the PI class, future epidemiologic studies examining CVD risk in HIV need to consider the effects of individual PIs.

Dyslipidemic effects of NRTIs
Antiretroviral treatment regimens containing NRTIs have also been associated with metabolic alterations, particularly changes in serum triglyceride concentrations (**Table 2**).[9,39,52–61] Replacement of NRTIs such as stavudine with tenofovir is a strategy to reduce the cardiovascular risk and improve the lipid profile of patients with dyslipidemia.[9,39] Currently, the association between abacavir and excess CVD risk remains controversial. Several studies have found a consistent association[52,57]; however, others have not,[55,56] and the mechanism underlying this association remains unclear.[58] Switching from multidrug class-suppressive regimens to triple therapy containing 2 NRTIs showed increases in plasma lipids.[62] Overall, within the NRTI class, tenofovir and lamivudine/emtricitabine seem to be the drugs that are not associated with dyslipidemia.

Table 1 Main studies investigating the effects of PIs on lipids	
PIs	**Main Findings**
Lopinavir/ritonavir and indinavir	D:A:D study: increased risk of MI with longer duration of treatment compared with other treatments.[20]
Lopinavir/ritonavir and ritonavir-boosted fosamprenavir	The French Hospital Database: increased risk of MI with longer duration of treatment compared with other treatments.
PI-treated patients switched to atazanavir-containing regimens	Several randomized trials: improvement of lipid parameters, while the immunologic and virologic efficacy of the regimen was maintained.[47]
Ritonavir-boosted atazanavir and darunavir	Different studies: pls recommended for the initial treatment of HIV infection because each has shown better lipid effects and overall tolerability than ritonavir-boosted lopinavir.[50,51]
Darunavir/ritonavir or atazanavir/ritonavir plus tenofovir-emtricitabine	Pilot study, Aberg and colleagues[48]: similar 48-wk lipid changes between darunavir and atazanavir.
Darunavir/ritonavir or atazanavir/ritonavir compared with raltegravir	Ofotokun and colleagues[49]: 96-wk trial found no difference in lipid profiles with atazanavir/ritonavir and darunavir/ritonavir. Raltegravir had more favorable lipid profile than both PIs.

Dyslipidemic effects of NNRTIs

In patients who have initiated NNRTIs as first-line therapy, increases in the serum concentrations of TC, HDL, LDL, and triglycerides have been observed (**Table 3**).[11,63–70] Many studies have reported that NNRTI may induce greater increases in HDL levels compared with PIs, hence, balancing out the overall lipid risk profile.[70] Patients treated with efavirenz had increases of TC (at least 3% mean relative increase in levels) and triglyceride (at least 10% mean relative increase in levels) concentrations.[63] Switching from a PI to efavirenz may improve the lipid profile, depending on the specific PI used.[71] With regard to other agents, the newer NNRTIs, rilpivirine and etravirine, have more favorable lipid profiles than efavirenz.[72]

Dyslipidemic effects of integrase inhibitors and C-C chemokine receptor type 5 antagonists

The integrase inhibitors, raltegravir, elvitegravir, and dolutegravir, and the C-C chemokine receptor type 5 (CCR5) receptor antagonist, maraviroc, appear to have little or no impact on lipid parameters, even in long-term use.[73,74] Switching to these agents in patients who are well suppressed on first-line therapy may benefit many HIV-infected patients by improving their lipid profiles (**Table 4**).[74–85] Preliminary studies support the beneficial lipid profile of unboosted integrase inhibitors.[79] Recent data suggest that elvitegravir-cobicistat-tenofovir-emtricitabine induced similar changes in lipids compared with atazanavir/ritonavir and had less prominent effects on total and LDL cholesterol compared with efavirenz.[83,84] Data from 2 independent studies confirms that the boosted PIs, atazanavir and darunavir, are associated with greater increases in TC and triglycerides compared with raltegravir.[48,49]

Table 2 Studies investigating the effects of different NRTIs on lipids	
NRTIs	**Comments**
Stavudine	Stavudine is still used in some developing countries and at full doses induces significant metabolic abnormalities compared with other ART such as tenofovir.[53] No association between stavudine use and risk of MI was found in the D:A:D study.[57]
Tenofovir	Regimens containing tenofovir are associated with lower serum concentrations of LDL-c, TC, and triglycerides compared with regimens using other NRTIs, suggesting a lipid-lowering action of tenofovir, which differs from that of other NRTIs.[54] No association between tenofovir use and risk of MI was found in the D:A:D study.[52] Several studies[100] found maintained virologic suppression and improved cholesterol concentrations in patients with increased lipid concentrations on ritonavir-boosted, PI-based regimens that included abacavir who were switched to tenofovir.
Abacavir and didanosine	The use of the NRTIs abacavir and didanosine was found to be an independent risk factor for myocardial infarction in the D:A:D study.[52,57] Several analyses with conflicting results have been performed in an attempt to better understand the association between abacavir and, to a lesser extent, didanosine and CVD events.[55,56] In a meta-analysis based on 52 clinical trials and a total 14,174 HIV-infected adults who received abacavir (n = 9502) or not (n = 4672), baseline demographics and HIV disease characteristics, including lipids values, MI rates were similar.[58] Further data are needed to evaluate any association between abacavir and increased risk of MI.
Tenofovir-emtricitabine vs abacavir-lamivudine	In the ACTG 5202 study, changes in lipid concentrations were generally greater with abacavir-lamivudine than tenofovir-emtricitabine (when combined with either efavirenz or atazanavir/ritonavir); however, researchers found no differences in the TC:HDL-c ratios.[59] In a study examining lipid subfractions, a more atherogenic LDL profile was noted in patients switched to abacavir-lamivudine compared with tenofovir-emtricitabine, including a decrease in LDL level in the abacavir group.[60] Of note, in the SPIRAL study,[61] no significant differences in lipid concentrations were identified between the tenofovir and abacavir recipients who switched from a ritonavir-boosted PI to raltegravir, suggesting that the combination of a ritonavir-boosted PI and abacavir might have distinct lipid effects.

LIPID CHANGES DURING TREATED HIV DISEASE MAY CONTRIBUTE TO IMMUNE ACTIVATION IN HIV INFECTION

A hallmark of HIV infection is activation of the immune system, which persists to some degree even after the initiation of effective ART.[19] Although the exact mechanisms that drive this immune activation are unclear, residual HIV replication, microbial transloca-tion, and inflammatory lipids are potential contributors. Modified lipoproteins such as oxidized LDL carry oxidized lipids and may regulate immunity.[86] We recently showed that HIV-infected subjects have dysfunctional HDL that is associated with biomarkers of T-cell activation.[87] We also showed that among HIV-infected subjects but not con-trols that dysfunctional HDL was significantly associated with circulating levels of the macrophage activation marker, soluble CD163.[45] The temporal relationship between these observations remains unclear. Among HIV-infected patients, studies suggest that after the initiation of ART, salutary changes to HDL structure occur, possibly caused by improvements in immune activation.[8] Data suggesting that oxidized forms of LDL are present in atherosclerotic lesions and constitute major epitopes for natural antibodies show that these lipids may be a stimulus for monocytes from HIV-infected subjects.[38,88,89] Modified lipoproteins may also directly activate immune cells such as macrophages and T cells.[90] Further studies are needed to elucidate the interplay between immune activation, ART, HDL structure/function of modified lipoproteins, and CVD risk in HIV.

MANAGEMENT OF LIPID DISORDERS
Diagnosis of Lipid Disorders in the Context of CVD

Current HIV treatment recommendations emphasize the importance of CVD risk screening in all patients starting ART and throughout the course of treatment.[91,92] Fasting lipid levels should be obtained at initiation of care for HIV-infected subjects and before and within 1 to 3 months after starting ART.[91] In addition, screening for other metabolic abnormalities should also be performed. For example, fasting blood glucose or hemoglobin A1c should be obtained before and within 1 to 3 months after starting ART.[91,92] When triglycerides are greater than 500 mg/dL, the measurements of non–HDL-c, apoB, or both may be useful because measurement of LDL-c may underestimate the CVD risk.[9,41] However, although fasting lipid levels determine well-established quantitative lipid abnormalities, there are no established diagnostic methods to determine qualitative abnormalities of lipids and lipoproteins.

Treatment of Dyslipidemia in HIV Infection

Management of dyslipidemia in patients with HIV follows recommendations for the general population according to the National Cholesterol Education Program Guidelines (**Table 5**).[9,39,91–94]

Lifestyle changes are the initial step in management of dyslipidemia and CVD risk in HIV-infected subjects. Lifestyle modifications including diet, exercise, and smoking cessation should be the first step in management, whereas lipid-lowering therapy and ART changes should be considered for patients at high risk of CVD.[91] Diet and exercise improved lipid profile in patients on ART with hypertriglyceridemia[95]; however, a recent meta-analysis of dietary intervention studies in patients with HIV reported only slight effects on triglyceride concentrations.[96]

Lipid-lowering therapy should be prescribed with caution in HIV-infected patients. There are significant drug interactions between lipid-lowering agents and PIs most notably among the statin drugs simvastatin and lovastatin.[9] HIV guidelines recommend the use of statins that have fewer interactions with ART, such as pravastatin and atorvastatin,[91] whereas use of newer statins such as pitavastatin may further reduce these interactions.[91] Treating hypertriglyceridemia may be challenging in HIV-infected patients. In a recent study, fibrates were more effective than fish oil or atorvastatin at lowering plasma triglycerides in HIV-infected patients with hypertriglyceridemia,[93] suggesting that fibrates should be the first choice.

Switch strategies that deploy newer antiretrovirals with more favorable lipid profile (integrase inhibitors, second-generation NNRTIs, and newer PIs) are increasingly used as an intervention for ART-related dyslipidemia. Improvements in lipids have been seen when patients with dyslipidemia on ritonavir-boosted PIs were switched from abacavir to tenofovir[97] or when the PI was switched to another agent.[98] The

Table 3	
Studies investigating the effects of different NNRTIs on lipids	
NNRTIs	**Comments**
Efavirenz	Patients treated with efavirenz presented a significant increase of TC and triglyceride concentrations[63] compared with baseline. In the ACTG study 5202[64] participants randomly assigned to efavirenz had statistically significantly greater increases in TC and LDL-c concentrations but not in TC:HDL-c ratios compared with participants receiving atazanavir/ritonavir (each in combination with abacavir-lamivudine or tenofovir-emtricitabine). A recent meta-analysis compared the effects of the NNRTI, efavirenz, and various ritonavir-boosted PIs (including darunavir/ritonavir) on lipid levels using data from 15 clinical trials of first-line antiretroviral therapy in which standardized 48-wk lipids data were reported (n = 6368).[65] In this study, efavirenz and the more recently introduced PIs, such as DRV and atazanavir, had only a modest impact on serum lipids and their pattern of effect differed. In a substudy of a trial in 91 antiretroviral-naïve patients randomly assigned to tenofovir + emtricitabine + atazanavir/ritonavir or EFV (patients assigned to EFV had greater increases in TC, LDL-c, and HDL-c and in large HDL particles, but not in TC:HDL-c ratio or indication for lipid-lowering interventions relative to patients assigned to atazanavir and ritonavir.[66]
Nevirapine	ART regimens containing nevirapine are associated with a favorable lipid profile, mainly because they provide higher serum concentrations of HDL-c.[63]
Etravirine	Switching from efavirenz or ritonavir-boosted PIs to etravirine led to a significant improvement of lipids irrespective of the presence of previous hyperlipidemia and type of ART.[67]
Rilpivirine	Two phase 3 trials (ECHO[68] and THRIVE[69]) of similar design, with the exception of the background NRTI regimen, compared rilpivirine with efavirenz in ART-naive patients with HIV. After 48 wk, TC, HDL-c, LDL-c and triglyceride concentrations were significantly greater in the patients randomly assigned to efavirenz than those receiving rilpivirine; however, the TC:HDL-c ratio did not change significantly between the treatment groups because of a greater HDL increase in the patients given efavirenz.

SWITCHMRK study[98] found that switch from a lopinavir/ritonavir-based regimen to a raltegravir-based regimen had favorable effects on the lipid profile in patients. However, clinicians should consider prior treatment history before switching antiretrovirals, as higher rates of virologic failure have been noted among those with prior failure who were switched from a boosted PI to a raltegravir based regimen.

Strategies to increase HDL cholesterol levels and HDL function in HIV-infected individuals should be investigated. Although there are available therapies for elevated LDL-c levels, therapeutic strategies to increase HDL levels are limited and of unclear clinical significance.[99] In general, treatment with NNRTI-based regimens appears to increase HDL levels more so than therapy with other classes of drugs. The clinical significance of this effect is unclear. Thus, therapies that may also improve HDL function in HIV infection need further study as a CVD prevention strategy.

SUMMARY

As the HIV population ages, it is important to prevent development of long-term comorbidities such as CVD. The mechanisms of atherosclerosis in HIV remain to be fully elucidated. Host, virus, immune deficiency, and ART factors have a major role in the increased risk for CVD in HIV and lipid changes may both be a consequence and a driver of these interactions (**Fig. 2**). During untreated HIV infection, lipid

Table 4
Studies investigating the effects of different NNRTIs on lipids

New Antivirals	Comments
Maraviroc	In a mouse model of genetic dyslipidemia, maraviroc reduced atherosclerotic progression by interfering with inflammatory cell recruitment into plaques and by reversing the proinflammatory profile.[75] Switching from PIs or NNRTIs to maraviroc, decreased TC and triglycerides in a small, randomized, clinical trial.[76] MacInnes and colleagues[74] investigated treatment-naive patients randomly assigned to receive either maraviroc or efavirenz in combination with zidovudine-lamivudine for up to 96 wk. The investigators reported that of the patients with baseline TC and LDL-c less than the National Cholesterol Education Programme treatment thresholds, more patients receiving efavirenz than those treated with maraviroc exceeded the thresholds for TC and LDL-c. Additionally, among participants with baseline lipid concentrations exceeding National Cholesterol Education Programme thresholds, 84% of patients on efavirenz vs 50% of those on maraviroc still exceeded the thresholds at 96 wk.
Raltegravir	In the STARTMRK trial, Rockstroh and colleagues[77] compared raltegravir with efavirenz in treatment-naive adults, and identified that 240-wk increases in fasting triglycerides and TC, LDL-c, and HDL-c were significantly greater in those receiving efavirenz than raltegravir. Additionally, 9% of adults given raltegravir vs 34% given efavirenz needed initiation of lipid-lowering treatment during follow-up. Switching from different class-suppressive regimens to raltegravir and tenofovir and emtricitabine or abacavir and lamivudine led to improvements in plasma lipids after 48 wk.[78] In virologically suppressed aging HIV-positive patients, there are promising results from small, short-term studies assessing dual therapy with raltegravir and a nonnucleoside reverse inhibitor such as etravirine or nevirapine.[79,80]
Dolutegravir	Dolutegravir is a once-daily integrase inhibitor that does not need a boosting drug. In the SPRING-2 trial,[81] a 96-wk, phase 3, randomized, double-blind, noninferiority study comparing dolutegravir with raltegravir in treatment-naive patients, no significant changes in lipid measures were shown in either treatment group.
Elvitegravir-cobicistat-emtricitabine-tenofovir DF	The fixed-dose combination of elvitegravir-cobicistat-emtricitabine-tenofovir DF, has been compared with efavirenz-tenofovir-emtricitabine and ritonavir plus atazanavir plus emtricitabine-tenofovir DF in treatment-naive adults, and statistically similar overall changes in lipid profiles among the 3 regimens were found.[82] Rockstroh and colleagues[83] compared elvitegravir-cobicistat with atazanavir/ritonavir in treatment-naive patients and reported that after 96 wk, changes in TC were greater with elvitegravir-cobicistat; but triglyceride increases were greater with atazanavir/ritonavir, and no difference in the TC:HDL-c ratio was noted between the 2 treatment groups. Sax and colleagues[84] compared treatment of efavirenz-tenofovir DF-emtricitabine with elvitegravir-cobicistat-tenofovir DF-emtricitabine and showed that mean changes in TC, HDL-c, and LDL-c were greater in the efavirenz than elvitegravir-cobicistat group, whereas the TC:HDL-c ratio was the same in both groups. In another study, Elion and colleagues[85] randomly assigned treated patients to either elvitegravir or raltegravir combination with a ritonavir-boosted PI and a third active drug. No differences in lipid concentrations were reported between the 2 treatment groups. Collectively, these results suggest that elvitegravir-cobicistat-tenofovir DF-emtricitabine has a similar lipid profile to ritonavir-atazanavir, and has less severe TC and LDL-c perturbations (but also less HDL improvement) than does efavirenz.

Table 5
Treatment of dyslipidemia in the context of CVD in HIV infection

Therapeutic Intervention	Comments
Lifestyle modifications	Diet, exercise, and smoking cessation.
Lipid-lowering therapy	
Statins that have minimal interactions with ART	PIs and ritonavir mainly inhibit cytochrome P and could increase the toxicity of some statins. NNRTIs (eg, efavirenz) are inducers of cytochrome P and could reduce statin efficacy. In the HIV-infected patient taking a PI, statins with a low risk for interaction with PIs should be preferred, such as pravastatin, fluvastatin, low-dose atorvastatin, or low-dose rosuvastatin.[9,91,92]
Fibrates	Fibrates should be prescribed when the triglyceride concentration is >500 mg/d.[9]
Fish oil	Limited evidence on the role of omega-3 fatty acids on the management and prevention of the metabolic abnormalities in HIV-infected patients but randomized, controlled clinical trials have not shown a clear benefit.[93]
Switch strategies	
Switch PI to an NNRTI or to a new drug such as integrase or CCR5 inhibitors	See evidence presented in **Tables 1–4**.
Switch first-generation NRTIs (eg, stavudine) to second-generation NRTIs (eg, tenofovir)	See evidence presented in **Table 2**.
Switch first-generation NNRTIs (eg, efavirenz) to new NNRTI (eg, etravirine, rilpivirine)	See evidence presented in **Table 3**.
Switch first-generation NNRTIs (eg, efavirenz) to a new drug such as integrase inhibitors (eg, raltegravir)	See evidence presented in **Tables 2 and 4**.
Manage other comorbidities that may contribute to CVD	Regarding hypertension, blockers of the rennin-angiotensin system should be the first therapy because of their protective effects on the vasculature, kidney function, and favorable metabolic effects.[9] Telmisartan is being evaluated for favorable effects on visceral adiposity in HIV-infected subjects.[39] Antiplatelet drugs such as aspirin, clopidogrel, prasugrel, and ticagrelor should be given according to the guidelines for the general population.[9] Diabetes and insulin resistance should be managed according to the guidelines for the general population and HIV-infected subjects.[91,92]

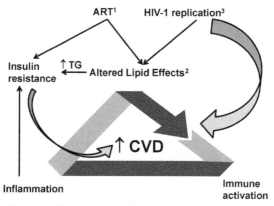

Fig. 2. Factoring influencing dyslipidemia and CVD risk in HIV. ART directly alters lipid meta-bolism and may increase the risk of insulin resistance (1). The lipid effects of ART include elevated triglycerides and for some agents elevations in TC. The elevations in triglycerides may also contribute to insulin resistance and to CVD risk (2). HIV replication per se increases immune activation and may have a direct effect on CVD risk (3). In addition HIV replication may indirectly alter HDL function via indirect effects on inflammation. These altered lipids may have direct and indirect immunoregulatory effects and induce further activation of im-mune cells (T cells and monocytes/macrophages), which may further increase systemic inflam-mation. Inflammation also contributes to insulin resistance, which, in turn, may increase CVD risk. Thus, there are complex interactions between these pathophysiologic processes that are at least partially driven by altered lipids that are formed during HIV infection and that may directly or indirectly contribute to increased CVD in HIV-infected subjects. TG, triglycerides.

alterations are associated with the virus and its effects on the immune system. These are characterized by a decrease of TC, LDL-c, and HDL-c and by an increase of tri-glyceride levels. In contrast, ART regimens promoted distinct alterations in the lipid metabolism of these patients and vary by individual agents. Thus, it is critical to address traditional risk factors for CVD, such as dyslipidemia, in the HIV-infected pop-ulation. Clinicians need to focus on improved methods for screening and treatment of lipid disorders while taking into consideration potential drug-drug interactions, partic-ularly with statins and ART. Newer HIV drugs, such as etravirine, rilpivirine, raltegravir, dolutegravir, and elvitegravir, are metabolically well-tolerated drug options and may be particularly useful for aging HIV-infected patients. As our understanding of genetic predisposition to dyslipidemia in HIV-infected patients improves, these findings should translate from research to clinical care. Further research is needed to fully elucidate the pathophysiology of dyslipidemia in HIV-infected patients, with particular emphasis on defining the roles of lipids in inflammation, immune activation, and CVD.

REFERENCES

1. Sackoff JE, Hanna DB, Pfeiffer MR, et al. Causes of death among persons with AIDS in the era of highly active antiretroviral therapy: New York City. Ann Intern Med 2006;145(6):397–406.
2. Currier JS, Lundgren JD, Carr A, et al. Epidemiological evidence for cardiovas-cular disease in HIV-infected patients and relationship to highly active antiretro-viral therapy. Circulation 2008;118(2):e29–35.
3. Triant VA, Lee H, Hadigan C, et al. Increased acute myocardial infarction rates and cardiovascular risk factors among patients with human immunodeficiency virus disease. J Clin Endocrinol Metab 2007;92(7):2506–12.

4. Triant VA, Meigs JB, Grinspoon SK. Association of C-reactive protein and HIV infection with acute myocardial infarction. J Acquir Immune Defic Syndr 2009; 51(3):268–73.

5. Baker JV, Neuhaus J, Duprez D, et al. Changes in inflammatory and coagulation biomarkers: a randomized comparison of immediate versus deferred antiretroviral therapy in patients with HIV infection. J Acquir Immune Defic Syndr 2011;56(1):36–43.

6. El-Sadr WM, Lundgren J, Neaton JD, et al. CD4+ count-guided interruption of antiretroviral treatment. N Engl J Med 2006;355(22):2283–96.

7. Grunfeld C, Delaney JA, Wanke C, et al. Preclinical atherosclerosis due to HIV infection: carotid intima-medial thickness measurements from the FRAM study. AIDS 2009;23(14):1841–9.

8. Baker JV, Neuhaus J, Duprez D, et al. Inflammation predicts changes in high-density lipoprotein particles and apolipoprotein A1 following initiation of antiretroviral therapy. AIDS 2011;25(17):2133–42.

9. Boccara F, Lang S, Meuleman C, et al. HIV and coronary heart disease: time for a better understanding. J Am Coll Cardiol 2013;61(5):511–23.

10. Choi AI, Li Y, Deeks SG, et al. Association between kidney function and albuminuria with cardiovascular events in HIV-infected persons. Circulation 2010;121(5): 651–8.

11. Friis-Moller N, Thiebaut R, Reiss P, et al. Predicting the risk of cardiovascular disease in HIV-infected patients: the data collection on adverse effects of anti-HIV drugs study. Eur J Cardiovasc Prev Rehabil 2010;17(5):491–501.

12. Duprez DA, Neuhaus J, Kuller LH, et al. Inflammation, coagulation and cardiovascular disease in HIV-infected individuals. PLoS One 2012;7(9):e44454 [Important reference for key points].

13. Kaplan RC, Landay AL, Hodis HN, et al. Potential cardiovascular disease risk markers among HIV-infected women initiating antiretroviral treatment. J Acquir Immune Defic Syndr 2012;60(4):359–68.

14. Gresele P, Falcinelli E, Sebastiano M, et al. Endothelial and platelet function alterations in HIV-infected patients. Thromb Res 2012;9(3):301–8.

15. Kelesidis T, Kendall MA, Yang OO, et al. Biomarkers of microbial translocation and macrophage activation: association with progression of subclinical atherosclerosis in HIV-1 infection. J Infect Dis 2012;206(10):1558–67.

16. Burdo TH, Lo J, Abbara S, et al. Soluble CD163, a novel marker of activated macrophages, is elevated and associated with noncalcified coronary plaque in HIV-infected patients. J Infect Dis 2011;204(8):1227–36.

17. Subramanian S, Tawakol A, Burdo TH, et al. Arterial inflammation in patients with HIV. JAMA 2012;308(4):379–86.

18. Blodget E, Shen C, Aldrovandi G, et al. Relationship between microbial translocation and endothelial function in HIV infected patients. PLoS One 2012;7(8): e42624.

19. Brenchley JM, Price DA, Schacker TW, et al. Microbial translocation is a cause of systemic immune activation in chronic HIV infection. Nat Med 2006;12(12): 1365–71.

20. Friis-Moller N, Weber R, Reiss P, et al. Cardiovascular disease risk factors in HIV patients–association with antiretroviral therapy. Results from the DAD study. AIDS 2003;17(8):1179–93.

21. Egana-Gorrono L, Martinez E, Cormand B, et al. Impact of genetic factors on dyslipidemia in HIV-infected patients starting antiretroviral therapy. AIDS 2013; 27(4):529–38.

22. Nicholaou MJ, Martinson JJ, Abraham AG, et al. HAART-associated dyslipidemia varies by biogeographical ancestry in the multicenter AIDS cohort study. AIDS Res Hum Retroviruses 2013;29(6):871–9 [Important reference for key points].
23. Cassol E, Misra V, Holman A, et al. Plasma metabolomics identifies lipid abnormalities linked to markers of inflammation, microbial translocation, and hepatic function in HIV patients receiving protease inhibitors. BMC Infect Dis 2013;13:203.
24. Grunfeld C, Feingold KR. The role of the cytokines, interferon alpha and tumor necrosis factor in the hypertriglyceridemia and wasting of AIDs. J Nutr 1992; 122(3 Suppl):749–53.
25. Grunfeld C, Pang M, Doerrler W, et al. Lipids, lipoproteins, triglyceride clearance, and cytokines in human immunodeficiency virus infection and the acquired immunodeficiency syndrome. J Clin Endocrinol Metab 1992;74(5): 1045–52 [Important reference for key points].
26. Drozd DR, Nance RM, Delaney JA. et al. Lower CD4 Count and Higher Viral Load Are Associated With Increased Risk of Myocardial Infarction. Centers for AIDS Research Network of Integrated Clinical Systems (CNICS) Cohort. 21st Conference on Retroviruses and Opportunistic Infections. Boston (MA), March 3–6, 2014. [abstract: 739].
27. Riddler SA, Smit E, Cole SR, et al. Impact of HIV infection and HAART on serum lipids in men. JAMA 2003;289(22):2978–82 [Important reference for key points].
28. Grunfeld C, Kotler DP, Hamadeh R, et al. Hypertriglyceridemia in the acquired immunodeficiency syndrome. Am J Med 1989;86(1):27–31.
29. Duprez DA, Kuller LH, Tracy R, et al. Lipoprotein particle subclasses, cardiovascular disease and HIV infection. Atherosclerosis 2009;207(2):524–9.
30. Enkhmaa B, Anuurad E, Zhang W, et al. HIV disease activity as a modulator of lipoprotein(a) and allele-specific apolipoprotein(a) levels. Arterioscler Thromb Vasc Biol 2013;33(2):387–92.
31. Khovidhunkit W, Memon RA, Feingold KR, et al. Infection and inflammation-induced proatherogenic changes of lipoproteins. J Infect Dis 2000;181(Suppl 3): S462–72.
32. Rose H, Hoy J, Woolley I, et al. HIV infection and high density lipoprotein metabolism. Atherosclerosis 2008;199(1):79–86.
33. Khera AV, Cuchel M, Llera-Moya M, et al. Cholesterol efflux capacity, high-density lipoprotein function, and atherosclerosis. N Engl J Med 2011;364(2): 127–35.
34. Mujawar Z, Rose H, Morrow MP, et al. Human immunodeficiency virus impairs reverse cholesterol transport from macrophages. PLoS Biol 2006;4(11):e365 [Important reference for key points].
35. Feeney ER, McAuley N, O'Halloran JA, et al. The expression of cholesterol metabolism genes in monocytes from HIV-infected subjects suggests intracellular cholesterol accumulation. J Infect Dis 2013;207(4):628–37.
36. Van Lenten BJ, Hama SY, de Beer FC, et al. Anti-inflammatory HDL becomes pro-inflammatory during the acute phase response. Loss of protective effect of HDL against LDL oxidation in aortic wall cell cocultures. J Clin Invest 1995; 96(6):2758–67.
37. Grinspoon S, Carr A. Cardiovascular risk and body-fat abnormalities in HIV-infected adults. N Engl J Med 2005;352(1):48–62.
38. Holvoet P, Lee DH, Steffes M, et al. Association between circulating oxidized low-density lipoprotein and incidence of the metabolic syndrome. JAMA 2008; 299(19):2287–93.

39. Lake JE, Currier JS. Metabolic disease in HIV infection. Lancet Infect Dis 2013; 13(11):964–75.

40. Haubrich RH, Riddler SA, DiRienzo AG, et al. Metabolic outcomes in a randomized trial of nucleoside, nonnucleoside and protease inhibitor-sparing regimens for initial HIV treatment. AIDS 2009;23(9):1109–18 [Important reference for key points].

41. Navab M, Reddy ST, Van Lenten BJ, et al. HDL and cardiovascular disease: atherogenic and atheroprotective mechanisms. Nat Rev Cardiol 2011;8(4): 222–32.

42. Kelesidis T, Currier JS, Huynh D, et al. A biochemical fluorometric method for assessing the oxidative properties of HDL. J Lipid Res 2011;52(12):2341–51.

43. Kelesidis T, Yang OO, Currier JS, et al. HIV-1 infected patients with suppressed plasma viremia on treatment have pro-inflammatory HDL. Lipids Health Dis 2011;10:35.

44. Kelesidis T, Yang OO, Kendall MA, et al. Dysfunctional HDL and progression of atherosclerosis in HIV-1-infected and -uninfected adults. Lipids Health Dis 2013; 12:23.

45. Zanni MV, Kelesidis T, Fitzgerald ML, et al. HDL redox activity is increased in HIV-infected men in association with macrophage activation and noncalcified coronary atherosclerotic plaque. Antivir Ther, in press.

46. Carr A, Samaras K, Chisholm DJ, et al. Pathogenesis of HIV-1-protease inhibitor-associated peripheral lipodystrophy, hyperlipidaemia, and insulin resistance. Lancet 1998;351(9119):1881–3 [Important reference for key points].

47. Lang S, Mary-Krause M, Cotte L, et al. Increased risk of myocardial infarction in HIV-infected patients in France, relative to the general population. AIDS 2010; 24(8):1228–30.

48. Aberg JA, Tebas P, Overton ET, et al. Metabolic effects of darunavir/ritonavir versus atazanavir/ritonavir in treatment-naive, HIV type 1-infected subjects over 48 weeks. AIDS Res Hum Retroviruses 2012;28(10):1184–95.

49. Ofotokun I, Ribaudo H, Na L, et al. Darunavir or atazanavir vs raltegravir lipid changes are unliked to ritonavir exposure: ACTG 5257. Presented at the 21st Conference on Retroviruses and Opportunistic Infections. Boston (MA), March 3–6, 2014. [abstract: #746].

50. Mobius U, Lubach-Ruitman M, Castro-Frenzel B, et al. Switching to atazanavir improves metabolic disorders in antiretroviral-experienced patients with severe hyperlipidemia. J Acquir Immune Defic Syndr 2005;39(2):174–80.

51. Mills AM, Nelson M, Jayaweera D, et al. Once-daily darunavir/ritonavir vs. lopinavir/ritonavir in treatment-naive, HIV-1-infected patients: 96-week analysis. AIDS 2009;23(13):1679–88.

52. Worm SW, Sabin C, Weber R, et al. Risk of myocardial infarction in patients with HIV infection exposed to specific individual antiretroviral drugs from the 3 major drug classes: the data collection on adverse events of anti-HIV drugs (D: A:D) study. J Infect Dis 2010;201(3):318–30 [Important reference for key points].

53. Menezes CN, Crowther NJ, Duarte R, et al. A randomized clinical trial comparing metabolic parameters after 48 weeks of standard- and low-dose stavudine therapy and tenofovir disoproxil fumarate therapy in HIV-infected South African patients. HIV Med 2014;15(1):3–12.

54. Crane HM, Grunfeld C, Willig JH, et al. Impact of NRTIs on lipid levels among a large HIV-infected cohort initiating antiretroviral therapy in clinical care. AIDS 2011;25(2):185–95.

55. Ribaudo HJ, Benson CA, Zheng Y, et al. No risk of myocardial infarction associated with initial antiretroviral treatment containing abacavir: short and long-term results from ACTG A5001/ALLRT. Clin Infect Dis 2011;52(7):929–40.
56. Lang S, Mary-Krause M, Cotte L, et al. Impact of individual antiretroviral drugs on the risk of myocardial infarction in human immunodeficiency virus-infected patients: a case-control study nested within the French Hospital Database on HIV ANRS cohort CO4. Arch Intern Med 2010;170(14):1228–38.
57. Sabin CA, Worm SW, Weber R, et al. Use of nucleoside reverse transcriptase inhibitors and risk of myocardial infarction in HIV-infected patients enrolled in the D: A:D study: a multi-cohort collaboration. Lancet 2008;371(9622): 1417–26.
58. Brothers CH, Hernandez JE, Cutrell AG, et al. Risk of myocardial infarction and abacavir therapy: no increased risk across 52 GlaxoSmithKline-sponsored clinical trials in adult subjects. J Acquir Immune Defic Syndr 2009;51(1):20–8.
59. Sax PE, Tierney C, Collier AC, et al. Abacavir/lamivudine versus tenofovir DF/emtricitabine as part of combination regimens for initial treatment of HIV: final results. J Infect Dis 2011;204(8):1191–201.
60. Saumoy M, Ordonez-Llanos J, Martinez E, et al. Low-density lipoprotein size and lipoprotein-associated phospholipase A2 in HIV-infected patients switching to abacavir or tenofovir. Antivir Ther 2011;16(4):459–68.
61. Martinez E, d'Albuquerque PM, Perez I, et al. Abacavir/lamivudine versus tenofovir/emtricitabine in virologically suppressed patients switching from ritonavir-boosted protease inhibitors to raltegravir. AIDS Res Hum Retroviruses 2013; 29(2):235–41.
62. Guaraldi G, Zona S, Cossarizza A, et al. Randomized trial to evaluate cardiometabolic and endothelial function in patients with plasma HIV-1 RNA suppression switching to darunavir/ritonavir with or without nucleoside analogues. HIV Clin Trials 2013;14(4):140–8.
63. Williams P, Wu J, Cohn S, et al. Improvement in lipid profiles over 6 years of follow-up in adults with AIDS and immune reconstitution. HIV Med 2009;10(5): 290–301.
64. Daar ES, Tierney C, Fischl MA, et al. Atazanavir plus ritonavir or efavirenz as part of a 3-drug regimen for initial treatment of HIV-1. Ann Intern Med 2011;154(7): 445–56.
65. Hill A, Sawyer W, Gazzard B. Effects of first-line use of nucleoside analogues, efavirenz, and ritonavir-boosted protease inhibitors on lipid levels. HIV Clin Trials 2009;10(1):1–12.
66. Gotti D, Cesana BM, Albini L, et al. Increase in standard cholesterol and large HDL particle subclasses in antiretroviral-naive patients prescribed efavirenz compared to atazanavir/ritonavir. HIV Clin Trials 2012;13(5):245–55.
67. Casado JL, de los Santos I, Del Palacio M, et al. Lipid-lowering effect and efficacy after switching to etravirine in HIV-infected patients with intolerance to suppressive HAART. HIV Clin Trials 2013;14(1):1–9.
68. Molina JM, Cahn P, Grinsztejn B, et al. Rilpivirine versus efavirenz with tenofovir and emtricitabine in treatment-naive adults infected with HIV-1 (ECHO): a phase 3 randomised double-blind active-controlled trial. Lancet 2011;378(9787): 238–46.
69. Cohen CJ, Andrade-Villanueva J, Clotet B, et al. Rilpivirine versus efavirenz with two background nucleoside or nucleotide reverse transcriptase inhibitors in treatment-naive adults infected with HIV-1 (THRIVE): a phase 3, randomised, non-inferiority trial. Lancet 2011;378(9787):229–37.

70. van der Valk M, Kastelein JJ, Murphy RL, et al. Nevirapine-containing antiretroviral therapy in HIV-1 infected patients results in an anti-atherogenic lipid profile. AIDS 2001;15(18):2407–14.

71. Vigano A, Aldrovandi GM, Giacomet V, et al. Improvement in dyslipidaemia after switching stavudine to tenofovir and replacing protease inhibitors with efavirenz in HIV-infected children. Antivir Ther 2005;10(8):917–24.

72. Fatkenheuer G, Duvivier C, Rieger A, et al. Lipid profiles for etravirine versus efavirenz in treatment-naive patients in the randomized, double-blind SENSE trial. J Antimicrob Chemother 2012;67(3):685–90.

73. Rockstroh JK, Lennox JL, DeJesus E, et al. Long-term treatment with raltegravir or efavirenz combined with tenofovir/emtricitabine for treatment-naive human immunodeficiency virus-1-infected patients: 156-week results from STARTMRK. Clin Infect Dis 2011;53(8):807–16.

74. MacInnes A, Lazzarin A, Di Perri G, et al. Maraviroc can improve lipid profiles in dyslipidemic patients with HIV: results from the MERIT trial. HIV Clin Trials 2011; 12(1):24–36.

75. Cipriani S, Francisci D, Mencarelli A, et al. Efficacy of the CCR5 antagonist maraviroc in reducing early, ritonavir-induced atherogenesis and advanced plaque progression in mice. Circulation 2013;127(21):2114–24.

76. Bonjoch A, Pou C, Perez-Alvarez N, et al. Switching the third drug of antiretroviral therapy to maraviroc in aviraemic subjects: a pilot, prospective, randomized clinical trial. J Antimicrob Chemother 2013;68(6):1382–7.

77. Rockstroh JK, DeJesus E, Lennox JL, et al. Durable efficacy and safety of raltegravir versus efavirenz when combined with tenofovir/emtricitabine in treatment-naive HIV-1-infected patients: final 5-year results from STARTMRK. J Acquir Immune Defic Syndr 2013;63(1):77–85.

78. Fabbiani M, Mondi A, Colafigli M, et al. Safety and efficacy of treatment switch to raltegravir plus tenofovir/emtricitabine or abacavir/lamivudine in patients with optimal virological control: 48-week results from a randomized pilot study (Raltegravir Switch for Toxicity or Adverse Events, RASTA Study). Scand J Infect Dis 2014;46(1):34–45.

79. Monteiro P, Perez I, Laguno M, et al. Dual therapy with etravirine plus raltegravir for virologically suppressed HIV-infected patients: a pilot study. J Antimicrob Chemother 2014;69(3):742–8.

80. Reliquet V, Chirouze C, Allavena C, et al. Nevirapine-raltegravir combination, an NRTI and PI/r sparing regimen, as maintenance antiretroviral therapy in virologically suppressed HIV-1-infected patients. Antivir Ther 2014;19(1):117–23.

81. Raffi F, Rachlis A, Stellbrink HJ, et al. Once-daily dolutegravir versus raltegravir in antiretroviral-naive adults with HIV-1 infection: 48 week results from the randomised, double-blind, non-inferiority SPRING-2 study. Lancet 2013;381(9868):735–43.

82. FDA notifications. Ongoing safety review of abacavir, possible MI risk. AIDS Alert 2011;26(5):58–9.

83. Rockstroh JK, DeJesus E, Henry K, et al. A randomized, double-blind comparison of coformulated elvitegravir/cobicistat/emtricitabine/tenofovir DF vs ritonavir-boosted atazanavir plus coformulated emtricitabine and tenofovir DF for initial treatment of HIV-1 infection: analysis of week 96 results. J Acquir Immune Defic Syndr 2013;62(5):483–6.

84. Sax PE, DeJesus E, Mills A, et al. Co-formulated elvitegravir, cobicistat, emtricitabine, and tenofovir versus co-formulated efavirenz, emtricitabine, and tenofovir for initial treatment of HIV-1 infection: a randomised, double-blind, phase 3 trial, analysis of results after 48 weeks. Lancet 2012;379(9835):2439–48.

85. Elion R, Molina JM, Ramon Arribas LJ, et al. A randomized phase 3 study comparing once-daily elvitegravir with twice-daily raltegravir in treatment-experienced subjects with HIV-1 infection: 96-week results. J Acquir Immune Defic Syndr 2013;63(4):494–7.
86. Tsimikas S, Miller YI. Oxidative modification of lipoproteins: mechanisms, role in inflammation and potential clinical applications in cardiovascular disease. Curr Pharm Des 2011;17(1):27–37.
87. Kelesidis T, Flores M, Tseng CH, et al. HIV-infected adults with suppressed viremia on antiretroviral therapy have dysfunctional HDL that is associated with T cell activation. Abstract 662; Presented at IDWeek 2012. San Diego (CA), October 17–21, 2012.
88. Bjorkbacka H, Fredrikson GN, Nilsson J. Emerging biomarkers and intervention targets for immune-modulation of atherosclerosis - a review of the experimental evidence. Atherosclerosis 2013;227(1):9–17.
89. Yilmaz A, Jennbacken K, Fogelstrand L. Reduced IgM levels and elevated IgG levels against oxidized low-density lipoproteins in HIV-1 infection. BMC Infect Dis 2014;14:143.
90. Graham LS, Parhami F, Tintut Y, et al. Oxidized lipids enhance RANKL production by T lymphocytes: implications for lipid-induced bone loss. Clin Immunol 2009;133(2):265–75.
91. Aberg JA, Gallant JE, Ghanem KG, et al. Primary care guidelines for the management of persons infected with HIV: 2013 update by the HIV Medicine Association of the Infectious Diseases Society of America. Clin Infect Dis 2014;58(1): 1–10 [Important reference for key points].
92. Lundgren JD, Battegay M, Behrens G, et al. European AIDS Clinical Society (EACS) guidelines on the prevention and management of metabolic diseases in HIV. HIV Med 2008;9(2):72–81.
93. Munoz MA, Liu W, Delaney JA, et al. Comparative effectiveness of fish oil versus fenofibrate, gemfibrozil, and atorvastatin on lowering triglyceride levels among HIV-infected patients in routine clinical care. J Acquir Immune Defic Syndr 2013;64(3):254–60.
94. Grinspoon SK, Grunfeld C, Kotler DP, et al. State of the science conference: Initiative to decrease cardiovascular risk and increase quality of care for patients living with HIV/AIDS: executive summary. Circulation 2008;118(2): 198–210.
95. Wooten JS, Nambi P, Gillard BK, et al. Intensive lifestyle modification reduces Lp-PLA2 in dyslipidemic HIV/HAART patients. Med Sci Sports Exerc 2013; 45(6):1043–50.
96. Stradling C, Chen YF, Russell T, et al. The effects of dietary intervention on HIV dyslipidaemia: a systematic review and meta-analysis. PLoS One 2012;7(6): e38121.
97. Campo R, DeJesus E, Bredeek UF, et al. SWIFT: prospective 48-week study to evaluate efficacy and safety of switching to emtricitabine/tenofovir from lamivudine/abacavir in virologically suppressed HIV-1 infected patients on a boosted protease inhibitor containing antiretroviral regimen. Clin Infect Dis 2013;56(11): 1637–45.
98. Eron JJ, Young B, Cooper DA, et al. Switch to a raltegravir-based regimen versus continuation of a lopinavir-ritonavir-based regimen in stable HIV-infected patients with suppressed viraemia (SWITCHMRK 1 and 2): two multicentre, double-blind, randomised controlled trials. Lancet 2010;375(9712): 396–407 [Important reference for key points].

99. Singh IM, Shishehbor MH, Ansell BJ. High-density lipoprotein as a therapeutic target: a systematic review. JAMA 2007;298(7):786–98.

100. Behrens G, Maserati R, Rieger A, et al. Switching to tenofovir/emtricitabine from abacavir/lamivudine in HIV-infected adults with raised cholesterol: effect on lipid profiles. Antivir Ther 2012;17(6):1011–20.

Coronary Artery Calcium Scanning

The Key to the Primary Prevention of Coronary Artery Disease

Harvey S. Hecht, MD, FACC, FSCCT

KEYWORDS

- Calcium scanning • Atherosclerosis • Coronary artery disease

KEY POINTS

- The potential impact of coronary artery calcium scanning (CAC) on primary prevention cannot be overestimated because it eliminates the guesswork implicit in extrapolating risk from guidelines derived from large population bases to individual patients and provides a snapshot of the cumulative effect of an individual's life on the coronary circulation.
- The role of risk factors is most important in identifying treatable therapeutic targets after risk has been established by a test that is 100% specific for atherosclerosis and far superior to any risk factor–based paradigm.
- The remaining barriers include physician education to overcome instinctive clinging to the old established paradigms, patient education to increase awareness of the widespread availability and low radiation of CAC, and more widespread insurance reimbursement.

INTRODUCTION

Despite the overwhelming peer reviewed data supporting the role of CAC in the primary prevention of coronary artery disease (CAD), its penetration into clinical practice has been inexplicably low. Screening for lung, breast, and colon cancer has been officially endorsed by the US Preventive Services Task Force, whereas CAD, which kills more than all cancers combined, is not likely to be approved for screening by CAC in the near future. Instead, reliance is placed on risk assessment by various risk factor–based paradigms, all of which have proved inferior to CAC. **Fig. 1** illustrates the essential flaw in risk factor–based evaluations. In more than half a million patients presenting with their first myocardial infarction, almost half had less than 2 risk factors and 80% had less than or equal to 2. Moreover, mortality was inversely related to the number of risk factors.[1]

This article originally appeared in Endocrinology and Metabolism Clinics, Volume 43, Issue 4, December 2014.
Disclosure/Conflict of Interest Statement: Philips Medical Systems consultant.
Department of Cardiology, Mount Sinai Medical Center, Icahn School of Medicine at Mount Sinai, One Gustave L. Levy Place, Box 1030, New York, NY 10029-6574, USA
E-mail address: harvey.hecht@mountsinai.org

RF: hypertension, smoking, dyslipidemia, diabetes, and FH (<60)
542,008 patients with first MI

| | # RF | | | | | |
	0	1	2	3	4	5
N	14.4%	34.1%	31.6%	15.4%	4.1%	0.4%
Age	71.5	68.6	64.	61.7	58.8	56.7
Hosp Mortality	14.9%	10.9%	7.9%	5.3%	4.2%	3.6%

Mortality OR 1.54: inverse # RF

"The high prevalence of the same risk factors mong patients without CHD decreases the discriminatory power of these risk factors to accurately predict which patients will develop MI or even clinically significant atherosclerosis."

Fig. 1. The number of risk factors and mortality in patients with first MI. MI, myocardial infarction; OR, odds ratio; RF, risk factors. (*Reproduced with permission* of Wiley from Hecht HS, Narula J. Coronary artery calcium scanning in asymptomatic patients with diabetes mellitus: A paradigm shift. J Diab 2012;4:342–50.)

THE CORONARY ARTERY CALCIUM SCAN

CAC is a noncontrast, limited chest CT scan acquired with an approximate 3- to 5-second breath hold that automatically quantitates calcified coronary plaque, providing both an absolute Agatston unit (AU) score and a percentile normalized for age, gender, and ethnicity. Radiation exposure has progressively declined to approximately 1 mSv, comparable to mammography (0.8 mSv). Newer reconstruction algorithms decrease this dose to approximately 0.5 mSv. Examples of CAC scans displaying varying degrees of plaque are displayed in **Fig. 2**.

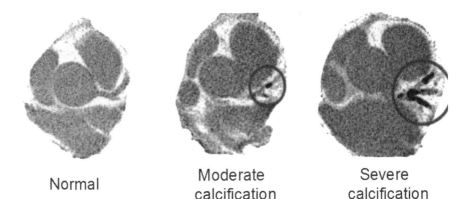

Normal   Moderate calcification   Severe calcification

Fig. 2. Examples of coronary artery scans.

THE PROGNOSTIC DATA

Every prognostic study, whether prospective or retrospective, population-based, or self-referred, has demonstrated the power of CAC, with relative risks (**Table 1**) far exceeding all risk factors, whether individually or collectively, in risk factor–based paradigms.[2–17]

Moreover, CAC has consistently added to the receiver operating characteristic (ROC) curve for risk factors and has always been superior to risk factors by themselves (**Fig. 3**).

Amalgamation of data from 5 large prospective randomized studies[9,11,14–16] yields 10-year event rates that can be translated into Framingham Risk Score (FRS) equivalents (**Table 2**).

Table 1
The prognostic power of coronary artery calcium in asymptomatic patients

	N	Mean Age (y)	Follow-up (y)	Calcium Score Cutoff	Comparator Group for RR Calculat	Relative Risk Ratio
Arad et al,[2] 2000	1173	53	3.6	CAC >160	CAC <160	20.2
Park et al,[3] 2002	967	67	6.4	CAC >142.1	CAC <3.7	4.9
Raggi et al,[4] 2000	632	52	2.7	Top quartile	Lowest quartile	13
Wong et al,[5] 2000	926	54	3.3	Top quartile (>270)	First quartile	8.8
Kondos et al,[6] 2003	5635	51	3.1	CAC	No CAC	10.5
Greenland et al,[7] 2004	1312	66	7.0	CAC >300	No CAC	3.9
Shaw et al,[8] 2003	10,377	53	5	CAC ≥400	CAC ≤10	8.4
Arad et al,[9] 2005	5585	59	4.3	CAC ≥100	CAC <100	10.7
Taylor et al,[10] 2005	2000	40–50	3.0	CAC >44	CAC = 0	11.8
Vliegenthart et al,[11] 2002	1795	71	3.3	CAC >1000 CAC 400–1000	CAC <100 CAC <100	8.3 4.6
Budoff et al,[12] 2007	25,503	56	6.8	CAC >400	CAC 0	9.2
Lagoski et al,[13] 2007	3601	45–84	3.75	CAC >0	CAC 0	6.5
Becker et al,[14] 2008	1726	57.7	3.4	CAC >400	CAC 0	6.8 Men 7.9 Women
Detrano et al,[15] 2008	6814	62.2	3.8	CAC >300	CAC 0	14.1
Erbel et al,[16] 2010	4487	45–75	5	>75th %	<25th %	11.1 Men 3.2 Women
Taylor et al,[17] 2010	1634	42	5.6	CAC >0	CAC 0	9.3

Reproduced with permission of Wiley from Hecht HS, Narula J. Coronary artery calcium scanning in asymptomatic patients with diabetes mellitus: A paradigm shift. J Diab 2012;4:342–50; and *Data from* Refs.[2,3,5–17]

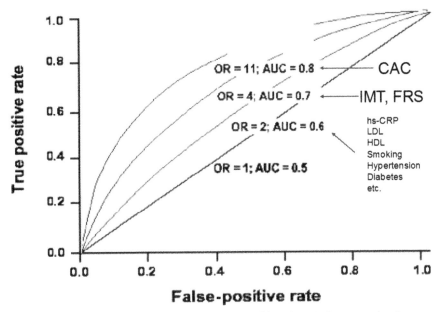

False-positive rate

Fig. 3. The ROC curve, its AUC, and corresponding odds ratios. AUC, area under the curve; HDL, high-density lipoprotein; OR, odds ratio.

CAC greater than 400 is a CAD equivalent, with 10-year event rates exceeding 20% in asymptomatic patients. The absence of calcified plaque conveys an extraordinarily low 10-year risk (1.1%–1.7%), irrespective of the number of risk factors (**Fig. 4**).[18]

Of critical importance is the net reclassification index (NRI) conferred by CAC in the asymptomatic population by 3 major prospective population-based studies (**Table 3**).[11,15,16] The percentage of patients with FRS risk estimate correctly reclassified by CAC based on outcomes ranged from 52% to 65.6% in the intermediate-risk population, 34% to 35.8% in the high-risk group, and 11.6% to 15% in the low-risk cohort, with NRIs for the entire study population from 19% to 25%.

Comparison of CAC in the intermediate-risk population with risk markers other than those included in the FRS revealed its overwhelming superiority to ankle-brachial index, brachial flow–mediated dilation, carotid intima media thickness (IMT), family history (FH) of premature CAD, and high-sensitivity C-reactive protein (hs-CRP) (**Fig. 5**).[19]

In addition, multiple blood biomarkers, including hs-CRP, interleukin 8, myeloperoxidase, B-type natriuretic peptide; and plasminogen activator type 1, did not add to the

Table 2
Event rates of CAC scores in asymptomatic patients and their FRS equivalents

CAC	10-y Event Rate (%)	FRS Risk
0	1.1–1.7	Very low
1–100	2.3–5.9	Low
100–400	12.8–16.4	Intermediate
>400	22.5–28.6	High
>1000	37	Very high

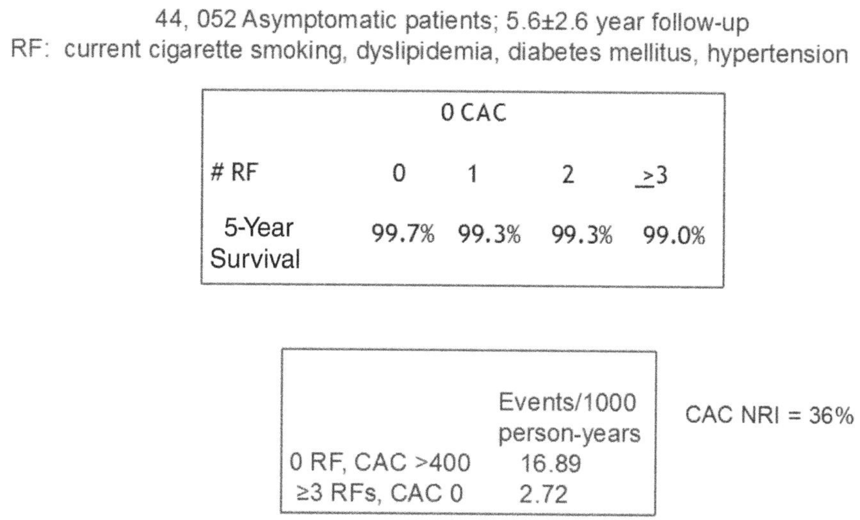

44, 052 Asymptomatic patients; 5.6±2.6 year follow-up
RF: current cigarette smoking, dyslipidemia, diabetes mellitus, hypertension

	0 CAC			
# RF	0	1	2	≥3
5-Year Survival	99.7%	99.3%	99.3%	99.0%

	Events/1000 person-years	CAC NRI = 36%
0 RF, CAC >400	16.89	
≥3 RFs, CAC 0	2.72	

Fig. 4. Interplay of CAC and traditional risk factors for prediction of all-cause mortality in asymptomatic patients. RF, risk factors. (*Data from* Nasir K, Rubin J, Blaha MJ, et al. Interplay of coronary artery calcification and traditional risk factors for the prediction of all-cause mortality in asymptomatic individuals. Circ Cardiovasc Imaging 2012;5:469.)

Table 3
Reclassification of FRS risk by CAC: primary prevention outcome studies

Study	Reclassified (%)	N	Age (y)	Follow-up (y)
MESA		5878	62.2	5.8
FRS 0%–6%	11.6			
FRS 6%–20%	54.4			
FRS >20%	35.8			
NRI	25			
Heinz Nixdorf		4487	45–75	5.0
FRS <10%	15.0			
FRS 10%–20%	65.6			
FRS >20%	34.2			
NRI	22.4			
Rotterdam		2028	69.6	9.2
FRS <10%	12			
FRS 10%–20%	52			
FRS >20%	34			
NRI	19			

Abbreviation: N, number of patients.
    Reproduced with permission of Wiley from Hecht HS, Narula J. Coronary artery calcium scanning in asymptomatic patients with diabetes mellitus: A paradigm shift. J Diab 2012;4:342–50.

6814 MESA participants
1330 Intermediate FRS (5-20%) without DM
7.6-Year follow-up, 94 CHD, 123 CVD events

Risk Markers and CVD

Marker	Multivariate HR	P	NRI vs FRS
ABI	0.79	.01	.036
Brachial FMD	0.82	.52	.024
CAC	2.60	<.001	.659
Carotid IMT	1.33	.13	.102
Family history	2.18	.001	.160
hs-CRP	1.26	.05	.079

Fig. 5. Comparison of novel risk markers for improvement in cardiovascular risk assessment in intermediate-risk individuals. ABI, ankle-brachial index; CVD, cardiovascular disease; DM, diabetes mellitus; FMD, flow-mediated dilation; HR, hazard ratio. (*Data from* Okwuosa TM, Greenland P, Ning H, et al. Yield of screening for coronary artery calcium in early middle-age adults based on the 10-year Framingham risk score: The CARDIA Study. JACC Cardiovasc Imaging 2012;5(9):923–30.)

C statistic for CAD outcomes of CAC and the FRS, whereas CAC increased the FRS C statistic from 0.73 to 0.84 (**Fig. 6**).[20]

PATIENT SUBGROUPS
Inflammatory Diseases

Inflammation as the common pathway of atherosclerosis is one of the tenets of cardiovascular disease. Nonetheless, with the exception of diabetes mellitus, the focus of early identification of risk by CAC scanning has been on intermediate-risk patients irrespective of associated disease states. It is now clearly understood that cardiovascular risk is high and is often the leading cause of death in a broad spectrum of diseases with the common link of inflammation, which has been evaluated to varying degrees by CAC. There is sufficient evidence to warrant consideration of CAC scanning for patients with the inflammatory diseases shown in **Fig. 7** who may not otherwise be in the intermediate-risk category.

Diabetes

The 2010 American College of Cardiology Foundation (ACCF)/American Heart Association (AHA) Guideline for Assessment of Cardiovascular Risk in Asymptomatic Adults awarded a class IIa recommendation for all adults older than 40 with diabetes.[21] Although the initial reasoning was to identify the high-risk patients with CAC greater than 400 for further evaluation to rule out obstructive disease, CAC prognostic data have challenged the ingrained concept of diabetes mellitus as a CAD disease equivalent. Patients with diabetes and CAC have higher risks than those without diabetes and similar CAC, but the absence of CAC conveys a similar low risk in both groups (**Table 4**).[22–26] Therefore, the more appropriate rationale is for straightforward risk classification as with any other risk factor, allowing for the possibility of downgrading risk.

1,286 Asymptomatic patients (59 + 8 years)
Follow-up 4.1 y; 35 events

Biomarkers:
CRP
Interleukin 6
Myeloperoxidase
BNP
Plasminogen activator type 1

	c statistic	P
FRS	.73	
FRS + all bio	.75	.32
FRS + CAC	.84	.003
FRS + CAC + all bio	.84	NS

Fig. 6. Comparative value of CAC and multiple blood biomarkers for prognostication of cardiovascular events. BNP, beta natriuretic protein; CRP, C-reactive protein. (*Data from* Rana JS, Gransar H, Wong ND, et al. Comparative value of coronary artery calcium and multiple blood biomarkers for prognostication of cardiovascular events. Am J Cardiol 2012;109:1450.)

Family History of Premature Coronary Artery Disease

Many articles have documented the strong association between FH and both clinical and subclinical CAD.[27]

In the younger population (<45 for men and <55 for women), however, these patients are an overlooked higher-risk group who would not qualify for treatment based on the FRS or any other paradigm. In recognition of this problem, the 2009 CAC Appropriate Use Criteria[28,29] considered CAC "appropriate" for asymptomatic patients with an FH of premature CAD and a low global risk estimate. The best approach

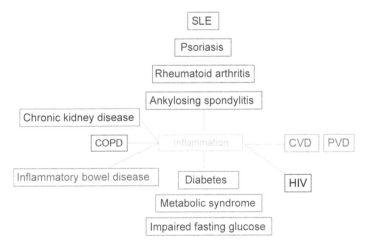

Fig. 7. Inflammatory diseases associated with a higher risk of CAD. COPD, chronic obstructive pulmonary disease; CVD, cardiovascular disease; PVD, peripheral vascular disease; SLE, systemic lupus erythematosis.

Study	N	Prevalence	Hazard Ratio	AUC	Event Rates/year

Table 4
Relationship between coronary artery calcium and events in asymptomatic diabetic patients

Study	N	Prevalence	Hazard Ratio	AUC	Event Rates/year
Wong et al,[22] 2003	1823	Any CAC No DM: 53% DM: 73.5%			0 CAC: 0.2% CAC >400: 5.6%
Becker et al,[23] 2008	716 DM	0 CAC: 15% CAC >400: 42%		CAC: 0.77 FRS: 0.68 UKPDS: 0.71 P<.01	
Elkeles et al,[24] 2008	589 DM		Compared with CAC 0–10 CAC >1000: 13.8 CAC 401–1000: 8.4 CAC 101–400: 7.1 CAC 11–100: 4.0	CAC: 0.73 UKPDS: 0.63 P<.03	CAC <10: 0%
Anand et al,[25] 2006	510 DM	CAC <10: 53.7%	Compared with CAC <100: CAC >1000: 58 CAC 401–1000: 41 CAC 101–400: 10	CAC: 0.92 UKPDS: 0.74 FRS: 0.60 P<.001	
Malik et al,[26] 2011	881 DM1 4036 No DM		Increasing CAC: 2.9–6.5 Increasing CAC: 2.6–9.5	CAC + RF: 0.78–0.80 RF: 0.72–0.73 P<.001	1.5% 0.5%

Abbreviations: AUC, area under curve; DM, diabetes mellitus.
Reproduced with permission of Wiley from Hecht HS, Narula J. Coronary artery calcium scanning in asymptomatic patients with diabetes mellitus: A paradigm shift. J Diab 2012;4:342–50.

is to start with CAC scanning. If any calcified plaque is detected, high risk has been established. If the CAC is 0, a low radiation dose (approximately 1 mSv) prospectively gated coronary CT angiography to evaluate for noncalcified plaque may be considered. With the progressive decrease in radiation dose, coronary CT angiography in patients as young as the 20s may be reasonable in selected cases. Repeat scanning in 4 to 5 years is appropriate if the initial test is entirely normal.

Young Patients

FH aside, the incidence of CAC greater than 0 in the 33- to 45-year age group is 9.9%; the percentages increase with increasing FRS (**Table 5**). Although CAC scanning is not guideline recommended in this age group, it can be helpful in decision making on starting statin usage in these younger individuals.

CORONARY ARTERY CALCIUM SCANNING AND ADHERENCE

Reviewing the CAC images with asymptomatic patients has consistently led to increased adherence to acetylsalicylic acid (aspirin) (ASA), statins, diet, and exercise (**Table 6**).[30–32]

Table 5
Yield of screening for CAC in middle-aged adults based on the 10-year FRS: the CARDIA study

FRS	>0 (%)	NNS	>100 (%)	NNS
Total	9.9		1.8	
0%–2.5%	7.3	14	1.3	79
2.6%–5%	20.2	5	2.4	41
5.1%–10%	19.1	5	3.5	29
>10%	44.8	2	17.2	6
>5%	22.7	3.6		
>2.5%	23.0	4.3		

Asymptomatic patients: 2831; 33–45 years.
Abbreviations: CARDIA, Coronary Artery Risk Development in Young Adults; NNS, number needed to scan.
Reproduced with permission of Wiley from Hecht HS, Narula J. Coronary artery calcium scanning in asymptomatic patients with diabetes mellitus: A paradigm shift. J Diab 2012;4:342–50.

In the Early Identification of Subclinical Atherosclerosis by Noninvasive Imaging Research (EISNER) trial, asymptomatic patients were randomized to using CAC to guide treatment or employing usual care.[33] CAC-directed care produced significant improvement in systolic blood pressure, low-density lipoprotein cholesterol (LDL-C), weight, and waist size compared with usual care, without an increase in downstream testing. Patients with CAC greater than 400 had greater improvement than those with 0 CAC (**Table 7**).

SERIAL CORONARY ARTERY CALCIUM SCANNING

After the initial CAC scan, repeat scanning may be used to determine the response to treatment. A significant increase in plaque burden, as opposed to not achieving a specific LDL-C goal, defines treatment failure. Without tracking subclinical atherosclerosis, the only method for assessing treatment failure is the occurrence of an event or the development of symptoms, at which point it may be too late. The ability to identify treatment nonresponders by progressive excessive increases in CAC offers the opportunity to intervene with more aggressive treatment and possibly affect outcomes. The validity of this reasoning depends on demonstrating adverse outcomes

Table 6
Effect of coronary calcium on patient adherence

Author	N	Follow-up (y)	CAC	Statin	ASA	Diet	Exercise	Statin + ASA
Kalia et al,[30] 2006	505	3.6	>400	90%				
			100–400	75%				
			1–99	63%				
			0	44%				
Orakzai et al,[31] 2008	980	3	>400			61%	67%	56%
			0			29%	33%	44%
Schmermund et al,[32] 2008	1640	6	>0 vs 0	OR 3.5	OR 3.1			OR 7.0

Abbreviation: OR, odds ratio.
Data from Refs.[30–32]

Table 7 EISNER trial			
Parameters	CACS = 0	CACS >400	P
Change in LDL-C	−12 mg/dL	−29 mg/dL	<.001
Change in SBP	−4 mm Hg	−9 mm Hg	<.001
Exercise	32%	47%	.03
New lipid Rx	19%	65%	<.001
New BP Rx	20%	46%	<.001
New ASA Rx	5%	21%	<.001
Lipid adherence	80%	88%	.04

Middle-aged patients (2137; 45–79 years) without CVD; 4-year follow-up; CAC treatment-directed versus usual care.

Abbreviations: BP, blood pressure; Rx, prescription; SBP, systolic blood pressure.

From Rozanski A, Gransar H, Shaw LJ, et al. Impact of coronary artery calcium scanning on coronary risk factors and downstream testing: the EISNER (Early Identification of Subclinical Atherosclerosis by Noninvasive Imaging Research) prospective randomized trial. J Am Coll Cardiol 2011;57:1627; with permission.

with plaque progression. Otherwise, calcification of preexisting noncalcified plaque could be invoked to explain an absence of increased risk. The data uniformly support the significant direct relationship between CAC progression and coronary events. In the Multi-Ethnic Study of Atherosclerosis (MESA), development of CAC in patients with 0 baseline scores and increases in CAC in those with greater than 0 baseline scores were associated with a poorer prognosis directly related to the extent of CAC progression (**Fig. 8**).[34] Although there is greater average CAC progression on statins versus no statins, those who start with a 0 CAC score and progress at a rate of 5 AU/year or those starting with a score greater than 0 AU and progress at a rate of greater than or equal to 15%/year have a 40% to 60% increase in event rates versus those who progress at lower rates over a 7.5-year follow-up.

The deleterious effects of CAC progression are more pronounced in patients with diabetes; similar progression yielded greater decreases in event-free survival in those with compared with those without diabetes (**Fig. 9**).[35]

The CAC progression-related risk is more pronounced in patients with diabetes and the metabolic syndrome compared with those with the metabolic syndrome alone (**Fig. 10**).[36]

Greater progression in patients on statins (see **Fig. 8**)[34] might have suggested greater conversion of noncalcified to calcified plaque by the drug, but greater progression in patients with events on statins negates this theory and implies a therapeutic failure of statins to sufficiently halt the atherosclerotic process. This emphasizes the fallacy in conventional thinking that statin treatment must slow progression because it is well known that "statins save lives." Statin monotherapy, however, produces no greater than a 44% event reduction compared with placebo,[37–40] and there are no data demonstrating differences in attained LDL-C between treated patients with and without events.

Inadequate treatment is demonstrated in **Fig. 11**, with excessive progression of CAC despite dramatic improvement in lipid values.

Even for patients on moderate or high statin doses, there is usually room for improvement, whether by further increases in LDL-C–lowering drugs, or intensifying lifestyle modification, the need for which can only be determined by repeat scanning.

6778 Patients, 45-84 years old
2 Scans: baseline and 2.5 years later
7.6-Year follow-up: 343 total, 206 hard events

Hazard Ratio				Progression (AU)	
0 Baseline CAC n = 3396					
Events	Total	Hard		No statins	46.2/y
Per 5 AU/y	1.4	1.5		Statins	60.0/y
				P	<.001
>0 Baseline CAC n = 3382					
Per 100 AU/y	1.2	1.3		Events	
>300 AU/y	3.8	6.3		No statins	55.7/y
				Statins	119.3/y
<5%/y	1.0	1.0			
5%–14%/y	1.1	1.0			
15%–29%/y	1.6	1.4			
>30%/y	1.5	1.4			

Fig. 8. Coronary calcium progression and incident CHD events in MESA. (*Data from* Budoff MJ, Young R, Lopez VA. Progression of coronary calcium and incident coronary heart disease events: MESA [Multi-Ethnic Study of Atherosclerosis]. J Am Coll Cardiol 2013;61(12):1236, 1237.)

296 Asymptomatic patients with DM
300 Controls
59±6 years, 29% women
Scan interval 1–2 years
Follow-up 56±11 months

Event-Free Survival		
ΔCAC	DM	No DM
<10%	97.9%	100%
10%–20%	95.9%	97.2%
21%–30%	92.7%	94%
>30%	79.6%	90.6%

Death HR: DM vs Controls (N=596)			
ΔCAC	Matched Control Group	DM	P
10%–20% vs <10%	1.0	1.88	0.0001
21%–30% vs <10%	1.0	2.29	0.0001
>30% vs <10%	1.0	6.95	0.0001

*Adjusted for age, gender, HTN, HLP, FH of CHD, baseline CAC, and smoking

Fig. 9. Impact of CAC progression on outcome in subjects with and without diabetes. DM, diabetes mellitus; HLP, hyperlipidemia; HTN, hypertension. (*Data from* Kiramijyan S, Ahmadi N, Isma'eel H, et al. Impact of coronary artery calcium progression and statin therapy on clinical outcome in subjects with and without diabetes. Am J Cardiol 2013;111:358, 359.)

5662 Patients, 51% Female, 61.0 + 10.3 years, 4.9-year follow-up
2 Scans 2.4 years apart: 2927—0 baseline CAC
2735—>0 baseline CAC

RR for Events Related to CAC Progression			
	o Prog	2nd Tertile	3rd Tertile
+MetS/–DM	1	2.3	4.1
+MetS/+DM	1	4.1	8.5
P		<.05	<.05

Fig. 10. Metabolic syndrome, DM, and incidence and progression of CAC: MESA. DM, diabetes mellitus; MetS, metabolic syndrome. (*Data from* Wong ND, Nelson JC, Granston T, et al. Metabolic syndrome, diabetes, and incidence and progression of coro-nary calcium: the Multiethnic Study of Atherosclerosis [MESA]. JACC Cardiovasc Imaging 2012;5:363, 364.)

Continued progression in the setting of truly maximal treatment serves to identify patients who should be educated regarding the warning signs of acute coronary syndromes.

Asymptomatic patients with a 0 CAC score should not undergo repeat scanning for at least 4 years. The average time to conversion to a greater than 0 CAC was 4.1 ± 0.9 years and the average score at the time of conversion was 19 ± 19.[41]

The repeat scanning interval in patients with greater than 0 CAC is not data determined. Rather, logic dictates that the greater the concern, the shorter should be the interval. It seems reasonable to rescan after 2 years for CAC greater than 400 or greater than 75th percentile, with 3- or 4-year intervals for lower scores. The low radiation dose makes repeat scanning less problematic.

POST–CORONARY ARTERY CALCIUM SCANNING TESTING

The appropriateness of stress testing after CAC scanning in asymptomatic patients is directly related to the CAC score. The data indicate that the incidence of abnormal

43-year-old asymptomatic man, father, MI 41

		Baseline	2 y
Lipids:	TC	244	163
	LDL	149	92
	HDL	39	52
	TG	280	94
Plaque:	Calcium score	12	56
	Calcium percentile	**75**	**89**
Treatment:	Statin	None	20 mg
	Niacin	None	2000 mg

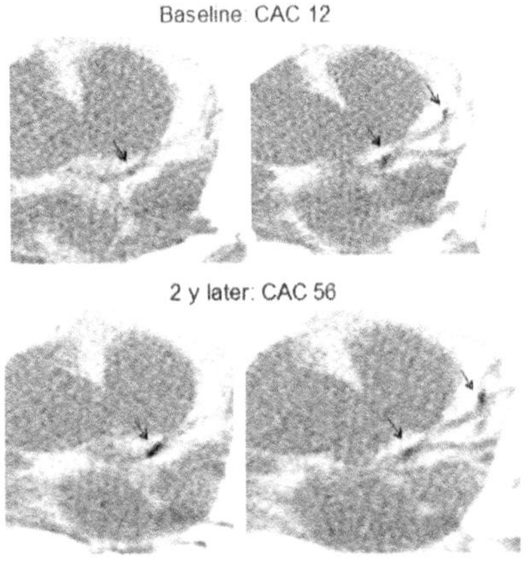

Baseline CAC 12

2 y later: CAC 56

Fig. 11. Progression of coronary artery calcium demonstrating inadequate treatment. MI, myocardial infarction.

nuclear stress testing is 1.3%, 11.3%, and 35.2% for CAC scores of less than 100, 100 to 400, and greater than 400, respectively.[42–46] It is only in the greater than 400 group that the pretest likelihood is sufficiently high to warrant further evaluation with functional testing. Coronary CT angiography is appropriate in patients with CAC less than 1000; higher CAC scores may preclude accurate evaluation. It is never appropriate to proceed directly to the catheterization laboratory in asymptomatic patients.

Evaluation of incidental findings, in particular lung nodules, should follow standard radiology guidelines.[47]

CORONARY ARTERY CALCIUM SCANNING AND THE 2013 GUIDELINES

The 2010 ACCF/AHA Guideline for Assessment of Cardiovascular Risk in Asymptomatic Adults appropriately assigned a class IIa recommendation to CAC for evaluation of the asymptomatic intermediate-risk population and for all patients older than 40 with diabetes mellitus.[21] The 2013 American College of Cardiology (ACC)/AHA Guideline on the Treatment of Blood Cholesterol to Reduce Atherosclerotic Cardiovascular Risk in Adults[48] and the 2013 ACC/AHA Guideline on the Assessment of Cardiovascular Risk[49] have reversed course and downgraded CAC to a class IIb recommendation. Assuming that the goal of guidelines is to use the most powerful predictors of risk to direct treatment, it is difficult to understand how the most powerful risk predictor (ie, CAC) has been downgraded from earlier documents rather than further upgraded based on robust data published after the 2010 ACCF/AHA guideline.[21] The explanations for the downgrading of CAC to class IIb can only be understood as follows:

1. The outcomes on which the 2013 guidelines were based were changed by the addition of stroke, for which the investigators believed there was not sufficient CAC data, even though the Heinz Nixdorf Recall Study of 4180 patients demonstrated hazard ratios of CAC for stroke to be similar to age, hypertension, and smoking (**Table 8**).[50]

Consequently, the CAC data for coronary risk was essentially discarded and the recommendation lowered to IIb.

Table 8
Coronary artery calcium is an independent predictor of stroke in the general population: the Heinz Nixdorf Recall Study

	CAC	
	CVA	No CVA
Median	104.8	11.2
Q1;Q3	14.0;482.2	0;106.2
P		<.001

	Hazard Ratio	P
log10 (CAC + 1)	1.52	.001
Age/5 y	1.35	<.001
SBP/10 mm	1.25	<.001
Smoking	1.75	.025

Patients: 4180; 45–75 years; 47.1% men; 94.9 ± 19–month follow-up.
Data from Hermann DM, Gronewold J, Lehmann N, et al, Heinz Nixdorf Recall Study Investigative Group. Coronary artery calcification is an independent stroke predictor in the general population. Stroke 2013;44:1008–13.

2. Erroneous cost and radiation exposure concerns were also invoked to justify the IIb classification. In reality, the cost of CAC scanning has dramatically decreased to the approximately $100 level, and a recent analysis demonstrated that treating 7.5% 10-year risk patients with statins at a $1/pill cost who had CAC greater than 0 resulted in cost per quality-adjusted life year saved of $18,000 compared with $78,000 for risk factor assessment alone.[51] The radiation issue has become less relevant as the dosage has progressively decreased to 1 mSv or less.

3. The guidelines noted that the class IIb recommendation is consistent with the recommendations in the 2010 ACCF/AHA guideline for patients with a 10-year coronary heart disease (CHD); risk of less than 10%.[21] It is totally inconsistent, however, with the class IIa 2010 guideline recommendation for the 10% to 20% group,[21] which is now excluded from CAC evaluation because they will all receive statins by the new recommendations. It is precisely this large group for which the NRI by CAC in 3 major population-based prospective outcome studies[11,15,16] has ranged from 52% to 66% (see **Table 3**). Moreover, as demonstrated in every outcome study comparing CAC to conventional risk factor–based assessment, CAC is superior to risk factors.

4. The most persistent criticism of CAC has been the absence of randomized controlled trials (RCTs) that demonstrate its ability to improve outcomes. The 2013 guidelines acknowledge, however, that their new risk assessment paradigm has also not been formally evaluated in randomized controlled trials.

In summary, the 2013 guidelines, under the mantle of dedication to RCTs, have presented a non–RCT-validated risk assessment paradigm, which is erroneous in at least 50% of the 7.5% to 20% 10-year risk group, and have downgraded CAC to a IIb recommendation for whom only those few patients who are not in their 4 primary risk categories will be eligible. Consequently, with respect to CAC, the 2010 guideline, rather than the 2013 guidelines, should be implemented.

CORONARY ARTERY CALCIUM SCANNING LIMITATIONS

1. CAC is not a perfect test and events do occur in the setting of a 0 CAC. Only 5% of acute myocardial infarctions or unstable angina occur, however, in both younger (mean age 47 years) and older (mean age 57 years) patients with a 0 CAC (**Fig. 12**).[52,53]
   In asymptomatic patients with 0 CAC, the incidence of obstructive CAD is less than 1%; in patients with chest pain and 0 CAC, it is approximately 5%.

2. Radiation is no longer a significant issue because the absorbed radiation dose falls to the level of mammography. Unfortunately, irresponsible scare tactics have magnified public concern; education is needed to counter these negative effects.

3. Cost has also become less of a concern as the price of CAC scanning has plummeted to approximately $100. As discussed previously, cost-effectiveness analyses highly favor CAC.

4. Incidentalomas and their subsequent evaluation have generated negative sentiments. The frequency of clinically significant findings is 1.2%, with indeterminate findings at 7.0%.[54] The associated costs do not have a negative impact on the cost effectiveness of CAC.[51] Standard guidelines on how to handle these findings may reassure patients and physicians.[47]

5. Patient anxiety related to CAC findings has also been cited as a negative. Anxiety is not an intended consequence but a certain amount is appropriate and inevitable

114 Patients: MI (97) or UA (17)
Age: 57 ± 11 y

102 Patients < 60 with MI
Age: 41 ± 7 y

% of ASHD Patients

Calcium Present

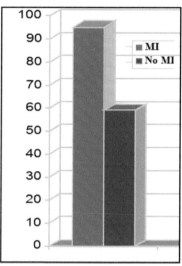

Fig. 12. Coronary calcium in patients with first myocardial infarction (MI) or unstable angina (UA). (*Data from* Schmermund A, Baumgart D, Görge G, et al. Coronary artery calcium in acute coronary syndromes: a comparative study of electron-beam computed tomography, coronary angiography, and intracoronary ultrasound in survivors of acute myocardial infarction and unstable angina. Circulation 1997;96:1465, with permission; and Pohle K, Ropers D, Mäffert R, et al. Coronary calcifications in young patients with first, unheralded myocardial infarction: a risk factor matched analysis by electron beam tomography. Heart 2003;89:627.)

when informed of increased cardiac risk and may motivate increased adherence. On the other hand, for those with high anxiety of early arteriosclerotic cardiovascular disease (ASCVD) based on a severe FH or a high calculated ASCVD risk score, concern can often be calmed when reclassified toward significantly less risk by CAC.

SUMMARY

The potential impact of CAC on primary prevention cannot be overestimated. It eliminates the guesswork implicit in extrapolating risk from guidelines derived from large population bases to individual patients and provides a snapshot of the cumulative effect of an individual's life on the coronary circulation. The role of risk factors is most important in identifying treatable therapeutic targets after risk has been established by a test that is 100% specific for atherosclerosis and far superior to any risk factor–based paradigm. The remaining barriers include physician education to overcome instinctive clinging to the old established paradigms, patient education to increase awareness of the widespread availability and low radiation of CAC, and more widespread insurance reimbursement.

REFERENCES

1. Canto JG, Kiefe CI, Rogers WJ, et al. Number of coronary heart disease risk factors and mortality in patients with first myocardial infarction. JAMA 2011;306: 2120–7.
2. Arad Y, Spadaro LA, Goodman K, et al. Prediction of coronary events with electron beam computed tomography. J Am Coll Cardiol 2000;36:1253–60.
3. Park R, Robert Detrano R, Xiang M, et al. Combined use of computed tomography coronary calcium scores and C-reactive protein levels in predicting cardiovascular events in nondiabetic individuals. Circulation 2002;106:2073–7.
4. Raggi P, Callister TQ, Cooil B, et al. Identification of patients at increased risk of first unheralded acute myocardial infarction by electron beam computed tomography. Circulation 2000;101:850–5.
5. Wong ND, Hsu JC, Detrano RC, et al. Coronary artery calcium evaluation by electron beam compute tomography and its relation to new cardiovascular events. Am J Cardiol 2000;86:495–8.
6. Kondos GT, Hoff JA, Sevrukov A, et al. Electron-beam tomography coronary artery calcium and cardiac events: a 37-month follow-up of 5,635 initially asymptomatic low to intermediate risk adults. Circulation 2003;107:2571–6.
7. Greenland P, LaBree L, Azen SP, et al. Coronary artery calcium score combined with Framingham score for risk prediction in asymptomatic individuals. JAMA 2004;291:10.
8. Shaw LJ, Raggi P, Schisterman E, et al. Prognostic value of cardiac risk factors and coronary artery calcium screening for all- cause mortality. Radiology 2003; 28:826–33.
9. Arad Y, Goodman KJ, Roth M, et al. Coronary calcification, coronary risk factors, and atherosclerotic cardiovascular disease events. The St Francis Heart Study. J Am Coll Cardiol 2005;46(1):158–65.
10. Taylor AJ, Bindeman J, Feuerstein I, et al. Coronary calcium independently predicts incident premature coronary heart disease over measured cardiovascular risk factors mean three-year out- comes in the Prospective Army Coronary Calcium (PACC) project. J Am Coll Cardiol 2005;46:807–14.
11. Vliegenthart R, Oudkerk M, Song B, et al. Coronary calcification detected by electron-beam computed tomography and myocardial infarction. The Rotterdam Coronary Calcification Study. Eur Heart J 2002;23:1596–603.
12. Budoff MJ, Shaw LJ, Liu ST, et al. Long-term prognosis associated with coronary calcification. Observations from a registry of 25, 253 patients. J Am Coll Cardiol 2007;49:1860–70.
13. Lakoski SG, Greenland P, Wong ND, et al. Coronary artery calcium scores and risk for cardiovascular events in women classified as "Low Risk" based on Framingham risk score. The Multi-Ethnic Study of Atherosclerosis (MESA). Arch Intern Med 2007;167(22):2437–42.
14. Becker A, Leber A, Becker C, et al. Predictive value of coronary calcifications for future cardiac events in asymptomatic individuals. Am Heart J 2008;155: 154–60.
15. Detrano R, Guerci AD, Carr JJ, et al. Coronary calcium as a predictor of coronary events in four racial or ethnic groups. N Engl J Med 2008;358:1336–45.
16. Erbel R, Möhlenkamp S, Moebus S, et al. Coronary risk stratification, discrimination, and reclassification improvement based on quantification of subclinical coronary atherosclerosis. The Heinz Nixdorf Recall Study. J Am Coll Cardiol 2010;56:1397–406.

17. Taylor AJ, Fiorillia PN, Hongyan W, et al. Relation between the Framingham risk score, coronary calcium, and incident coronary heart disease among low-risk men. Am J Cardiol 2010;106:47–50.

18. Nasir K, Rubin J, Blaha MJ, et al. Interplay of coronary artery calcification and traditional risk factors for the prediction of all-cause mortality in asymptomatic individuals. Circ Cardiovasc Imaging 2012;5:467–73.

19. Yeboah J, McClelland RL, Polonsky TS, et al. Comparison of novel risk markers for improvement in cardiovascular risk assessment in intermediate-risk individuals. JAMA 2012;308:788–95.

20. Rana JS, Gransar H, Wong ND, et al. Comparative value of coronary artery calcium and multiple blood biomarkers for prognostication of cardiovascular events. Am J Cardiol 2012;109:1449–53.

21. Greenland P, Alpert JS, Beller GA, et al. 2010 ACCF/AHA Guideline for assessment of cardiovascular risk in adults. A report of the American College of Cardiology Foundation/American Heart Association Task Force on Practice Guidelines. J Am Coll Cardiol 2010;56:e50–103.

22. Wong ND, Sciammarella MG, Polk D, et al. The metabolic syndrome, diabetes, and subclinical atherosclerosis assessed by coronary calcium. J Am Coll Cardiol 2003;41:1547–53.

23. Becker A, Leber A, Becker B, et al. Predictive value of coronary calcifications for future cardiac events in asymptomatic patients with diabetes mellitus: prospective study in 716 patients over 8 years. BMC Cardiovasc Disord 2008;27:1–8.

24. Elkeles R, Godsland IF, Feher MD, et al. Coronary cal- cium measurement improves prediction of cardiovascular events in asymptomatic patients with type 2 diabetes: the PREDICT study. Eur Heart J 2008;29:2244–51.

25. Anand DV, Lim E, Hopkins D, et al. Risk stratification in uncomplicated type 2 diabetes: prospective evaluation of the combined use of coronary artery calcium imaging and selective myocardial perfusion scintigraphy. Eur Heart J 2006;27:713–21.

26. Malik S, Budoff M, Katz R. Impact of subclinical atherosclerosis on cardiovascular disease events in individuals with metabolic syndrome and diabetes: the multi-ethnic study of atherosclerosis. Diabetes Care 2011;34:2285–90.

27. Kashani M, Eliasson A, Vernalis M, et al. Improving assessment of cardiovascular disease risk by using family history. J Cardiovasc Nurs 2013;28:E18–27.

28. Taylor A, Cerqueira M, Hodgson JM, et al. Appropriate use criteria for cardiac computed tomography. J Am Coll Cardiol 2010;56:1864–94.

29. Okwuosa TM, Greenland P, Burke GL, et al. Prediction of coronary artery calcium progression in individuals with low Framingham risk score: the multi-ethnic study of atherosclerosis. JACC Cardiovasc Imaging 2012;5:923–30.

30. Kalia NK, Miller LG, Nasir K, et al. Visualizing coronary calcium is associated with improvements in adherence to statin therapy. Atherosclerosis 2006;185:394–9.

31. Orakzai RH, Nasir K, Orakzai SH, et al. Effect of patient visualization of coronary calcium by electron beam computed tomography on changes in beneficial lifestyle behaviors. Am J Cardiol 2008;101:999–1002.

32. Schmermund A, Baumgart A, Taylor AJ, et al. Community-based provision of statin and aspirin after the detection of coronary artery calcium within a community-based screening cohort. J Am Coll Cardiol 2008;51:1337–41.

33. Rozanski A, Gransar H, Shaw LJ, et al. Impact of coronary artery calcium scanning on coronary risk factors and downstream testing: the EISNER (Early Identification of Subclinical Atherosclerosis by Noninvasive Imaging Research) prospective randomized trial. J Am Coll Cardiol 2011;57:1622–32.

34. Budoff MJ, Young R, Lopez VA, et al. Progression of coronary calcium and incident coronary heart disease events: MESA (Multi-Ethnic Study of Atherosclerosis). J Am Coll Cardiol 2013;61:1231–9.

35. Kiramijyan S, Ahmadi N, Isma'eel H, et al. Impact of coronary artery calcium progression and statin therapy on clinical outcome in subjects with and without diabetes. Am J Cardiol 2013;111:356–61.

36. Wong ND, Nelson JC, Granston T, et al. Metabolic syndrome, diabetes, and incidence and progression of coro- nary calcium: the Multiethnic Study of Atherosclerosis (MESA). JACC Cardiovasc Imaging 2012;5:358–66.

37. Scandinavian Simvastatin Survival Study Group. Randomised trial of cholesterol lowering in 4444 patients with coronary heart disease: the Scandinavian SimvastatinSurvival Study (4S). Lancet 1994;344:1383–9.

38. Sacks FM, Moyé LA, Davis BR, et al. Relationship between plasma LDL concentrations during treatment with pravastatin and recurrent coronary events in the cholesterol and recurrent events trial. Circulation 1998;97:1446–52.

39. Prevention of cardiovascular events and death with pravastatin in patients with coronary heart disease and a broad range of initial cholesterol levels. The Long-Term Intervention with Pravastatin in Ischaemic Disease (LIPID) study group. N Engl J Med 1998;339:1349–57.

40. Ridker PM, Danielson E, Fonseca FA, et al. Rosuvastatin to prevent vascular events in men and women with elevated C-reactive protein. N Engl J Med 2008;359:2195–207.

41. Min JK, Lin FY, Gidseg DS, et al. Determinants of coronary calcium conversion among patients with a normal coronary calcium scan. What is the "warranty period" for remaining normal? J Am Coll Cardiol 2010;55:1110–7.

42. He ZX, Hedrick TD, Pratt CM, et al. Severity of coronary artery calcification by electron beam computed tomography predicts silent myocardial ischemia. Circulation 2000;101:244–51.

43. Moser KW, O'Keefe JH, Bateman TM, et al. Coronary calcium screening in asymptomatic patients as a guide to risk factor modification and stress myocardial perfusion imaging. J Nucl Cardiol 2003;10:590–8.

44. Berman DS, Wong ND, Gransar H, et al. Relationship between stress-induced myocardial ischemia and atherosclerosis measured by coronary calcium tomography. J Am Coll Cardiol 2004;44:923–30.

45. Anand DJ, Lim E, Raval U, et al. Prevalence of silent myocardial ischemia in asymptomatic individuals with subclinical atherosclerosis detected by electron beam tomography. J Nucl Cardiol 2004;11:450–7.

46. Su Min Chang SM, Faisal Nabi F, Xu J, et al. The coronary artery calcium score and stress myocardial perfusion imaging provide independent and complementary prediction of cardiac risk. J Am Coll Cardiol 2009;54:1872–82.

47. MacMahon H, Austin JH, Gamsu G, et al. Guidelines for management of small pulmonary nodules detected on CT scans: a statement from the Fleischner Society. Radiology 2005;237:395–400.

48. Stone NJ, Robinson J, Lichtenstein AH, et al. 2013 ACC/AHA guideline on the treatment of blood cholesterol to reduce atherosclerotic cardiovascular risk in adults. J Am Coll Cardiol 2013. http://dx.doi.org/10.1016/j.jacc.2013.11.002.

49. Goff DC Jr, Lloyd-Jones DM, Bennett G, et al. 2013 ACC/AHA guideline on the assessment of cardiovascular risk. J Am Coll Cardiol 2013. http://dx.doi.org/10.1016/j.jacc.2013.11.005.

50. Hermann DM, Gronewold J, Lehmann N, et al. Coronary artery calcification is an independent stroke predictor in the general population. Stroke 2013;44: 1008–13.
51. Pletcher MJ, Pignone M, Earnshaw S, et al. Using the coronary artery calcium score to guide statin therapy. A cost-effectiveness analysis. Circ Cardiovasc Qual Outcomes 2014;7:276–84.
52. Schmermund A, Baumgart D, Görge G, et al. Coronary artery calcium in acute coronary syndromes: a comparative study of electron-beam computed tomography, coronary angiography, and intracoronary ultrasound in survivors of acute myocardial infarction and unstable angina. Circulation 1997;96:1461–9.
53. Pohle K, Ropers D, Mäffert R, et al. Coronary calcifications in young patients with first, unheralded myocardial infarction: a risk factor matched analysis by electron beam tomography. Heart 2003;89:625–8.
54. MacHaalany J, Yeung Y, Ruddy TD, et al. Potential clinical and economic consequences of noncardiac incidental findings on cardiac computed tomography. J Am Coll Cardiol 2009;54:1533–4.

Dyslipidemia in Special Ethnic Populations

Jia Pu, PhD[a],*, Robert Romanelli, PhD[a], Beinan Zhao, MS[a],
Kristen M.J. Azar, RN, MSN, MPH[a], Katherine G. Hastings, BA[b],
Vani Nimbal, MPH[a], Stephen P. Fortmann, MD[c],
Latha P. Palaniappan, MD, MS[b]

KEYWORDS

- Dyslipidemia • Racial/ethnic differences • Prevalence • Mortality • Treatment
- Lifestyle modification

KEY POINTS

- Among racial/ethnic groups, Asian Indians, Filipinos and Hispanics are at greater risk for dyslipidemia, which is consistent with the higher coronary heart disease (CHD) mortality rates.
- Compared with other racial/ethnic groups, statins may have a higher efficacy for Asians. Studies suggest lower starting dosage in Asians, but the data are mixed.
- Genetic differences in statin metabolism can in part explain this racial/ethnic difference in statin sensitivity and adverse effects.
- Lifestyle modification is recommended as part of dyslipidemia control and management; African Americans and Hispanics have more sedentary behavior and a less favorable diet profile.

INTRODUCTION

Dyslipidemia, including high levels of low-density lipoprotein cholesterol (LDL-C; $\geq$130 mg/dL), total cholesterol ($\geq$200 mg/dL), and triglycerides (TG; $\geq$150 mg/dL), or low levels of high-density lipoprotein cholesterol (HDL-C; <40 [men] and <50 [women] mg/dL), is among the leading risk factors for coronary heart disease (CHD) and stroke.[1] A report of the National Health and Nutrition Examination Survey

This article originally appeared in Cardiology Clinics, Volume 33, Issue 2, May 2015.

Conflicts of Interest: All authors declare they have no conflicts of interest.

[a] Palo Alto Medical Foundation Research Institute, Ames Building, 795 El Camino Real, Palo Alto, CA 94301, USA; [b] Stanford University School of Medicine, 1265 Welch Road, Stanford, CA 94305, USA; [c] Kaiser Permanente Center for Health Research, 3800 North Interstate Avenue, Portland, OR 97227, USA

* Corresponding author.

E-mail address: puj@pamfri.org

(NHANES) from 2003 to 2006 estimated that 53% (105.3 million) US adults have at least one lipid abnormality: 27% (53.5 million) have high LDL-C, 23% (46.4 million) have low HDL-C, and 30% (58.9 million) have high TG. In addition, 21% (42.0 million) of US adults have mixed dyslipidemia, defined as the presence of high LDL-C combined with at least one other lipid abnormality.[2]

Significant heterogeneity in patterns of dyslipidemia prevalence, its relation to CHD and stroke mortality rates, and response to lipid-lowering agents has been observed across racial/ethnic groups.[3] These differences in dyslipidemia provide important information that may in part explain the variation in cardiovascular disease (CVD) burden observed across racial/ethnic subgroups. Better understanding of dyslipidemia in special racial/ethnic populations is needed to guide prevention, screening, and treatment efforts.

PREVALENCE OF DYSLIPIDEMIA SUBTYPES AMONG SPECIAL RACIAL/ETHNIC GROUPS

The NHANES is the primary data source for national prevalence rates of dyslipidemia in the United States, sampling mainly non-Hispanic whites (whites), non-Hispanic blacks (blacks), and Mexican Americans. The NHANES has very limited samples from the Asian subgroups.[4] Other data sources, such as primary care settings and observational studies, contribute to a comprehensive picture of racial/ethnic differences in dyslipidemia by providing important information about races and ethnicities that are less represented in the NHANES. One should be aware that the prevalence of dyslipidemia varies by data source. The observed differences in the prevalence rates of dyslipidemia between studies can be attributable to factors such as study design, sampling methods, time period, geographic variation, and participants' characteristics.

Low-Density Lipoprotein Cholesterol

NHANES data in 2013 showed that the prevalence rate of high LDL-C was highest among Mexican men (40%) and women (30%), followed by non-Hispanic black men (33%) and women (31%). Non-Hispanic white men (30%) and women (29%) had the lowest prevalence of high LDL-C among the 3 racial/ethnic groups.[5]

Similarly, data from a clinic-based cohort in northern California from 2008 to 2011 showed that 63% of black men and 57% of black women had high LDL-C, which were slightly higher than the prevalence rates among non-Hispanic white men (62%) and women (53%).[3] Further, Mexican American men (66%) and women (57%) also had higher prevalence of high LDL-C compared with non-Hispanic whites.[3] Filipino men (73%) and women (63%) had the highest prevalence rates of high LDL-C among Asian subgroups, non-Hispanic whites, non-Hispanic blacks, and Hispanics.[3]

Several other studies provide further estimates for variation in prevalence among race/ethnic minority subgroups. Data from the Hispanic Community Health Study (HCHS)/Study of Latinos (SOL), an observational study in San Diego, Chicago, New York City, and Miami, showed variations among Hispanic subgroups with particularly high prevalence of dyslipidemia among Central American men (55%) and Puerto Rican women (41%).[6] The Study of Health Assessment and Health Risk in Ethnic groups (SHARE) investigated the prevalence of CHD risk factors for a multiethnic cohort from 3 Canadian cities. They found that South Asians, mainly Asian Indians, had an increased prevalence of higher total and LDL cholesterol compared with Europeans and Chinese.[7]

High-Density Lipoprotein Cholesterol

NHANES data in 2013 showed that 20% of black men and 10% of black women had low HDL-C, defined as less than 40 mg/dL in both men and women, which were lower than the prevalence rates among non-Hispanic white men (33%) and women (12%).[5] NHANES data also showed Mexican American men (34%) and women (15%) had higher prevalence of low HDL-C compared with non-Hispanic whites.[5] According to NHANES data from 2011 to 2012, 25% of Asian American men and 5% of Asian American women had low HDL-C.[8]

Although NHANES data showed Asian Americans had the lowest prevalence of low HDL-C as an aggregated group, data from a clinic-based cohort with disaggregated Asian ethnic groups in northern California between 2008 and 2011 found that Asian Indian men (53%) and women (55%) had the highest prevalence of low HDL-C among Asian American subgroups; their prevalence was also higher than Mexican American men (48%) and women (51%), non-Hispanic black men (34%) and women (40%), and non-Hispanic white men (36%) and women (31%).[3] Similarly, data from the SHARE study showed South Asians including Asian Indians had an increased prevalence of low HDL-C compared with Europeans and Chinese.[7]

Triglycerides

NHANES data from 1999 through 2008 showed 35% of Mexican Americans had high TG, followed by 33% among non-Hispanic whites, and 16% among non-Hispanic blacks.[9] Data from a clinic-based cohort in northern California from 2008 to 2011 found that Filipino men (60%) and Mexican women (45%) had the highest prevalence of high TG, compared with Mexican men (56%) and Filipino women (42%), Asian Indian men (55%) and women (37%), non-Hispanic white men (43%) and women (28%), and non-Hispanic black men (30%), and women (18%).[3] Data from the SHARE study showed South Asians had the highest prevalence of high TG among South Asians, Chinese, and Europeans.[7]

Potential explanations for racial/ethnic differences in dyslipidemia prevalence have been explored by several studies. In the Multi-Ethnic Study of Atherosclerosis (MESA), researchers found that ethnic disparities were substantially attenuated by adjusting for access to health care.[10] The racial/ethnic differences could also be related to lifestyle, genetic, and cultural differences associated with total and LDL-C concentrations.[11] For example, the predilection of South Asians to have lower HDL-C levels has been attributed to the higher prevalence of insulin resistance and related metabolic abnormalities, which may be the consequence of a combination of genetic predisposition, physical inactivity, and a high carbohydrate diet.[12–14]

DYSLIPIDEMIA-RELATED MORTALITY IN SPECIAL RACIAL/ETHNIC GROUPS

Dyslipidemia often results in an increased risk of premature atherosclerosis, a major risk factor for CHD.[15] CHD is the leading cause of mortality for both men and women in the United States and worldwide, with increasing evidence of gender and racial/ethnic minority disparities in CHD morbidity and mortality.[16–19] Despite declines in CHD death rates over the past decades, CHD contributes to more than one-third of all deaths for those over the age of 35 years.[20]

Differences in mortality rate from CHD have been found across races/ethnicities. In the United States, CHD mortality rates are highest in blacks, intermediate in whites and Hispanics, and lowest in some Asian subgroups.[15,21,22] These CHD rates are paralleled with observed racial/ethnic disparities in dyslipidemia prevalence, with higher

CHD rates seen in Hispanics and blacks, potentially owing to limited health care access and other less favorable behavioral factors seen in these groups.[10]

Meanwhile, although traditionally known as the "model minority," disproportionate mortality burden owing to CHD and stroke has been shown among certain Asian subgroups, such as Asian Indians, Filipinos, and Japanese.[23,24] Of note, the landmark Ni-Hon-San study showed increased CHD mortality rates and decreased stroke rates among Japanese-American men compared with rates in Japan, suggesting a differential disease impact of acculturation to Westernized lifestyles.[25] A recent study found higher proportional mortality owing to CHD among Asian Indians, especially in younger age groups, compared with all other racial/ethnic groups.[17] Increased burden from CHD mortality has been well-documented in both native and immigrant Asian Indian populations.[7,26,27] This observation is consistent with the higher prevalence rates of dyslipidemia (especially low HDL-C) in Asian Indians compared with other Asian subgroups and non-Hispanic whites in the United States.[3,7,28]

Environmental and social factors (eg, acculturation, socioeconomic status, diet) have been known to increase CHD mortality risk.[29,30] Cultural diets high in fat, increasing the risk for dyslipidemia, are also of concern.[31] Differences in susceptibility to CHD may also have a genetic basis, although this has not been determined adequately yet. Thus, it is critical for clinicians to modify lipid management appropriately among these rapidly growing populations.

TREATMENT OF DYSLIPIDEMIA
Overview

There are several US Food and Drug Administration (FDA)-approved 3-hydroxy-3-methyl-glutaryl-coenzyme A reductase inhibitors (statins) and a variety of nonstatin therapies available for the treatment of dyslipidemia, including bile acids sequestrants, cholesterol absorption inhibitors, fibrates, niacin, and omega-3 fatty acids. Statins are the most widely prescribed treatment for dyslipidemia, and one of the most commonly prescribed drugs in the United States.[32] In the most recent national cholesterol treatment guidelines, published in November 2013 by the American College of Cardiology (ACC)/American Heart Association (AHA),[1] the Expert Panel determined from robust clinical trial data that statins have the most acceptable CVD risk reduction benefit and side effect profile, and that the addition of nonstatin therapy does not seem to provide further benefit in reducing CVD. Clinical trials on which cholesterol treatment guidelines are based have often underrepresented racial/ethnic minority groups. Accordingly, our knowledge of optimal statin treatment regimens, and the effectiveness, tolerability, and safety of these regimens in clinical practice, is limited across diverse racial/ethnic populations.

Racial/Ethnic Differences in Risk Stratification

The most recent ACC/AHA guidelines expand the criteria for patients who would benefit from statin treatment, and more than 80% of newly eligible patients are expected to have no prior CVD.[33] Therefore, they would be assessed for optimal statin treatment based on the new Atherosclerotic CVD (ASCVD) Risk Estimator.[33] This estimator is intended to improve on previous CVD risk estimators, including the Framingham[34] and Adult Treatment Panel III[35] risk algorithms. It was derived from several longitudinal epidemiologic cohort studies of non-Hispanic whites and blacks, and was validated externally in 2 cohort studies with similar populations (MESA and REGARDS),[36] as well as in contemporary samples of the derivation cohorts. However, studies among other race/ethnic minority groups are lacking. The ACC/AHA Work

Group, which developed the algorithm for the ASCVD Risk Estimator, acknowledges that it should be used only in men and women of non-Hispanic white or non-Hispanic black decent, and that it may not accurately predict risk in other racial/ethnic groups.[37] Specifically, there is concern of overestimation of risk in Mexican Americans and East Asians and underestimation of risk in other groups, such as Puerto Ricans and South Asians.[37,38] Other countries with diverse racial/ethnic minority populations, such as the United Kingdom, have validated algorithms predicting risk for more than 9 specific racial/ethnic subpopulations (available at: http://qrisk.org/).[39]

Race/Ethnic Differences in Statin Response

Statin metabolism and drug sensitivity

Much of the data on race/ethnic differences in statin metabolism have shown that some Asian subgroups are slower to metabolize statins compared with non-Hispanic whites, which leads to higher systemic drug concentrations. Pharmacokinetic studies indicate rosuvastatin plasma concentrations are 2-fold higher in Japanese relative to non-Hispanic white individuals. Rosuvastatin plasma concentrations have been shown to be elevated similarly in other Asian subgroups; these included Chinese, Malay, and Asian Indians, whose rosuvastatin concentrations were approximately 2 times higher relative to Caucasians.[40]

There are several genetic variants associated with altered statin metabolism. Such variants include, but are not limited to, single nucleotide polymorphisms in the genes that encode the organic anion-transporting polypeptide (OATP)1B1 (521T> C), which regulates hepatic uptake of statins, and the adenosine triphosphate-binding cassette G2 (ABCG2) transporter (421C> A), which regulates hepatic efflux.[41,42] Variants of both genes are associated with increased statin plasma concentrations within multiple race/ethnic groups.[41–44] 421C> A has been found to be a single nucleotide polymorphism candidate to explain the observed racial differences in statin metabolism: the allelic frequency of 421C> A in ABCG2 is higher in Chinese ($\sim$35%) relative to Caucasians (9%–14%).[43,45]

Higher plasma levels of statins in Asians compared with non-Hispanic whites has led to concern about increased risk for statin-induced side effects in this population. Such concerns have led to a revised package insert recommending lower starting doses of rosuvastatin in this population (5 vs 10 mg for non-Hispanic whites).[46] Notably, in Japan, starting doses for most statins are one-half of what is recommended in the United States.[47]

There is less information on statin metabolism in other racial/ethnic minority groups. We are aware of 1 study that evaluated the pharmacokinetics of single-dose pravastatin in non-Hispanic blacks versus European Americans.[44] In this study, the OATP1B1 521T> C polymorphism was associated significantly with higher statin plasma concentrations in subjects of European versus African ancestry.[44] This may be explained by the low allelic frequency of OATP1B1 521T> C in non-Hispanic blacks ($\sim$1%)[44] relative to non-Hispanic whites. To our knowledge, no studies have been published on the pharmacokinetics of statins in Hispanics.

Myalgia (muscle pain) is one of the most commonly observed side effects associated with statins, but has been reported to occur at varying frequencies (5%–20%) in randomized controlled trials (RCT) and observational studies.[48–50] More severe but rare muscle side effects have also been reported, including myopathy (0.01%–0.3%) and rhabdomyolysis (0.003%–0.01%).[51] To date, high-dose simvastatin (80 mg) is the only statin to receive a US FDA warning for increased risk of muscle damage.[52] The use of statins in combination with other drugs has also been shown to increase the risk of adverse events.[53,54] In HPS2-THRIVE, which included 25,673 adults from Europe and China on simvastatin 40 mg/d, a higher risk of adverse events, including myopathy, were reported in patients randomized to niacin–laropiprant relative to placebo.[55] Furthermore, the relative risk of musculoskeletal events (mostly myopathy) in the niacin–laropiprant versus placebo group was markedly higher among Chinese participants than European participants.[55] To our knowledge no safety concerns have been raised for statins alone or in combination with agents in non-Hispanic blacks or Hispanics.

Statin efficacy in Asian populations

Studies conducted in Asian countries have documented that lower statin doses can achieve similar therapeutic effects in Asian populations.

- In an open-label study of Japanese patients receiving simvastatin (initial dose 5 mg/d), LDL-C decreased by 26% over 6 months, an effect that corresponds with simvastatin 20 mg/d in Western studies[56]
- In a multicenter, double-blind, RCT in 6 Asian countries, patients randomized to receive 10 mg simvastatin or atorvastatin daily over 8 weeks had an average LDL-C reduction of 35% and 43%, respectively, with more than 80% of patients achieving a National Cholesterol Education Program LDL-C target.[57] To see similar effects in non-Hispanic whites would generally require at least double this dose of simvastatin.
- In a prospective RCT of the primary prevention of CVD in Japan, pravastatin 10 to 20 mg/d reduced LDL-C by only 18% but reduced CHD by 33% relative to diet-alone[58]; this level of risk reduction in CVD is similar to trials of predominantly non-Hispanic white populations taking higher daily doses of pravastatin (40 mg)[59] or a higher potency statin (atorvastatin 10 mg/d).[60]

It is tempting to speculate that the apparently increased effect of statins in Asians relative to non-Hispanic whites is owing to genetic differences in statin metabolism; however, because comparisons in these studies were indirect and were conducted on ethnic populations outside of the United States or Europe, underlying cultural differences in diet and lifestyle cannot be ruled out as a causal factor.

In addition, other studies have failed to demonstrate differences in response to statins in Asian and non-Hispanic white populations.

- In a combined analysis of 2 small multicenter open-label studies, GOALLS (included non-Asian and Asian participants) and STATT (included Asians only), the authors compared cholesterol outcomes among patients with CHD treated with simvastatin for 14 weeks.[61] There were no differences in changes in LDL-C among Asians in the STATT study (n = 133; −45.4 mg/dL) relative to Asians (n = 15) or non-Asians (n = 183) in the GOALLS study (−41.1 and −41.2 mg/dL, respectively)[61]
- In an observational, prospective study in Canada, no difference in the magnitude of LDL-C lowering was observed among non-Hispanic whites and South Asians (−41% vs −43%, respectively; $P = .40$), taking atorvastatin or simvastatin (20 mg median dose for each) for more than 3 years in the secondary prevention of CVD[62]
- Using data from an RCT evaluating atorvastatin versus placebo in a multiethnic population in the UK, Chapman and colleagues[63] matched White (n = 198) and South Asian (n = 76) cohorts receiving atorvastatin to evaluate the effects of statins across race/ethnic groups. The authors again found no difference in

the percent reduction in LDL-C among whites and South Asians (-40% vs -39%; $P = .92$)[63]

To our best knowledge, no existing studies have shown differences in statin efficacy in non-Hispanic blacks, Hispanics, and non-Hispanic whites.[63–65]

Lifestyle Modification in Special Racial/Ethnic Groups

Lifestyle modification has been recommended to treat dyslipidemia and to reduce ASCVD risk, both before and in addition to the use of lipid-lowering agents.[1] These lifestyle risk factors include unhealthy diet, overweight and obesity, and physical inactivity. The AHA has the following specific recommendations for individuals with dyslipidemia[66]:

- Diet: increase the intake of vegetables, fruits, and whole grains and limit intake of sweets; reduce the intake of saturated fat and trans fat.
- Physical activity: engage in aerobic physical activity; three to four 40-minute sessions per week; moderate-to-vigorous intensity physical activity.

Racial/ethnic disparities also exist in these lifestyle risk factors. According to data from the Behavioral Risk Factor Surveillance System in 2002, non-Hispanic whites had more fruits and vegetables in their diet compared with Hispanics and non-Hispanic blacks.[6,67] According to the National Health Interview Survey for 2008 through 2010, 71% of Hispanics were overweight or obese, followed by non-Hispanic blacks (70%), non-Hispanic whites (62%), and Asian Americans (42%). In addition, National Health Interview Survey for 2008 through 2010 also found that, compared with non-Hispanic whites (20%), non-Hispanic black (17%), Asian American (16%), and Hispanic (13%) adults were less likely to meet the 2008 guidelines for aerobic and muscle strengthening through leisure time activity.[68] All these data indicate that both non-Hispanic blacks and Hispanics are at higher risk for having both diet and lifestyle risk factors, and Asian Americans are more likely to be physically inactive.

A recent systematic review included nutrition and physical activity intervention studies in adult African Americans, from 2000 to 2011.[69] This study found both diet and physical activity interventions for weight loss improved cholesterol clinical outcomes among African Americans.[69] In particular, it provided evidence to support interventions in community-based settings among African Americans. A 2011 systematic review included intervention studies that promote physical activity in Hispanic adults published between 1988 and 2011.[70] This study concluded that physical activity interventions in Hispanics should include community-based settings, social support strategy, culturally sensitive intervention design, and staff from the same ethnic group. A systemic review of RCTs of lifestyle interventions for Asian Americans published between 1995 and 2013 concluded that lifestyle interventions improved physical activity, healthy diet, and weight control in Asian Americans.[71] However, the studies included in this review were limited in cultural appropriateness. In particular, Asian subgroups were aggregated together although they have different cultures and health behavior patterns. Other recommendations include individual tailoring, education and modeling of lifestyle behaviors, and providing support during a maintenance phase.

Immigration and acculturation have a profound impact on lifestyle in both Hispanics and Asians in the United States. For example, traditional Hispanic diets contain high levels of fiber. However, studies found US-born Hispanics had a hard time retaining traditional diets and consumed more fat and sugar compared with their counterparts in their home countries.[72,73] They have less access to high nutritional quality foods and are at risk for overweight/obesity.[72,74] Similarly, traditional East Asian diets contain less total and saturated fat but more sodium intake compared with Western diets and Asian Indian diets.[75,76] However, Chinese immigrants who have lived in the United States for longer than 10 years had a more unhealthy diet and less physical activity compared with recent immigrants.[30] In contrast, higher acculturation levels were associated with more physical activity among Korean Americans.[77] Future studies should consider providing culturally tailored, ethnic-specific interventions to these diverse immigrant populations.

SUMMARY

There are significant racial/ethnic differences in dyslipidemia prevalence, dyslipidemia-related mortality rates, and response to lipid-lowering agents. Among all racial/ethnic groups, Asian Indians, Filipinos and Hispanics are at most elevated risk for dyslipidemia, which is consistent with the higher CHD mortality rates in these groups. More attention should be paid to these at-risk groups for screening and treatment purposes. Compared with other racial/ethnic groups, statins may have a higher efficacy for Asians, which may potentially be explained by genetic differences in statin metabolism, but overall the data are mixed. At present it may be wise to start with a lower statin dose in an individual with Asian ancestry until the treatment and adverse effects can be determined. In addition, racial/ethnic differences in health behavior patterns should be taken into consideration when promoting lifestyle modification among individuals with dyslipidemia. In particular, Hispanic subgroups (Mexican, Puerto Rican, etc) and Asian (Chinese, South Asian, etc) subgroups should be disaggregated in lifestyle interventions. Further studies are needed to better understand racial/ethnic-specific risk factors contributing to the observed differences in dyslipidemia, CHD, and stroke. Culturally tailored prevention and intervention should be provided to the minority populations with elevated risk for dyslipidemia and considerably more research is needed to determine the best approaches to helping specific subgroups.

REFERENCES

1. Stone NJ, Robinson J, Lichtenstein AH, et al. 2013 ACC/AHA guideline on the treatment of blood cholesterol to reduce atherosclerotic cardiovascular risk in adults: a report of the American College of Cardiology/American Heart Association task force on practice guidelines. Circulation 2014;129:S1–45.
2. Toth PP, Potter D, Ming EE. Prevalence of lipid abnormalities in the United States: the National Health and Nutrition Examination Survey 2003-2006. J Clin Lipidol 2012;6(4):325–30.
3. Frank AT, Zhao B, Jose PO, et al. Racial/ethnic differences in dyslipidemia patterns. Circulation 2014;129(5):570–9.
4. Holland AT, Palaniappan LP. Problems with the collection and interpretation of Asian-American health data: omission, aggregation, and extrapolation. Ann Epidemiol 2012;22(6):397–405.
5. Statistical fact sheet 2013 update: high blood cholesterol & other lipids. 2013. Available at: http://www.heart.org/idc/groups/heart-public/@wcm/@sop/@smd/documents/downloadable/ucm_319586.pdf. Accessed November 15, 2014.
6. Rodriguez CJ, Allison M, Daviglus ML, et al. Status of cardiovascular disease and stroke in Hispanics/Latinos in the United States: a science advisory from the

American Heart Association. Circulation 2014;130:593–625 (1524-4539 [Electronic]).

7. Anand SS, Yusuf S, Vuksan V, et al. Differences in risk factors, atherosclerosis and cardiovascular disease between ethnic groups in Canada: the Study of Health Assessment and Risk in Ethnic groups (SHARE). Indian Heart J 2000; 52(7 Suppl):S35–43.

8. Aoki Y, Yoon SS, Chong Y, et al. Hypertension, abnormal cholesterol, and high body mass index among non-Hispanic Asian adults: United States, 2011-2012. NCHS Data Brief 2014;(140):1–8.

9. Miller M, Stone NJ, Ballantyne C, et al. Triglycerides and cardiovascular disease: a scientific statement from the American Heart Association. Circulation 2011; 123(20):2292–333.

10. Goff DC Jr, Bertoni AG, Kramer H, et al. Dyslipidemia prevalence, treatment, and control in the Multi-Ethnic Study of Atherosclerosis (MESA): gender, ethnicity, and coronary artery calcium. Circulation 2006;113(5):647–56.

11. Huang MH, Schocken M, Block G, et al. Variation in nutrient intakes by ethnicity: results from the Study of Women's Health Across the Nation (SWAN). Menopause 2002;9(5):309–19.

12. McKeigue PM, Miller GJ, Marmot MG. Coronary heart disease in South Asians overseas: a review. J Clin Epidemiol 1989;42(7):597–609.

13. Chambers JC, Kooner JS. Diabetes, insulin resistance and vascular disease among Indian Asians and Europeans. Semin Vasc Med 2002;2(2):199–214.

14. Radhika G, Ganesan A, Sathya RM, et al. Dietary carbohydrates, glycemic load and serum high-density lipoprotein cholesterol concentrations among South Indian adults. Eur J Clin Nutr 2009;63(3):413–20.

15. Enas EA. Clinical implications: dyslipidemia in the Asian Indian population. 2002. Available at: https://southasianheartcenter.org/docs/AAPImonograph.pdf. Accessed November 15, 2014.

16. Roger VL, Go AS, Lloyd-Jones DM, et al. Heart disease and stroke statistics—2011 update: a report from the American Heart Association. Circulation 2011; 123(4):e18–209.

17. Jose PO, Frank AT, Kapphahn KI, et al. Cardiovascular disease mortality in Asian Americans (2003 to 2010). J Am Coll Cardiol 2014;64(23):2486–94.

18. Palaniappan L, Wang Y, Fortmann SP. Coronary heart disease mortality for six ethnic groups in California, 1990-2000. Ann Epidemiol 2004;14(7):499–506.

19. Keppel KG, Pearcy JN, Heron MP. Is there progress toward eliminating racial/ethnic disparities in the leading causes of death? Public Health Rep 2010; 125(5):689–97.

20. Farnier M, Chen E, Johnson-Levonas AO, et al. Effects of extended-release niacin/laropiprant, simvastatin, and the combination on correlations between apolipoprotein B, LDL cholesterol, and non-HDL cholesterol in patients with dyslipidemia. Vasc Health Risk Manag 2014;10:279–90.

21. Enas E, Yusuf S, Mehta J. Meeting of international working group on coronary artery disease in South Asians. Indian Heart J 1996;48:727–32.

22. Hoyert DL. 75 years of mortality in the United States, 1935-2010. NCHS Data Brief 2012;(88):1–8.

23. Ye J, Rust G, Baltrus P, et al. Cardiovascular risk factors among Asian Americans: results from a national health survey. Ann Epidemiol 2009;19(10):718–23.

24. Klatsky AL, Tekawa IS, Armstrong MA. Cardiovascular risk factors among Asian Americans. Public Health Rep 1996;111(Suppl 2):62–4.

25. Marmot MG, Syme SL, Kagan A, et al. Epidemiologic studies of coronary heart disease and stroke in Japanese men living in Japan, Hawaii and California: prevalence of coronary and hypertensive heart disease and associated risk factors. Am J Epidemiol 1975;102(6):514–25.
26. Balarajan R. Ethnic differences in mortality from ischaemic heart disease and cerebrovascular disease in England and Wales. BMJ 1991;302(6776): 560–4.
27. Enas EA, Garg A, Davidson MA, et al. Coronary heart disease and its risk factors in first-generation immigrant Asian Indians to the United States of America. Indian Heart J 1996;48(4):343–53.
28. Karthikeyan G, Teo KK, Islam S, et al. Lipid profile, plasma apolipoproteins, and risk of a first myocardial infarction among Asians: an analysis from the INTER-HEART Study. J Am Coll Cardiol 2009;53(3):244–53.
29. Marmot MG, Syme SL. Acculturation and coronary heart disease in Japanese-Americans. Am J Epidemiol 1976;104(3):225–47.
30. Taylor VM, Yasui Y, Tu SP, et al. Heart disease prevention among Chinese immigrants. J Community Health 2007;32(5):299–310.
31. Gupta M, Brister S. Is South Asian ethnicity an independent cardiovascular risk factor? Can J Cardiol 2006;22(3):193–7.
32. Bartholow M. Rx focus: top 200 drugs of 2012. Pharm Times 2012.
33. Pencina MJ, Navar-Boggan AM, D'Agostino RB Sr, et al. Application of new cholesterol guidelines to a population-based sample. N Engl J Med 2014; 370(15):1422–31.
34. D'Agostino RB Sr, Vasan RS, Pencina MJ, et al. General cardiovascular risk profile for use in primary care: the Framingham heart study. Circulation 2008;117(6): 743–53.
35. National Cholesterol Education Program (NCEP) Expert Panel on Detection, Evaluation, and Treatment of High Blood Cholesterol in Adults (Adult Treatment Panel III). Third report of the national cholesterol education program (NCEP) expert panel on detection, evaluation, and treatment of high blood cholesterol in adults (Adult treatment panel III) final report. Circulation 2002;106(25):3143–421.
36. Goff DC Jr, Lloyd-Jones DM, Bennett G, et al. 2013 ACC/AHA guideline on the assessment of cardiovascular risk: a report of the American College of Cardiology/American Heart Association Task Force on Practice Guidelines. J Am Coll Cardiol 2014;63(25 Pt B):2935–59.
37. Goff DC Jr, Lloyd-Jones DM. 2013 Report on the assessment of cardiovascular risk: full work group report supplement. 2013. Available at: http://jaccjacc.cardiosource.com/acc_documents/2013_FPR_S5_Risk_Assesment.pdf. Accessed May 22, 2014.
38. Stone NJ, Robinson JG, Lichtenstein AH. 2013 Report on the treatment of blood cholesterol to reduce atherosclerotic cardiovascular disease in adults: full panel report supplement. 2013. Available at: http://www.kcumb.edu/uploadedFiles/Content/Academics/_Assets/CME_Presentations/Moriarty12_5_full.pdf. Accessed May 23, 2014.
39. Hippisley-Cox J, Coupland C, Vinogradova Y, et al. Predicting cardiovascular risk in England and Wales: prospective derivation and validation of QRISK2. BMJ 2008;336(7659):1475–82.
40. Lee E, Ryan S, Birmingham B, et al. Rosuvastatin pharmacokinetics and pharmacogenetics in white and Asian subjects residing in the same environment. Clin Pharmacol Ther 2005;78(4):330–41.

41. Nishizato Y, Ieiri I, Suzuki H, et al. Polymorphisms of OATP-C (SLC21A6) and OAT3 (SLC22A8) genes: consequences for pravastatin pharmacokinetics. Clin Pharmacol Ther 2003;73(6):554–65.

42. Niemi M. Transporter pharmacogenetics and statin toxicity. Clin Pharmacol Ther 2010;87(1):130–3.

43. Zhang W, Yu BN, He YJ, et al. Role of BCRP 421C>A polymorphism on rosuvastatin pharmacokinetics in healthy Chinese males. Clin Chim Acta 2006;373(1–2): 99–103.

44. Ho RH, Choi L, Lee W, et al. Effect of drug transporter genotypes on pravastatin disposition in European- and African-American participants. Pharmacogenet Genomics 2007;17(8):647–56.

45. Keskitalo JE, Zolk O, Fromm MF, et al. ABCG2 polymorphism markedly affects the pharmacokinetics of atorvastatin and rosuvastatin. Clin Pharmacol Ther 2009; 86(2):197–203.

46. AstraZeneca. CRESTOR (rosuvastatin) prescribing information. 2014. Available at: http://www1.astrazeneca-us.com/pi/crestor.pdf. Accessed November 12, 2014.

47. Liao JK. Safety and efficacy of statins in Asians. Am J Cardiol 2007;99(3):410–4.

48. Bruckert E, Hayem G, Dejager S, et al. Mild to moderate muscular symptoms with high-dosage statin therapy in hyperlipidemic patients–the PRIMO study. Cardiovasc Drugs Ther 2005;19(6):403–14.

49. Stewart A. SLCO1B1 polymorphisms and statin-induced myopathy. PLOS Currents Evidence on Genomic Tests December 4, 2013. Edition 1. http://dx.doi.org/10.1371/currents.eogt.d21e7f0c58463571bb0d9d3a19b82203.

50. Fung EC, Crook MA. Statin myopathy: a lipid clinic experience on the tolerability of statin rechallenge. Cardiovasc Ther 2012;30(5):e212–8.

51. Law M, Rudnicka AR. Statin safety: a systematic review. Am J Cardiol 2006; 97(8A):52C–60C.

52. FDA drug safety communication: new restrictions, contraindications, and dose limitations for Zocor (simvastatin) to reduce the risk of muscle injury. 2011. Available at: http://www.fda.gov/Drugs/DrugSafety/ucm256581.htm. Accessed November 15, 2014.

53. Thompson PD, Clarkson P, Karas RH. Statin-associated myopathy. JAMA 2003; 289(13):1681–90.

54. Pasternak RC, Smith SC Jr, Bairey-Merz CN, et al. ACC/AHA/NHLBI clinical advisory on the use and safety of statins. J Am Coll Cardiol 2002;40(3):567–72.

55. Group HT, Landray MJ, Haynes R, et al. Effects of extended-release niacin with laropiprant in high-risk patients. N Engl J Med 2014;371(3):203–12.

56. Matsuzawa Y, Kita T, Mabuchi H, et al. Sustained reduction of serum cholesterol in low-dose 6-year simvastatin treatment with minimum side effects in 51,321 Japanese hypercholesterolemic patients. Circ J 2003;67(4):287–94.

57. Wu CC, Sy R, Tanphaichitr V, et al. Comparing the efficacy and safety of atorvastatin and simvastatin in Asians with elevated low-density lipoprotein-cholesterol–a multinational, multicenter, double-blind study. J Formos Med Assoc 2002;101(7): 478–87.

58. Nakamura H, Arakawa K, Itakura H, et al. Primary prevention of cardiovascular disease with pravastatin in Japan (MEGA Study): a prospective randomised controlled trial. Lancet 2006;368(9542):1155–63.

59. Shepherd J, Cobbe SM, Ford I, et al. Prevention of coronary heart disease with pravastatin in men with hypercholesterolemia. West of Scotland coronary prevention study group. N Engl J Med 1995;333(20):1301–7.

60. Colhoun HM, Betteridge DJ, Durrington PN, et al. Primary prevention of cardiovascular disease with atorvastatin in type 2 diabetes in the Collaborative Atorvastatin Diabetes Study (CARDS): multicentre randomised placebo-controlled trial. Lancet 2004;364(9435):685–96.

61. Morales D, Chung N, Zhu JR, et al. Efficacy and safety of simvastatin in Asian and non-Asian coronary heart disease patients: a comparison of the GOALLS and STATT studies. Curr Med Res Opin 2004;20(8):1235–43.

62. Gupta M, Braga MF, Teoh H, et al. Statin effects on LDL and HDL cholesterol in South Asian and white populations. J Clin Pharmacol 2009;49(7):831–7.

63. Chapman N, Chang CL, Caulfield M, et al. Ethnic variations in lipid-lowering in response to a statin (EVIREST): a substudy of the Anglo-Scandinavian Cardiac Outcomes Trial (ASCOT). Ethn Dis 2011;21(2):150–7.

64. Albert MA, Glynn RJ, Fonseca FA, et al. Race, ethnicity, and the efficacy of rosuvastatin in primary prevention: the justification for the use of statins in prevention: an intervention trial evaluating rosuvastatin (JUPITER) trial. Am Heart J 2011; 162(1):106–14.e102.

65. Lipworth L, Fazio S, Kabagambe EK, et al. A prospective study of statin use and mortality among 67,385 blacks and whites in the Southeastern United States. Clin Epidemiol 2014;6:15–25.

66. Eckel RH, Jakicic JM, Ard JD, et al. 2013 AHA/ACC guideline on lifestyle management to reduce cardiovascular risk: a report of the American College of Cardiology/AMERICAN HEART ASSOCIATION Task Force on Practice Guidelines. J Am Coll Cardiol 2014;63:2960–84 (1524–4539 (Electronic)).

67. Behavioral risk factor surveillance system: BRFSS 2002 survey data and documentation. Available at: http://www.cdc.gov/brfss/annual_data/annual_2002. htm. Accessed November 15, 2014.

68. Schoenborn CA, Adams PF, Peregoy JA. Health behaviors of adults: United States, 2008-2010. Vital Health Stat 10 2013;(257):1–184.

69. Lemacks J, Wells BA, Ilich JZ, et al. Interventions for improving nutrition and physical activity behaviors in adult African American populations: a systematic review, January 2000 through December 2011. Prev Chronic Dis 2013;10:E99.

70. Ickes MJ, Sharma M. A systematic review of physical activity interventions in Hispanic adults. J Environ Public Health 2012;2012:156435.

71. Bender MS, Choi J, Won GY, et al. Randomized controlled trial lifestyle interventions for Asian Americans: a systematic review. Prev Med 2014;67:171–81.

72. Dhokarh R, Himmelgreen DA, Peng YK, et al. Food insecurity is associated with acculturation and social networks in Puerto Rican households. J Nutr Educ Behav 2011;43:288–94 (1878–2620 [Electronic]).

73. Mainous AG 3rd, Diaz VA, Geesey ME. Acculturation and healthy lifestyle among Latinos with diabetes. Ann Fam Med 2008;6:131–7 (1544–1717 [Electronic]).

74. Lin H, Bermudez OI, Tucker KL. Dietary patterns of Hispanic elders are associated with acculturation and obesity. J Nutr 2003;133:3651–7 (0022–3166 [Print]).

75. Palaniappan LP, Araneta MR, Assimes TL, et al. Call to action: cardiovascular disease in Asian Americans: a science advisory from the American Heart Association. Circulation 2010;122(12):1242–52.

76. Zhou BF, Stamler J, Dennis B, et al. Nutrient intakes of middle-aged men and women in China, Japan, United Kingdom, and United States in the late 1990s: the INTERMAP study. J Hum Hypertens 2003;17:623–30 (0950–9240 [Print]).

77. Song YJ, Hofstetter CR, Hovell MF, et al. Acculturation and health risk behaviors among Californians of Korean descent. Prev Med 2004;39:147–56 (0091–7435 [Print]).

Printed and bound by CPI Group (UK) Ltd, Croydon, CR0 4YY

03/10/2024

01040398-0015